Comprehensive Healthcare Simulation

Series Editors

Adam I. Levine
Department of Anesthesiology
Mount Sinai Medical Center
New York, NY
USA

Samuel DeMaria Jr.
Department of Anesthesiology
Mount Sinai Medical Center
New York, NY
USA

More information about this series at http://www.springer.com/series/13029

Bryan Mahoney • Rebecca D. Minehart
May C. M. Pian-Smith
Editors

Comprehensive Healthcare Simulation: Anesthesiology

Springer

Editors
Bryan Mahoney
Department of Anesthesiology
Perioperative and Pain Medicine
Mount Sinai St. Luke's and West Hospitals
Mount Sinai St. Luke's & Roosevelt Hospital
Icahn School of Medicine at Mount Sinai
New York
NY
USA

May C. M. Pian-Smith
Department of Anesthesia
Critical Care and Pain Medicine
Massachusetts General Hospital
Boston
MA
USA

Harvard Medical School
Boston
MA
USA

Rebecca D. Minehart
Department of Anesthesia
Critical Care and Pain Medicine
Massachusetts General Hospital
Boston
MA
USA

Harvard Medical School
Boston
MA
USA

ISSN 2366-4479 ISSN 2366-4487 (electronic)
Comprehensive Healthcare Simulation
ISBN 978-3-030-26848-0 ISBN 978-3-030-26849-7 (eBook)
https://doi.org/10.1007/978-3-030-26849-7

This Springer imprint is published by the registered company Springer Nature Switzerland AG
The registered company address is: Gewerbestrasse 11, 6330 Cham, Switzerland

Foreword

The Truth About Simulation: Beyond the Obvious

Readers of this text are perhaps already well-familiar with the ways in which simulation training can improve individual technical skills, nontechnical skills, and team performance. But the as-yet underappreciated truth about simulation training is this: simulation fundamentals are actually leadership fundamentals. The educator or clinician who masters the simulation content in this book will also be a master of difficult communication, institutional change management, emotional intelligence, strategic planning, decision-making, and other core skills identified ubiquitously by authorities on leadership development.

Simulation as Play

Although medical simulation is serious in nature, simulation itself may be viewed as a form of play. Play activities confer many benefits, which may include strengthened relationships, enhanced problem-solving, and heightened creativity, which combine to create more flexible, adaptive, and effective responses to tough situations. As well, simulation activities by nature are a kind of role-play activity, which offers opportunities to experiment with event management or communication styles in low-state environments. Feedback on these approaches, including an understanding of how others are likely to think and feel, enhances participants' emotional intelligence and therefore prepares participants to respond most effectively, and quickly, during real critical events. Play also strengthens social bond, which is a critical component to resilience and the combat of burnout. In the setting of inter-professional simulation, play builds a stronger sense of community and trust, which benefits healthcare professionals, healthcare organizations, and patients. Finally, improvisation (either during a scenario or as used in a debriefing exercise) fosters mindfulness. One definition of mindfulness is the state of being attentive to and aware of what is happening in the present moment. Clearly, anesthesiology requires vigilant attention and sharp situation awareness, which mirrors the definition of mindfulness exactly. And, improv training is an increasingly popular tool for leadership development.

Simulation as Organizational Change

Many pioneers of simulation education and developers or champions of new simulation centers over the past two decades share a common experience. They identify with the "build it and they will come" evolution of interest and resourcing of their intended activities, physical and logistical needs, and personnel requirements. These leaders faced tough challenges and by necessity have developed great elevator pitches and value propositions. Simulation training is characterized by an often elusive and somewhat intangible return on investment, especially when it is in the early stages of development. But simulation has been studied as a major tool for effecting cultural change (adopting or improving organizational safety culture), including safety strategies and responses to error or adverse events. The increasing demand for interprofessional and multidisciplinary simulation training that is sweeping medical centers across the nation is indeed the result of early wins by simulation pioneers and subsequent organizational change.

Simulation as Strategic Planning

Designing, building, stocking, and staffing a new clinical care center (whether small outpatient procedure center or major hospital) are no small feat. Simulation allows for provocation of workflow models, internal systems, and environmental vulnerabilities while there is still an opportunity to modify those elements without jeopardizing patient safety. A principle of adaptive leadership (as outlined by Travis Bradberry in *Leadership 2.0*) is *organizational justice*, which includes decision fairness and outcome concern. Simulations for strategic planning inform where and why specific resources should be allocated and prioritized. This not only strengthens the safety and effectiveness of the new clinical care environment but also provides transparency and justification to the organization as a whole. Even if there are groups who are disappointed with the eventual decisions, it will be clear that leaders care about how such decisions and system designs impact the work of everyone involved and have performed highly visible, thoughtful analysis of competing priorities.

Simulation as Communication Training

High-stakes communications occur every day in every operating room, intensive care unit, or pain management clinic setting. Even routine cases are characterized by multiple opportunities for communication failure, and communication failure is noted as a root cause in The Joint Commission's review of sentinel events year after year. Communication challenges are frequent and can be magnified if relationships are threatened or authority gradients exist. Widely adopted debriefing models (such as the "advocacy/inquiry" approach) include an exploration of the "frames" of all participants, mirroring the classic advice from Stephen Covey in *The 7 Habits of Highly Effective People*: "seek first to understand, then to be understood." Many debriefing paradigms also include elements of psychological safety, exploring others' perspectives, and acknowledging that one's own interpretation of observed behavior is augmented (perhaps erroneously) by past experience. These elements are among those featured in Kerry Patterson's *Crucial Conversations: Tools for Talking When Stakes Are High*. As important as understanding these techniques, if not more so, is the repeated opportunity to *practice* language models that facilitate critical communication in time-pressured, high-stakes situations.

Simulation as Team Management Training

Leaders of clinical emergencies must be facile in timely decision-making, delegation of roles, monitoring of performance, mobilizing resources, and anticipating and planning for future patient states. Simulation allows for practice in each of these areas. Emergency management paradigms (including crisis resource management) include elements of leveraging differences – what can people do, how can we be sure that all necessary items get done, and who is best to do what. These questions inform optimal role assignment, task delegation, and resource management. Although typically not characterized by the same level of urgency, classic leadership skills for managing individuals and teams include optimizing outcomes by understanding and valuing the differences among team members and putting them to best use.

As you read the text, notice these themes. Decision-making, team training, event management, communication, and other major leadership skills are highly represented in every chapter.

Simulation educators not only teach leadership skills but also use those same skills as they navigate difficult debriefing situations, design curricula creatively in low-resource environments, and add value to their institutions by contributing to patient safety initiatives and strategic planning. In every element of simulation training design, implementation, and evaluation, you will see core leadership principles at play.

Simulation fundamentals are leadership fundamentals.

Raleigh, NC, USA Marjorie Podraza Stiegler, MD

Preface

Simulation technology has been with us for decades, and as early adopters, anesthesiologists have played a major role in integrating this tool not only into our own training and assessment but throughout healthcare pedagogy. A goal of this text was to avoid an over-reliance on an esoteric narrative or descriptive approach to the use of simulation technology in the field of anesthesiology. While those looking to create a report or historical account on this topic may find something of utility in these pages, our intended audience has been, from the outset, *educators*. What we hope to have accomplished, to the extent possible, is the creation of a practical tool for those tasked with implementing a curriculum that is simulation-based or that incorporates simulation. We have, by necessity, included the requisite background information regarding the history of this technology and its associated pedagogy in order to equip the novice simulation educator with baseline knowledge and familiarity. What follows, however, is meant to be practical in its composition, providing our audience with a "how to" manual for integrating simulation into a variety of settings involving anesthesiology education, assessment, and practice.

In this text, you will find insights and tools provided by the leading simulation experts in the field of anesthesiology. In the first section, you will find a tripartite introduction to simulation in anesthesiology consisting of the application of the basics of education theory and practice to simulation, the context in which simulation is applied in the field of anesthesiology, and a review of the modalities through which simulation can be applied. The next section provides a review and a practical guide to the application of simulation to different populations of learners within the field of anesthesiology. In the third section, our authors provide a review and practical guide to simulation in the subspecialties of anesthesiology. The prospective (or experienced) simulationist/anesthesiologist can turn to these pages as a first resource when tasked with creating a curriculum for any level of learner and in any subspecialty of the field. Each chapter provides instructions, examples, and further resources for those looking to incorporate simulation into their educational toolkit.

We have bookended this text with a historic perspective on simulation in the field of anesthesiology and a look into the future of the application of this technology. A strong theme that runs through both chapters is one of the increasing incorporations of simulation into the training, assessment, and even practice of the anesthesiology. It is a privilege to provide you, our readers, with this "first of its kind" practical guide aimed to facilitate education in the field that blazed the trail for the incorporation of simulation in healthcare and seems likely to maintain this role in the future. Like all technology, the past and future of simulation in healthcare is highly dynamic and rapidly evolving, and this text will likely hold a modest shelf life barring future revisions. However, we have provided lessons from experts in the field, so our readers will be unburdened from "recreating the wheel" and will instead have the opportunity to contribute their own novel approaches in the application of this exciting technology to improving the training of tomorrow's providers and the quality of care our patients receive.

Acknowledgments

Bryan Mahoney, MD, FASA: I would like to thank the editors of the original *The Comprehensive Textbook of Healthcare Simulation* who invited us to prepare this text, my coeditors who have joined me on this amazing journey, the Mount Sinai Health System Department of Anesthesiology for its support in time and resources, and my family for its patience with many extra nights and weekends spent preparing this text.

Rebecca D. Minehart, MD, MSHPEd: I am honored to have been given the opportunity to be an editor for this text and am grateful to Drs. Adam Levine and Bryan Mahoney, who first offered me the chance to work alongside them. I am eternally grateful to my other coeditor, Dr. May Pian-Smith, for being an incredible mentor for many years. Last, but never least, I would like to thank my family for their love and support throughout this journey.

May C. M. Pian-Smith, MD, MS: I am grateful to Dr. Adam Levine and my coeditors for the opportunity to have partnered on this special project. As with the simulations we teach, this has been an experiential learning scenario unto itself, for which the teaming process has been hard, fun, and rewarding. I thank my simulation mentors, Drs. Jeff Cooper and Dan Raemer, and my family for their support.

New York, NY, USA — Bryan Mahoney
Boston, MA, USA — Rebecca D. Minehart
Boston, MA, USA — May C. M. Pian-Smith

Contents

Contributors

Alexander F. Arriaga, MD, MPH, ScD Department of Anesthesiology and Pain Medicine, Brigham and Women's Hospital, Boston, MA, USA

Harvard Medical School, Boston, MA, USA

Arna Banerjee, MBBS Department of Anesthesiology, Division of Critical Care, Medical Education and Administration, Simulation in Medical Education, Vanderbilt University Medical Center, Vanderbilt University School of Medicine, Nashville, TN, USA

Jeanette R. Bauchat, MD, MS Department of Anesthesiology, Vanderbilt University Medical Center, Vanderbilt University School of Medicine, Nashville, TN, USA

Wendy K. Bernstein, MD, MBA, FASA, FAMWA Division of Cardiac Anesthesiology, Department of Anesthesiology and Perioperative Medicine, University of Rochester Medical Center, Rochester, NY, USA

Kimberly R. Blasius, MD Department of Anesthesiology, University of North Carolina Children's Hospital, Chapel Hill, NC, USA

Amanda Burden, MD Department of Anesthesiology, Clinical Skills and Simulation, Cooper Medical School of Rowan University, Cooper University Hospital, Camden, NJ, USA

Y. Melissa Chan, MD Department of Anesthesiology, University of Mississippi Medical Center, Jackson, MS, USA

Erik Clinton, MD Department of Obstetrics and Gynecology, Massachusetts General Hospital, Boston, MA, USA

Harvard Medical School, Boston, MA, USA

Jeffrey B. Cooper, PhD Department of Anaesthesia, Harvard Medical School, Boston, MA, USA

Department of Anesthesia, Critical Care and Pain Medicine, Massachusetts General Hospital, Boston, MA, USA

Center for Medical Simulation, Boston, MA, USA

Christopher Cropsey, MD Cardiovascular Anesthesiologists, P.C., Nashville, TN, USA

Priti G. Dalal, MD, FRCA Department of Anesthesiology and Perioperative Medicine, Penn State Health Hershey Medical Center, Hershey, PA, USA

Samuel DeMaria, MD Department of Anesthesiology, Perioperative and Pain Medicine, Icahn School of Medicine at Mount Sinai, New York, NY, USA

Mary DiMiceli, MD Anesthesia Medical Group, Inc., Nashville, TN, USA

David A. Edwards, MD, PhD Department of Anesthesiology, Vanderbilt University Medical Center, The Vanderbilt Clinic, Nashville, TN, USA

Michaela Kristina Farber, MD, MS Department of Anesthesiology, Perioperative, and Pain Medicine, Brigham and Women's Hospital, Boston, MA, USA

Harvard Medical School, Boston, MA, USA

Idalid Franco, MD, MPH Harvard T.H. Chan School of Public Health, Boston, MA, USA

Harvard Medical School, Boston, MA, USA

Department of Radiation Oncology, Massachusetts General Hospital, Boston, MA, USA

Roxane Gardner, MD, MSHPEd, DSc Department of Obstetrics & Gynecology, Brigham and Women's Hospital, Boston, MA, USA

Harvard Medical School, Boston, MA, USA

Department of Anesthesia, Critical Care and Pain Medicine, Massachusetts General Hospital, Boston, MA, USA

Center for Medical Simulation, Boston, MA, USA

Kristina L. Goff, MD Department of Anesthesiology and Pain Management, University of Texas Southwestern Medical Center, Dallas, TX, USA

Andrew Goldberg, MD Department of Anesthesiology, James J Peters VA Medical Center, New York, NY, USA

Oren T. Guttman, MD, MBA Department of Anesthesiology, Health System Vice President For High Reliability and Patient Safety, Jefferson Health, Philadelphia, PA, USA

Maryann Henry, CRNA, MS Department of Anesthesiology and Critical Care, University of Pennsylvania Health System, Philadelphia, PA, USA

Bryan Hill, MD Department of Anesthesiology, The Ohio State University Wexner Medical Center, Columbus, OH, USA

Jesse T. Hochkeppel, MD Interventional Pain Management, Connecticut Pain Care/ OrthoConnecticut, Danbury, CT, USA

Michelle Lee Humeidan, MD, PhD Department of Anesthesiology, The Ohio State University Wexner Medical Center, Columbus, OH, USA

Daniel Katz, MD Department of Anesthesiology, Perioperative and Pain Medicine, Icahn School of Medicine at Mount Sinai, New York, NY, USA

January Kim, BS Institute of Behavioral Medicine Research, The Ohio State University Wexner Medical Center, Columbus, OH, USA

Sang Kim, MD Department of Anesthesiology, Critical Care & Pain Management, Hospital for Special Surgery, New York, NY, USA

Amanda H. Kumar, MD Department of Anesthesiology, Regional Anesthesia and Acute Pain Management, Duke University, Duke University Medical Center, Durham, NC, USA

Michael Kushelev, MD Department of Anesthesiology, The Ohio State University Wexner Medical Center, OSU East Hospital, Columbus, OH, USA

Samsun Lampotang, PhD, FSSH Center for Safety, Simulation & Advanced Learning Technologies, Simulation Innovation, Office of Educational Affairs/Office of Medical Education, Simulation Core, Clinical & Translational Science Insitute, University of Florida, Gainesville, FL, USA

Adam I. Levine, MD Department of Anesthesiology, Perioperative and Pain Medicine, Department of Otolaryngology and Pharmacological Sciences, Icahn School of Medicine at Mount Sinai, New York, NY, USA

Jonathan Lipps, MD Department of Anesthesiology, The Ohio State University Wexner Medical Center, Columbus, OH, USA

Bryan Mahoney, MD Department of Anesthesiology, Perioperative and Pain Medicine, Mount Sinai St. Luke's and West Hospitals, Mount Sinai St. Luke's & Roosevelt Hospital, Icahn School of Medicine at Mount Sinai, New York, NY, USA

Christine Lan Mai, MD, MS-HPEd Department of Anesthesia, Critical Care and Pain Medicine, Massachusetts General Hospital, Boston, MA, USA

Harvard Medical School, Boston, MA, USA

Joshua A. Marks, MD, FACS Department of Surgery, Sidney Kimmel Medical College at Thomas Jefferson University Hospitals, Philadelphia, PA, USA

Matthew D. McEvoy, MD Division of Multispecialty Anesthesia, Department of Anesthesiology, CIPHER (Center for Innovation in Perioperative Health, Education, and Research), Vanderbilt University School of Medicine, Vanderbilt University Medical Center, Nashville, TN, USA

Carlene McLaughlin, CRNA, MSN, PhD Department of Anesthesiology and Critical Care, University of Pennsylvania Health System, Philadelphia, PA, USA

Lori Meyers, MD Department of Anesthesiology, The Ohio State University Wexner Medical Center, Columbus, OH, USA

Rebecca D. Minehart, MD, MSHPEd Department of Anesthesia, Critical Care, and Pain Medicine, Massachusetts General Hospital, Boston, MA, USA

Harvard Medical School, Boston, MA, USA

Kenneth R. Moran, MD Department of Anesthesiology, The Ohio State University Wexner Medical Center, Columbus, OH, USA

Andrés T. Navedo, MD, MS-HPEd Department of Anesthesiology, Critical Care and Pain Medicine, Boston Children's Hospital, Boston, MA, USA

Harvard Medical School, Boston, MA, USA

Deborah D. Navedo, PhD, MSN STRATUS Center for Medical Simulation, Brigham and Women's Hospital, Boston, MA, USA

Jordan L. Newmark, MD Department of Anesthesiology, Division of Pain Medicine, Alameda Health System, Oakland, CA, USA

Department of Anesthesiology, Perioperative & Pain Medicine, Stanford University School of Medicine, Palo Alto, CA, USA

Mark W. Newton, MD Department of Anesthesiology and Pediatrics, Vanderbilt University Medical Center, Nashville, TN, USA

Cesar Padilla, MD Anesthesiology and Pain Management, Cleveland Clinic, Pepper Pike, OH, USA

Christine S. Park, MD Graham Clinical Performance Center, University of Illinois College of Medicine, University of Illinois at Chicago, Anesthesiology and Medical Education, Chicago, IL, USA

Shivani Patel, MBBS Department of Pediatric Anesthesiology and Critical Care Medicine, Johns Hopkins University, Baltimore, MD, USA

Jeremy T. Rainey, DO Center for Critical Care Medicine, Anesthesiology Institute, Cleveland Clinic, Cleveland, OH, USA

Cortessa Russell, MD Department of Anesthesiology, New York Presbyterian – Columbia University Medical Center, New York, NY, USA

Daniel Saddawi-Konefka, MD, MBA Harvard Medical School, Boston, MA, USA

Department of Anesthesia, Critical Care and Pain Medicine, Massachusetts General Hospital, Boston, MA, USA

Migdalia H. Saloum, MD Department of Anesthesiology, Perioperative and Pain Medicine, Mount Sinai St. Luke's and West Hospitals, Mount Sinai St. Luke's & Roosevelt Hospital, Icahn School of Medicine at Mount Sinai, New York, NY, USA

Jacob Schaff, MD Department of Anesthesiology, New York Presbyterian – Columbia University Medical Center, New York, NY, USA

Maricela Schnur, MD, MBA Interventional Pain Management, St. Luke's, Duluth, MN, USA

Department of Anesthesiology, Perioperative and Pain Medicine, Department of Otolaryngology, and Pharmacological Sciences, Icahn School of Medicine at Mount Sinai, New York City, NY, USA

David L. Schreibman, MD Department of Anesthesiology, University of Maryland School of Medicine, University of Maryland Medical Center, Baltimore, MD, USA

Michael Seropian, MD, FRCPC, FSSH Department of Anesthesiology and Perioperative Medicine, Oregon Health & Science University, Portland, OR, USA

Anjan Shah, MD Department of Anesthesiology, Perioperative and Pain Medicine, Icahn School of Medicine at Mount Sinai, New York, NY, USA

Alan Julius Sim, MD Department of Anesthesiology, Perioperative and Pain Medicine, Icahn School of Medicine at Mount Sinai, New York, NY, USA

Devika Singh, MS, MD Department of Anesthesiology and Critical Care, The Children's Hospital of Philadelphia, Philadelphia, PA, USA

Elizabeth Sinz, MD, MEd Department of Anesthesiology and Perioperative Medicine, Penn State Health Hershey Medical Center, Hershey, PA, USA

Agathe Streiff, MD Department of Anesthesiology, Montefiore Medical Center, Bronx, NY, USA

Rachel E. Sweeney, BA Department of Anesthesiology and Critical Care, University of Pennsylvania Health System, Philadelphia, PA, USA

Perelman School of Medicine, University of Pennsylvania, Philadelphia, PA, USA

Ankeet D. Udani, MD, MS.Ed Department of Anesthesiology, Duke University Medical Center, Durham, NC, USA

Rashmi Vandse, MD Department of Anesthesiology, Loma Linda University Medical Center, Loma Linda, CA, USA

Scott C. Watkins, MD Department of Anesthesiology and Critical Care Medicine, Johns Hopkins University School of Medicine, Johns Hopkins All Children's Hospital, Saint Petersburg, FL, USA

Chelsea Willie, MD Department of Anesthesiology, Medical College of Wisconsin/Children's Hospital of Wisconsin, Milwaukee, WI, USA

Miguel A. Yaport, MD Department of Anesthesiology and Critical Care, University of Pennsylvania Health System, Philadelphia, PA, USA

Jeron Zerillo, MD Department of Anesthesiology, Perioperative and Pain Medicine, Icahn School of Medicine at Mount Sinai, New York, NY, USA

Part I

Introduction to Simulation for Anesthesiology

Anesthesia and Simulation: An Historic Relationship

1

Daniel Saddawi-Konefka and Jeffrey B. Cooper

Introduction

While the rise of simulation in healthcare in general appears to be fairly recent, simulation of many forms has actually been used for well over a thousand years. Owen, in his book *Simulation in Healthcare Education: An Extensive History*, goes back to 500 AD for the first documented use of simulation in healthcare education [1]. This was described in the *Sushruta Samhita*, where students were urged to practice incisions on items that resembled parts of the human body (e.g., gourds, leather bags filled with fluid, or dead animals). Students were encouraged to practice "so that they could be quick, which was important when operating on patients without the benefit of anesthesia" [1]. In its long history since, simulation spread across many geographies and disciplines, including surgery, obstetrics and gynecology, ophthalmology, urology, dentistry, trauma, and nursing. What is remarkable is that Owen's historical textbook of over 400 pages ends its story at about 1950! All of those working in the modern world of simulation who think they have started something new may in fact have much to learn from earlier generations.

Use of simulation in anesthesiology is now widespread, and anesthesiologists are seen as pioneers of the modern era of simulation. Interestingly, however, the term "anesthesia" is mentioned only a few times in Owen's text, and even then only as it related to practice of intubation (not involving anesthesiologists). This may not be too surprising since anesthesiology as an independent field only developed its footing in the early 1900s, and simulation's first major introduction in anesthesiology did not occur until the 1960s and took over two decades to gain any serious national attention. In telling the story of the now widespread uses of simulation in anesthesiology, we can learn much from why it took so long for this now-obvious patient safety and educational tool to take hold in anesthesiology and the rest of health care. What does it take to spread an idea? It is an inspiring story, but not without some fits and starts. There are pioneers and innovative technologies. There are lessons to be learned that can be applied to the patient safety challenges that still face us. And there is an unfinished story that needs to be continued.

In this chapter, we pick up the story in the 1960s, shortly after Owen left off, focusing on simulation in anesthesiology. Due to anesthesiology's central place in the development of modern simulation, this history has been discussed in several other writings. We draw on two of these key references more heavily in this chapter and recommend them to interested readers [2, 3]. Because of the foundational role patient safety played in the dissemination of simulation in anesthesiology, we begin by describing the relationship between anesthesiology, simulation, and patient safety.

Chapter Objectives

Readers will learn about the earliest "modern" simulators in anesthesiology and the challenges that these pioneers faced in trying to establish the role of simulation in anesthesiology education. They will also learn about the critical drivers that led to the successful dissemination of simulation in the field. In particular, they will read about the critical role of patient safety to establish a successful value proposition for simulation. Finally, they will learn about the scholars whose work propelled simulation to the central stage it currently holds in anesthesiology.

D. Saddawi-Konefka (✉)
Harvard Medical School, Boston, MA, USA

Department of Anesthesia, Critical Care and Pain Medicine, Massachusetts General Hospital, Boston, MA, USA
e-mail: dsaddawi-konefka@mgh.harvard.edu

J. B. Cooper
Department of Anaesthesia, Harvard Medical School, Boston, MA, USA

Department of Anesthesia, Critical Care and Pain Medicine, Massachusetts General Hospital, Boston, MA, USA

Center for Medical Simulation, Boston, MA, USA
e-mail: JCOOPER@mgh.harvard.edu

B. Mahoney et al. (eds.), *Comprehensive Healthcare Simulation: Anesthesiology*, Comprehensive Healthcare Simulation,
https://doi.org/10.1007/978-3-030-26849-7_1

Anesthesiology, Simulation, and Patient Safety

Anesthesiology is rooted in patient safety. Because anesthesia is not generally therapeutic by itself, there is even more than the usual motivation to do no harm, or, in the words of the original mission and now vision of the Anesthesia Patient Safety Foundation (APSF) , "To ensure that no patient is harmed by anesthesia" [4]. In this chapter, we will trace how those roots are responsible for the leading role that anesthesiology has played in the development and dispersion of simulation in health care.

Anesthesiology simulation, as we have come to know it, grew independently and convergently from the interests of different individuals in both medical education and patient safety. In the 1960s, Dr. Stephen Abrahamson, an educator, led the first relatively modern introduction of full-scale simulation in anesthesiology [5]. His foray into medical education came from his interest in using early-stage computers to enhance the educational experience. It was somewhat serendipitous that he teamed with an anesthesiologist for his simulation project. Their focus was on education, not patient safety, and as a result, they struggled to "find a market" for their work – there was no recognized unmet need.

It was not until the second modern wave of simulation (starting in the mid-1980s) that simulation in healthcare began to take hold. This wave was driven not just to develop physiologic models of anesthesia that could enhance teaching but also from full-scale simulation environments created to address patient safety issues. Five simulation pioneers in anesthesiology (each developing some aspect of simulation for different reasons) were James Philip, Howard Schwid, David Gaba, and the mentor/mentee team of J.S. Gravenstein and Michael Good [6–10].

In between these two waves, Jeffrey Cooper and Ellison Pierce championed an increased focus on patient safety [11–13], fertilizing the grounds from which simulation would grow. This focus on patient safety was key to simulation's success, as simulation became a powerful tool to combat a widely appreciated problem. Figure 1.1 illustrates how some specific landmark events aligned with the growth of interest in anesthesiology (as gauged by the number of peer-reviewed publications on simulation in anesthesiology). The clear inflection that occurred in the 1980s was in large part a result of the research program of the APSF and other activities it promoted to enhance dissemination.

Stephen Abrahamson and Judson Denson: Sim One's Attempt to Establish a New Educational Paradigm [14]

"Sim One," the first computer-controlled simulation mannequin, was a remarkably capable device, with features that surpass some of those in technologies found today. It was developed by Drs. Stephen J. Abrahamson and Judson S. Denson at the University of Southern California and publicly revealed in 1967 – only 20 years after the first

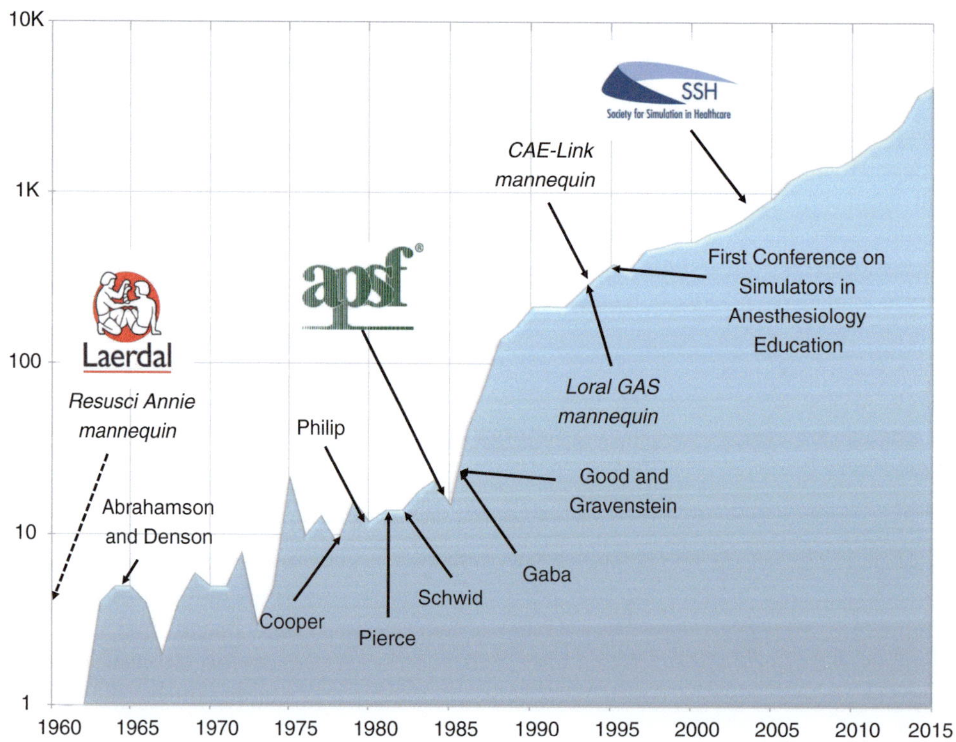

Fig. 1.1 The graph is a semilog plot showing the number of PubMed-indexed citations for "anesthesia and simulation" or "anesthesiology and simulation" from 1965 through 2015. Overlaid on top of this graph are the approximate years that each of the pioneers in the field first made their work public. Relevant societies are also shown. Major commercial mannequin releases are shown in italics

computer (ENIAC) was developed. This impressive feat of technology proposed a drastic and expensive change from the teaching paradigm of the day, and this is likely why it received limited acceptance from academic medical education.

Abrahamson earned his Ph.D. in Education from New York University in 1951 with post-doctoral work concentrating on evaluation. In 1952, he joined the faculty at the University of Buffalo and soon became the head of the Education Research Center. In 1963, he was recruited by the University of Southern California to lead its Department of Medical Education. One of his early charges was to partner with an engineer, Tullio Ronzoni, to explore uses for computing in medical education. Typical uses for computers in medicine at the time were for data storage, retrieval, and some analysis. Using a computer for simulation or interactive scenarios was uncommon, if done at all, but that is exactly what they set out to do. More specifically, their idea was to use computers to present anesthesiology trainees with simulated data reflecting what they might see during a typical anesthetic (e.g., pulse, respiratory rate), and have them react to that data. The operator of the simulator could manipulate the data in real time, and trainees would then have to decide what actions to take in response.

Because he had essentially no knowledge of anesthesia, Abrahamson approached Dr. Judson "Sam" Denson, the chief anesthesiologist at Los Angeles County Hospital. Over time, the idea grew, and they decided to mock up an entire body, "life-like and life-size," complete with plastic skin that could become cyanotic, chest wall and diaphragm movement for breathing, heart sounds, palpable pulses (temporal and radial), teeth that could be broken with laryngoscopy, eyes that closed with variable force, pupils that constricted, and more. They used variably magnetized needles with flow sensors to identify which "drugs" were being injected into the simulator and in what quantities. Despite multiple failures to obtain funding from the NIH, Abrahamson was ultimately able to secure a grant of $272,000 from the US Office of Education's Cooperative Research Project to fund a 2-year feasibility study. Abrahamson developed measurement and assessment tools for performance and ultimately compared trainees who had used the simulator versus those who had not [5, 15].

Though several lay publications reported on Sim One [16], the medical community strongly resisted adopting this model for training. It is likely that the cost and limitations of the rudimentary computer technology made it impractical for replication at the time. It is also likely that the technology threatened to undermine traditional education methods that were widely accepted and in use. This is supported by anecdotal reports that the reaction to Sim One was at times viscerally unfavorable. For example, when being moved from one location to another, someone deliberately and unnecessarily cut off one of Sim One's arms, which contained much of its electronics, to fit the simulator through a doorway. It has been suggested that Sim One was simply a disruptive technology far ahead of its time [3].

Ellison "Jeep" Pierce and Jeffrey Cooper: Galvanizing the Focus on Patient Safety in Anesthesiology

The Patient Safety Movement in healthcare began years before the oft-cited 1999 publication of the influential Institute of Medicine report "To Err is Human", which catalyzed a widespread Patient Safety Movement in the USA and throughout the world. Early work in anesthesiology started in 1978, with a publication by Dr. Jeffrey Cooper (an engineer) and colleagues that brought attention to the role of human error in preventable adverse outcomes [11]. His later publication in 1984 expanded on that work [17].

Jeff Cooper completed his Bachelor's in Chemical Engineering and Master's in Biomedical Engineering from Drexel University before completing a Ph.D. in Chemical Engineering at the University of Missouri. In 1972, he joined the Anesthesia Bioengineering Unit of the Department of Anesthesia at the Massachusetts General Hospital (MGH). In 1974, leading an interdisciplinary team, he set out to learn about how errors in using anesthesia equipment contributed to adverse outcomes. In so doing, his team stumbled onto the "critical incident" technique and used it to learn about the broader topic of errors in anesthesiology, with a focus on human factors [11, 17, 18].

The work of the MGH team shifted the focus to human error. Coupled with relatively high malpractice insurance premiums and some media attention about anesthesia-related deaths, this work created fertile ground for change and innovation. But, an effective clinical leader was still needed to make the topic visible and palatable. Dr. Ellison C. Pierce, Jr. was that leader. At the time, he was the Chair of the Department of Anesthesia at the Deaconess Hospital. Affectionately called by his nickname "Jeep" by all his colleagues, Pierce met with Cooper when he volunteered his department for participation in the critical incident studies. Pierce and Cooper found common ground in their interest in preventing accidental deaths and serious injuries related to anesthesia. As President of the American Society of Anesthesiologists in 1983, Pierce spoke about the importance of injury prevention as the best way to address the malpractice crisis.

In 1984, Pierce, Cooper, and Richard J. Kitz, Chairman of the Anesthesia Department at the MGH, organized the International Symposium on Preventable Anesthesia Mortality and Morbidity in 1984 [18]. During the conference, Pierce conceived the idea of a foundation dedicated to preventing adverse outcomes. Working with a few colleagues, he founded the APSF in 1986 to accomplish this goal [12, 19]. Cooper, seeing the need for funding to support patient safety research, instigated the creation of the APSF's research program. In its first 3 years, 1987–1989, APSF awarded four grants for work that involved simulation by three of the pioneers whom we highlight below. Later, the APSF sponsored conferences to explore and support the use of simulation throughout anesthesiology.

James Philip: Development of a Digital Pharmacokinetic Simulator [20, 21]

Dr. James "Jim" Philip earned Bachelor's and Master's Degrees in Electrical Engineering from Cornell University before completing medical school at SUNY in Syracuse. He completed his anesthesiology residency and then joined the faculty at the Peter Bent Brigham Hospital (now the Brigham and Women's Hospital, or BWH) in 1978. Because his contributions to simulation have been limited to anesthesiology (and more specifically to digital simulation of volatile anesthetic kinetics), he is not often mentioned in general simulation history texts. As this book is devoted to the history of simulation in anesthesiology, Jim Philip's contributions are certainly relevant. In 1978, when he was first on faculty, his department chair, Leroy D. Vandam, M.D., challenged him to become an expert in inhalation anesthetic agent kinetics and teach it to their residents; Philip accepted the challenge (Fig. 1.2).

To this end, he assembled a device composed of tubing sections and containers to simulate the lungs, cardiac output, tissues, etc. By adjusting stopcocks and roller clamps, he could dynamically alter each variable (e.g., decrease venous return by partially closing one of the roller clamps). Infusing colored liquids into the system completed the effect; he had created a dynamic, tangible simulation of inhaled anesthetic agent kinetics. This model was met with wonderful reviews from faculty and residents. After accidentally spilling a copious quantity of the blue dyed liquid on his shirt, he realized that he needed a much more convenient and sustainable model.

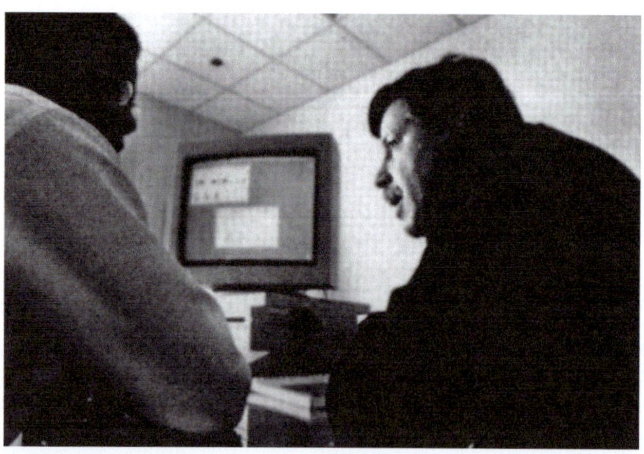

Fig. 1.2 James Philip (right) and Roger Russell with early version of Gasman, 1991

Philip turned to computers for a solution. In August of 1980, he successfully applied for a grant from the Apple Educational Foundation to use Apple II computers to graphically display the compartment model of inhaled anesthetic agent kinetics. Through incredible dedication, he was able to design, code, and test the program, which he ultimately called "Gas Man™." Gas Man™ received positive reviews at the 1982 American Society of Anesthesiologists Annual Meeting and won a Special Award for Innovation at the New York State Society of Anesthesiologists Post Graduate Assembly.

Over the next few years, Philip successfully obtained the full title to Gas Man™ and published his work with Addison-Wesley. Though this was commercially fairly successful, Addison-Wesley dropped its entire medical publishing division in 1986, including Gas Man™. In 1991, Philip contracted with H. M. Franklin Associates (HMFA) to perform all further programming and updates to Gas Man™; that relationship has continued. Currently, this form of educational simulation is being used to teach inhaled anesthetic agent uptake and distribution at over 100 institutions including anesthesiology residency programs, medical schools, manufacturers, and veterinary schools. Philip was one of the founding members of the Society for Technology in Anesthesia (STA) and served as its President from 1999 to 2000.

Howard Schwid: Moving Physiology Simulation to the Personal Computer

In the 1970s, Dr. N. Ty Smith and Dr. Yasuhiro Fukui developed computerized models to simulate physiology and its response to medications [22]. This work would form the foundation for Dr. Howard A. Schwid's contributions to simulation [3]. After developing an early interest in computer programming and artificial intelligence, Schwid studied biomedical engineering at the University of Wisconsin-Madison. He spent much of his elective time in computer and electrical engineering, with a special interest in mathematical modeling of physiological processes, including those earlier developed by Fukui. During medical school at the University of Washington, he found physiology classes (that included lectures and a dog lab) much less satisfying than the complete mathematical models he could seamlessly manipulate during his engineering days. Though his clinical years would teach him that "physicians are seldom able to measure everything," [3] he maintained his passion for modeling physiological processes with computers (Fig. 1.3).

Schwid was drawn to anesthesiology because of its emphasis on monitors, data, physiology, and pharmacology. In 1982, during his final year in medical school, he began the development of a computerized model of inhalational anesthetic agent uptake and distribution using the computer programming language Fortran. He continued his work during his anesthesiology residency, adding the cardiovascular system and capability of simulating the pharmacokinetic and dynamic responses to intravenous agents as well. This robust system could reasonably predict responses to many anesthetic agents under several pathophysiological conditions.

After completing the computer modeling system, Schwid turned his attention to developing a physical complement to make it seem real. He joined Dr. N. Ty Smith at the University of California San Diego as a fellow and began working with a flight simulator company (Rediffusion Simulation Incorporated) to develop a simulator on a Sun workstation. Though this simulator was met with some interest (it won the "Best Instructional Exhibit" at the 1985 New York State Society of Anesthesiologists Postgraduate Assembly), it did not become a commercial success. That was likely due in part to its requiring an expensive workstation. Also, as with Sim One, the field was not yet ready to accept computers over traditional models of training. Indeed, Schwid commented that when he was applying for full time positions where he could further his work, "most believed there was no future in medical simulation, and some even went so far as to counsel me to do something else with my career."

He was given a chance to pursue this passion by Dr. Tom Hornbein at the University of Washington, and he joined the faculty in 1986. He advanced the computer modeling of his simulator and published numerous articles on various aspects of it [9, 10, 23–27]. Since Schwid was unable to secure sufficient funding to further develop his simulation ideas, he formed his own company with the aim of disseminating his training concepts. He recognized that for the product to be practical for individual clinicians to use themselves, it would have to run on personal computers. He thus developed a program that ran on DOS machines. Further developments (including a scoring and debriefing tool) were developed using profits from his company and a grant from the APSF. This offering was eventually sold under the name "Anesthesia Simulator" through the company he founded in 1987, Anesoft. Interestingly, though Schwid had assumed that sales of his program would be driven by educational demand, residency programs and medical schools were the smallest fraction of purchasers, whereas private practice groups comprised the largest market. It was eventually folded into the CAE-Link Patient Simulator (which is discussed in the "Dissemination since 1990" section below).

David Gaba: Simulation for Crisis Resource Management and the Study of Human Performance

Dr. David Gaba's interest in simulation grew from a passion for patient safety [3]. Gaba's undergraduate education was in biomedical engineering. He had a keen interest in what he termed "intelligent responsive systems." Being drawn to the clinical aspects of biomedical engineering, he pursued medicine and found a natural home for his passions in anesthesiology, ultimately taking a faculty position at Stanford University (Fig. 1.4).

In a memoir, Gaba wrote that the book *Normal Accidents: Living with High-Risk Technologies* by Charles Perrow transformed the way he viewed patient safety in anesthesiology [28]. The book detailed the Three Mile Island nuclear power plant accident (among other famous accidents), suggesting that some accidents are unavoidable because of the "tight coupling" in complex systems. In 1987, Gaba applied

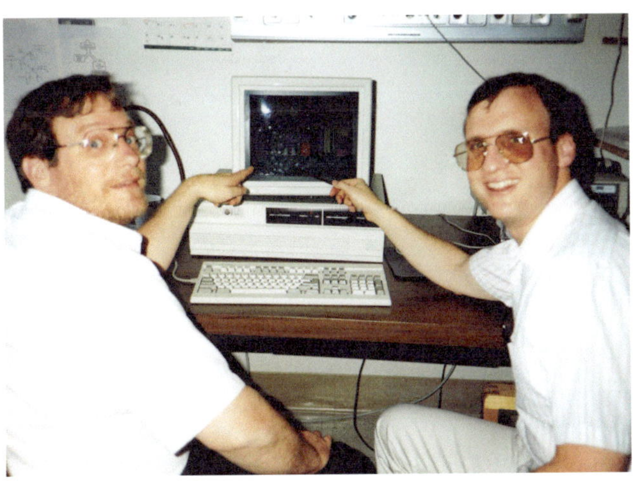

Fig. 1.3 Howard Schwid and Dan O'Donnell with Anesoft Anesthesia Simulator, 1989

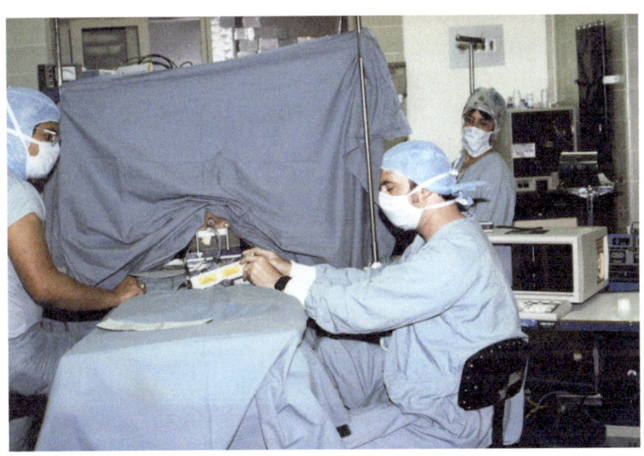

Fig. 1.4 David Gaba, Abe DeAnda, and Mary Maxwell, with pre-prototype simulator (CASE 0.5), 1986

Perrow's principles to anesthesiology in a landmark paper, "Breaking the Chain of Accident Evolution in Anesthesia" [29]. Gaba set about creating a laboratory in which he could subject anesthesiologists to critical situations and study how they responded. He believed that simulating critical events could also help train clinicians, improve their decision-making, and avoid some errors.

With no commercially available simulators at the time, Gaba and his team developed their own technology. Initially, they did so by combining an airway intubation trainer with an endotracheal tube (to serve as the extension of the simulated trachea) that was connected to a reservoir bag (to simulate the lungs). They used virtual devices to produce pulse oximeter, EKG, and blood pressure readings. Finally, they developed a scenario – a pneumothorax, which was simulated by altering the displayed vital signs and partially clamping the simulated trachea to increase airway pressures. To test the scenario, an anesthesiologist unaware of the scenario participated while Gaba recorded and analyzed her think-aloud responses to the events as they unfolded.

Gaba used this preliminary work to successfully apply for a $35,000 grant from the APSF to develop a more sophisticated prototype. Gaba called the more sophisticated prototype CASE (Comprehensive Anesthesia Simulation Environment), which was first described in 1988 [7]. The studies he and his team performed over the following years had some interesting and sometimes unexpected results. For example, he found that experience alone was not a reliable predictor of accident avoidance [30].

Perhaps Gaba's greatest contribution to simulation in anesthesiology was the development of Anesthesia Crisis Resource Management (ACRM) [31, 32]. Gaba had learned that the aviation industry used Cockpit Resource Management (later called Crew Resource Management, CRM) to focus on and develop decision-making and teamwork skills for pilots – not just "stick-and-rudder" technical skill) [3]. He had the insight to bring this practice to anesthesiology. Via a second grant from the APSF, Gaba developed a curriculum, course syllabus, and a set of four simulation scenarios that have since evolved in the now widely taught ACRM paradigm. Pivotal to current ACRM is debriefing after each scenario. Debriefing is generally accepted as the most critical and challenging aspect of simulation-based training. That concept is now widely accepted as a standard throughout the world wherever simulation is implemented. The first ACRM course was ran with a dozen anesthesiology residents in 1990. The book, Crisis Management in Anesthesiology, containing descriptions and management processes for eighty anesthesiology-based critical event scenarios, was another landmark, published in 1994 and updated in 2015 [33, 34].

Michael Good and J.S. Gravenstein: Simulation for the Avoidance of Errors

As an anesthesiology resident, Dr. Michael Good was frustrated that he would only care for two or three patients per day. He felt his exposure to critical events and opportunities to develop necessary skills was too small, and that the "surgery" part of the case was not conducive to more efficient mastery learning. In a memoir, he wrote that the "aha" moment that launched him into simulation came to him in 1985, as he practiced in a batting cage, attempting to hit ball after ball in a devoted effort to develop mastery [3].

Good graduated from the University of Michigan with a bachelor's degree in computer and communication science and completed medical school there. Completing his anesthesiology residency and fellowship at the University of Florida in Gainesville, he began his collaboration with Dr. Joachim S. "Nik" Gravenstein, a medical technology guru and patient safety leader, to develop a patient simulator. The two began regular meetings and wrote original code on a personal computer for digital analogs of the cardiovascular system. Gravenstein had connections with the Eindhoven University of Technology in the Netherlands, a group that worked on (among other things) computer modeling of a Bain breathing circuit (known as the "Bain team"). In 1987, Good and Gravenstein recruited Samsun "Sem" Lampotang, who had been a member of the Bain team, and was then a graduate research assistant at the University of Florida Department of Anesthesiology (Fig. 1.5).

Lampotang had expanded on his previous work and developed a mechanical lung that could interact with an actual ventilator and respiratory circuit in a realistic fashion. Based on this advance, the team approached Ohmeda, then one of the two leading manufacturers of anesthesia machines in the US,

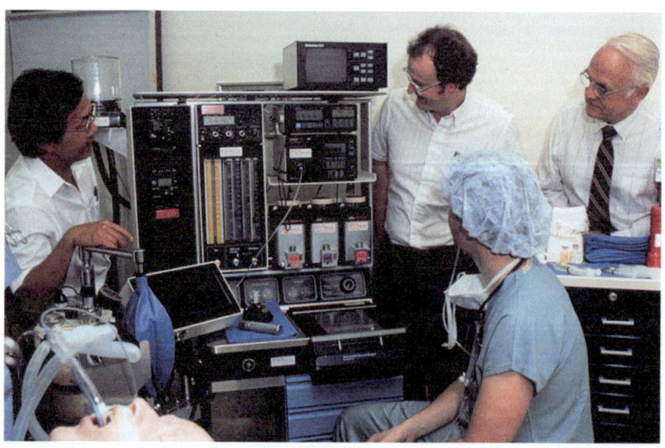

Fig. 1.5 Left to right: Samsun Lampotang, Gordon Gibby, Michael Good (seated), and JS Gravenstein, with GAS, c 1987

for funding to develop an anesthesia simulator that interacted directly with a ventilator. Ohmeda agreed, and Lampotang began developing what became known as the Gainesville Anesthesia Simulator (GAS I) during a summer externship at Ohmeda in 1987. Subsequent enhancements to their design included a computer-controlled vital signs display and the ability to physically consume and excrete anesthetic vapors.

With the funding from APSF, Good's team was able to add substantially to the simulator (now called the "Human Patient Simulator" or HPS). The simulator gained palpable pulses, responsiveness to a twitch monitor, the ability to detect volumes of medications injected, airway resistors, and more. Good's team also hired Ron Caravano, who served as a business administrator for the team. Caravano's business expertise contributed to the market success of the HPS and funding for further developments (e.g., the lung's ability to autoregulate respiratory rate in order to maintain a particular carbon dioxide level). The group's first purchase order came in 1993 from the Icahn School of Medicine at Mount Sinai Department of Anesthesiology, where Drs. Richard Kayne (then the residency program director) and Adam I. Levine installed the first HPS.

Dissemination Since 1990: How Did Simulation in Anesthesiology Propagate?

What were the key factors that enabled the diffusion of simulation since 1990? Clearly, technological advances (with less expensive and more accessible computers) were critical. As we have noted, patient safety seems to have been a main driver of dissemination. The early mannequin simulators (after Sim One) addressed patient safety concerns (e.g., how to discover anesthesia machine faults, how to prepare clinicians to manage critical events). But even in anesthesiology, with the demand to offer a more systematic and controlled process of learning, simulation is seen to have some advantages over the purely apprenticeship form of training. We describe here some important processes that have contributed to the slow growth of simulation in anesthesiology since the initial works of Schwid, Gaba, Good, and Gravenstein.

In 1991, the APSF Executive Committee made site visits to both the Stanford University's and University of Florida, Gainesville's simulation programs to learn about the progress each had made. From these visits, the APSF leadership concluded that simulation was a potentially powerful tool for patient safety. To help promote and disseminate it, the APSF proposed that the three simulation grant awardees collaborate to build a commercial simulator. Such cooperation was ultimately too difficult to achieve, and early dissemination thus took two routes.

CAE-Link, a large Canadian company that worked in flight simulation, worked with Gaba and Schwid to develop the CAE-Link Patient Simulator. They relied heavily on Gaba's CASE simulator and some of Schwid's mathematical modeling for pulmonary mechanics. The simulator was aimed primarily at management of critical incidents, following the CRM concepts that Gaba had adapted from aviation. CAE-Link sold the business to Eagle Corporation, which later sold it to MedSim Corporation. Although it was widely used in the early years of mannequin simulation, ultimately the technology did not survive market competition.

The Gainesville program partnered with the Loral Corporation, a defense contractor, to commercially develop the Human Patient Simulator (HPS). In 1996, the HPS was spun off into its own company, called Medical Education Technologies Inc. (METI), which was acquired 25 years later (in 2011) by CAE Healthcare. This simulator is still in wide use today.

Another aspect of dissemination came in the form of application of the simulators and their intended use by one early adopter. Jeff Cooper was one of the APSF Executive Committee members who had visited both the sites of both awardees of grants for mannequin simulators. Especially impressed by Gaba's ACRM program, he returned to Boston excited and determined to put together a similar offering [18]. Cooper organized the anesthesiology departments at the five major academic hospitals associated with Harvard Medical School to send a contingent of eleven anesthesiologists to Stanford to experience Gaba's ACRM training. The departments funded the travel and tuition, and the participants came away impressed.

Serendipitously, Gaba was preparing for a sabbatical; Cooper invited him to bring his simulator to Boston for 3 months to expose a larger group of anesthesiology providers to the ACRM experience. Seventy-two anesthesiologists, residents, and certified registered nurse anesthetists (CRNAs) participated in the event in the fall of 1992, and feedback was almost uniformly positive. This led to a collaboration of the five hospitals to build the Boston Anesthesia Simulation Center in downtown Boston. It was equipped with the first CAE-Link production mannequin. The Boston Anesthesia Simulation Center (BASC) was renamed the Center for Medical Simulation (CMS) in 1996. This first educational program outside of the centers that developed the first mannequins likely gave further credibility that the idea of simulation had value.

Shortly after the Harvard-affiliated hospitals' simulation program was established, simulation was adopted in New York in the Anesthesia Department at Mt. Sinai Hospital. After hearing about the human patient simulator from Dr. Richard Kayne, and after visiting the University of

Florida, Gainesville to see the GAS simulator, the department's chair, Dr. Joel Kaplan, quickly developed interest in using simulation [3]. Mt. Sinai was the first beta test site for the METI HPS. In 1994, under the directorship of Dr. Adam I. Levine, they formed their first simulation center. This initiative morphed and expanded to become the HELPS (Human Emulation, Education, and Evaluation Lab for Patient Safety) Center Program in 2002, where they currently perform educational simulations, MOCA simulations, and simulation for reentry to anesthesia practice after extended time away from clinical duties [35].

Many other applications of simulation to the practice of anesthesiology have been developed. We describe many of these in Table 1.1.

Table 1.1 Varied uses of simulation in anesthesiology and when they first were introduced

Activity	Description
Resident training in crisis management	One of the very first uses of simulation was for residents managing acute events, based on the principles of Anesthesia Crisis Resource Management [33]. Virtually all anesthesiology programs now have such programs of various types
Trainee training in procedures	Partial task training (e.g., intubation mannequins) predated the modern era of mannequin-based simulation. More recently, task trainers for regional anesthesia and central line insertion (with or without ultrasound guidance) have become popular [38, 39]
Use of simulation in training of nurse anesthetists	Not too long after simulation mannequins became available commercially, training for procedures and managing critical events were adopted in schools of nurse anesthesia. Joanne Fletcher, EdD, CRNA and John O'Donnell, DrPH, CRNA, at the University of Pittsburgh and Alfred Lupien, CRNA, Ph.D., then at the Medical College of Georgia, were early pioneers [40]
Research in human performance	One of the first uses of mannequin-based simulation was in the study of human performance in anesthesiology to develop better prevention of initiating events and improved responses to events [41–43]. The work by this group has been followed over the years by the use of simulation for many different aspects of human performance, teamwork, educational methods, etc.
Introducing new clinical techniques	In 1998, Murray and colleagues demonstrated how simulation can be used for training in the use of a new drug or technology, in this case the introduction of remifentanil [44]
Resident performance assessment	Devitt and colleagues and Gaba and colleagues both reported on the use of simulation for performance assessment in 1998 [45–47]. Later, deeper work in developing assessment processes for technical skills and rating rubrics was reported by anesthesiologist David Murray and his psychometrician colleague, John Boulet [48, 49]. They demonstrated that reliable scoring can be produced through careful development of the scoring instruments and effective rater training. More recently, Blum and colleagues demonstrated that reliable rating instruments can be created for identifying behavioral performance weaknesses early in residency [50]. That assessment via simulation has come of age is evidenced by the American Board of Anesthesiology's (ABA) use of a low-fidelity OSCE in its licensing exam, beginning in 2017 [51]
Perioperative teamwork (TOMS)	Almost all early uses of simulation in anesthesiology involved only anesthesiologists or only CRNAs as learners. One notable exception is the Team-Oriented Medical Simulation (TOMS) program started in Switzerland in 1995 by Drs. Hans Schaefer, Robert Helmreich, and Daniel Scheidegger. Using a pig liver-based simulation scenario, they trained teams of surgeons, anesthesiologists, and nurses in teamwork skills [52]
Training practicing anesthesiology providers	The first decade of the modern era of anesthesiology simulation focused mostly on trainee education. In 2001, a program for attending anesthesiologists was created among the hospitals affiliated with Harvard Medical School, catalyzed by an incentive from their insurance company, CRICO (Controlled Risk Insurance Company) [53, 54]. CRICO offered a $500 rebate from the approximately $10,000 annual premium for those who participated in this training at least once every 3 years. Virtually all attending anesthesiologists did so between 2001 and 2003, and the program became permanently established. Over a few years, this training became a requirement for hospital credentialing
Maintenance of Certification in Anesthesiology (MOCA®)	In 2008, the ABA adopted a requirement of a 1-day, CRM program every 10 years for maintenance of certification of anesthesiologists [55] licensed starting in that year. A process was created to endorse anesthesia simulation programs to conduct the courses; the American Society of Anesthesiologists' Simulation Education Network currently includes 49 centers. However, vocal anesthesiologists pushed back against the requirement, and it was made optional starting in 2015
Reentry into practice	Simulation has been used to evaluate providers whose clinical skills are in question or who are returning to practice after an extended hiatus. Such a program was developed at Mt. Sinai Hospital around 2002 [56, 57]

After the initial introduction of simulation in what we might called the "modern" era that started in the late 1980s, simulation in anesthesiology, typical of most technology innovations, had slow growth through the 1990s. We summarize here many of the new applications of simulation that appeared either first in anesthesiology or were introduced into anesthesiology from elsewhere. Most of these topics are given deeper discussion in other chapters of this book

Society for Simulation in Healthcare

An important milestone in the growth of simulation in anesthesiology, and later for all of healthcare, was the formation of the Society for Simulation in Healthcare [36]. This organization grew out of anesthesiology over several years. It started in 1995 with the *First Conference on Simulators in Anesthesiology Education* at the University of Rochester in New York, with fewer than 100 attendants. Daniel Raemer, Ph.D., attended the second conference. He was a biomedical engineer who had developed various clinical technologies while working in the Department of Anesthesia at BWH, and was introduced to simulation by Jeff Cooper, who brought him onto the BASC team in 1995. Raemer, as President of the Society for Technology in Anesthesia (STA), steered the topic of the 1998 annual meeting to "Simulation in Anesthesiology." The meeting drew an unusually large turnout. In 2000, the leadership of STA convened the first International Meeting on Medical Simulation (IMMS) in Scottsdale. Based on growing attendance, an independent society, the Society for Medical Simulation (SMS), was formed in 2003. Raemer became the first President of the Board of Overseers at its first meeting in January 2004, in Albuquerque, New Mexico. Raemer was elected as its first Chairman. In 2005, Ms. Beverlee Anderson (widely acknowledged as having been critical to the success of the society) was hired as the first Executive Director.

It is a testimony to the wisdom of anesthesiology as a field and its simulation leaders that the society it spearheaded was deliberately designed to be ecumenical and interprofessional. This is unusual since so many healthcare specialties have traditionally leaned toward independence. The society's organizing documents required a diversity of healthcare professions to be members of the Board. But, it was not until 2006 that SMS changed its name to the Society for Simulation in Healthcare (SSH) [36]; SSH renamed its meeting to the International Meeting for Simulation in Healthcare (IMSH), recognizing the truly interprofessional spirit and collaboration that is vital to patient care effectiveness and patient safety. The society membership is currently broadly distributed among physicians, nurses, allied health professionals, educators, and scientists.

Dan Raemer advocated for SSH to start its own journal. And thus, another milestone for simulation internationally was SSH's creation of its first journal, *Simulation in Healthcare* in 2005. Its first Editor-in-Chief was anesthesiologist and healthcare simulation pioneer, David Gaba. Gaba retired from the position in 2016. He is widely credited with leadership that enabled growth in research and practice of healthcare simulation [37].

Analysis and Conclusions

Technologies and pedagogical frameworks for the modern era of simulation were catalyzed and enabled by innovative applications in anesthesiology. Yet, the core of this story is not about technology- it is about pioneers, their passions, and the dissemination of a new idea that arose at a time when unmet needs were ready for it. One common theme from these stories is that all the pioneers had some education in engineering or computer science. And, in most of the stories, there were close collaborations of interprofessional teams, including engineers. Perhaps there is a familiar message here about the critical contribution of engineering to many medical advances and the power of interprofessional teams.

Also interesting is that, from what we can tell, the pioneers who simultaneously developed their applications of simulation did so independently. We might expect that the early work of Abrahamson and Denson, while before its time, would have informed the ideas of Philip, Schwid, Gaba, Good, and Gravenstein, but that does not appear to be the case. Rather, each instantiation of simulation emerged from different driving goals and without knowledge of Sim One – a form of "convergent evolution". Philip was driven by an educational interest in one topic that was especially challenging to teach without the aid of simulation of mathematical models; Schwid was similarly interested in education as it related to physiology, pharmacology, and resuscitation; Gaba started out of interest in understanding human performance in managing critical events generically and improving it; Good's and Gravenstein's objectives were to improve mastery performance. These different drivers led to several successful implementations of simulation and, together, spread of the technology through different means.

Competition and market pressure between several companies also helped spread simulation technologies. We discussed the two companies that arose specifically to address anesthesiology-related needs. One succeeded; the other failed (those stories are not well enough documented yet to be understood). The other current market leader, Laerdal, had a different origin (i.e., in resuscitation). While that has some relationship to anesthesiology, anesthesiology was not the source of the company's entry into the market.

There is no one truth about how any idea propagates to become mainstream [58]. For simulation, there were several drivers, including development of enabling technologies, unmet needs in education, and the factor that we believe catalyzed simulation's explosive growth – a growing focus on patient safety. In many (but not all) cases, grant funding enabled dissemination.

The pattern of simulation's trajectory of dissemination is not unusual. With any innovation, there are early adopters who are willing to take a risk on something new, and the speed of dissemination varies after that. Passionate pioneers who use these technologies to address the needs they identify most with likely accelerate the spread; this has been the case with simulation. There is much credit to be given to those who developed the many pioneering applications of simulation in anesthesiology and contributed to its spread throughout healthcare around the world. Those who benefit from simulation, most of all the patients, should be thankful to those who took the challenges and risk and had the passion and perseverance to see their ideas succeed.

References

1. Owen H. Simulation in healthcare education: an extensive history: Springer, Switzerland. 2016. p. 16.
2. Cooper JB, Taqueti VR. A brief history of the development of mannequin simulators for clinical education and training. Qual Saf Health Care. 2004;13(Suppl 1):i11–8.
3. Rosen K. The history of simulation. In: Levine AI, Jr. DeMaria S, Schwartz AD, Sim AJ, editors. The comprehensive textbook of healthcare simulation. New York: Springer Science+Business Media; 2013. p. 5–48.
4. Stoelting RK. About APSF: Foundation History. Available from: http://apsf.org/about_history.php.
5. Abrahamson S, Denson J, Wolf R. A computer-based patient simulator for training anesthesiologists. Educational Technol. 1969;9(10).
6. Gaba D. Anesthesia simulations in an actual operating room environment. Anesthesiology. 1987;67(3A):A467.
7. Gaba DM, DeAnda A. A comprehensive anesthesia simulation environment: re-creating the operating room for research and training. Anesthesiology. 1988;69(3):387–94.
8. Good M, Lampotang S, Gibby G, Gravenstein J. Critical events simulation for training in anesthesiology. J Clin Monit Computing. 1988;4:140.
9. Schwid HA. A flight simulator for general anesthesia training. Comput Biomed Res. 1987;20(1):64–75.
10. Schwid HA, O'Donnell D. The anesthesia simulator-recorder: a device to train and evaluate anesthesiologists' responses to critical incidents. Anesthesiology. 1990;72(1):191–7.
11. Cooper JB, Newbower RS, Long CD, McPeek B. Preventable anesthesia mishaps: a study of human factors. Anesthesiology. 1978;49(6):399–406.
12. Pierce EC Jr. The 34th Rovenstine Lecture. 40 years behind the mask: safety revisited. Anesthesiology. 1996;84(4):965–75.
13. Pierce EC Jr, Cooper JB. Analysis of anesthesia mishaps. Int Anesthesiol Clin. Boston: Little Brown; 1984.
14. Gaba DM, Abrahamson SJ. Dr. Stephen Abrahamson – Profile of a Pioneer Youtube https://www.youtube.com/watch?v=grz1cI7QN2s2014.
15. Abrahamson S. Human simulation for training in anesthesiology. In: Glasser, editor. Medical physics; 1970.
16. Anonymous. Deathproof patient for student doctors. Life. 1967;1967:87–9.
17. Cooper JB, Newbower RS, Kitz RJ. An analysis of major errors and equipment failures in anesthesia management: considerations for prevention and detection. Anesthesiology. 1984;60(1):34–42.
18. Cooper JB. Patient safety and biomedical engineering. In: Kitz RJ, editor. This is no humbug: reminiscences of the Department of Anesthesia at the Massachusetts General Hospital. Boston: Department of Anesthesia and Critical Care, Massachusetts General Hospital; 2002. p. 377–420.
19. Cooper JB, Pierce EC Jr. The anesthesia patient safety foundation (editorial). APSF Newsletter. 1986;1(1):1.
20. Gas Man. Available from: http://www.gasmanweb.com/.
21. Philip JH. Personal communication with J Philip. November 2016.
22. Fukui Y, Smith NT. Interactions among ventilation, the circulation, and the uptake and distribution of halothane--use of a hybrid computer multiple model: II. Spontaneous vs. controlled ventilation, and the effects of CO2. Anesthesiology. 1981;54(2):119–24.
23. Schwid HA. Electrocardiogram simulation using a personal computer. Comput Biomed Res. 1988;21(6):562–9.
24. Schwid HA. Frequency response evaluation of radial artery catheter-manometer systems: sinusoidal frequency analysis versus flush method. J Clin Monit. 1988;4(3):181–5.
25. Schwid HA. Semiautomatic algorithm to remove resonance artifacts from the direct radial artery pressure. Biomed Instrum Technol. 1989;23(1):40–3.
26. Schwid HA, Buffington CW, Strum DP. Computer simulation of the hemodynamic determinants of myocardial oxygen supply and demand. J Cardiothorac Anesth. 1990;4(1):5–18.
27. Schwid HA, Taylor LA, Smith NT. Computer model analysis of the radial artery pressure waveform. J Clin Monit. 1987;3(4):220–8.
28. Perrow C. Normal accidents- living with high-risk technologies. New York: Basic Books, Inc; 1984.
29. Gaba DM, Maxwell M, DeAnda A. Anesthetic mishaps: breaking the chain of accident evolution. Anesthesiology. 1987;66(5):670–6.
30. DeAnda A, Gaba DM. Role of experience in the response to simulated critical incidents. Anesth Analg. 1991;72(3):308–15.
31. Gaba D, Howard S, Fish K, Smith B, Sowb Y. Simulation-based training in anesthesia crisis resource management (ACRM): a decade of experience. Simul Gaming. 2001;32:175–93.
32. Howard SK, Gaba DM, Fish KJ, Yang G, Sarnquist FH. Anesthesia crisis resource management training: teaching anesthesiologists to handle critical incidents. Aviat Space Environ Med. 1992;63(9):763–70.
33. Gaba D, Fish K, Howard S. Crisis management in anesthesiology. Philadelphia: Churchill Livingstone; 1994. 294 p.
34. Gaba D, Fish K, Howard S, Burden A. Crisis management in anesthesiology. 2nd ed. Philadelphia: Saunders; 2015.
35. Mount Sinai Simulation HELPS Center [November 27, 2016]. Available from: http://msmc.affinitymembers.net/simulator/main.html.
36. Raemer D. Society for simulation in healthcare. In: Riley R, editor. Manual of simulation in healthcare. New York: Oxford University Press, Inc.; 2006. p. 529–32.
37. Cooper JB, Issenberg BS, DeVita MA, Glavin R. Tribute to David Gaba on the occasion of his retiring as editor-in-chief of simulation in healthcare. Simul Healthc. 2016;11(5):301–3.
38. Ma IW, Brindle ME, Ronksley PE, Lorenzetti DL, Sauve RS, Ghali WA. Use of simulation-based education to improve outcomes of central venous catheterization: a systematic review and meta-analysis. Acad Med. 2011;86(9):1137–47.
39. Niazi AU, Haldipur N, Prasad AG, Chan VW. Ultrasound-guided regional anesthesia performance in the early learning period: effect of simulation training. Reg Anesth Pain Med. 2012;37(1):51–4.
40. O'Donnell JM, Phrampus PE. Simulation in nurse anesthesia education and practice. In: Henrichs B, Thompson J, editors. A resource for nurse anesthesia educators. 2nd ed: Elsevier; 2017. (in press).
41. Gaba DM, DeAnda A. The response of anesthesia trainees to simulated critical incidents. Anesth Analg. 1989;68(4):444–51.

42. Gaba D, editor. Dynamic decision-making in anesthesiology: use of realistic simulation for training. Nato Advanced Research Workshop: advanced models for cognition for medical training and practice; 1991.
43. Gaba D. Human work environment and simulators. In: Miller R, editor. Anesthesia. New York: Churchill-Livingstone; 1994. p. 2635–79.
44. Murray W, Good M, Gravenstein J, Brasfield W. Novel application of a full human simulator: training with remifentanil prior to human use. Anesthesiology. 1998;89(3A):A56.
45. Devitt JH, Kurrek M, Cohen M. Can a simulator-based performance be used to assess anesthesiologists? Anesthesiology. 1998;89(3A):A1173.
46. Devitt JH, Kurrek MM, Cohen MM, Fish K, Fish P, Noel AG, et al. Testing internal consistency and construct validity during evaluation of performance in a patient simulator. Anesth Analg. 1998;86(6):1160–4.
47. Gaba DM, Howard SK, Flanagan B, Smith BE, Fish KJ, Botney R. Assessment of clinical performance during simulated crises using both technical and behavioral ratings. Anesthesiology. 1998;89(1):8–18.
48. Murray D, Boulet J, Ziv A, Woodhouse J, Kras J, McAllister J. An acute care skills evaluation for graduating medical students: a pilot study using clinical simulation. Med Educ. 2002;36(9):833–41.
49. Boulet JR, Murray D, Kras J, Woodhouse J, McAllister J, Ziv A. Reliability and validity of a simulation-based acute care skills assessment for medical students and residents. Anesthesiology. 2003;99(6):1270–80.
50. Blum RH, Boulet JR, Cooper JB, Muret-Wagstaff SL. Simulation-based assessment to identify critical gaps in safe anesthesia resident performance. Anesthesiology. 2014;120(1):129–41.
51. Rathmell JP, Lien C, Harman A. Objective structured clinical examination and board certification in anesthesiology. Anesthesiology. 2014;120(1):4–6.
52. Schaefer HG, Helmreich RL, Scheidegger D. TOMS- Team Oriented Medical simulation (safety in the operating theatre- part 1: interpersonal relationships and team performance). Current Anaesth Crit Care. 1995;6:48–53.
53. Blum R, Cooper JB, Feinstein D, Raemer D, Russell R, Sunder N. Sustaining development of crisis resource management training for academic faculty: a new approach to continuing education. Anesth Analg. 2003;97(S2):S10.
54. Hanscom R. Medical simulation from an insurer's perspective. Acad Emerg Med. 2008;15(11):984–7.
55. The American Board of Anesthesiology – MOCA 2.0 Part 4. Available from: http://www.theaba.org/MOCA/MOCA-2-0-Part-4.
56. DeMaria S, Levine AI, Bryson EO. The use of multi-modality simulation in the retraining of the physician for medical licensure. J Clin Anes. 2010;22:294–9.
57. DeMaria S Jr, Samuelson ST, Schwartz AD, Sim AJ, Levine AI. Simulation-based assessment and retraining for the anesthesiologist seeking reentry to clinical practice: a case series. Anesthesiology. 2013;119(1):206–17.
58. C. M. Disruptive innovation: In need of better theory. J Prod Innov Manag. 2005;23:19–25.

Education and Learning Theory

2

Deborah D. Navedo and Andrés T. Navedo

Introduction

"See one; Do one; Teach one…" While this approach worked well for generations, we now live in a world in which evidence-based medicine is the expectation. Similarly, calls for educational reform across the health professions compel us to practice evidence-based education. In this chapter, we will review the evolution of educational theories and practices, from the Flexner era through current educational best practices (see Table 2.1).

Evolution of Perspectives on Teaching and Learning

Education across the health professions shifted significantly in the past 50 years, away from the simple application of teaching and learning principles that apply to children as honed in primary and secondary schools (pedagogy) to teaching and learning principles uniquely effective for the adult learners (*andragogy*). Most learners in the health professions are considered adult learners for the purpose of designing educational experiences not only because of their age but also because of their cognitive and social level of maturation.

Adult learners have fairly well described learning needs. Malcolm Knowles [1], who built on earlier European models of adult learning, described six major assumptions related to motivation in adult learners:

D. D. Navedo (✉)
STRATUS Center for Medical Simulation, Brigham and Women's Hospital, Boston, MA, USA
e-mail: DNAVEDO@MGH.harvard.EDU

A. T. Navedo
Department of Anesthesiology, Critical Care and Pain Medicine, Boston Children's Hospital, Boston, MA, USA

Harvard Medical School, Boston, MA, USA

Table 2.1 Teaching in a New Era

	Flexner-era focus	The twenty-first century best practices
Focus of field	Teacher centric	Learner centric
Mode of learning	Content delivery	Content discovery
Learner engagement	Passive (lecture, readings)	Active (multimodal)
Social context	In isolation	In groups and teams
Learning	Time on task based	Competency based
Epistemological view	Cognition as objective and rational	Cognition as context dependent and bounded
Clinical decision-making	Decisions as logical	Subject to unconscious bias
Teacher role	Expert that gives knowledge	Facilitator that guides learning

For additional readings, see L D Fink, (2013) [11] Creating Significant Learning Experiences

1. Need to know: Adults need to know the reason why and how they are learning.
2. Self-concept: Adults learn value through autonomous self-directed learning.
3. Prior experience: Adults prefer learning that is connected to available resources and mental models.
4. Readiness: Adults prefer learning that is immediately connected to their own work or personal lives.
5. Orientation: Adults learn better when problem-based rather than content-based.
6. Motivation: Adults respond better to internal rather than external motivations.

Understanding and capitalizing on these motivators can help the educator design effective learning experiences.

When mapping the topics for learning, there are three domains of Bloom's taxonomy [2] of learning: *cognitive, psychomotor, and affective*. These are often referred to as knowledge, skills, and attitudes/behaviors, or "KSA," across the health professions' education literature [3, 4]. Each of the domains is described as having levels of increasing complexity (see Table 2.2).

B. Mahoney et al. (eds.), *Comprehensive Healthcare Simulation: Anesthesiology*, Comprehensive Healthcare Simulation,
https://doi.org/10.1007/978-3-030-26849-7_2

Table 2.2 Bloom's taxonomy and levels of competency

	Cognitive	Psychomotor	Affective
More complex	Creating	Naturalizing	Characterizing
	Evaluating	Articulation	Organizing
	Analyzing	Precision	Valuing
	Applying	Manipulation	Responding
	Understanding		
Less complex	Remembering	Imitation	Receiving

Adopted from Anderson and Krathwohl (2001) [5]

First, *cognitive learning* of knowledge can take many forms. Knowledge is often defined as content, information, or protocols, and usually takes the form of materials that are given to the learner. Examples of learning within this domain might include the memorization of anatomical nomenclature and structures, function and use of equipment, or a series of criteria and decision points within a resuscitation protocol. The updated version of Bloom's taxonomy and its application to learning was described by Anderson and Krathwohl (2001) [5], in which they further defined four subcategories of knowledge as factual, conceptual, procedural, and metacognitive. While discussion of these is beyond the scope of this introductory chapter, the domains are useful for defining the levels of outcomes expected from the learning.

The most common model used to identify the developmental levels of learning in medical education is *Miller's model* (1990) [6], in which a learner gains progressing competencies toward independent practice.

1. Knows: Can report definitions, identify landmarks, or discuss the underlying physics
2. Knows how: Can describe the detailed steps in a procedure either written or orally
3. Shows how: Can accurately complete a skill according to a checklist
4. Does: Can complete a skill within the complexities of clinical environment

The cognitive domain of Bloom's taxonomy is considered the standard framework for writing learning objectives for a given learning activity. We should note that charts of sample objectives, or "verbs," are often based on only the cognitive domain and omit the psychomotor and affective domains. If simulation session goals include learning in domains beyond the cognitive, appropriate objectives should be defined in these areas as well (see also Chap. 3).

Assessment of cognitive learning has been oversimplified in the past. Multiple choice questions and "fill in the blank"-type text questions have been used to assess the learner's ability to recall definitions, identify structures, and recognize patterns [7]. In the clinical context, there are many more contextual factors affecting procedural decision-making and metacognition that require more sophisticated approaches to assessment, such as case studies, direct observation, or portfolios (see Assessment section below).

Second, *psychomotor learning* of skills may occur in various forms and progresses through an anticipatable sequence of developmental stages. While not limited to psychomotor learning, deliberate practice as described by K Anders Ericsson [8] has been the standard theory for skills acquisition in the health professions. The basic premise rests with the notion that expert performance is primarily the result of expert practice, not innate talent or natural abilities, meaning how one practices matters most.

The four critical characteristics of effective *deliberate practice* are:

1. Motivation: Learners must attend to the task and exert effort to improve.
2. Link to the known: Learners must understand the mechanism and purpose of the task easily in the context of preexisting knowledge.
3. Immediate feedback: Learners must receive immediate formative feedback.
4. Repetition: Learners must repeatedly perform the same task accurately.

Many simulation centers invest in partial task trainers, which are models in which the learner may perform a focused portion of a skill repeatedly, for deliberate practice. Examples of such equipment include intravenous arms, central line torsos, or phantom models for ultrasonography. Skills acquisition in the context of simulation-based learning is most effectively accomplished through separate deliberate practice on task trainers, prior to integration into a scenario.

Assessment of psychomotor learning is often accomplished by accuracy measures, such as percentage of errors in repeated performances or time to completion [9].

Finally, *affective learning* of attitudes, beliefs, and behaviors is often more complex requiring thoughtful staging by the educator and more effort by the learners. Krathwohl (1964) [2] described levels of learning with increasing sophistication, from basic to complex:

1. Receiving: Awareness of (and willing to tolerate) the existence of ideas, materials, or phenomena
2. Responding: Commitment (in some manner) to the ideas, materials, or phenomena by taking action to respond to them
3. Valuing: Willingness to be perceived by others as valuing the ideas, materials, or phenomena
4. Organization: Integration of the value with those already held into an internally consistent philosophy
5. Characterization: Takes action consistently according to the internalized values

For example, a department may decide to integrate principles of team communication from Team STEPPS including the two challenge rule, in which team members are empowered to "stop the line" if they sense or discover an essential safety breach. This may be a difficult change of organizational culture, especially in places where challenges to traditional authority may not be welcome. Learners at the Receiving level will tolerate the notion that those with authority may need to be challenged, but may not want to speak up. The Responding level learners might be able to speak up during a simulation, while those at the Valuing level are willing to encourage others to speak up in the clinical environment. Those at the Organization stage will become comfortable with a changing culture of respectful cross-monitoring and open discussion of safety issues, and those at the Characterization stage will be able to consistently role model the new behaviors as part of their professional practice.

While assessment of effective or attitudinal learning has been often neglected completely, this domain has recently received fresh attention and scrutiny [10]. Observable behaviors were used as proxies for non-observable values and intentions. These may only indicate a Responding level of isolated action, and not an integration of new values into a cohesive approach to professional practice. Reflective writing or authentic (in situ) assessment by peers can be informative in this context.

In the following sections, the additional theories that help define the individual learners' needs are summarized.

Learner Centric Approaches

Recognition that the quality of teaching and learning is best assessed in the learners, not in the actions of the person at the lectern, drawings on the board, or in the slides on the screen, has shifted the approaches in the field of health professions education from focus on improving teaching skills to focus on creating meaningful learning environments and individual learner activities and outcomes. This shift from teaching-centric to learner-centric approaches is the keystone that defines current best practices in adult education, with broad implications from higher education to professional and clinical education [11]. Additionally, the learner is now seen as having learner characteristics associated with specific developmental stages.

Developmental models within the clinical settings are readily visible, especially in the discipline of pediatrics. Erik Erikson's stages of psychosocial development guide clinical assessment and care, and education's developmental models serve similar purposes of better understanding the learners. The *novice to expert model* (Dreyfus and Benner) [12, 13] describes stages of professional development and skills acquisition.

1. Novice: Rigid adherence to rules with no discretionary judgment
2. Advanced beginner: Limited situational awareness, without ability to prioritize
3. Competent: Deliberate planning with some awareness of actions and effect on goals
4. Proficient: Holistic view and prioritizes, applies heuristics meaningfully
5. Expert: Intuitively transcends guidelines in treating whole and can be analytical when needed

Understanding the learner through these stages helps in designing effective learner centric experiences. A novice is not ready to think about complex prioritizations and can only follow rules. The *zone of proximal development* (ZPD) (Vygotsky in Chaiklin 2003) [14] describes the area of growth that is immediately beyond the current abilities of the learner, but within reach with support of scaffolding, which is a teaching method designed to increasingly promote the learner's independence in understanding over time. For example, optimal learning for the novice might be to start focusing on the situation as a whole, with the recognition that some rules can uniformly apply across contexts. Similarly, the competent learner may still need to be learning about how actions affect the overall goal of patient care.

Similarly, by understanding the individual learner's developmental stage, learning environments or simulation sessions can be tailored to include just enough, but not too much, realistic environmental factors. *Cognitive load theory* (Sweller, 1988 [15]) refers to the brain's ability to sort through and focus on certain stimuli, while becoming overwhelmed when overburdened with stimuli. Initially described in the context of multimedia-based instructional design, cognitive burden was primarily derived from sorting out portions of the media that were important to attend to for successful learning. With regard to education, cognitive load has a number of varieties that warrant consideration, given their influences on a learner's ability to learn effectively:

1. Intrinsic cognitive load: The inherent difficulty of a topic or task. Calculus has more intrinsic cognitive load than simple addition.
2. Extraneous cognitive load: This depends on the manner in which information is presented to the learner, and is the portion controlled by the instructor.
3. Germane cognitive load: The cognitive activity devoted to processing, construction, and automation of information and activities. This is where learning occurs.

Simulation environments may contain multiple extrinsic cognitive load factors as distractions, such as crying family members. The mental effort required to suppress the non-educative factors may adversely affect the learning outcome.

For the novice to advanced beginner learners, a crying family member may present an overload, in which the learners cannot effectively prioritize the needs of the patient.

A robust and simulation-based educational program will consider the learning needs of the learner through these various theoretical lenses, and each session will be designed as appropriate to the learner's level of training and predefined learning outcomes for that session.

Experiential and Reflective Learning

Once the learning needs of the individual learners have been assessed, education theory and best practices can inform how to create meaningful learning environments.

First, Knowles' reminds us that adults prefer to learn through problem solving and *experiential learning*, and any learning is optimized by *activating the learner*. The evidence supporting neuroplasticity in learning and the role of catecholamines is resounding (Reinis and Goldman, 2013 [16]). The excited and activated learners appear to have increased adrenergic and dopaminergic activities, which have been tied to longer duration of learning. *Russell's circumplex model of emotion* presents a framework for describing learner emotion. Activated learners will be in the upper right quadrant of the model (see Fig. 2.1).

Many traditional content delivery-focused lectures left students in the lower quadrants, resulting in them choosing to review the lecture by watching the recording at double speed to save time, and skipping the actual lecture completely.

Simulation, on the other hand, has the built-in benefit of requiring the learner to engage the experience and problem-solve from the beginning of the session. Knowing that the activated learner can be in either the positive or negative side of the model with regard to emotional valence, the instructor will need to monitor the learner's affect and actively manage the experience to avoid destructive environments leading to unintended outcomes from excessively negative experiences that cause the learner to feel distressed, disgusted, or miserable [17]. Extreme cases might lead to symptoms similar to post-traumatic stress disorder, in which the learner refuses to engage in simulation-based learning in the future. (See section below on Psychological Safety, also covered in Chap. 4.)

While there may be preferences for more pleasant learning experiences, there appear to be divergent preferences between learners regarding mode of learning. For example, some learners prefer to read and fully understand the skills being taught before touching the equipment, while others prefer to handle the equipment first before reading about its features. David *Kolb's learning styles* model has been applied to health professions and is

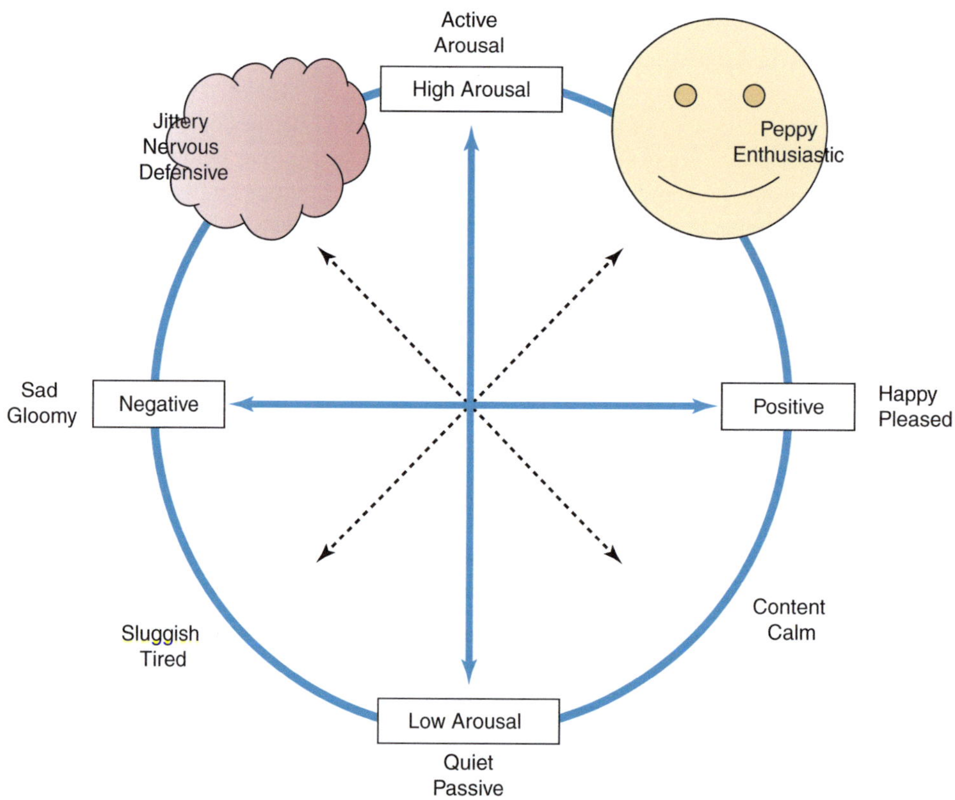

Fig. 2.1 Russell's circumplex model of emotion https://blog.biopac.com/circumplex-model-affect-motivational-state/

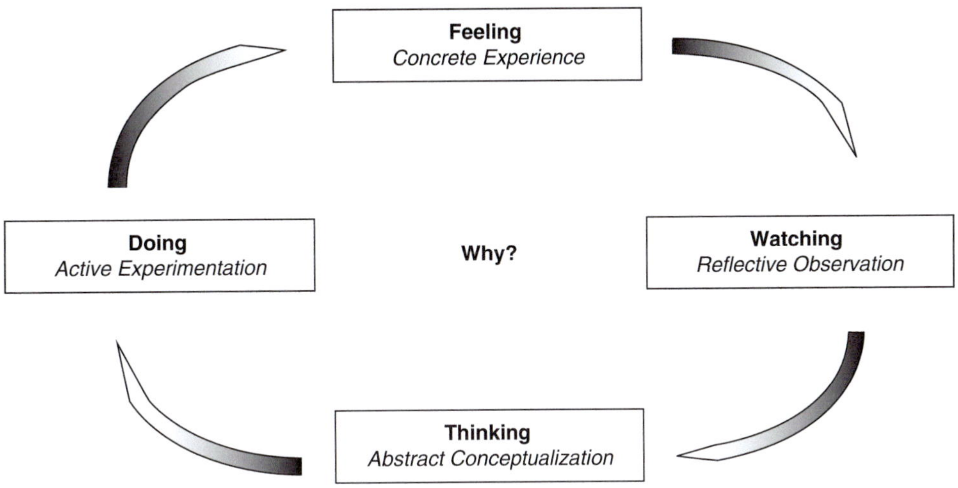

Fig. 2.2 Kolb's learning styles http://www.businessballs.com/kolblearningstyles.htm

useful in understanding that learners may prefer certain learning activities over others (Kolb 1984 [18]). The categories of learning activities are:

1. Feeling: concrete experiencing
2. Reflecting: reflective observation
3. Thinking: abstract conceptualization
4. Doing: active experimentation

The learning styles and preferences rest between the learning activities (see Fig. 2.2).

1. Diverging (feeling and watching): Learners are able to take on various perspectives easily. They are idea generators and brainstormers.
2. Assimilating (watching and thinking): Learners prefer concise and logical ideas, even when broad ranging thinking is needed, and they are skilled at seeing common threads and overarching goals.
3. Converging (doing and thinking): Learners prefer technical tasks and practical applications of theories and like to experiment with new ideas.
4. Accommodating (doing and feeling): Learners are hands-on and prefer intuition to logic, preferring to rely on other people's analyses, and like to be on teams.

These learning preferences are not considered static, and some shifting of preferences may occur over time. However, a deep appreciation for one's own preferences will help the educator to better engage learners of differing learning preferences.

The *Kolb's learning cycle* model is an integrated and inclusive approach for instructional design. Learning activities are sequentially presented through the four quadrants in a specific order for maximal learning impact. Doing is followed by feeling, reflection, and thinking in this order. The premise is that while each learner will be engaged in their preferred learning activity at some point, all learners can benefit from engaging in learning in all quadrants, especially in the health professions (Armstrong, 2005 [19]).

While the point of entry into the learning cycle can be flexible, the adult learner needs to know why he or she is learning, and this is the common starting point. Some prefer to read the chapters before engaging the simulation, preferring to have a strong understanding of the content before being asked to perform. Others may be very happy to jump into the simulation without much guidance, knowing that the chapters will be far more meaningful reading once they have the experience or a context. This variation in learner preference within any given group of learners requires thoughtful oversight to assure meaningful learning for all.

Paired with experiential learning, *reflective learning* is increasingly recognized as the second essential element in effective simulation-based learning. The theoretical foundation of reflective learning can be found in Donald Schon's work on *reflection-in-action* and *reflection-on-action.* Skillful debriefers invite the learners, following the simulation scenario, to recall and explore their thoughts and actions during the simulation and to openly consider how it went (reflection-on-action). Reflection and accurate self-assessment are not as intuitive as one may believe. Self-assessments have been widely discredited in the past decades due to the lack of understanding surrounding the wide variation in validity across contexts [20]. Accurate self-assessment is increasingly described as an acquired skill, and simulation facilitators are encouraged to examine the characteristics of the master learner as described by Schumacher [21].

Simulation experiences without the benefit of thoughtfully facilitated debriefing with reflective learning can be not only less effective, but, on occasion, harmful [22]. *Psychological safety* is a core requirement for an effective debriefing to occur. Also described as emotional safely, this is a shared agreement among participants and facilitators that values behaviors such as "seeking feedback, sharing information, asking for help, talking about errors, and experimentation" [23]. For additional discussion of creating the safe learning environment, see Chap. 4.

Simulation as an Educational Modality

Simulation is the ideal environment for advantaging both experiential and reflective learning and the application of sound educational practices. In this section, we review how principles of instructional design and assessment can be applied to simulation-based learning.

Instructional Design in Simulation

The field of education has shifted from *content-focused design* to results-focused design. Historically, the curriculum was mapped according to the topics that were to be taught, and lecturers were scheduled. Current approaches to instructional design begin with the results or learning outcomes in mind before choosing the activities. The focus has shifted from the content to be taught to the competencies to be demonstrated. This perspective is particularly useful when designing simulation sessions.

There are two common problems with content-focused classes that can be seen in poorly designed simulation sessions as well, called the "twin sins" of content-focused education by authors Wiggins and McTighe [24].

- Hands-on without being minds-on: Activities that were fun and interesting, but were not designed for and did not lead to new insights or achievements.
- Coverage of content: Students are marched through chapters of texts or procedural details in sequential order to touch on all of the material in a prescribed time. An example might include a simulation scenario that was packed with teaching points to the extent that the learners become overwhelmed passive listeners in the debriefing.

In *results-focused design, or "backwards design,"* learning activities are designed with the outcomes in mind. A well-designed simulation session or curriculum will be designed with the final learning goals and objectives being defined first (Wiggins and McTighe, 2005 [24]):

- Stage 1—Identify the desired results: What should learners know, understand, and be able to do at the end of the session? Which established standards or curricula inform this (e.g., milestones)? Is this at the appropriate priority and level for the learners?
- Stage 2: Determine acceptable evidence: How will we know that learners have achieved the desired learning results? Plan the assessments first.
- Stage 3: Plan [simulation] session: What enabling knowledge or skills will the learners need ahead of time to engage the simulation effectively? What clinical problems would reasonably trigger the desired self-assessments and behaviors, which will evidence the successful learning? Are there too many nonrelevant distracters within the case that will muddle the learning for the novice learner?

Tied to this design approach is the *flipped classroom*, in which much of the content exposure or acquisition is pushed out to the learners prior to attending case discussion or the simulation session. The goal of this approach is to maximize learning in the simulation session by focusing on application and management level activities, such as case discussion and problem analysis, rather than on the review of basics. Many simulation centers now have online modules, which the learners complete prior to attending the simulation session. These may include readings, videos, and even quizzes.

Finally, there are two guides that inform the instructional design of and educational best practices in simulation-based learning. *Gagne's Nine Events of Instruction* describe the elements of a well-run educational session [25]:

1. Gain attention of the learner.
2. Inform learners of the objectives.
3. Stimulate recall of prior learning.
4. Present the content.
5. Provide learning guidance.
6. Elicit performance.
7. Provide feedback.
8. Assess performance.
9. Enhance retention and transfer to the job.

Similarly, the *Debriefing Assessment for Simulation in Healthcare (DASH)* instrument describes elements of a well-run simulation and debriefing [26]:

1. Establishes engaging learning environment (prebriefing)
2. Maintains engaging learning environment
3. Structures debriefing in an organized way
4. Provokes engaging discussions
5. Identifies and explores performance gaps
6. Helps trainees achieve or sustain good future performance

These two can be combined to inform the design and implementation of a theory-driven simulation-based learning experience. The common characteristics for the orientation, scenario, and debriefing can be derived (see Table 2.3).

Table 2.3 Instructional design in simulation

Simulation component	Gagne's model	DASH model
Orientation	1. Gain attention 2. Informing learner of objectives	1. Establishes an engaging learning environment
Scenario	3. Stimulating recall of prerequisite learning 4. Presenting the stimulus materials 6. Eliciting the performance	2. Maintains engaging learning environment
Debriefing	5. Providing learning guidance 7. Providing feedback 8. Assessing performance 9. Enhancing retention and transfer	3. Structures debriefing in an organized way 4. Provokes engaging discussions 5. Identifies and explores performance gaps 6. Helps trainees achieve or sustain good future performance

Data from: https://harvardmedsim.org/media/DASH.handbook.2010.Final.Rev.2.pdf

Thoughtful design of the simulation scenario, based on accurate understanding of learning needs, is key to the effectiveness of simulation as an educational modality. See Chap. 3 regarding essentials of scenario building.

Assessment of Learning Outcomes

In the context of simulation-based education, there are three types of assessment that are used in specifically different contexts. All assessments involve the judgment by an expert or facilitator, who gives some form of feedback or report on their evaluation of the learning outcome (Svinicki, 2014 [27]).

1. *Formative assessment*: For learning purposes only. Often in the form of feedback that is shared with the learner only. Assessment results are never kept by the facilitator or the department and have no influence on future decisions around learner progression, graduation, or employment.
2. *Summative assessment*: For grading purposes. The results of these assessments are documented and recorded and become part of the learner's educational or employment record. Summative assessments that are shared with the learner for continued learning can have formative components, but are not purely formative.
3. *High-stakes assessment*: For direct decision-making around progression, graduation, or employment. Any simulation assessment that will affect the school's or department's decision regarding completion of training program or continued employment is considered high stakes, and there may be other contexts as well.

Clarity around the purpose of the simulation session and how the results will be used is a key element of session planning and implementation. If a learner believes that a simulation session is for formative purposes only and is very candid about self-criticism in the debriefing and then later discovers that his or her disclosures of lack of knowledge or clinical uncertainty were used to change scheduling assignments or progression, decisions can be destructive to the trusting relationships needed for effective debriefing. See Chap. 4 for additional discussion of the safe learning environment.

While many approaches to assessment in simulation-based learning exist, the following four approaches are commonly seen: quizzes that might include multiple choice questions, checklists, behaviorally anchored scales, and expert global rating scales (Scalese and Hatala 2013 [28]).

First, the traditional quizzes based on *multiple choice questions* (MCQs), with paper and pencil or electronic means, were the gold standard for assessment of learning during the industrial era (Krathwohl, 1964 [2]). The underlying assumption is that if learners can retain and apply knowledge on paper, then they are at least ready to start applying this knowledge in clinical practice. As discussed earlier, this often assesses only the learning in the cognitive domain, and limitedly so. Writing valid and reliable MCQs takes time and expertise, and creating a list of plausible but definitely incorrect distracters to accompany the one correct answer often requires specific training. MCQs are often used today to assure learner readiness by checking for prerequisite knowledge prior to the simulation session.

Second, the *checklist* is broadly used within simulation-based learning. The purpose is to standardize the elements to be assessed. Direct observations by a trained examiner and use of a checklist have improved assessments in both simulation and clinical settings. While some educators have access to established and well-studied checklists, others may need to create their own, based on their own expert understanding of the practice [29]. Others may find an instrument with a checklist that has been implemented before. A common criticism of checklists is that these fail to recognize individual patient or clinical contexts and factors, leading to the broad application of rules-based practice in complex cases that require additional assessment. Consulting an education specialist or research methodologist is highly recommended before implementing checklists, especially in high-stakes assessments.

Third, *behaviorally anchored scales* are a combination of checklists with descriptions of observable behaviors for each developmental level. For example, the ACGME Milestones project is based on descriptions of commonly observable behaviors as characteristic of developmental levels within graduate medical education. A milestone is defined as a coherent group of competency-based developmental outcomes (e.g., knowledge, skills, attitudes, and performance) that can be demonstrated progressively by residents/fellows from the beginning of their education through graduation to the unsupervised practice of their specialties. The *Debriefing Assessment in Healthcare Simulation (DASH)* is another example of an anchored scale, related to assessing quality of debriefings (as described earlier). The users can be easily oriented to the common definitions, improving inter-rater reliability. Many well-established instruments for assessment take the form of behaviorally anchored scales and have been implemented in various contexts. Establishment of validity and reliability of these instruments is somewhat easier than of checklists or open rating scales.

Finally, *expert global ratings* are often open scales, which do not include a significant amount of description of the passing or failing points. Global rating scales rely on the expert perspectives of experienced clinicians and educators. Sessions are observed as a whole, and the experts report their perspectives regarding the quality of the performance, often on a numeric scale of high quality performance to poor quality performance. Benefits include fairly easy application of these types of assessments. Experts are assumed to have the insight to differentiate excellent performances from those in which additional learning is required. The reports can be in the form of a pass/fail or a general point in development, such as "performing at the level commonly seen in second year learners." Pitfalls include the very real concern that one expert rater may not agree with another expert rater. Some raters may become known as "doves" (those who consistently score more favorably) and others as "hawks" (those who consistently score more harshly). This inconsistency in inter-rater reliability may go unchecked if not identified early and rater training sessions instituted to mitigate the variance.

There is considerable disagreement in the field of health professions education and assessment regarding the reliability of using simulation as a sole determinant of the high-stakes academic or employment decision. Both the nursing education [30, 31] and medical literature [32, 33] have significant findings questioning the reliability of simulation use for high stakes purposes. For further reading, see the Competency Assessment chapter in Levine's Comprehensive text (2013) [34].

In the following sections, we will apply these educational theories into the context of simulation-based learning in anesthesiology.

Simulation in Anesthesiology as Seen Through Learning Theory

Just as formal training in the practice of anesthesia prepares individuals to become expert clinicians, formal training in the science of learning is essential to becoming expert educators.

Simulation-based education in anesthesiology at the undergraduate, graduate, and continuing education stages presents different contexts in which learners of varying knowledge, skills, and attitudes may have distinct needs. Simulation-based educators would reasonably be expected to offer educational opportunities tailored to each combination of factors even in the presence of similar scenarios.

Undergraduate education in anesthesiology, required in most Canadian medical schools (Brull) [35], is not required in the United States (Euliano) [36], or by the Royal College of Anaesthetists in the United Kingdom. Application of the learning theories will be influenced by the learner's life experiences. For example, a recent high school graduate enrolled in a 6-year program of medical education, who may be 17 or 18 years of age, would be expected to have a different zones of proximal development (ZPD) as compared to the entry-level resident, who may be in his or her mid- to late twenties.

While there is no requirement for simulation-based education in anesthesiology at the undergraduate medical education level, the ACGME does require residents to participate in at least one simulated clinical experience each year (ACGME). It is of note that the Review Committee in Anesthesiology encourages training programs to incorporate surgeons and nurses into the simulation (FAQs). This is consistent with the emphasis on interprofessional education and practice also encouraged by the Institute of Medicine (IOM) and the World Health Organization (WHO).

Learning Outcomes and Session Objectives

Learning outcomes and session objectives will vary by participant level of practice or training. For example, the early trainee may be offered a simulation session on airway management in an otherwise healthy asthmatic adult, while a more advanced anesthesiologist may be offered a session on airway management in the context of conjoined twins.

The practice of anesthesia across clinical contexts requires mastery of complex actions guided by understanding or familiarity across the domains of knowledge, skills, and attitudes/behaviors. The ACGME has a defined roadmap of competencies and milestones that inform the learning outcomes (see Chap. 14).

Skill training in anesthesiology would be expected to be more prevalent where learners are in the early phases of training. Skills such as intravenous catheter insertion, airway intubation, and regional nerve block placement are examples of such skills.

As we move from time-based education, promotion, and maintenance of certification to competency-based criteria, the educational system should become more responsive to individual needs and strengths. Recent advances in clinical technology highlight examples such as the experienced practitioner seeking to add ultrasound to his or her practice. Similarly, a practitioner/trainee may return to practice/training after an extended absence. Educators familiar with educational theories and models would be better suited to identify appropriate learning outcomes and to guide such learners.

Case Study

Let us look at a sample scenario and how the learning theories and concepts can help inform the implementation of a scenario for second year anesthesia residents. For the clinical context, we can use the premise of the healthy patient who develops anaphylaxis after routine preoperative administration of antibiotic prophylaxis.

Such a scenario presents multiple possible learning outcomes. Some objectives are in the knowledge domain (appropriate epinephrine dosage, significance of tryptase level), some in the skills domain (setting up of infusion pumps, intubation), and others in the attitude domain (prioritization of interventions, communication with team members to clarify each member's roles).

Miller's model of clinical competence would guide us to assess the learner's cognition (*knows* the doses) and behavior (*shows* adequate cardiopulmonary resuscitation, or CPR, when asked or *does* CPR appropriately without being prompted).

Adding complexity to the scenario (such as comorbidities, emergency setting, or electrical failure) would increase cognitive load and make the simulation more challenging for proficient participants (see Dreyfus developmental model above) and achieve a scenario difficulty within the ZPD for the participants, depending on the learning objectives. However, the novice learner might be overwhelmed by the increasing complexity and cognitive load pushing the scenario well beyond the ZPD for this learner.

Content presented prior to the simulation session can follow the principles of the flipped classroom technique, presenting content or activities that focus the learner's attention on the educational goals for which the simulation has been designed.

While debriefing after the simulation is the first part of reflection-on-action, pauses for discussion during a given simulation can expand the time for participants to benefit from reflection-in-action.

Conclusion

In conclusion, this exciting field of simulation-based learning has grown in sophistication as we better understand the complexity of the human mind and how clinicians think and make decisions that affect the quality and safety of patient care. All simulation-based instructors are encouraged to both consult education specialists and to seek further opportunities for continued professional development in the field of education.

References

1. Knowles MS, Holton EFIII, Swanson RA. The adult learner. 7th ed. New York: Routledge; 2012.
2. Krathwohl DR, Bloom BS, Masia MD. Taxonomy of educational objectives: book 2 – affective domain. New York/London: Longman; 1964.
3. Quinones MA, Ehrenstein A, editors. Training for a rapidly changing workplace: applications of psychological research. 1st ed. Washington, DC: Amer Psychological Assn; 1996.
4. Institute of Medicine (US) Committee on the Health Professions Education Summit. Health professions education: a bridge to quality. (Greiner AC, Knebel E, eds.). Washington (DC): National Academies Press (US); 2003. http://www.ncbi.nlm.nih.gov/books/NBK221528/. Accessed 21 May 2018.
5. Anderson LW, Krathwohl DR, et al., editors. A taxonomy for learning, teaching, and assessing: a revision of Bloom's taxonomy of educational objectives. Boston: Allyn & Bacon/Pearson Education Group; 2001.
6. Miller GE. The assessment of clinical skills/competence/performance. Acad Med. 1990;65(9 Suppl):S63–7.
7. Norcini JJ. Setting standards on educational tests. Med Educ. 2003;37(5):464–9.
8. Ericsson KA. Deliberate practice and acquisition of expert performance: a general overview. Acad Emerg Med Off J Soc Acad Emerg Med. 2008;15(11):988–94. https://doi.org/10.1111/j.1553-2712.2008.00227.x.
9. Norcini J, Burch V. Workplace-based assessment as an educational tool: AMEE Guide No. 31. Med Teach. 2007;29(9):855–71. https://doi.org/10.1080/01421590701775453.
10. Norcini JJ, Blank LL, Duffy FD, Fortna GS. The mini-CEX: a method for assessing clinical skills. Ann Intern Med. 2003;138(6):476–81.
11. Fink LD. Creating significant learning experiences: an integrated approach to designing college courses, revised and updated, p. 13. Second.; 2013.
12. Dreyfus HL, Dreyfus SE. Mind over machine. New York: The Free Press; 1986. p. 16–51.
13. Benner P. From novice to expert. Upper Saddle River: Prentice Hall; 2001.
14. Chaiklin S. The zone of proximal development in Vygotsky's analysis of learning and instruction; 2003. doi:https://doi.org/10.1017/CBO9780511840975.004.
15. Sweller J. Cognitive load during problem solving: effects on learning. Cogn Sci. 1988;12(2):257–85. https://doi.org/10.1207/s15516709cog1202_4.
16. Reinis and Goldman. The chemistry of behavior: a molecular approach to neuroplasticity. London: Plenuem Press; 2013. p. 336.

17. Rudolph JW, Foldy EG, Robinson T, Kendall S, Taylor SS, Simon R. Helping without harming: the instructor's feedback dilemma in debriefing – a case study. Simul Healthc J Soc Simul Healthc. 2013;8(5):304–16. https://doi.org/10.1097/SIH.0b013e318294854e.
18. Kolb DA. Experiential learning: experience as the source of learning and development. Englewood Cliffs: Prentice Hall; 1984.
19. Armstrong E, Parsa-Parsi R. How can physicians' learning styles drive educational planning? Acad Med. 2005;80(7):680–4.
20. Davis DA, Mazmanian PE, Fordis M, Van Harrison R, Thorpe KE, Perrier L. Accuracy of physician self-assessment compared with observed measures of competence: a systematic review. JAMA. 2006;296(9):1094–102. https://doi.org/10.1001/jama.296.9.1094.
21. Schumacher DJ, Englander R, Carracio C. Developing the master learner: applying learning theory to the learner, the teacher, and the learning environment. Acad Med. 2013;88(11):1635–45.
22. Rudolph JW, Simon R, Rivard P, Dufresne RL, Raemer DB. Debriefing with good judgment: combining rigorous feedback with genuine inquiry. Anesthesiol Clin. 2007;25(2):361–76.
23. Edmondson A. Psychological safety and learning behavior in work teams. Adm Sci Q. 1999;44(2):350–83. https://doi.org/10.2307/2666999.
24. Wiggins G, McTighe J. Understanding by design. Alexandria: ASCD; 2005.
25. Gagné RM, Briggs LJ, Wager WW. Principles of instructional design. Fort Worth: Harcourt Brace Jovanovich College Publishers; 1992. http://catalog.hathitrust.org/api/volumes/oclc/24219317.html. Accessed 21 May 2018.
26. DASH_handbook_2010_Rev2.pdf. https://harvardmedsim.org/wp-content/uploads/2016/10/DASH_handbook_2010_Rev2.pdf. Accessed 21 May 2018.
27. Svnicki M, McKeachie WJ, editors. Teaching tips: strategies, research, and theory for college and university teachers. 14th ed. Belmont: Wadsworth Cengage Learning; 2014.
28. Scalese and Hatala. Levine et al, comprehensive textbook on simulation in healthcare. Ch 11 competency assessment. New York: Springer; 2013.
29. Gawande AA. The checklist manifesto: how to get things right. New York: Metropolitan Books; 2010.
30. McWilliam PL, Botwinski CA. Identifying strengths and weaknesses in the utilization of Objective Structured Clinical Examination (OSCE) in a nursing program. 2012;33(1):35–9.
31. Rutherford-Hemming T, Kardong-Edgren S, Gore T, Ravert P, Rizzolo MA. High-stakes evaluation: five years later. Clin Simul Nurs. 2014;10(12):605–10. https://doi.org/10.1016/j.ecns.2014.09.009.
32. Boulet JR, Murray DJ. Simulation-based assessment in anesthesiology: requirements for practical implementation. Anesthesiology. 2010;112(4):1041–52. https://doi.org/10.1097/ALN.0b013e3181cea265.
33. Schott M, Kedia R, Promes SB, et al. Direct observation assessment of milestones: problems with reliability. West J Emerg Med. 2015;16(6):871–6. https://doi.org/10.5811/westjem.2015.9.27270.
34. Scalese RJ, Hatala R. Competency assessment. In: Levine AI, Jr SD, Schwartz AD, Sim AJ, editors. The comprehensive textbook of healthcare simulation. New York: Springer; 2013.
35. Brull R, Bradley JW. The role of anesthesiologists in Canadian undergraduate medical education. Can J Anaesth J Can Anesth. 2001;48(2):147–52. https://doi.org/10.1007/BF03019727.
36. Euliano TY, Robicsek SA, Banner MJ. The value of anesthesiology in undergraduate medical education as assessed by medical school faculty. J Educ Perioper Med JEPM. 2010;12(2). http://www.ncbi.nlm.nih.gov/pmc/articles/PMC4719531/. Accessed 8 Jan 2017.

3 Essentials of Scenario Building

Y. Melissa Chan, Jeremy T. Rainey, and Christine S. Park

Introduction

Merriam-Webster Dictionary defines the word scenario as "a sequence of events especially when imagined." [1] However, in healthcare simulation, a scenario is more than simply an "outline or synopsis"; [1] it is a comprehensive document. As defined by the Society for Simulation in Healthcare Dictionary, a simulation scenario describes "the goals, objectives, debriefing points, narrative description of the clinical simulation, staff requirements, simulation room set up, simulator, props, simulator operation and instructions for [standardized patients]." [2] Broadly speaking, a simulation scenario resembles a screenplay; both have not only a script that delineates a story, but also production directions for the cast and crew. An immersive simulation experience also has been described as a "serious game". Since games are by nature participatory, a scenario must be more than a screenplay, as a scenario must anticipate and plan for the intrinsic variability and dynamism of the experience. At its best, to design an immersive simulation scenario is to commit to an iterative process of drafting and refinement while thoughtfully adhering to principles and best evidence behind adult education theories and simulation research. Adhering to evidence-based instructional design features ensures the most effective educational experience for learners [3, 4]. In their review, Issenberg et al. listed ten features of high-fidelity simulation that can lead to effective learning when simulation is used as an education intervention: feedback, repetitive practice, curriculum integration, range of difficulty level, multiple learning strategies, capture clinical variation, controlled environment, individualized learning, defined outcomes or benchmarks, and simulator validity [5]. Developing an effective simulation educational experience is often a complicated task because of the sheer number of choices available to the instructional designer. To start, the definition of "scenario" above, taken from the Healthcare Simulation Dictionary, includes ten elements. In healthcare, the application of simulation activity similarly has been described in terms of 12 dimensions by Rall et al. [6] Some of these dimensions are categorically scaled while others are in gradients, so the possible combination of simulation current and future application is on the order of millions.

A well-written scenario is central to creating an effective experience and reflective practice that leads to knowledge and skills transfer, along with changed attitudes and values after training. Simulation experience, "in and of itself," does not automatically lead to learning no matter how much participants may enjoy the experience or feel as if they achieved the objectives. The simulation experience is the acknowledged pretext for debriefing [5, 7]. However, a haphazardly constructed and poorly produced simulation can not only sabotage learning but also create what Dieckmann et al. called "negative learning" by instilling the wrong "frame" (or perspective, which can influence subsequent judgments) in novices if the simulated scenario is their first exposure to that clinical problem [8].

Planning

Purpose and Goals

"Form ever follows function" is an often-quoted modernist design principle attributed to Louis Sullivan, who believed

Y. M. Chan (✉)
Department of Anesthesiology, University of Mississippi Medical Center, Jackson, MS, USA
e-mail: ychan@umc.edu

J. T. Rainey
Center for Critical Care Medicine, Anesthesiology Institute, Cleveland Clinic, Cleveland, OH, USA
e-mail: jrainey@umc.edu

C. S. Park
Graham Clinical Performance Center, University of Illinois College of Medicine, University of Illinois at Chicago, Anesthesiology and Medical Education, Chicago, IL, USA
e-mail: cpark1@uic.edu

B. Mahoney et al. (eds.), *Comprehensive Healthcare Simulation: Anesthesiology*, Comprehensive Healthcare Simulation,
https://doi.org/10.1007/978-3-030-26849-7_3

that the style of an architecture or object should reflect its intended purpose. This precept holds true to many design projects, including simulation scenarios. The simulation scenario should be written with a clear purpose in mind – the reason why the experience is being planned at all [9, 10]. This broad purpose, in turn, influences the selection of learning objectives. Learning objectives are the knowledge, skills/behaviors, and attitudes/values the participants are meant to acquire by the end of the learning exercise and should align with the purpose and goal of the learning exercise [11]. As with any instructional tool, for a simulation experience to be effective, regardless of the exact design technique or framework used, writing specific, realistic and achievable learning objectives is foundational. Goals and learning objectives should be edited for clarity and attainability. Bloom's taxonomy (see also Chap. 3) is a broadly accepted framework for categorizing learning goals often used in medical education [12]. Of the literature available on the topic of simulation scenario design, the words "educational rationale," [13] "goals," "outcomes," [14] "purpose," "broad objectives," or "competencies" are often used interchangeably [15]. Despite the lack of uniformity in terminology, the authors generally agree on a tiered approach where specific learning objectives are culled from a higher level or broader tier (e.g., purpose/goals/needs assessments). When there is more than one purpose and goal, the goals must be prioritized. As we will discuss later in this chapter, some script choices may undermine scenario goal(s) creating confusion for the learner when goals and objectives are not prioritized. The selection and prioritized goals ultimately drive the decisions behind learning objectives, script writing, and production management.

Some good starting questions to ask include the following: Is the scenario being created for teaching, training, or research? [9] What are the needs of the learners or institution? Is the scenario designed for a novice beginning a career in anesthesiology, an advanced trainee, or for maintenance of certification? Immersive scenarios often include both clinical and nontechnical competencies. In general, we find it useful to think of the scenario goals in two categories: clinical conundrums or managerial conundrums. A clinical conundrum primarily focuses on cognitive medical knowledge and skills (e.g., central line placement, peripheral nerve block placement), whereas a managerial conundrum tends to spotlight nontechnical issues like interpersonal skills, human factors and ergonomics, decision-making, and situational awareness. For example, arriving at the correct diagnosis is often the point of a clinical conundrum scenario, whereas in a management conundrum scenario, the diagnosis can be obvious but with competing "people problems." A "malignant hyperthermia scenario" can have goals directed either at learning the treatment algorithm or at the team's effectiveness in crisis management, or it can address both. Although we like to think in terms of these two categories, by no means should one conundrum exclude the other from a scenario as some simulation educators (who we will call "simulationists") intentionally design scenarios that blend the two. Immersive simulations may not be the most appropriate tools for accomplishing certain teaching goals such as training the initial exposure to new processes or equipment. If the goal is to teach nothing else but a discrete bit of medical knowledge (e.g., initial dose of dantrolene) or train a psychomotor skill in isolation (e.g., hand motion of an ultrasound probe while scanning neck anatomy), another educational modality may be equally effective and less costly.

Perhaps the goal of the scenario is meant to identify a gap, assessing the learner in either summative or formative evaluation (see also Chaps. 3 and 6). Immersive simulation written for research or assessment purposes must be planned and staged with more rigor, minimizing flexibility and adaptive dynamism to argue for validity and reliability. Simulation designed for summative assessment purposes will likely require standardization of templates, pre-brief, debrief, and scenario delivery, like those created by the Royal College of Surgeons and Physicians in Canada as part of their transition to competence-based education in anesthesiology [16]. On a whole, using immersive simulation for summative assessment of anesthesiology trainees should be approached with caution [17].

Other possible goals may be to monitor organizational issues via a process-oriented simulation where workflow and efficiency can be evaluated and patient safety issues like systemic latent threats can be discovered [18]. Perhaps the scenario goal is to expose clinicians and non-clinicians to the complexity of systems-wide crisis such as those involving weapons of mass destruction and terrorism [19]. Optimizing team performance is integral to achieving high reliability in healthcare organization [20]. Simulation provides an opportunity to conduct research or teach a unit's response to infrequent but high impact events in a controlled practice environment (e.g., emergent cesarean sections after fetal umbilical cord prolapse, or extracorporeal membrane oxygenation emergencies) [21, 22]. Perhaps the goal is to train a newly formed team or a team of stable composition; the goal may be to observe an ad hoc team in a surprise in situ drill. The goal may also be to "elicit reflection about patient safety, about the team's usual style of interaction among its members, or about their individual and collective leadership." [23] Organizational simulation goals can be internally driven and include identifying gaps or analyzing sentinel events (e.g., root cause analysis), or externally driven (e.g., an Accreditation Council of Graduate Medical Education, or ACGME, requirement). Simulation scenarios have also been written as a departmental project to reduce malpractice insurance premiums [24].

Participants

A central tenant of andragogy is that the instructional experience should be learner-centered. To maximize the experience, a simulationist should take account into individual participant characteristics as well as group dynamics. The scenario objectives should be relevant and appropriately challenging; underestimating or overestimating learners' prior knowledge and abilities can impede learning. This requires some basic knowledge of the participants' job descriptions as well as an understanding of the daily responsibilities of each participant. Some instructional design strategies that minimize cognitive load in novices may show no effect or even backfire on experts [25]. If the scenario is judged too simplistic by the participants, they may become bored. If the scenario is overwhelming, the participants may find it vague or unintelligible and dismiss the experience as irrelevant. It is noted that scenarios and their associated debriefs tend to focus on different aspects of the same scenario as the participant's level of expertise rises. Novices tend to focus more on the medical management rather than on nontechnical skills or systems issues [7].

For any given group, the participant characteristics may range from being relatively homogenous to quite diverse in expertise in a single domain or multiple domains (e.g., a team of anesthesiology interns vs. an interprofessional or interdisciplinary team). Scenario difficulty should be adjusted to accommodate novices (e.g., discrete activities like mock code drills) or tailored to advanced learners (e.g., complex cases requiring global integration of knowledge/skills/attitudes, or KSA, in multiple domains). There may be medical students or residents, or even clinicians with different experiences post-training, all involved in the same scenario. The group may be comprised of participants well-known to each other outside of the simulation (e.g., anesthesiology residents within one residency), or they may be acquaintances or complete strangers. Participants may have no prior exposure to immersive simulation, while others may be credentialed simulation instructors. Enthusiasm of the participants can also vary where some are volunteering their time for the purpose of acquiring new knowledge or refresh a skill set, while others attend only because they are compelled.

When providing care, anesthesiology providers rarely work independently of other professions or disciplines. If the goal of the simulation does not match the current composition of the participants, either the goal or the group composition should be modified. For example, if the goal is to evaluate and train the process of perimortem cesarean delivery and the simulation is to be staged in situ, it may be ideal to gather a team that could realistically respond to the event. Collaboration with interprofessional or interdisciplinary teams opens an entire new area of design consideration. Some questions to consider include the following: Should we invite colleagues to take part as actors, as participants (e.g., "combined-team training), or as the production crew? Should they be included as consultants or debriefers? If participants are scheduled to help in a scenario as embedded actors (EA), unless they volunteered and were forewarned, it is imprudent to ask them to commit obvious errors or mistakes, "creating a no-win situation for the participant who was invited to 'join' but was ambushed ... and was restricted and used as a prop." [26] When possible, we recommend using standardized patients to play key roles.

Broadly speaking, if the group is heterogeneous, consider creating a scenario with learning objectives around a managerial conundrum. Learning objectives focused on managerial conundrums tend to apply widely across different groups. To lend credibility to the experience, it is advisable to include a debriefer whom the participants will perceive as a subject content expert, particularly if the topic is in a niche, e.g., medical management of a rapidly decompensating toddler with Fontan physiology. Sometimes, this necessitates inviting multiple debriefers so that each discipline or profession is represented. Particularly when participants are skeptical or resentful of having to attend simulation-based training, or if they are apprehensive and feel at risk of embarrassment before colleagues and direct reports, the presence of an experienced senior simulation debriefer is desirable who will attend to structuring a "safe container for learning" (see also Chap. 4).

Learning Objectives

Each simulation scenario should be structured around learning objectives as they are indispensable to good instructional design [11, 27, 28]. Learning objectives are most germane when derived from a needs analysis through careful consideration of the curriculum and overall goals and tailored to the characteristics of the participants [29]. Each goal may have several subordinate learning objectives [30]. Depending on the time allocated to the scenario, the total number of learning objectives may vary. Keep in mind that the duration of a debriefing session is typically twice as long as the scene itself, so that writing too many learning objectives is counterproductive. When taken together, the set of goals and learning objectives pinpoint the exact KSA that participants are expected to acquire at the end of the event [31–33].

Well-written learning objectives are learner-centered using action verbs to describe specific cognitive processes that are broken down into measurable tasks [11]; however, Fanning and Gaba recognize that learning objectives "may be emergent and evolve within the simulation." [7] Learning objectives guide the reorientation and rescue the scene when staging goes awry (e.g., participant improvisation, equipment failure) [34]. Just as with goals, when there are more than one learning objective, these should be ranked in priority. Some design choices during script writing and scenario production are self-evident from the learning objectives, particularly when the goal is medical knowledge- or technical skill-oriented. The goal and learning objectives determine where to establish the scene, whether to advance the narrative and when to mark the beginning and end of the scenario [28]. For example, if the novice learner is to treat a pediatric patient in laryngospasm during emergence from general anesthesia, the scene should be established in the typical and expected setting like an operating room. By contrast, if the goal is to challenge advanced trainees to work under the condition of limited resources, then for the same patient, perhaps the scene should be placed in an endoscopy suite or some other remote location. Process-oriented simulation, particularly when created to assess, evaluate, or troubleshoot existing workflow, or to develop new systems processes, may find additional value when staged in situ [2].

When appropriate, learning objectives should be underpinned by a theoretical framework. In their review, Issenberg et al. found that clearly defined outcomes contributed to an increased probability of skill acquisition by learners [5]. Specific and actionable feedback, based on well-articulated objectives, allows for the identification and improvement of performance gaps [35]. When the goals of the simulation are broad like those pertinent to nontechnical skills (e.g., interpersonal communication), concrete learning objectives rooted in a theoretic or conceptual framework help participants organize interrelated concepts by providing context. This is especially true if the scenario is not integrated into an overall curriculum. Take, for example, the goal of improving teamwork. Theoretical frameworks on teamwork can be approached from a social psychological, sociotechnical, ecological, human resource, technological, lifecycle, functional/task-oriented, or integrative perspective [36]. It is highly unlikely that a single scenario or even a day's worth of immersive simulation would address these concepts in totality, much less permanently alter complex behaviors. Without organizing these interrelated concepts and anchoring them to something concrete, and then surrounding them with context, the learning objectives can feel abstract or disconnected.

Before EACH Each Immersive Simulation

The Presimulation Preparation

It is a good practice to standardize a presimulation process (also known as a "prebrief" or an "in-brief") delivered immediately before every immersive simulation event. Typically, this process includes setting expectations for participant and facilitators' attitudes and behavior as well as orientating the participants to the area where the simulation will be held and equipment to be used. Participants are introduced to the mannequins and shown the limits of their engineering. Proper orientation minimizes the possibility that the lack of familiarity with a mannequin's functions will hinder the effectiveness of learning experience. To avoid accidental damage to expensive equipment, many simulation centers will also show participants what can and cannot be done to a particular mannequin (e.g., cricothyroidotomy) and the exact location a procedure (if any) should be performed (e.g., chest tube insertion site on the mannequin).

Case Construction

Introduction

While background preparation is critical to focusing the purpose and objectives of the simulation scenario first, now comes the case construction phase where the instructional designer must commit to a story and create a cohesive and credible context for these learning objectives. When designed wisely, the scenario creates an opportunity for participants to exhibit and practice targeted knowledge, skills, and attitudes. The simulated environment, responses, and interactions must be plausible using realistic and familiar equipment so that the scenario makes sense to the participants [31].

Given the parallel between simulation and participatory theater, it is useful to borrow some terminology from the latter. A *story* is the headline topic, while a *plot* is story with causality. For practical reasons, the *title* of the scenario should not give away the story or the plot. The simulation scenario, like a play, should include the story, plot, characters, as well as stage directions for the cast and crew. Decisions need to be made on set design as well as props and moulage. The mannequin needs to be able to handle the script requirements, or an alternative solution should be planned. The flow of the scenario in terms of passage of time, the selection of triggering events, and the resolution of the scenario are also critical design elements. To aid the process of writing, various script templates or planning worksheets are available in the literature or as online resources [13, 37, 38]. These templates vary in length and depth and may be originally designed for other disciplines or professions. Benishek et al. provided a useful comparison of features of five readily accessible healthcare simulation templates [39]. Other simulationists choose to write out the entire scene like a screenplay. In either case, common elements include the following: (1) demographics data for the mannequin such as age, gender, weight, and height (in addition to accompanying paperwork to be shared with participants, such as the history and physical exam, consents, laboratory, and imaging study results); (2) estimated time allotted for the scene and debriefing; (3) description of the target audience in terms of education background; (4) goals and learning objectives; and (5) a list of events with associated vital signs trends. Typical advice is to allow two to three times as much time for debriefing as the actual simulated scenario is proposed to run. The description of the target audience may be as limited as the year of training (e.g., postgraduate year 1, "PGY1") or may be as detailed as a list of prerequisite knowledge, cognitive, and psychomotor skills. Other components of the script will be discussed later in this chapter. Some templates include a section to write out "debriefing points" [38] or "teaching points" and "instructor's notes." [40]

The full script is reserved for the nonparticipant cast, crew, and instructors. The participants receive only enough information to prepare them for the scenario. Typically, this includes a case stem [13], also known as case briefing or the preliminary situation. This is analogous to the "exposition" piece of a play with the background information needed for the audience to understand the story including an introduction of the characters and settings. It is reasonable to withhold specific learning objectives from the participants until debriefing if disclosure would spoil the surprise, particularly if the scenario is a diagnostic conundrum [28].

Selecting the Story and Plot

For any given set of goals and objectives, there are often more than one appropriate choice for the story and plot. For straightforward goals and objectives, the narrative possibilities are bound only by imagination. Accordingly, we believe it is useful to point out the pitfalls during case construction and will comment on such throughout this section.

The plot declares the causality relationships of the story, meaning that a plot makes explicit what caused what. If the story is local anesthetic systemic toxicity (LAST), then the plot may be LAST caused by accidental intravenous injection of a local anesthetic during an axillary nerve block. A *critical event* is a plot point that must transpire to create the learning environment. *Triggers* are "time, drugs," and learner actions or inactions that shift the mannequin physiology from one state to another [13] including those that push the scenario narrative into the critical event (Fig. 3.1). In a medically oriented LAST scenario, the critical event is the physiologic decompensation of the patient, while the trigger would be the intravenous injection of a local anesthetic. During the initial design phase, it is useful to select the critical event first as this is likely to be directly linked to the learning objectives. We will discuss more on this later in the chapter.

Although controversial, some simulationists suggest the "answer" to the scenario need not be assigned every time. For example, if the scenario goal is to train novice residents on the initial *management* of a hypoxic patient in the postanesthesia care unit (PACU), it is not necessarily relevant (and can be distracting) to assign a definitive cause of the hypoxemia to the patient. Furthermore, the simulationist may choose to not assign a cause to the event because in real life, the primary cause of the hypoxemia may remain indefinitely unknown. However, having some plausible initiating events (e.g., reasons for the hypoxia) are crucial to the credibility of the scenario and must be considered.

Some crisis scenarios have "answers" or diagnosis that are end points themselves (e.g., LAST or malignant hyperthermia), while other crisis scenarios are designed around symptoms (e.g., hypotension, bradycardia). Although many plotlines can be structured sufficiently to be credible forums to showcase the goals and objectives, the best scenarios allow the participants to interact with the situation so that the learning objectives are elicited organically. For example: a scenario is constructed for senior anesthesiology residents with the goal of preparing them for independent practice in a care-team model. The learning objective is: formulate a strategy for gathering information when paged into a crisis event in the operating room. In this instance, although any generic "crisis" would probably do, it is better to have a story that

Fig. 3.1 Nomenclature for case construction

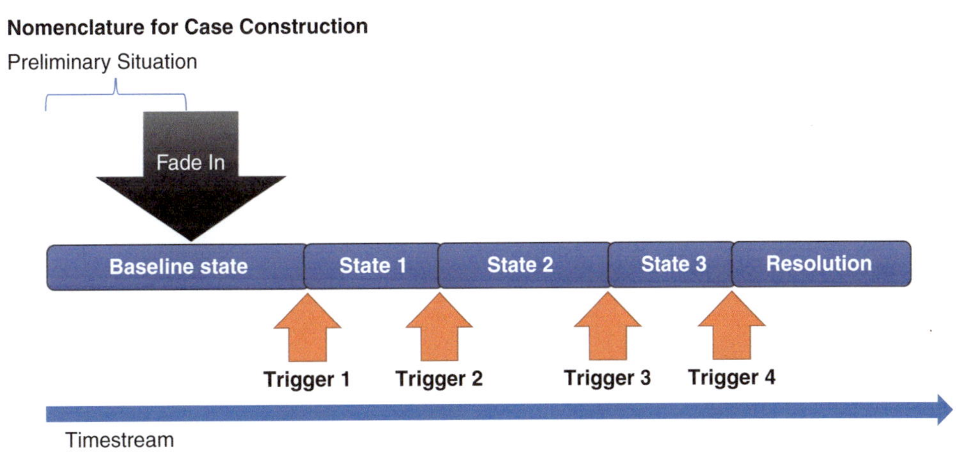

is about a symptom, like hypoxemia, as opposed to something specific like malignant hyperthermia. The differential diagnosis for hypoxemia is long, so it is more likely that the learners will have to think on their feet and come up with a plan to elicit information from the embedded actors (EAs) or other participants when it is not immediately apparent. On the other hand, inserting a "malignant hyperthermia scenario" into the learning objectives gives a diagnosis that may be too obvious so that there is not much need to obtain information from the team, which may fail to meet the larger goal of preparing the residents to work together with their team members to diagnose and treat a decompensating patient.

Sometimes, simulationists construct the plot de novo; at other times, they are inspired by a noteworthy misadventure. Both are appropriate techniques as long as the plot creates a situation that logically allows for the demonstration of learning objectives. Scenarios based on real-life events, particularly those that experts find memorable, run the risk of being too complicated to stage or too exotic to be credible, especially with novice learners. Judicious editing and culling of the script to align with the learning objectives is prudent. Strategies include adjusting the number of issues, adding or subtracting distractions, providing or withholding context, highlighting or hiding clues. For instance, a senior provider may be expected to secure a difficult airway while maintaining hemodynamic stability of the patient, which is an integrated skill set that a novice is unlikely to be able to perform well. It may be helpful to first identify the basic elements of the scenario, sketch out the basic plot and then come back to add or subtract complexity [14]. On a whole, any element in the script that adds cognitive load, intentionally or not, will increase complexity, possibly too overwhelming for learning to take place [41]. Fraser et al. discussed in detail the interplay between cognitive load principles and instructional design in simulation education [42]. Particularly during the review and revision phases of scenario writing, their points are worth considering. For example, it has been recommended that all adult patients who require medication dosing in a scenario should weight 70 kg so that standard medication doses can be used – unless the purpose of the scenario requires the added complexity of arithmetic [43].

Suggested strategies for adjusting the difficulty of a scenario are listed in Table 3.1. One approach is to modify the amount, type, and availability of information to the participants to distract, confound, or hint at the diagnosis [44]. Subtle misdirection aside, another approach is to adjust the availability of resources, in term of personnel and equipment in a credible way. For example, if participants ask for a cardiologist to join them in the operating room, that cardiologist may be occupied elsewhere or on his or her way – indefinitely. Time can be compressed by adding patient comorbidities forcing faster physiologic decompensation, necessitating quicker decision-making (e.g., a difficult airway scenario in a young healthy patient with excellent pulmonary reserve, as opposed to a cystic fibrosis patient who is on the lung transplant list). In a medical conundrum scenario, another idea to increase difficulty would be to present the same diagnosis under different physiologic conditions. For example, if written for novices, a scenario involving a patient with a saddle pulmonary embolus would be scripted so that the vital signs trend in a manner consistent with a textbook description. However, if the scenario is written for more experienced providers, that same diagnosis can present atypically, say in a patient with an undiagnosed patent foramen ovale. The first "novice" scenario may have learning objective that requires participants to recall facts whereas the latter scenario obliges higher-order thinking, and at the least, the application of medical knowledge to a new situation.

Table 3.1 Ideas for adjusting complexity of scenario

I. General availability of additional people or equipment
(a) Scene may be set at a remote and unfamiliar place or vice versa
(b) Additional helpers may or may not be available
(c) Amount and quality of "help" from the embedded actors
(d) Take away obvious solutions (e.g., Glidescope is unavailable)
II. Time
(a) Change the speed at which the events unfold
(b) Consider pauses in the scenario to embed discussion or practicing for learners
III. Information
(a) Amount of information revealed during the presimulation preparation
(b) Embedded misdirection
(c) Participant witnesses unfolding of event versus entering into the scenario after the triggering event
IV. Combine medical issues with nontechnical challenges
(a) Ethical dilemmas
(b) Teamwork
(c) Communication
(d) Decision-making
V. Presence of more complex physiology
(a) Increasing number and/or severity of comorbidities
(b) Presence of a PFO
(c) Neonatal/pediatric scenario

It may be best to resist the temptation to add more complexity than necessary to achieve the learning objectives [14, 45]. Some problematic script choices are listed in Table 3.2. One scheme was assigned the following four categories: "too much," "too fast," "find the details," and "props and whistles." [37] The "too much" scenario is complicated by too many major events, subplots, or plot twists. The simulation is unlikely to be effective if the mannequin endured first major bleeding, then anaphylaxis and a pulmonary embolus all in one scenario, as any one of those events can take a great deal of effort to manage and treat. The "too fast" scenario suffers from unrealistically rapid shifting physiology, and can frustrate learners who feel helpless to intervene. The "find the

Table 3.2 Some problematic design choices for immersive simulation scenario

1. "Trigger" event is difficult to observe either by design or cannot be seen or heard by the facilitators
2. "Trigger" event is dependent on a trainee's action or inaction
3. Scenario relies heavily on equipment
4. Scenario relies heavily on differentiating between obscure physical finding
5. Scenario relies heavily on external resources or personnel
6. Scenario forces trainees into unfamiliar roles or tasks
7. "Trigger" event relies on trainee violating their ethics
8. Too many learning objectives for allotted time

detail" scenario physically hides critical props or information from the participants to the extent of being distracting, and lends an air of trickery to the scenario. The "props and whistles" scenario is full of gimmicks that may erode the perceived relevance of the simulation exercise.

The author of a Society for Pediatric Anesthesiology workshop determined another classification system of problematic scripts [46]: (1) when the scenario is dependent "heavily on equipment or obscure physical findings" that cannot be trusted to be reliably produced by the mannequin (e.g., having to distinguish between rales vs. wheezing), (2) when the scenario relies "heavily on external resources and personnel," (3) when the scenario "forces people into unfamiliar roles or tasks" (e.g., first year medical student asked to be a scrub technician), or (4) when the scenario has events "secondary to environmental/simulator failure." These should be avoided when possible.

Mannequin technology has undergone many cycles of development, but limitations still exist. Scripts that depend heavily on the nuances of human facial expression, skeletal muscle and neurological exams may require preplanned work-arounds. Creative use of props or dialogue by EAs can overcome some constraints. Clinical photographs or videos may better display some physical findings, such as mottled skin and paradoxical breathing, as well as distinguish between the subtleties of rashes. When in doubt, an operations specialist is a good consultant resource.

Beginning the Scripting Process

Practically speaking, we like to begin the scripting process by writing an overview; an overview creates a shared mental model for the simulation development team. In a template, this section may be labeled as "ideal scenario flow," [47] "narrative description," "brief summary," the "situation," or the "backstory" [7]. We try to give context to the story by providing not only a synopsis of the plot, setting and events, but also the preliminary situation or the exposition of what was happening before the "hot seat" participant walks into the scene and what is about to transpire as the scene opens. One template asks for a description of the "anticipated management mistakes" in narrative format [47] which may help the development team to focus on the most likely branches in the storyline.

Next, we identify the critical event in the scenario that must occur. For a LAST scenario, the critical event could be decompensation of the mannequin triggered by the administration of local anesthetic in a manner that can plausibly cause systemic toxicity. The scene is crafted so that trigger and critical events will absolutely come to pass. Typically, this means writing in a way that takes the trigger out of the participants' control. We eliminate any opportunity for a scenario to come to a halt because of a participant's action or inaction. If the goal is to medically manage a patient with a "high spinal," the participants should not be given the opportunity to refuse placing a spinal anesthetic. A possible solution would be that an EA performs the spinal anesthesia with the participant present. Another solution is to open the scene (or to "*fade in*") after the trigger event already occurred where the "hot seat" participant enters the scenario after the procedure, perhaps receiving a handoff from the EA. Or, perhaps the participant is called in to help after the mannequin decompensates. On the other hand, going back to the goals, if the goal of the scenario is to identify that a patient has an allergic reaction to penicillin for the first time, without anyone (including the patient) aware of this possibility,, then the script may be left open to the participants to give penicillin themselves.

Another pitfall we avoid is the conundrum unintentionally inserted in the plot – one that distracts from the planned goals and objectives. Often, it is a dilemma accidentally built into a medically oriented scenario. Unless the objective is to address both clinical conundrum *and* the dilemma, it is best to avoid increasing complexity by creating unintended discussion points during debriefing. For example: the scenario goal is to teach the medical management of anaphylaxis. The administration of penicillin is the planned trigger event. If the case stem clearly states that the mannequin has a penicillin allergy and the participant is aware of it, it is expected that the participant will not administer penicillin. However, by refusing to administer penicillin, the participant brings the entire production to a halt. From this point, there are three possible responses for the stage manager (also known as the scenario director), none of them ideal. Option one: abort the scene and the scenario ends. Option two: an EA attempts or successfully administers penicillin, which is commission of an error. Option three: an EA tries to coerce the participant into giving penicillin. This weak plot construction can send the wrong cues thus creating confusion for the participants as to the goal of the scenario. With options two and three, learning objectives of the nontechnical variety emerged unintentionally. If the learning objective is purely medically related, the scenario is better designed if the participant arrives into the operating room with a bag of penicillin, half-empty, already hanging on the IV pole and connected to the mannequin.

Structuring the Flow of the Narrative

Each scenario has a beginning and an end connected by a chain of events along a time continuum. In its simplest form, events occur serially and chronologically with time passing at a constant and realistic rate. During the scenario, we may choose to speed up time (e.g., immediate return of lab result) or we may choose to slow down time (e.g., a piece of equipment that is perpetually "on its way"). Notice that in the above examples, the timestreams for the "lab result" and the "equipment" flow independently of the timestream of the scene itself. Mapping the flow of the narrative may be a complicated and laborious affair depending on the number of "skips" or "branches" designed into the main timeline. Particularly for the end of the scenario, these branches can become quite intricate.

"Master Event List" (MEL) is the portion of the script that accounts for and anticipates possible participant decisions [48]. Ideally, the scenario progression is mapped out so it includes not only all of the discrete events (or "states") that will occur when the participants perform perfectly, but also a list of likely/possible participant mistakes that would trigger a skip or branch from the main plotline. Dubrowski et al. described the use of scenario frames, tables, and "if-then" formats in the literature as some strategies to present the scenario's evolution [49]. For example, an "if-then" statement could be: if chest compressions are inadequately performed, then the mannequin will not respond to epinephrine administered – and will remain at its current physiologic state.

Another common strategy is to think of the scenario timestream as individual "states" connected by different triggers. Like a sequence of cause-and-effect, what happens during the scene in one state will transition into a different state depending on the nature of the trigger. The script catalogues the common triggers and their resulting states. In the Duke University template, they give an example of five states: baseline, mild, moderate, severe, and resolution [13]. For a story of acute trauma with massive blood loss, these five states may correspond to one baseline state of normal physiology plus four states each representing the classes of hemorrhagic shock. At a minimum, the description for each state typically includes vital signs and physical exam findings (e.g., heart, lung, bowel sounds, eye-opening, pupils), and instructions for the mannequin operator to transition into the next state with triggers. There may also be a list of expected participant actions and anticipated mistakes, along with directions for how to respond to them. It is common for the scenario to include some references and basic background information on the subject at hand to minimize variation in content expertise. Instructions for the behind-the-scenes crew member playing the voice of the mannequin include dialogue or vocalizations for the mannequin during that state. In the script, all triggers should be specific and observable. During the presimulation preparation, we ask our residents to verbalize their intended behavior so that there is no confusion or misunderstanding (e.g., "I'm listening to the lungs, and I hear no breath sounds on the right").

Too many branch points in a script can distract from the intended/prioritized goal. When writing these branch points, we caution against creating a "moving target" or a "punishment" scenario. A "moving target" scenario is one where the diagnosis changes and the narrative travels down a different branch every time the learner "gets it right." A "punishment" scenario is where the mannequin goes into ventricular fibrillation every time the learner "gets it wrong." Neither type of these scripts seem likely to foster the development of planned learning objectives.

Considerations Related to People

The *crew* refers to behind-the-scene staff, such as operation specialists, necessary to the staging of a production. A *character* is a role in the scenario played by a cast member or the mannequin. The *cast* refers to the list of people, both participants and embedded actors (EAs), who will play the characters on stage.

In simulation-based education, "not all learning requires direct participation" [50]. For any given scenario, a participant may be an active participant or an observer; vicarious learning occurs best with observers being given tasks while observing, such as noticing when vital signs change, or noting communication between participant and EA [51]. Of the active participants, they may begin the scenario "in the hot seat" or begin in a secluded room with no knowledge of the unfolding event. For example, a secluded participant may enter the scene when help is requested during the scenario. Of the participants who purely observe, some simulation centers have adjacent viewing rooms where they watch the scenario broadcast live. Typically, all participants will attend the debriefing since alternative perspectives provided by the observers often furnishes new insights into the discussion. This design decision should be discussed early in the planning phase as it is often dictated by logistics of the simulation-learning event (e.g., number of sessions, time allotted, number of scenarios, group composition).

In the simulation literature, planted cast members may be referred to as actors, confederates, embedded participants, role players, simulated persons, or standardized patients. Scenario challenges can be circumvented not only with imaginative script writing but also with a trained cast. In this chapter, we have been referring to them as embedded actors (EA). EAs can be played by anyone, from standardized patients to clinicians, simulation center personnel and professional actors. EAs can confirm key physical findings, give additional information or clarify a history. After the participants listens to the lungs, an EA can pick up the stethoscope, auscultate, and verbally corroborate that it is rales and not wheezing. EAs can spur the unfolding of a scenario by declaring physical/environmental findings (e.g., "is that a rash?," "is that smoke?").

When writing out the scenario, it is helpful to list the staff requirements, such as whether there are specific needs. Perhaps a critical event hinges on skillful, evocative acting (e.g., a "breaking bad news" scenario). Some content experts may have trouble accurately under-performing a specific task or convincingly faking mismanagement. Despite the additional cost, some simulation centers hire professional actors to play roles that may be potentially embarrassing (e.g., a clumsy, incompetent clinician) or stereotyped (e.g., drug-addicted anesthesiologist). On the other hand, for those scenarios designed to have a more fluid storyline, where emergent learning objectives and sophisticated improvisation is anticipated, it is advantageous to have healthcare providers portray EAs as their reactions are more likely to be realistic and appropriate. For controversial scenarios that may be emotionally charged (e.g., use of deceptive methodology) or potentially threaten psychological safety (e.g., mock codes that end in mannequin death despite optimal resuscitation), the presence of an expert facilitator is prudent.

Some simulationists recommend that the script devotes a section itemizing each character's motivations along with key stage directions [52]. If a character is responsible for a trigger event, this should be unmistakably highlighted in the script. Depending on the familiarity of an EA with a specific character's role, we also point out the cues to avoid improvisation by the EA that can confuse the participants and detract from the learning objectives. At some centers, the control room communicates with EAs live during the scene via two-way radio and headsets to address participant improvisation or staging hiccups.

Each character, including the mannequin, should have a backstory flushed out to the depth appropriate for the goals. For example, in a scenario focused on clinical conundrum, the patient-character should have a complete and thorough history, including past, present, family, and social histories as well as physical findings. Relevant labs and other test results should be included not only for the initial situation but also those that need to be made available as the scenario unfolds. On the other hand, with a story focused on managerial conundrum (e.g., disruptive physician), the physician-character's personality and motivation would be more pertinent than the details of medical history. Specificity is key. In assertiveness skills training, the strategy for dealing with difficult people depends on the personality type. It is more useful to describe the exact behavior, affect, or mannerism, rather than simply assigning a label. A "disruptive physician" can be openly aggressive or quietly hostile. Is this character prone to verbal outbursts, physical threats, or snide, condescending remarks? Does this character tend to gesture wildly, or sigh loudly and roll his or her eyes?

The participants and cast members may be asked to take on their real-life roles or asked to play a character from a different specialty, profession, or even from a different time (e.g., resident asked to pretend it is the first day of a new private practice job). This is potentially problematic if a lack of familiarity with the role generates fidelity issues.

Considerations Related to the Setting

The environmental conditions created for the scenario, or *set design*, as well as the props and moulage, will influence participants' learning. Together, the set design, props, and moulage help participants place the event in the right mental frame. Metaphysical locations are "death on stage" [6], and this adage applies to immersive simulation as well. Since anesthesiology personnel provide services across the hospital, consider the entire range of possible environments; a code can be set in the operating room, an intensive care unit, in the labor and delivery suite, postanesthetic care unit, or the cafeteria. At least in terms of achieving high fidelity in set design, it may be tempting to think of in situ simulation as the epitome of immersive simulation to which we should all aspire. Generally, although there is value to in situ simulation, it is accompanied by its own set of staging challenges as articulated by Patterson and colleagues, along with "no-go" considerations for when in situ simulation is inappropriate, described by Bajaj et al. [18, 53]

To help the crew set the stage, the script should describe the simulation set in detail using concrete and precise terms including the location, time of day, and the characters present at "fade in" or initiation of the scenario. In their article on the theoretical framework of scenarios in social practice, Dieckmann et al. discussed the difference in mental frames between novices and the more experienced people. Those with more experience in any given domain will have elaborate frames from which decisions are made so more detail is required. For example, a participant's decision-making process when securing the airway in a decompensating patient with angioedema is arguably different if the scene is set in a 750-bed university hospital on a Monday at 9:00 am as opposed to a small ambulatory surgery center in a rural location on New Year's Day, where resources are likely to be scarce. Practically speaking, a scenario targeted for expert learners will need more attention paid toward construction details not only in script writing but also during production.

A prop such as an empty syringe on an anesthesia cart carries certain implications. An unintentional swap, say a 30 mL for 3 mL syringe, may wreck a simulation on local anesthetic systemic toxicity by sending the wrong reality cue, confusing the participants and sabotaging the suspension of disbelief. A detailed equipment checklist may be helpful in this instance.

On the issue of fidelity, it is impossible to reproduce real-life on stage no matter how immersive or participatory the scenario, how cutting-edge the technology, or how realistic the moulage. Fidelity should be treated as a threshold phenomenon where the aim is to achieve "a critical mass of realism" enough to engage the learners and allow them to accept some of the fiction in the environment [44]. As Beaubien and Baker [54] pointed out: "High-fidelity simulations can enhance the perceived realism of well-designed team training programs, but cannot compensate for poorly designed ones." It does not follow that the higher the fidelity, the better the education [8]. Instead, evidence suggests that a range of fidelities may be incorporated into a "progressive training regimen" backed by theoretical principles. [55]

Dieckmann et al. proposed some cost-effective strategies to maintain overall fidelity of the scenario based on theoretical foundations in social practice [8]. Instead of a single-minded pursuit of maximizing physical fidelity, they suggested incorporating rituals like a change in costume or crossing a door to demarcate a transition in space and time signaling the beginning and end of a scenario [8]. It is important to write in as much details as possible into the script, particularly elements that may corrode the suspension of disbelief as oppose to details that reinforce it. On the flip side, too much realism may threaten the effectiveness of the scenario, e.g., fulfilling a participant request, like ordering a new chest x-ray, where accurate portrayal of the passage of time is impractical. At the minimum, the scenario should not violate the tenets professed during briefing. The environment, equipment, responses, and interaction of the scenario do not have to replicate real life, but they should be plausible. [31]

The script should also include a checklist of the props. Any critical elements should be bolded and highlighted with special instructions; e.g., stethoscope – stored somewhere clearly visible from where the participant will be standing. Props include those that are needed for setting the scene (e.g., IV pole), those for use during the scene (e.g., laryngoscope), and props that may be requested by the participants (e.g., chest x-ray, EKG). As mentioned earlier, we list the characters in the scene and develop their past and motivation as befitting the purpose of the simulation (e.g., scrub tech – appropriately helpful, reactive but not proactive; anesthesiology resident – follows concrete and specific instructions well but does not show backup behavior during crisis).

Conclusion

Scenario design is an iterative process of intentional decisions, thoughtful review and frequent revisions. Scenario templates are available in the literature to prompt and guide the design process. The strategic choices made regarding the essential elements of scenario building – the goals and learning objectives, identifying participant characteristics, and case construction – will determine the teaching impact and thus the value of a simulated scenario. Given the expense associated with immersive simulation, it is incumbent upon the simulationist to consider if the same goals and objectives can be achieved using a less costly tool. To be maximally effective, the simulation educator should clearly identify the one specific goal that is of priority, so that when decision-making become mired and complicated during the design process, choices are consistent with the prioritized goal in mind.

References

1. Scenario: Merriam-Webster Incorporated; [cited 2016 September 7]. Online Dictionary]. Available from: http://www.merriam-webster.com/dictionary/scenario.
2. Lopreiato JO, Downing D, Gammon W, Lioce L, Sittner B, Slot V, et al. Healthcare Simulation Dictionary 2016 January 3, 2017. Available from: http://www.ssih.org/dictionary.
3. Cook DA, Hamstra SJ, Brydges R, Zendejas B, Szostek JH, Wang AT, et al. Comparative effectiveness of instructional design features in simulation-based education: systematic review and meta-analysis. Med Teach. 2013;35(1):e867–98.
4. Hamstra SJ, Brydges R, Hatala R, Zendejas B, Cook DA. Reconsidering fidelity in simulation-based training. Acad Med. 2014;89(3):387–92.
5. Issenberg SB, McGaghie WC, Petrusa ER, Lee Gordon D, Scalese RJ. Features and uses of high-fidelity medical simulations that lead to effective learning: a BEME systematic review. Med Teach. 2005;27(1):10–28.
6. Rall M, Gaba D, Dieckmann P, Eich C. Patient Simulation. In: Miller RD, Ericcson LI, Fleisher LA, Wiener-Kronish JP, Young WL, editors. Miller's anesthesia. 7th ed. Philadelphia: Churchill Livingstone/Elsevier; 2010.
7. Fanning RM, Gaba DM. Debriefing. In: Gaba DM, Fish KJ, Howard SK, Burden AR, editors. Crisis management in anesthesiology. Philadelphia: Elsevier Saunders; 2015. p. 65–78.
8. Dieckmann P, Gaba D, Rall M. Deepening the theoretical foundations of patient simulation as social practice. Simul Healthc. 2007;2(3):183–93.
9. Benson DK, McMahon C, Sinnreich RH. Art of scenario design. Simul Games. 1972;3(4):439–63.
10. Stillsmoking KL. Simulation scenario building. In: Kyle R, Murray WB, editors. Clinical simulation: operations, engineering, and management. 1st ed. Burlington: Academic Press; 2007.
11. Ambrose SA, Bridges MW, DiPietro M, Lovett MC, Norma MK. How learning works: seven research-based principles for smart teaching. San Francisco: Jossey-Bass; 2010.
12. Armstrong P. Bloom's taxonomy [Internet]. Vanderbilt University; [cited 2017 May 20]. Available from: https://cft.vanderbilt.edu/guides-sub-pages/blooms-taxonomy/ - why.

13. Taekman JM. Template for simulation patient design: Duke University; 2003.
14. Bambini D. Writing a simulation scenario: a step-by-step guide. AACN Adv Crit Care. 2016;27(1):62–70.
15. McKimm J, Swanwick T. Setting learning objectives. Br J Hosp Med. 2009;70(7):406–9.
16. Chiu M, Tarshis J, Antoniou A, Bosma TL, Burjorjee JE, Cowie N, et al. Simulation-based assessment of anesthesiology residents' competence: development and implementation of the Canadian National Anesthesiology Simulation Curriculum (CanNASC). Can J Anaesth. 2016;63(12):1357–63.
17. Wen LY, Gaba DM, Udani AD. Summative assessments using Simulation requires safeguards. Anesth Analg. 2017;124(1):369.
18. Patterson MD, Blike GT, Nadkarini VM. *In Situ* simulation: challenges and results. In: Henriksen K, Battles JB, Keyes MA, editors. Advances in patient safety: new directions and alternative approaches. Agency for Healthcare Research and Quality (US): Rockville, MD; 2008. p. 3.
19. Kyle RR, Via DK, Lowy RJ, Madsen JM, Marty AM, Mongan PD. A multidisciplinary approach to teach responses to weapons of mass destruction and terrorism using combined simulation modalities. J Educ Perioper Med. 2004;6(1):E029.
20. Baker DP, Day R, Salas E. Teamwork as an essential component of high-reliability organizations. Health Serv Res. 2006;41(4 Pt 2):1576–98.
21. Anderson JM, Murphy AA, Boyle KB, Yaeger KA, Halamek LP. Simulating extracorporeal membrane oxygenation emergencies to improve human performance. Part II: assessment of technical and behavioral skills. Simul Healthc. 2006;1(4):228–32.
22. Sorensen JL, van der Vleuten C, Rosthoj S, Ostergaard D, LeBlanc V, Johansen M, et al. Simulation-based multiprofessional obstetric anaesthesia training conducted in situ versus off-site leads to similar individual and team outcomes: a randomised educational trial. BMJ Open. 2015;5(10):e008344.
23. Cooper JB, Singer SJ, Hayes J, Sales M, Vogt JW, Raemer D, et al. Design and evaluation of simulation scenarios for a program introducing patient safety, teamwork, safety leadership, and simulation to healthcare leaders and managers. Simul Healthc. 2011;6(4):231–8.
24. Blum RH, Raemer DB, Carroll JS, Sunder N, Felstein DM, Cooper JB. Crisis resource management training for an anaesthesia faculty: a new approach to continuing education. Med Educ. 2004;38(1):45–55.
25. van Merrienboer JJ, Sweller J. Cognitive load theory in health professional education: design principles and strategies. Med Educ. 2010;44(1):85–93.
26. Navedo DD, Reidy PA. Continuum of care. In: Palaganas J, Maxworthy J, Epps C, Mancini M, editors. Defining excellence in simulation programs. 1st ed: Wolters-Kluwer; 2015.
27. Sawyer T, Eppich W, Brett-Fleegler M, Grant V, Cheng A. More than one way to debrief: a critical review of healthcare simulation debriefing methods. Simul Healthc. 2016;11(3):209–17.
28. Alinier G. Developing high-Fidelity health care simulation scenarios: a guide for educators and professional. Simul Gaming. 2010;42(1):9–26.
29. Weaver SJ, Salas E, Lyons R, Lazzara EH, Rosen MA, Diazgranados D, et al. Simulation-based team training at the sharp end: a qualitative study of simulation-based team training design, implementation, and evaluation in healthcare. J Emerg Trauma Shock. 2010;3(4):369–77.
30. Arreola RA. Writing learning objectives 1998 [cited 2016 September 17]. Available from: https://www.uwo.ca/tsc/graduate_student_programs/pdf/LearningObjectivesArreola.pdf.
31. Seropian MA. General concepts in full scale simulation: getting started. Anesth Analg. 2003;97(6):1695–705.
32. Salas E, Cannon-Bowers JA. The science of training: a decade of progress. Annu Rev Psychol. 2001;52:471–99.
33. Nguyen N, Watson WD, Dominguez E. An event-based approach to design a teamwork training scenario and assessment tool in surgery. J Surg Educ. 2016;73(2):197–207.
34. Dieckmann P, Lippert A, Glavin R, Rall M. When things do not go as expected: scenario life savers. Simul Healthc. 2010;5(4):219–25.
35. Rudolph JW, Simon R, Raemer DB, Eppich WJ. Debriefing as formative assessment: closing performance gaps in medical education. Acad Emerg Med. 2008;15(11):1010–6.
36. Paris CR, Salas E, Cannon-Bowers JA. Teamwork in multi-person systems: a review and analysis. Ergonomics. 2000;43(8):1052–75.
37. Dieckmann P, Rall M. Designing a scenario as a clinical experience: the TuPASS scenario script. In: Kyle R, Murray WB, editors. Clinical simulation: operations, engineering, and management. 1st ed. Burlington: Academic Press; 2007.
38. Simulation Scenario Development Template [Internet]. University of Washington Center for Health Sciences Interprofessional Education, Research and Practice; [updated February 23, 2017; cited 2017 May 11]. Available from: https://depts.washington.edu/chsierp/wordpress/wp-content/uploads/2017/02/MedSurg_Ortho_Uro_2017_02_23_LB.pdf.
39. Benishek LE, Lazzara EH, Gaught WL, Arcaro LL, Okuda Y, Salas E. The template of events for applied and critical healthcare simulation (TEACH Sim): a tool for systematic simulation scenario design. Simul Healthc. 2015;10(1):21–30.
40. Scenario Template [Internet]. University of California Irvine: UC Irvine Medical Education Simulation Center, UC Regents; 2014 [cited 2017 May 11]. Available from: http://sites.uci.edu/medsim/files/2015/03/UCI-Scenario-template.docx.
41. Haji FA, Cheung JJ, Woods N, Regehr G, de Ribaupierre S, Dubrowski A. Thrive or overload? The effect of task complexity on novices' simulation-based learning. Med Educ. 2016;50(9):955–68.
42. Fraser KL, Ayres P, Sweller J. Cognitive load theory for the design of medical simulations. Simul Healthc. 2015;10(5):295–307.
43. Kyle R, Murray WB. Simulation scenario: telling the story – discussing the story. In: Kyle R, Murray WB, editors. Clinical simulation: operations, engineering, and management. 1st ed. Burlington: Academic Press; 2007.
44. Gaba DM, Fish KJ, Howard SK, Burden AR. Teaching anesthesia crisis resource management. In: Gaba DM, Fish KJ, Howard SK, Burden AR, editors. Crisis management in anesthesiology. Philadelphia: Elsevier Saunders; 2015. p. 54–64.
45. Torsher L, Craigo P. Simulation in anesthesiology. In: Levine A, Samuel DJ, Schwartz AD, Sim AJ, editors. The comprehensive textbook of healthcare simulation. New York: Springer; 2014. p. 257–87.
46. Hokanen A. SPA simulation workshop: designing your own scenario. Society for Pediatric Anesthesia 2012 Winter.
47. Educational Summary Report Template: Simulated cases. MedEdPORTAL Publications. 2016.
48. Focus on: Making crisis simulations matter [Internet]. 2015 [cited 2017 May 11]. Available from: https://www2.deloitte.com/content/dam/Deloitte/us/Documents/risk/us-risk-focus-making-crisis-simulations-matter-031615.PDF.
49. Dubrowski A, Alani S, Bankovic T, Crowe A, Pollard M. Writing technical reports for simulation in education for health professionals: suggested guidelines. Cureus. 2015;7(11):e371.
50. Gaba DM. The future vision of simulation in health care. Quality Safety Health Care. 2004;13(suppl_1):i2–i10.

51. Stegmann K, Pilz F, Siebeck M, Fischer F. Vicarious learning during simulations: is it more effective than hands-on training? Med Educ. 2012;46(10):1001–8.
52. Martin T, McIntosh CA. Preeclampsia in the delivery suite: a simulation scenario. Simul Healthc. 2013;8(3):183–90.
53. Bajaj K, Minors A, Walker K, Meguerdichian M, Patterson M. Simul Healthc. 2018; https://doi.org/10.1097/SIH.0000000000000301. [Epub ahead of print].
54. Beaubien JM, Baker DP. The use of simulation for training teamwork skills in health care: how low can you go? Qual Saf Health Care. 2004;13(Suppl 1):i51–6.
55. Brydges R, Carnahan H, Rose D, Rose L, Dubrowski A. Coordinating progressive levels of simulation fidelity to maximize educational benefit. Acad Med. 2010;85(5):806–12.

Essentials of Debriefing in Simulation-Based Education

4

Jeanette R. Bauchat and Michael Seropian

Introduction

Debriefing in healthcare is somewhat new but is well-established in other industries. It should be viewed as a process that utilizes a variety of established educational tools and strategies to enhance the learning and understanding of all participants, and can be applied to simulation-based educational encounters, or to real-life events. In this chapter, we focus on debriefing as it relates to the simulation-based educational encounter, but many principles discussed below apply equally to the debriefings after actual clinical encounters. Some types of debriefing activity, theoretically, can be applied to a variety of simulation-based educational encounters, from using drills to train critical steps in an algorithm, to procedural training, to immersive high-fidelity simulated clinical events, using the principles described in this chapter.

There are many schools of thought with respect to debriefing structure and technique. This is symbolic of an industry that is early in its development. This chapter will not present a "right" way to debrief but rather present a variety of objective tools that can be used across the spectrum of instruction. It is important to note that no one debriefing structure has been demonstrated to be superior to another. The choice of the technique should match the activity, learning objectives, learner profile, and educator preference. It is not uncommon to use multiple structures within a curriculum. The experienced debriefer will artfully and seamlessly navigate these structures.

As discussed in Chap. 2, experiential learning theory (ELT) defines learning as "the process whereby knowledge is created through the transformation of experience. Knowledge results from the combination of grasping and transforming experience" [1]. Experiential learning theory portrays two models of experience: a grasping experience of concrete experience (CE) and abstract conceptualization (AC) and a transforming experience of reflective observation (RO) and active experimentation (AE) [2]. David Kolb's ELT in its entirety is the process of interacting with the environment, processing these interactions, creating knowledge and then applying and adapting to the environment [1] (Fig. 4.1) [2]. Malcolm Knowles defined adult learning theory and

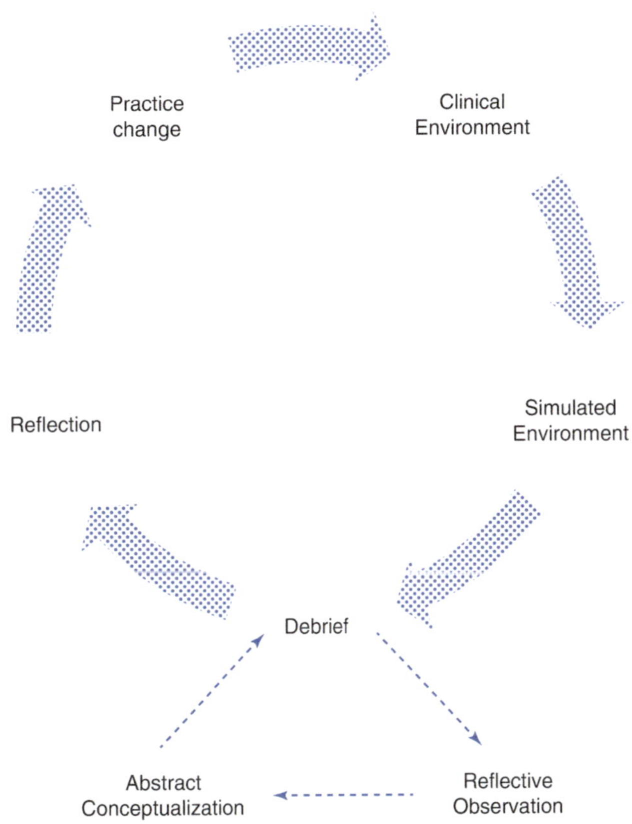

Fig. 4.1 The clinical learning cycle and Kolb's experiential learning theory framework. (Adapted from Stocker et al. [2])

J. R. Bauchat
Department of Anesthesiology, Vanderbilt University Medical Center, Vanderbilt University School of Medicine, Nashville, TN, USA

M. Seropian (✉)
Department of Anesthesiology and Perioperative Medicine, Oregon Health & Science University, Portland, OR, USA
e-mail: Seropian@ohsu.edu

B. Mahoney et al. (eds.), *Comprehensive Healthcare Simulation: Anesthesiology*, Comprehensive Healthcare Simulation,
https://doi.org/10.1007/978-3-030-26849-7_4

described adult learning as most effective if the learner was internally motivated, which most likely occurred when the new learning experiences are problem-centered and could be related to previous and future experiences [3]. In essence, adults learn best from relevant, experiential learning and use these experiences to make observations and reflect not only on the actual scenario but abstract and apply these concepts to future experiences [1]. Debriefing simply builds and leverages these concepts to provide learners with additional opportunities to maximize learning outcomes and effectiveness. Retention is similarly enhanced through learner engagement, understanding, analysis, and activation.

Feedback, Facilitation, Objectives, and Debriefing

Facilitation and debriefing are not synonymous. Effective debriefing pre-supposes the presence of an educator that may or may not use the tool of facilitation. Facilitation, or the use of guided questioning to help learners uncover and examine their own knowledge, attitudes, beliefs, and judgments, is not the only skill a debriefer may employ. A debriefer differs from a facilitator by additionally possessing expertise of the subject matter and the ability to judge when and how high-quality performance is achieved. Some simulation-based encounters are best-served by blending both the expertise of the debriefer with facilitation for a richer learning encounter.

Immersive simulation creates an environment where concrete experience and active experimentation occurs, but it is the debriefing session that facilitates the reflective observation and abstract conceptualization phases of Kolb's learning cycle [2]. Debriefing has been defined as a "facilitated or guided reflection in the cycle of experiential learning" [4]. Debriefing is erroneously and commonly equated purely to an instructor-guided session to facilitate the reflective observations and abstract conceptualizations by looking at and interpreting the events, actions, thoughts, and feelings of the learners within the simulated scenario [5]. Reflective observation describes observation and analysis of the simulation experience from the participants' perspectives with reference to events and problems that occurred during the simulated event. Abstract conceptualization is the process by which the lessons learned from the simulated event could be applied to the same event or different events in clinical care [1, 2, 6–8]. The former description by Gaba, Raemer, and Zigmont represent an interpretation of debriefing. Debriefing used within the context of education, assessment, and training is more simply a retrospective analysis of events and experiences that uses a variety of strategies to create understanding to be applied prospectively to future events. It is an effective learning strategy that enhances understanding, performance, and retention of technical, cognitive, and behavioral skills.

Debriefing is highly effective for learning in simulated and real clinical environments. A meta-analysis of 30 randomized controlled studies in the medical, aviation, and military literature has demonstrated that debriefing yields 25% improvement in performance compared with no debriefing. These findings were similar for both individual and team performance. Even more striking, when the debriefs were facilitated by an instructor, they were three times as effective as non-facilitated debriefs, though a majority of studies used instructor-facilitated debriefs [9, 10]. As a result, best practice in simulation-based healthcare education (SBHE) includes debriefing to maximize learning [11].

Debriefing and Feedback

Debriefs are a form of active self-learning where participants use self-discovery through reflection on their performance and experimentation with newly learned ideas to improve future performance [1, 12, 13]. Active learning is facilitated in a debrief through curiosity and exploration that encourage learner reflection, self-discovery, and discussion with other learners.

Debriefing often represents a conversation between learners and educator(s), whereas feedback is frequently a component of the debriefing conversation that is ideally, but not always, an objective observation of a performance compared to an ideal standard [14, 15]. Feedback is an important component of debriefing for performance improvement [9–11] and deliberate practice to promote expertise [16]. Feedback is generally construed as "formative" assessment (e.g., for the benefit of the learner, as opposed to "summative" assessment, which evaluates competency or skill acquisition), in which the learner may take corrective action. For feedback to be effective and lead to changes in behavioral, cognitive, and technical skills, it must contain several components [15, 17]. (Box 4.1) An effective debriefing allows for exploration of the intentions and reasoning behind the learners' behaviors and actions that stem from inference or frame of thought [18, 19]. Schön expanded on Kolb's ELT, arguing that the learner's conceptual framework must be questioned [20]. In the face of mistakes or even correct behaviors or actions, the learner's thought process should be elicited as incorrect frames can lead to incorrect actions in future clinical scenarios [18]. Effective feedback is an important but not the only component of debriefing. Feedback provides the opportunity for corrective action for behaviors and actions. Although a debriefer should be well-versed in giving effective feedback, an effective debriefing, but not feedback, elicits the frame of inference as a critical part of the learning process.

Box 4.1. Components of Constructive Feedback in the Medical Setting

- Instructor and learner as allies, working toward common goals
- Well-timed and expected
- Firsthand data
- Regulated in quantity and modifiable actions
- Descriptive
- Specific
- Nonjudgmental against the person's character
- Based on actions and decisions
- Based on standards/benchmark

An effective debrief allows for self-discovery and self-reflection, but also allows for instructor- and peer-based deepening of understanding and performance [21]. A meta-analysis of self-determination theory found that academic curriculum that creates an "autonomy supportive learning climate" which encourages *self-initiation*, promotes *volitional activities*, provides *rationale for the curriculum,* and uses *constructive feedback* increases self-motivation in learners [22, 23]. Tennanbaum spelled out the key components of debriefing, including active self-learning, developmental intent, clear learning objectives, and multiple perspectives [10, 21]. In fact, effective debriefing sessions are well aligned with the "autonomy supportive learning environment" which as "self-determination theory" argues is one of the modifiable factors that positively influences intrinsic motivation in learners [22] (Table 4.1).

Developmental Intent

It is important to give forethought to the developmental intent of any given educational session. Debriefs are typically effective to promote *learning* and *development*, and not for evaluation and judgment since performance rating affects how accurate or acceptable a learner perceives performance feedback to be [24, 25]. The debrief will be more acceptable and learners more motivated and honest about mistakes when they recognize the purpose of the activity is for the sake of their growth (formative) as clinicians and improved clinical practice [10]. Simulation sessions are being standardized and used more frequently for evaluative purposes (summative), and when this is the case, it must be recognized that both the rater and the learner alter their behaviors and as such the debrief. It is critically important to note that even summative assessments can still be given with respect, curiosity, and support of the learner, to promote continued learner growth.

Table 4.1 Comparing self-determination theory and components of debriefing

Self-determination theory	Components of debriefing
Self-initiation	Active self-learning
Volitional activities	Developmental intent
Rational for curriculum	Clear learning objectives
Constructive feedback	Multiple perspectives

Clear Learning Objectives

While debriefs can and should have some fluidity to allow for learner-directed objectives, having *specific learning objectives* affects motivational direction, intensity, and persistence in the learner [26, 27]. Having learning objectives provides the necessary rationale for the learner "buy-in" for the curriculum [22]. Furthermore, this may facilitate structure for the debriefs themselves which may make the debriefs more efficient and focused, improving learner performance [28].

Multiple Perspectives

Multiple learners in a learning episode allow for more information and perspectives of the learner's performance and thus allow more credibility of feedback and yield more accurate self-reflection and thus future learner objectives [22, 26, 29–31]. Self-assessment is notoriously inaccurate and multiple perspectives in an activity are likely one of the reasons inter-professional team training can be highly effective at inciting not only team learning, but individual learning as well [32–34]. High team performance requires regular reflections on teamwork; teams that reflect outperform teams that do not reflect [34]. Debriefs that include multiple perspectives are therefore particularly valuable in the learning process. Making explicit the notion that learners' single perspectives are not the only ones being held is a critical step in enhancing the perspective-taking process, as this additionally fosters curiosity and creativity, which are in themselves facilitators of learning [35].

Optimizing the Psychological Environment for Effective Learning

One of the first steps to promoting learning in the debriefing sessions is to optimize the psychological learning environment to promote learner engagement. The challenges for the debriefer is to engage the participants despite the psychological discomfort of "performing" in a simulation, with the potential of making "mistakes" and then going through the process of honest self-reflection and accepting feedback from instructors and peer learners.

Table 4.2 Optimizing the psychological environment for learning

Basic introductions	Introductions of personnel and learners Orientation to the location Orientation to the simulated environment Expectations for technology use
Setting expectations of curriculum	Academic content Developmental intent vs. assessment Scenarios designed to challenge
Setting expectation of learners	Fiction/learning contract Respect other learners Confidentiality of learners' performances and discussions
Skilled instructor	Deficiencies as learning opportunities Well-versed in feedback/debriefing methodologies

An essential concept to understand is that learners enter simulation with learner-specific psychological predispositions that will impact the type and effectiveness of learning. There are a variety of strategies that can better align the psychological state of learners with the simulation activity (Table 4.2). "Pre-briefs" is one example of a tool often used to create this alignment. It not only helps the learners but also gives the educators and other personnel insight into learner predisposition and frame of reference. A pre-briefing should "set the stage" with introductions of personnel and other learners, "ice-breaking" activities, orientation to the simulation area (i.e., location of restrooms), and orientation to the simulation environment to help increase the comfort level of the participants. Orientation to the simulation area should include locations for restrooms, break areas, availability of refreshments, and other such things, so participants feel empowered to care for their personal needs. Orientation to the simulated environment will increase the level of comfort and engagement of participants if they have a firm understanding of the capabilities of the mannequin (e.g., breath sounds, pulse check points) and the available equipment and medications (e.g., code cart, anesthesia cart). Respecting the adult learner's external commitments is important, but also requesting participants' respect for the learning environment for themselves and others by silencing technology and responding to phone calls, pagers, and other distractors only for urgent matters should be addressed. These expectations may vary with the intent of any given session, especially in an exam or assessment environment.

Setting clear expectations and having clear objectives for the debriefing sessions help participants know the process and curriculum, they will have a greater sense of control and are therefore more likely to engage [26, 27, 36]. Setting expectations and clear objectives related to the curriculum and the purpose of the academic activity is critical. It must be transparent if the simulation scenario and debriefing is to be used for formative or summative assessment [10, 37]. Although having one's simulated performance evaluated is never "comfortable," the debriefing environment must be optimized for the participant to decide to take a "risk" and feel comfortable enough to reflect on and explore their performance and accept constructive feedback in the presence of the instructor and potentially other learners [38]. Typically learners can and are willing to undertake this psychological "discomfort" as long as they feel there is a fair trade-off of learning, particularly if the learning is at the "edge" of their knowledge and will take them to the next level of competence [39–41]. Stating explicitly that the simulation experience is designed to challenge the participants and encourage them to work at the edge of their comfort level helps set the stage for the debriefing. The term "psychological safety" is often used to describe this trade-off, but this term is misleading; it is unrealistic to expect all individuals to feel "safe" in a learning environment. To be clear and explicit, the debriefer is critical to ensuring the learning environment is optimized to promote learning while reducing the "discomfort" of learning; this is the concept of "psychological safety."

Being upfront with expectations and intent for learning in the simulated environment can assist with learner engagement. Part of setting clear expectations also includes setting the expectations of the learners' behaviors including expectations of learner confidentiality, respect for other learners, and performing at their best in the simulated environment. Presuming the curriculum is being used with a formative intent, optimizing the learning environment should include a guarantee of the confidentiality of the learners' performance and asking all participants to hold to this standard. This is achieved through explicit dialogue and written affirmation of confidentiality. In addition, all participants should be asked to respect others' reflections and opinions and use respect as a grounding for their observations and feedback of others, as feedback given without respect can cause emotional distress [29, 42]. Acknowledging the simulation scenario is not "real" and that the participants may not act as they usually would in the clinical environment helps moderate and influence learners' willingness to engage despite the limitations of the simulated environment [38, 43]. Many debriefers use "the fiction contract" or "learning contract" where it is acknowledged that the simulation is not "real" but the instructor has done their best to make the learning experience valuable and in exchange; the learner will do their best to care for the simulated patient as they would in their clinical setting despite perceived gaps in realism [38, 43].

The skill and mindset of the debriefer, in making the participants' learning environment more comfortable and productive, cannot be overstated. In traditional education, errors are often ignored or corrected by instructors, and learners develop a fear of errors, perceived errors as "bad," and want to avoid them for risk of calling their clinical competency into question and diminishing their self-worth. Clinicians would agree that error avoidance is important in the clinical setting, but unfortunately, error avoidance principles should not be expanded into the learning environment, and the belief that by allowing learners to err or practicing incorrect behaviors and actions will lead to further error by strengthening these incorrect behaviors or actions should not be a guiding principle [44]. Unlike error avoidance theory, exploratory learning strategies, like simulation and debriefings, can be a highly beneficial way of learning, using and encouraging mistakes to promote corrective reflection and feedback [44–47]. In fact, errors committed with high confidence are more easily corrected than low confidence errors [44]. Therefore, debriefers may want to explicitly state that the simulation environment is a place to learn from errors and that both sub-optimal and optimal performances are expected and valuable opportunities for learning and growth.

Miettinen theorized that reflective thought and actions are driven by feelings of inadequacy and experiences that are outside of what feels "normal" and that people are intrinsically motivated to learn only if they perceive their performance was deficient [2, 48]. While a learner's motivation may be based on a sense of self-deficiency, instructors must be cautious to not equate what motivates the learner with a negative perception of learner themselves, as it can lead to anger and conflict between the learner and instructor and work against the intended outcomes of practice improvement and working toward common goals [29, 49, 50]. Debriefing requires a skilled facilitator who brings to light performance "deficiencies" and "normalizes" the commission of errors (without condoning the errors) without ascribing them to inherent deficiencies of the person and uses performance as an opportunity to promote reflection and learning for the entire learner group [18, 42, 45, 51]. When debriefers use effective debriefing structure and methodologies (including effective feedback techniques), they can help depersonalize and reduce the negative psychological effects of exploring deficiencies brought to light by the simulated scenario and maximize learning.

Structures for Effective Debriefing

Debriefing structure and methodology are not standardized and vary among institutions, disciplines and curricula [9, 11, 28, 52]. As discussed before, immersive educational activities should include a pre-briefing to set the stage for a safe learning environment as well as learner engagement, and most of these structures speak to this in the "introduction" or prior to the actual structured part of the educational session. There are a variety of standardized structures for debriefing that help organize and capture all necessary components of post-event debriefing (Table 4.3). These standardized structures contain common elements of allowing initial reactions, descriptions of events, an analysis and understanding of events, feedback from instructors or participants based on a benchmark performance and then summary of learning objectives and/or lessons learned from the analysis [7, 19, 45, 53–57].

Table 4.3 Post-scenario proposed debriefing structures

Title	Components
EXPRESS [55]	Introduction Reactions phase Understanding phase Summary
PEARLS [56]	Reaction Description Analysis Summary
The Diamond [52]	Description Analysis Application
TeamGAINS [44]	Reaction Debriefing Transfer from simulation to reality Benchmark standards Summarize Practice clinical skills (optional)
GAS [53]	Gather Analyze Summarize
Debriefing with Good Judgment (Rudolph 2006) [7]	Reaction Analysis Summary
AAR (Sawyer 2013) [55]	Define rules Explain learning objectives Benchmark performance Review what was supposed to happen Identify what happened Examine why Formalize learning
3D Model of Debriefing (Zigmont 2011) [6]	Diffusing Discovering Deepening

Many of the structures describe an initial reactions or a descriptive phase. This phase usually allows for venting of the emotions and stress from the scenario [19, 58]. Others do not believe a "venting" of feelings are a requirement as this may be determined by culture and clinician comfort with stressful situations [53]. The reactions/descriptive phase allows the revelation of underlying emotions and a description of the events that unfolded, so the instructor and learners have a shared mental model with respect to emotional state and about what occurred in the scenario. This allows instructors and learners alike to base the debriefing from a common or shared understanding [19, 21, 53–55]. This initial phase may also include clarification of the learning objectives or purpose of the activity [52].

Arguably, the most challenging phase for the debriefer involves the analysis, examining, discovery, and/or understanding phase(s). During this phase of the debrief, the debriefer must be skilled at using techniques to promote engagement and learning around the critical components related to the activity. These techniques include self-assessment, instructor-facilitated deepening of critical event reflection and understanding, and performance feedback from the instructor and other learners when possible [10, 21]. Specific techniques that facilitate these discussions are explained in further detail in the "debriefing techniques to promote discussion and learning" section of this chapter.

Lastly, the summary phase of the debriefing structure should ideally be grounded in the learning objectives of the activity but it is equally important to emphasize any additional relevant lessons learned. The summary phase should also include an opportunity for learner to forecast future learning objectives or goals in their clinical practice. Learners should be encouraged to describe how they will apply what was learned to future practice and performance. This last point is the critical bridge between the educational activity and the bedside.

Debriefing Techniques to Promote Discussion and Learning

At the core of debriefing, the debriefer must be able to promote critical reflection and analysis. There are several techniques the debriefer can use after the pre-briefing to promote an optimal learning environment while encouraging, what may be at times, uncomfortable conversation Table 4.4.

Table 4.4 Debriefing techniques

Open-ended questions	Open-ended questions begin: How What Why Please describe… Share with me… Help me understand… Tell me about…	Close-ended questions begin: Are/was Did/didn't Will/won't Aren't Would If
Active listening	Pay attention	Silence Full attention/avoid distractions Notice speaker's nonverbal communication
	Show you are listening	Silence Acknowledge (i.e., Hm, nodding) Open posture
	Verbal confirmation	Clarify Summarize
	Defer judgment	No interruptions Respond after listening
	Respond	Respectful Honest
Advocacy inquiry	Objective observation Subjective judgment Open-ended question	Example: "I noticed you didn't turn up the oxygen in this patient…. I was concerned that the patient needed oxygen supplementation with an oxygen saturation of 90%... In that moment, I'm wondering why you made that decision…"
Plus/delta	Plus	What went well?
	Delta	What would you do differently?
Guided team self-correction	Present the benchmark Allow the team to compare/contrast their performance Allow team to self-correct Facilitator shares observations/objectives	
Circular questioning	Question is directed at a third person who observed an interaction between two participants in a simulation	Example: "Person X, what did you think of the interaction between person Y and person Z?"
Role play	Two or more parties are asked to role play a situation or conversation for the purpose of making the learning and issue explicit	Example: "We discussed effective communication, now let's role play what that looks like. So this is what was said during the case, let's try to make it more specific, clear, and concise"
Directive	The debriefer has a specific issue that is to be addressed with little room for interpretation. It may be directed to a single individual or to many but has little room for misinterpretation	Example: "The code proceeded after the patient went into VF. Michael what are the protocol steps you should take and what are the essential team members you need?"

Open-ended questions can facilitate discussion. Open-ended questions are generally not intended to specifically elicit facts or lead someone to a correct answer. They tend to be perceived as less threatening when they are stated in the context of curiosity and receptivity, as they frequently are used to clarify or understand someone's perspective and are used to carry a conversation. Open-ended and closed questions tend to begin with specific question words Table 4.4. Open-ended questions are desirable when applied effectively. They can however also lead to a "guess what I am thinking" situation, reminiscent of more aggressive forms of "pimping" in the clinical environment. The questions must have relevance to the learner to elicit a response. Many theorists have diminished the value of close-ended questions. This may stem from their overuse (abuse) in educational settings. Questions that are closed have a real role in debriefing, but when they are overused or used for "testing" the learner, they can lead to a learning environment that discourages dialog, free thought, and expression.

Most debriefing instructors would agree that active listening skills are important in the instructor-learner relationship. Listening for the purpose of listening versus listening for the purpose of speaking is an important conceptual distinction. An important part of active listening is using silence to encourage your learner to speak and assist the instructor in listening. But active listening is not just about silence; it requires several skills Table 4.4 [59, 60]. Active listening is typically discussed in the context of the physician-patient relationship [61, 62]. The importance of active listening in the physician-patient relationship could be expanded to include the instructor-learner relationship. Active listening conveys to the speaker that the listener values and wants to understand what the person has to say. The instructor is listening to the verbal communication, noticing non-verbal communication and demonstrating a desire to understand the problems, needs, and perceptions of the speaker with their own body language and words [61–65]. Active listening fosters a relationship of growth, collaboration, and trust in the instructor-learner relationship.

Active listening and use of open-ended questions helps the instructor understand the learner-needs through understanding the learner's frame of reference for their behaviors and actions in the scenario. The advocacy-inquiry (also referred to as acknowledge/inquire) line of questioning requires the instructor to elicit the intent of behaviors and actions by asking, with genuine curiosity, about the learner's frame of reference during an objective action. Advocacy-inquiry may include honest judgment about the learner's performance [7]. This is often a point of confusion for debriefers. How can a debriefer be non-judgmental while offering judgment? The experienced debriefer is able to navigate this paradox. An example where judgment is included is "I heard multiple people talking at once without clear closed-loop communication. I was concerned because some of the things that were said were really important for patient care, like getting the code cart, but I wasn't sure everyone could hear those statements. What was going through your mind at the time?" The first part of the question includes an objective (hopefully) observation and honest judgment both from the debriefer's point of view that is quickly followed by exploration of the learners' frame of reference. This technique attempts to preserve the instructor-learner relationship through objective observation, an honest judgment and then eliciting the learner's frame with an open-ended question [7]. The objective observation and honest judgment components use the principles of constructive feedback discussed earlier in the chapter.

The Plus/Delta technique of debriefing uses self-assessment and objective differential assessment as a model for stimulating discussion [21, 55]. This method asks the participants to list actions, behaviors, or concepts that are relevant to the activity. This "benchmark" list is then juxtaposed to what actually occurred or to initial understanding. The delta is derived from the difference between what was done and what could/should have been done. This technique is often narrowly used as purely "What went well, and what would you change". The debriefer is effectively leading the learners to understand and recognize an ideal state or correct actions. The learner is prompted to recognize the appropriate alignment of their actions and understanding to a specific ideal or standard. The learner can then pivot to recognize differences and establish alternatives that may result in more effective performance or understanding. Although pure self-assessment has been shown to be inaccurate, this methodology works well to promote concrete understanding of concepts and actions. The technique can be quite effective for training multiple participants to provide "reality checks" for the team, as well as in time-limited debriefings [22, 26, 29–31].

Guided Team Self-Correction is a form of plus/delta that uses a pre-specified template for team behaviors as a benchmark, and the team is then asked to compare themselves to this benchmark [55, 66]. This technique is similar to the After-Action Review (AAR) used in the military which specifies the objectives and asks the group to compare themselves to a benchmark [55].

Circular questioning is a technique used in psychology which asks a third person perspective of a situation between other people [67]. This technique capitalizes on the "multiple perspectives" component of debriefing, for example, "Participant X. You witnessed the interaction between Participant Y and Z. How do you think Participant Y felt about the statement that Participant Z said in that interaction?" This method of questioning is sometimes used when there was a conflict between participants. A perceived "neutral" party (third party) can give an objective observation that may facilitate the resolution of the conflict. This also allows the instructor to step back and not be judgmental or a referee in an interaction between two participants.

Role-play is another technique that can be used by facilitators to emphasize and practice a benchmark behavior or action between two or more parties. This is a mini-simulation within the debriefing session that allows for the "active experimentation" part of the Kolb's learning cycle. This technique allows a deepening of understanding and promotion of explicit skills within the learners [68]. Role play can also be helpful as a demonstration of the benchmark through by either learners or instructors.

Directive debriefing is, as its name implies, directed. This technique can yield specific discussion around actions or concepts. The technique tends to use more close-ended questions or narrow inquiry and discourages free flow of thought. This may be appropriated with novice learners who simply lack the underlying knowledge and do not have a clinical context to draw from their experience. This technique, like any other, has a valid place in debriefing, especially when other techniques are not yielding success or progress. When overused or misapplied, it can devolve into the more instructor-centered traditional educational strategy.

Additional Techniques and Tools Used in Debriefing Sessions

There are several other tools and techniques that are commonly used by debriefers. These include restatement, role play, reflective journaling, checklists, and written prompts. A mixture of visual (video, writing surface), as well as spoken techniques will contribute to the common purpose of promoting understanding and growth. The use of video broadcasting and playback to demonstrate specific interactions, sequences, events, or actions is a common practice globally. Although studies have not shown performance improvement with instructor-facilitated + video debriefing compared to instructor-facilitated debriefing alone, video remains an important part of debriefing and post-event analysis in certain situations [69–72]. Video-assisted debriefing is particularly helpful in certain circumstances where participants in an event cannot recall, disagree, or lack clarity about what occurred in a simulation. Like any tool, it should be used when the debriefer feels that it will augment learning.

Co-debriefing, which uses multiple instructors during the debriefing sessions, has not been extensively explored in the healthcare literature but its advantages and uses can be derived from other industries. The potential advantages include the following: providing multiple instructor perspectives, additional subject expertise, complimenting styles of debriefing, more ability to manage learner expectations, model effective teamwork, and assist each other in managing challenging situations [60]. Co-debriefers can also help each other through feedback on their debriefing styles. For all these potential advantages, the disadvantages of co-debriefing can also be numerous. These disadvantages include the following: competing learning objectives, individual's expertise that is not used, one debriefer dominating or derailing their co-debriefer's points, or open disagreement between debriefers [60]. Creating clear expectations of who is the primary versus secondary debriefer for each simulated activity can help avoid many of these issues, in addition to planning how co-debriefers may invite each other to add to a discussion or ask permission to speak. Planning out the debriefing session objectives and who should cover each learning objectives helps facilitate a successful co-debrief as well.

Assessment Tools to Evaluate the Effectiveness of Debriefing

Due to the high variability in settings, objectives and learners in debriefing sessions, no two debriefing sessions are the same. There are highly specific validated assessment tools to assess the effectiveness of debriefing in the operating room [73], nursing [74], and surgical settings [75]. The DASH assessment tool for debriefing assessments can be applied broadly for any debriefing in the healthcare setting [76]. The DASH assessment tool includes the following elements: (1) establishes an engaging learning environment, (2) maintains an engaging learning environment, (3) structures debriefing in an organized way, (4) provokes engaging discussions, (5) identifies and explores performance gaps, and (6) helps trainees achieve or sustain good future performance [76]. The DASH is simply a singular example of a debriefer assessment tool that is generalizable. It, however, lacks many of the specific debriefing elements presented in this chapter. It takes a trained, skilled, and knowledgeable instructor familiar with simulation to use these tools to conduct debriefing assessments with feedback to the instructors. Ongoing research and work is needed to find a tool that is easy to use, perhaps even learner centered, that evaluates the effectiveness of the debriefing session.

Conclusion

Debriefing is an important educational strategy that requires skill and experience to deploy effectively. Healthcare education has used debriefing in a variety of settings over time, including the common nursing post conference. What has changed is the ability for multiple participants to not only share their experiences but to have peers critically evaluate each other in real time and asynchronously. The debrief session is intended to promote reflection and active learning with the outcome of learner growth and development. Ultimately this is intended to have impact on patient care, health, and system outcomes. Debriefing techniques share a common structure for the most part and an experienced debriefer will use a variety of different techniques as they flow through the structure. While the debrief is ultimately founded on creating and maintaining a safe learning environment and focusing on session learning objectives, instructors have the latitude to expand on significant elements that may be outside the specific objectives as the debrief process unfolds and learner-centered objectives emerge. Debriefing requires discipline and flexibility. While this seems contradictory, it is not. The discipline of understanding where the process needs to go, what needs to be achieved and addressed, and in what time-frame are requisite for success. The flexibility comes as the instructor leverages different strategies and techniques to achieve maximal learning from the simulated activity.

References

1. Kolb DA. Experiential learning: experience as the source of learning and development. Englewood Cliffs: Prentice Hall; 1984.
2. Stocker M, Burmester M, Allen M. Optimisation of simulated team training through the application of learning theories: a debate for a conceptual framework. BMC Med Educ. 2014;14:69.
3. Knowles MS. Application in continuing education for the health professions: chapter five of "andragogy in action". Mobius. 1985;5(2):80–100.
4. Fanning RM, Gaba DM. The role of debriefing in simulation-based learning. Simul Healthc. 2007;2(2):115–25.
5. Raemer D, et al. Research regarding debriefing as part of the learning process. Simul Healthc. 2011;6 Suppl:S52–7.
6. Zigmont JJ, Kappus LJ, Sudikoff SN. Theoretical foundations of learning through simulation. Semin Perinatol. 2011;35(2):47–51.
7. Rudolph JW, et al. There's no such thing as "nonjudgmental" debriefing: a theory and method for debriefing with good judgment. Simul Healthc. 2006;1(1):49–55.
8. Rudolph JW, et al. Debriefing as formative assessment: closing performance gaps in medical education. Acad Emerg Med. 2008;15(11):1010–6.
9. Issenberg SB, et al. Features and uses of high-fidelity medical simulations that lead to effective learning: a BEME systematic review. Med Teach. 2005;27(1):10–28.
10. Tannenbaum SI, Cerasoli CP. Do team and individual debriefs enhance performance? A meta-analysis. Hum Factors. 2013;55(1):231–45.
11. McGaghie WC, et al. A critical review of simulation-based medical education research: 2003–2009. Med Educ. 2010;44(1):50–63.
12. Darling MJ, Parry CS. From post-mortem to living practice: an in-depth study of the evolution of the after-action review. Boston: Signet Consulting Group; 2001.
13. Ellis S, Davidi I. After-event reviews: drawing lessons from successful and failed experience. J Appl Psychol. 2005;90(5):857–71.
14. van de Ridder JM, et al. What is feedback in clinical education? Med Educ. 2008;42(2):189–97.
15. Ende J. Feedback in clinical medical education. JAMA. 1983;250(6):777–81.
16. Ericsson KA. Deliberate practice and acquisition of expert performance: a general overview. Acad Emerg Med. 2008;15(11):988–94.
17. Johnson CE, et al. Identifying educator behaviours for high quality verbal feedback in health professions education: literature review and expert refinement. BMC Med Educ. 2016;16:96.
18. Rudolph JW, et al. Debriefing with good judgment: combining rigorous feedback with genuine inquiry. Anesthesiol Clin. 2007;25(2):361–76.
19. Zigmont JJ, Kappus LJ, Sudikoff SN. The 3D model of debriefing: defusing, discovering, and deepening. Semin Perinatol. 2011;35(2):52–8.
20. Schön DA. Toward a new design for teaching and learning in the professions. In: Educating the reflective practitioner. San Francisco: Jossey-Bass; 1987.
21. Eppich W, Cheng A. Promoting Excellence And Reflective Learning in Simulation (PEARLS): development and rationale for a blended approach to healthcare simulation debriefing. Simul Healthc. 2015;10(2):106Y115.
22. Orsini C, Evans P, Jerez O. How to encourage intrinsic motivation in the clinical teaching environment?: a systematic review from the self-determination theory. J Educ Eval Health Prof. 2015;12:8.
23. Kusurkar RA, Croiset G, Ten Cate TJ. Twelve tips to stimulate intrinsic motivation in students through autonomy-supportive classroom teaching derived from self-determination theory. Med Teach. 2011;33(12):978–82.
24. Jawahar IM, Williams CR. Where all the children are above average: the performance appraisal purpose effect. Pers Psychol. 1997;50:905–25.
25. Murphy KR, Cleveland JN. Understanding performance appraisal: social, organizational, and goal-based perspectives. Thousand Oaks: Sage; 1995.
26. Locke EA, Latham GP. A theory of goal setting and task performance. Englewood Cliffs: Prentice Hall; 1990.
27. Locke EA, Latham GP. Building a practically useful theory of goal setting and task motivation. A 35-year odyssey. Am Psychol. 2002;57(9):705–17.
28. Edelson DP, Lafond CM. Deconstructing debriefing for simulation-based education. JAMA Pediatr. 2013;167(6):586–7.
29. Kluger A, Denisi A. The effects of feedback interventions on performance: a historical review, a meta-analysis, and a preliminary feedback intervention theory. Psychol Bull. 1996;119:254.
30. Nicol DJ, MacFarlane-Dick D. Formative assessment and self regulated learning: a model and seven principles of good feedback practice. Stud High Educ. 2006;31:199–218.
31. Barrett A, et al. A BEME (Best Evidence in Medical Education) review of the use of workplace-based assessment in identifying and remediating underperformance among postgraduate medical trainees: BEME Guide No. 43. Med Teach. 2016;38(12):1188–98.
32. Davis DA, et al. Accuracy of physician self-assessment compared with observed measures of competence: a systematic review. JAMA. 2006;296(9):1094–102.
33. Schneider JR, et al. Patient assessment and management examination: lack of correlation between faculty assessment and resident self-assessment. Am J Surg. 2008;195(1):16–9.
34. Salas E, Rosen MA. Building high reliability teams: progress and some reflections on teamwork training. BMJ Qual Saf. 2013;22(5):369–73.
35. Parker SK, Axtell C. Seeing another viewpoint: antecedents and outcomes of employee perspective taking. Acad Manage J. 2001;44(6):1085–100.
36. Dismukes RK, McDonnell L, Jobe KK. Facilitating LOFT debriefings: instructor techniques and crew participation. Int J Aviat Psychol. 2000;10:35Y57.
37. Haefner J. National Institute for Learning Outcomes Assessment. The Transparency Framework 2012 December 10, 2012. Available from: http://www.learningoutcomeassessment.org/TransparencyFramework.htm.

38. Rudolph JW, Raemer DB, Simon R. Establishing a safe container for learning in simulation: the role of the presimulation briefing. Simul Healthc. 2014;9(6):339–49.
39. March JG. Exploration and exploitation in organizational learning. Org Sci. 1991;2(1):71Y87.
40. Elliot AJ, Dweck C. Handbook of competence and motivation. New York: Guilford; 2005.
41. Skinner EA, Belmont M. Motivation in the classroom: reciprocal effects of teacher behavior and student engagement across the school year. J Educ Psychol. 1993;85(4):572.
42. Lefroy J, et al. Guidelines: the do's, don'ts and don't knows of feedback for clinical education. Perspect Med Educ. 2015;4(6):284–99.
43. Dieckmann P, Gaba D, Rall M. Deepening the theoretical foundations of patient simulation as social practice. Simul Healthc. 2007;2(3):183–93.
44. Metcalfe J. Learning from errors. Annu Rev Psychol. 2017;68:6.1–6.25.
45. Kolbe M, et al. TeamGAINS: a tool for structured debriefings for simulation-based team trainings. BMJ Qual Saf. 2013;22(7):541–53.
46. Stevenson H, Stigler J. The learning gap: why our schools are failing and what we can learn from Japanese and Chinese education. New York: Simon and Schuster; 1994.
47. Keith N, Frese M. Effectiveness of error management training: a meta-analysis. J Appl Psychol. 2008;93(1):59–69.
48. Miettinen R. The concept of experiential learning and John Dewey's theory of reflective thought and action. Int J Lifelong Educ. 2000;19(1):54–72.
49. Baron RA. Negative effects of destructive criticism: impact on conflict, self-efficacy, and task performance. J Appl Psychol. 1988;73(2):199–207.
50. Sargeant J, et al. Understanding the influence of emotions and reflection upon multi-source feedback acceptance and use. Adv Health Sci Educ Theory Pract. 2008;13(3):275–88.
51. Loh V, et al. The moderating effect of individual differences in error-management training: who learns from mistakes? Hum Factors. 2013;55(2):435–48.
52. Sawyer T, et al. More than one way to debrief: a critical review of healthcare simulation debriefing methods. Simul Healthc. 2016;11(3):209–17.
53. Jaye P, Thomas L, Reedy G. 'The Diamond': a structure for simulation debrief. Clin Teach. 2015;12(3):171–5.
54. Phrampus P, O'Donnell J, Levine A, DeMaria S, Schwartz A, Sim A. Debriefing using a structured and supported approach. In: The comprehensive textbook of healthcare simulation. 1st ed. New York: Springer; 2013.
55. Sawyer T, Deering S. Adaptation of the U.S. Army's after-action review (AAR) to simulation debriefing in healthcare. Simul Healthc. 2013;8(6):388Y397.
56. Cheng A, et al. Examining pediatric resuscitation education using simulation and scripted debriefing: a multicenter randomized trial. JAMA Pediatr. 2013;167(6):528–36.
57. Eppich W, Cheng A. Promoting Excellence and Reflective Learning in Simulation (PEARLS): development and rationale for a blended approach to health care simulation debriefing. Simul Healthc. 2015;10(2):106–15.
58. Mitchell JT. When disaster strikes...the critical incident stress debriefing process. JEMS. 1983;8(1):36–9.
59. Boudreau JD, Cassell E, Fuks A. Preparing medical students to become attentive listeners. Med Teach. 2009;31(1):22–9.
60. Cheng A, et al. Co-debriefing for simulation-based education: a primer for facilitators. Simul Healthc. 2015;10(2):69–75.
61. Dean M, Street RL Jr. A 3-stage model of patient-centered communication for addressing cancer patients' emotional distress. Patient Educ Couns. 2014;94(2):143–8.
62. Ranjan P, Kumari A, Chakrawarty A. How can doctors improve their communication skills? J Clin Diagn Res. 2015;9(3):JE01–4.
63. Gerard E. The skilled helper: a problem-management approach to helping. 5th ed. Pacific Grove, California: Brooks/Cole; 1994.
64. Razavi D, Delvaux N. Communication skills and psychological training in oncology. Eur J Cancer. 1997;33(Suppl 6):S15–21.
65. Robbins JM, et al. Physician characteristics and the recognition of depression and anxiety in primary care. Med Care. 1994;32(8):795–812.
66. Smith-Jentsch KA, Cannon-Bowers J, Tannenbaum SI, Salas E. Guided team self-correction: impacts on team mental models, processes, and effectiveness. Small Group Resol. 2008;39(3):303Y327.
67. Kriz WC. A systematic-constructivist approach to the facilitation and debriefing of simulations and games. Simul Gaming. 2010;41:663Y680.
68. Jackson VA, Back AL. Teaching communication skills using role-play: an experience-based guide for educators. J Palliat Med. 2011;14(6):775–80.
69. Savoldelli GL, et al. Value of debriefing during simulated crisis management: oral versus video-assisted oral feedback. Anesthesiology. 2006;105(2):279–85.
70. Byrne AJ, et al. Effect of videotape feedback on anaesthetists' performance while managing simulated anaesthetic crises: a multicentre study. Anaesthesia. 2002;57(2):176–9.
71. Chronister C, Brown D. Comparison of simulation debriefing methods. Clin Simul Nurs. 2010;8(7):e281–8.
72. Sawyer T, et al. The effectiveness of video-assisted debriefing versus oral debriefing alone at improving neonatal resuscitation performance: a randomized trial. Simul Healthc. 2012;7(4):213–21.
73. Gururaja RP, et al. Examining the effectiveness of debriefing at the point of care in simulation-based operating room team training. In: Henriksen K, et al., editors. Advances in patient safety: new directions and alternative approaches, Performance and tools, vol. 3. Rockville: Agency for Healthcare Research and Quality (US); 2008.
74. Reed SJ. Debriefing experience scale: development of a tool to evaluate the student learning experience in debriefing. Clin Simul Nurs. 2012;8(6):211Y217.
75. Arora S, et al. Objective structured assessment of debriefing: bringing science to the art of debriefing in surgery. Ann Surg. 2012;256(6):982–8.
76. Brett-Fleegler M, et al. Debriefing assessment for simulation in healthcare: development and psychometric properties. Simul Healthc. 2012;7(5):288–94.

Crisis Resource Management and Interdisciplinary Team Training

5

Idalid Franco, Rachel E. Sweeney, Joshua A. Marks, Carlene McLaughlin, Maryann Henry, Miguel A. Yaport, and Alexander F. Arriaga

Introduction

The connections between crew/crisis resource management (CRM), interprofessional team training, and medicine have been written and studied extensively over the past several decades [1–6]. This is a testament to the interest on this topic and its relevance to healthcare practice. The purpose of this chapter is not to simply rewrite a story that has already been described at length elsewhere. Rather, the goal of this chapter is to give a brief summary of key topics within the field of CRM and interprofessional team training, followed by suggested practical approaches to teaching these topics in a simulation setting. The hope is that this chapter can be used together with other chapters in this book such that a comprehensive simulation program can be developed and delivered.

Supported by grants from the University of Pennsylvania Bach Fund and McCabe Fund.

Chapter Objectives

This chapter is divided into two sections. The first section will cover key domains within crew/crisis resource management, including references to illustrative studies, tables, and figures that a simulation instructor can use to draw parallels to events when delivering or debriefing a simulation session or as a vehicle to drive discussion. The second section will highlight the essentials of interprofessional team training in their application to medical simulation training, guiding the reader through specific curricular design, implementation, and evaluation.

CRM and interprofessional team training are large topics for which one can devote a career to understanding. Entire books have been written on these topics alone [1, 2, 7, 8]. This chapter aims to hit the highlights of these fields while acknowledging that due to time and space constraints, there will be domains and studies that will not be covered. This chapter should serve as a primer to get the reader interested in these topics in ways that foster integrating them into simulation efforts to improve healthcare. Once that interest exists, it is easier to explore further, and possibly develop studies of one's own, to advance the current knowledge on these topics.

I. Franco
Harvard T.H. Chan School of Public Health, Boston, MA, USA

Harvard Medical School, Boston, MA, USA

Department of Radiation Oncology, Massachusetts General Hospital, Boston, MA, USA

R. E. Sweeney
Department of Anesthesiology and Critical Care, University of Pennsylvania Health System, Philadelphia, PA, USA

Perelman School of Medicine, University of Pennsylvania, Philadelphia, PA, USA

J. A. Marks
Department of Surgery, Sidney Kimmel Medical College at Thomas Jefferson University Hospitals, Philadelphia, PA, USA

C. McLaughlin · M. Henry · M. A. Yaport
Department of Anesthesiology and Critical Care, University of Pennsylvania Health System, Philadelphia, PA, USA

A. F. Arriaga (✉)
Department of Anesthesiology and Pain Medicine, Brigham and Women's Hospital, Boston, MA, USA

Harvard Medical School, Boston, MA, USA
e-mail: aarriaga@post.harvard.edu

B. Mahoney et al. (eds.), *Comprehensive Healthcare Simulation: Anesthesiology*, Comprehensive Healthcare Simulation,
https://doi.org/10.1007/978-3-030-26849-7_5

For the purposes of setting a stable reference point, the frame for this chapter will be set within intraoperative anesthesiology. Nevertheless, many of the lessons and principles described here are applicable to the intensive care unit (ICU), obstetric anesthesiology, outpatient, out-of-operating room (OR), and the many other environments for which the anesthesiologist may practice over the course of a career. Anesthesiologists should take pride in the fact that many of the original studies that brought the principles of human factors, CRM, and team training into medicine came from studies of anesthesiologists and the operating room environment [9–12]. Our hope is that this tradition will continue to thrive through the next generation of anesthesiologists.

Crisis Resource Management

To begin the discussion, we will define "crisis resource management" using the words of Dr. David Gaba, a respected anesthesiologist on this topic and lead author of the book *Crisis Management in Anesthesiology*. He and colleagues describe crisis resource management as the ability to "command and control all the resources at hand in order to execute [care] as planned and to respond to problems that arise" [2]. It is important to note that this term is closely connected to the term "crew resource management" (formerly called "cockpit resource management"), which is embraced by many industries and gained popularity from much of its use in the aviation industry [1]. Many of the core principles are the same or similar, and we aim to leverage the strengths of crew/crisis resource management rather than expend time on subtle differences. Accordingly, for the purposes of this chapter, we will let the letters "CRM" serve as an abbreviation for crew/crisis resource management. Given the integral role that the aviation industry has had in the development of crew resource management, we will also give a very brief description of some of the origins of CRM in aviation for the novice reader. For the advanced reader, this will be supplemented by a description of key aviation accident reports that can have relevance to the anesthesiologist. These reports can be considered for drawing parallels to events that occur during simulation sessions or as a starting point to foster discussion in CRM principles. The remainder of the section will be devoted to a description of specific CRM principles that can be taught and integrated into simulation training and programming.

Origins of Crew Resource Management in Aviation and Selection of Key Incidents to Date

Several decades ago, there was a growing sentiment in the aviation industry that human error was contributing to serious plane accidents. There were two specific accidents in the late 1970s for which much attention on the topic was generated. In 1977, there was a collision of two Boeing 747 s (leading to 583 fatalities) on a runway on the Spanish island of Tenerife, where one of the flights took off without clearance from air traffic control [13, 14]. In 1978, United Airlines Flight 173 (UA173) crashed in Portland Oregon due to predictable fuel exhaustion, where the National Transportation Safety Board (NTSB) deemed that "…the probable cause of the accident was the failure of the captain to monitor properly the aircraft's fuel state and ... the failure of the other two flight crew members either to fully comprehend the criticality of the fuel state or to successfully communicate their concern to the captain." In the accident report for UA173, the NTSB formally recommended to the Federal Aviation Administration (FAA) an urgent call to ensure that "flight crews are indoctrinated in particulars of flight deck resource management" [15].

In 1979, a joint workshop was held by the National Aeronautics and Space Administration (NASA) and the aviation industry called *Resource Management on the Flight Deck*. The workshop included the presentation of an interview study conducted with pilots. This study found that, generally, those pilots who mentioned training were satisfied in the "technical aspects of flying and in flying skills." The difficulties that arose were related to issues on how to be a more effective leader and how to achieve more effective crew coordination and improved communication [16]. Prof. Robert Helmreich, a psychologist and one of the presenters at the workshop, noted in one of his articles that the term "cockpit resource management" was used as a label at this meeting to signify "the process of training crews to reduce 'pilot error' by making better use of the human resources on the flight deck" [17]. The word "cockpit" evolved into the word "crew" over a short period of time [1].

While the connection between CRM and aviation may appear intuitive, it was not initially universally accepted. At that time, efforts to promote CRM were sometimes referred to as "charm school, psychobabble, and attempted brainwashing" [1]. The acceptance was a gradual process that included CRM courses being taught and guidelines being initiated by the FAA [17, 18].

With this historical context, we present a table noting a selection of key aviation incidents containing CRM elements that have occurred over time, together with references to studies of analogous topics in the field of medicine (Table 5.1). The NTSB (noted above) is a United States Federal Agency "charged by Congress with investigating every civil aviation accident in the United States and significant accidents in other modes of transportation" [32]. The NTSB creates reports of these investigations that comment on the probable cause(s) of the incidents and contain safety recommendations. It is not uncommon for these reports to

Table 5.1 Illustrative Airline Incidents that Elucidate Important Crew/Crisis Resource Management (CRM) Principles in Aviation and Medicine

Flight number	Synopsis	Attributed cause of disaster	CRM principles	Medical simulation studies of relevant domains
1972: Eastern Air Lines 401 [19]	Jet crashed into the Florida Everglades.	Pilot error, controlled flight into terrain	Lack of situational awareness	*Situational awareness*: Graafland et al. (2015), Training Situational Awareness to Reduce Surgical Errors in the Operating Room [20]
1977: KLM Flight 4805/ Pan Am Flight 1736 [21, 22]	Fatal runway collision occurred between two Boeing 747 s at Los rodeos airport on the island of Tenerife.	Pilot error, runway incursion, heavy fog, limitations and failures in communication	Communication failure, lack of situational awareness	*Communication*: Minehart et al. (2012), Speaking Across the Drapes: Communication Strategies of Anesthesiologists and Obstetricians During a Simulated Maternal Crisis [23]
1978: United Airlines Flight 173 [24]	During the flight from Denver, CO, to Portland, OR, the aircraft ran out of fuel and crashed into a suburban neighborhood.	Fuel exhaustion due to pilot error (lack of situational awareness and maintenance error with landing gear)	Issues with assertiveness (inability of crew members to speak up to the captain), lack of situational awareness	*Assertiveness, speaking-up behavior*: Raemer et al. (2016), Improving Anesthesiologists' Ability to Speak Up in the Operating Room [25]
1997: Korean Air Flight 801 [26]	Aircraft crashed on approach to Antonio B. won pat International airport in the United States territory of Guam.	Insufficient pilot training, controlled flight into terrain, pilot error, captain fatigue, inhibition of the minimum safe altitude warning at Guam (agency failure to manage the system)	Communication failure, issues with assertiveness, absence of the use of checklists, insufficient training	*Checklists and preparation*: Just et al. (2015), The Effectiveness of an Intensive Care Quick Reference Checklist Manual – A Randomized Simulation-Based Trial [27]
2009: US Airways Flight 1549 [28]	Aircraft flying out of LaGuardia airport, NY, landed on the Hudson River upon experiencing engine failure shortly after takeoff.	Multiple bird strikes shortly after takeoff resulting to loss of power to engines and a rapid loss of altitude, controlled ditching by the captain resulted in successful landing	Strong leadership of the captain, use of reference handbook and checklists, informed decision making, presence of a culture of open communication	*Leadership*: Fernandez Castelao et al. (2015), Effect of CRM Team Leader Training on Team Performance and Leadership Behavior in Simulated Cardiac Arrest Scenarios [29]
2009: Air France Flight 447 [30]	Flight from Rio de Janeiro, Brazil to Paris, France, crashed into the Atlantic Ocean, killing everyone on board.	Aircraft entering high altitude stall and rapidly descending until impact with ocean, crew responding incorrectly to aerodynamic stall, resulting in crash	Communication failure, lack of situational awareness and assertiveness, ambiguous leader, poor decision making, failure to function as team	*Decision making*: Andrew et al. (2012), Development and Evaluation of a Decision-Based Simulation for Assessment of Team Skills [31]

have CRM principles that resonate well with a medical audience. Most notably to the reader interested in developing modules for teaching CRM principles, many of these reports are easily and publicly available, free of charge, through the NTSB website (http://www.ntsb.gov). Further, many of these incidents receive media attention, leading to items such as documentaries, newspaper articles, and other materials that may be well suited for a medical simulation session/debriefing. With decades of reports available, this table does not intend to be comprehensive or definitive. Rather, it serves as a primer to foster interest in the connections between aviation and anesthesiology, as well as an opportunity to consider a self-directed review of further aviation incidents for lessons most relevant to the reader's own objectives. We supply an additional table (Table 5.2) that gives a more detailed summary of one aviation incident that involved many CRM principles. For the advanced reader, one could consider also exploring incidents outside of aviation (such as the 2015 Amtrak train derailment near Philadelphia, PA [34]) or international incidents that are outside of the NTSB's purview. Further, a recent medical review article provides an additional historical discussion of the story of the parallel evolution of CRM in aviation and anesthesiology [35]. As we begin our discussion of *key domains commonly used in CRM and connections to anesthesiology/simulation*, we invite the reader to cross-reference these hybrid aviation/medical tables and consider whether these real incidents could be used to enhance an anesthesiology simulation program and ultimately to improve patient care.

Selection of Key Domains Commonly Used in CRM and Connections to Anesthesiology/Simulation

Although we list the key domains commonly used in CRM below, it is important to keep in mind that the list is not exhaustive of all domains utilized and studied within the field of CRM and should instead serve as a foundation to understand some of the core principles.

Table 5.2 Air France Flight 447 – Application of crew/crisis resource management (CRM) principles[a] [33]

CRM principle	Significance in Flight 447	Relevant transcript dialogue
Decision making	The captain, the most experienced pilot, takes a sleep break as weather begins to deteriorate. He leaves controls with the pilot of least experience (Copilot #1). His failure to respond to being called further extinguishes the possibility of recovering from aerodynamic stall.	*At 2:02 min the captain leaves to nap.* Copilot #1 to Copilot #2: "Did you sleep?" Copilot #2: "So-so." The Captain: "Well then I'm out of here." *At 2:10 min Copilot #2 summons the captain.* Copilot #2: "Where is he?" Copilot #2 (a minute later): "Is he coming or not?"
Situational awareness	The copilots both ignore the "stall" audio alarm, which sounds approximately 72 times. They are likely distracted by the strange electrical activity of the intertropical conversion zone, inundating their visual and olfactory systems.	*At 2:08 min Copilot #1 experiences additional weather-related stimuli.* Copilot #1: "Ah… you did something to the A/C." Copilot #2: "I didn't touch it." Copilot #1: "What's that smell, now?" Copilot #2: "It's ozone."
Leadership	The three pilots—The captain, copilot #2, and copilot #1—Have disparate levels of experience, from greatest to least respectively. The most novice pilot, copilot #1, was left to fly through the storm. When disaster strikes, no one emerges as a leader, no one delivers clear directives.	*At 2:11 min the Captain returns to the cockpit from his nap.* The Captain: "What the hell are you doing?" Copilot #1: "We've lost control of the plane!" Copilot #2: "We've totally lost control of the plane. We don't understand at all… We've tried everything… what do you think? What should we do?" The Captain: "Well, I don't know!"
Communication	Lapses in communication are pervasive throughout Air France Flight 447. The two copilots fail to engage in closed-loop communication and as a result are both operating the plane at the same time, copilot #1 pulling the aircraft's nose up while copilot #2 pulls it down.	*Copilot #1 and Captain #2 fail to communicate who is in control of the plane and the appropriate directives. At 2:13 min they realize their error.* Copilot #1: "But I've had the stick back the whole time!" Captain #2: "No, no, no… Don't climb… no, no." Copilot #1: "Descend then… Give me the controls… Give me the controls!"

[a]The names of the Captain and the two copilots were deidentified to "The Captain," "Copilot#1," and "Copilot#2." This table is presented in approximate chronological order of the transcripts, highlighting that failures of these principles do not necessarily occur in a particular sequence and are interrelated (rows may contain more than one domain)

Communication

Communication is defined as the transfer of information between (a) sender(s) and (b) receiver(s) (Fig. 5.1) [36].

Although communication may seem simple based on the definition, the practice and real-life applications of this principle, even those that we can recall from our personal experiences, illustrate the many ways in which communication can go wrong. Arriaga and colleagues point out that "Findings from both the American Society of Anesthesiologists (ASA) and the American College of Surgeons (ACS) closed claims studies have found poor communication both inside and outside the operating room to be a significant cause of preventable adverse events" [5]. Lorelei Lingard's work utilizes observational classification to describe the recurrent type of "communication failures" seen in the OR and their outcomes [3]. Four types of communication failures are discussed, which she states can compromise patient safety. These include (1) occasion failures, (2) content failures, (3) audience failures, and (4) purpose failures (Table 5.3).

Charles Vincent, in *Patient Safety*, describes communication errors as either "information that is not communicated, communicated with the wrong information, or communicated with incomplete information" [38]. Both models highlight the complex and interconnected network through which communication occurs and how it can become disrupted, ultimately compromising patient safety. The takeaway message for translating this principle into improved patient care is that once an understanding of these communication failures is achieved, teams can use this framework as a tool to describe the overall quality of team communication in the operating room. One important caveat is raised by Bowers and colleagues in their analysis of aviation team communication, where the authors point out that in addition to emphasizing *content*, an efficient *pattern* of information exchange is also crucial in successful team communication [39]. One particularly effective pattern observed, where information and questions are repeated by the receiver such that the sender is provided with appropriate feedback that the original message has been received and understood, was more frequently seen in the teams with good communication. Training and practice in this type of "closed-loop communication" can help team members improve and build more efficient communication strategies that are less susceptible to errors. As the reader progresses through this chapter, we will show how the breakdown in communication can occur within the context of each of the other domains. It is our goal

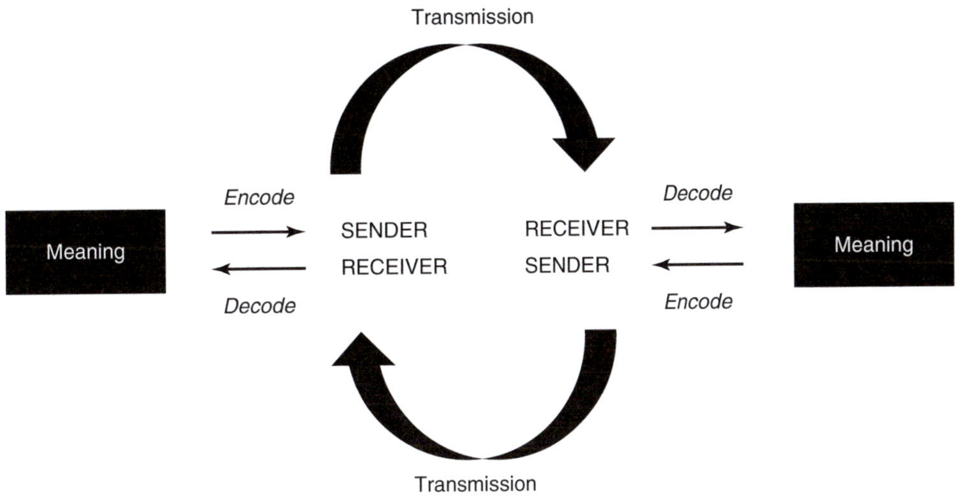

Fig. 5.1 Simplified model of two-way communication. (Reproduced with the permission of Flin et al., Fig. 4.2 [36])

Table 5.3 Definition of types of communication failure with illustrative examples and notes

Failure	Definition	Illustrative example and analytical note (in italics)
Occasion failures	Problems in the situation or context of the communication event	The staff surgeon asks the anesthesiologist whether the antibiotics have been administered. At the point of this question, the procedure has been underway for over an hour. *Since antibiotics are optimally given within 30 minutes of incision* [35], *the timing of this inquiry is ineffective both as a prompt and as a safety redundancy measure.*
Content failures	Insufficiency or inaccuracy apparent in the information being transferred	As this case is set up, the anesthesia fellow asks the staff surgeon if the patient has an ICU (intensive care unit) bed. The staff surgeon replies that the "bed is probably not needed, and there isn't likely one available anyways, so we'll just go ahead." *Relevant information is missing and questions are left unresolved: has an ICU bed been requested, and what will the plan be if the patient does need critical care and an ICU bed is not available? (Note: this example was classified as both a content and a purpose failure).*
Audience failures	Gaps in the composition of the group engaged in the communication	The nurses and anesthesiologist discuss how the patient should be positioned for surgery without the participation of a surgical representative. *Surgeons have particular positioning needs, so they should be participants in this discussion. Decisions made in their absence occasionally lead to renewed discussions and repositioning upon their arrival.*
Purpose failures	Communication events in which purpose is unclear, not achieved, or inappropriate	During a living donor liver resection, the nurses discuss whether ice is needed in the basin they are preparing for the liver. Neither knows. No further discussion ensues. *The purpose of this communication—to find out if ice is required – is not achieved. No plan to achieve it is articulated.*

Source: Lingard et al. [37]. Table 2. Used with permission

that readers begin to see how the domains are interrelated with each other and that in addressing one, others can also be improved.

Assertiveness

Assertiveness is defined as a *stance* of behavior that is in between "too passive" and "too aggressive" [36]. The range of passiveness and aggressiveness can be thought of as existing in a continuum where "too passive" is failing to stand up for oneself, or standing up for oneself in a way that is easily disregarded, and "too aggressive" as standing up for oneself with disregard to the opinions of others.

This principle has been studied within the field of anesthesiology in multiple ways. The first takes into account the inherent difficulty that comes from working in a hierarchical system [38]. Pian-Smith and colleagues point out that there is substantial difficulty in questioning the thought process for diagnosis and treatment or vocalizing disagreement with patient care or plans that can compromise patient safety, when these actions challenge the position of a superior [40]. The authors of the study utilized prior examples from the aviation industry in order to design and evaluate an intervention aimed at supporting the notion that all members of the team share in the responsibility for a safe outcome and are therefore obligated to speak up when actions do not seem right. They evaluated this intervention through a simulation-based operating room where anesthesiology trainees were presented with opportunities to challenge multiple members of the team. The "two challenge rule," taken from U.S. Army Aviation, was adapted to the clinical setting through the "advocacy-inquiry" approach from the discipline of organizational behavior. Trainees were encouraged to describe their position, by sharing data and making their thinking known (advocacy), and then asking an open-ended question to invite sharing of thoughts and opinions (inquiry), with the purpose of engaging in productive dialogue together. This process was done twice before the trainee called for reinforcement. The authors concluded that this intervention improved the trainees' ability to "speak up" to their superordinate physicians and therefore could serve as a route to reinforce assertiveness and address the difficulties inherent to the hierarchical healthcare system. Application of a framework that provides a structured pathway for "speaking up" can therefore help normalize and encourage such behavior, resulting in improved communication, increased assertiveness, and enhanced team dynamics that may lead to improvement in patient safety.

Raemer et al. also looked at assertiveness in a randomized controlled experiment of a simulation-based intervention of hurdles and enablers to improving anesthesiologists' ability to speak up in the OR [41]. Although they found no difference between the intervention and control group in their ability to speak up, they did identify common hurdles and enablers that impacted an individual's ability to speak up within an operating room setting. Interestingly, there were some similarities in reasoning between both, which included familiarity with the person in charge, which was categorized as both a hurdle and enabler. Other hurdles included uncertainty about the situation, stereotypes of others on the team, respect for the experience of the person in charge, and fear of repercussion. On the other hand, awareness of the problem, having a rubric, certainty about the consequences, and having a form of reinforcement either through a second opinion or someone to help were all cited as enablers.

Relating this back to what we have learned from aviation, Sexton et al. surveyed staff in the operating room and the intensive care unit about attitudes on error, stress, and teamwork and compared the results to those attitudes gathered from airline cockpit crews [42]. These surveys were administered in a diverse set of hospitals in the US, Israel, Germany, Switzerland, and Italy, as well as major airlines around the world. Not surprisingly, the authors found that surgeons were more likely to deny the effects of fatigue on performance, accept steep hierarchies in which senior team members were not open to input from junior members, and perceive higher levels of teamwork than other members of the team perceived. Medical staff was also more likely to report difficulty discussing mistakes, failure to acknowledge making errors, and feeling that errors were not handled appropriately in their hospital. Interestingly, pilots were less likely to deny the effects of fatigue on performance and were more likely to reject steep hierarchies. The authors pointed out that the aviation industry, similar to the field of medicine, is expected to function without error as both hold strong responsibility where outcomes in process are measured by human lives. Yet the difference in culture between the acceptance of human factors in aviation and healthcare may have played a large role in the differences that were seen in response to error. The authors concluded that much can be gained from implementing the lessons of crew resource management into healthcare safety through the implementation of training that allows individuals to recognize the role of stress, fatigue, and hierarchy in inducing error.

One effective communication tool that has been shown to play a role in improving communication and assertiveness by healthcare teams is the use of "C.U.S." words (Concerned, Uncomfortable, Safety). In their website, the Agency for Healthcare Research and Quality within the U.S. Department of Health and Human Services provides training as part of their TeamSTEPPS® system (Team Strategies & Tools to Enhance Performance & Patient Safety), which guides users through the use of these words to communicate the level of concern and action steps needed to address critical issues [43]. When a concerning issue occurs, team members are encouraged to use the phrase "I am Concerned about ___." In these situations, the word "Concern" serves as a cue to the team that they need to pay attention to the team member and the situation at hand. The statement can then be elevated to the next level with the phrase "I am Uncomfortable that___." This again brings attention to the situation, with the word "Uncomfortable" adding a higher level of urgency. Ultimately, if the statement needs an even higher level of awareness and action, the statement "This is a Safety issue" utilizes the word "Safety" to ensure that other providers stop the current activities in which they are engaged to evaluate the situation at hand and address the concern before returning to their previous tasks. These key words, when inserted into a medical situation, can create a common framework and vocabulary that simplifies communication between team members and underscores the degree of importance regarding the behavior that must be taken, clearly and efficiently prompting appropriate action when necessary. Simulation training can play a critical role in developing and fostering the assertiveness of all providers and promote a common framework that can be used to create a culture of safety that allows for the team as a whole to take responsibility for preventing errors and utilizes errors as a basis for learning and adapting improved strategies to approach patient care. Most importantly, communication techniques taught must include an emphasis on dialogue and moving from "who's right" to "what's right."

Situational Awareness

Situational awareness, a key component of CRM, can be defined as "the perception of the elements of one's environment, the comprehension of their meaning, and the projection of their status in the near future" [3]. This domain emphasizes the perceptual and anticipatory cognitive skills that are critical for patient safety and highlights the ease with which salient events are unintentionally missed and the harmful results.

By now, most people are familiar with the selective attention test, where a video of two groups of individuals, one group wearing white shirts and one group wearing black shirts, are passing around a basketball. The viewer is asked to count the number of times the team with the black shirts passes around the ball while ignoring the other team. Once the scene ends, the participants are asked how many times the ball was passed and numbers are yelled out, yet when the same group is asked if they saw the gorilla in the room the majority of observers stay quiet. A second viewing of the video clearly demonstrates a gorilla coming to the center of the room, pounding on his chest, and walking off. This is an example of selective attention or what is referred to in the field of psychology as "inattentional blindness." This experiment was done by Simons and Chabris in 1999, taken from a 1979 study by Neisser and colleagues, which used a woman with an umbrella [44]. You can see how missing salient events or facts in a high-stake stressful environment such as the operating room can increase opportunities for significant error and patient harm. Studies of inattentional blindness have typically involved naive observers engaged in an unfamiliar task, so one might question the implications when experts are exposed to similar situations, asking: would their content knowledge protect them from falling into the same trap as the more novice onlooker?

Look at Fig. 5.2 below. What do you see?

A study by Trafton Drew and colleagues at the Visual Attention Lab at Harvard Medical School found that when 24 expert radiologists were asked to perform a familiar lung nodule detection task, similar to the one presented above, 83 percent of the radiologists did not see the gorilla in the image [45]. Taking a second look, you can see that a gorilla, 48 times the size of an average lung nodule, has been inserted in the right upper corner. Eye tracking revealed that the majority of those that missed the gorilla looked directly at this location. This study illustrates the fact that even professionals operating within their area of expertise are susceptible to the effects of inattentional blindness. It is easy to see how the demanding tasks of working in the operating room can blind one's attention to the surrounding situations and negatively impact the situational awareness that is required for effective performance.

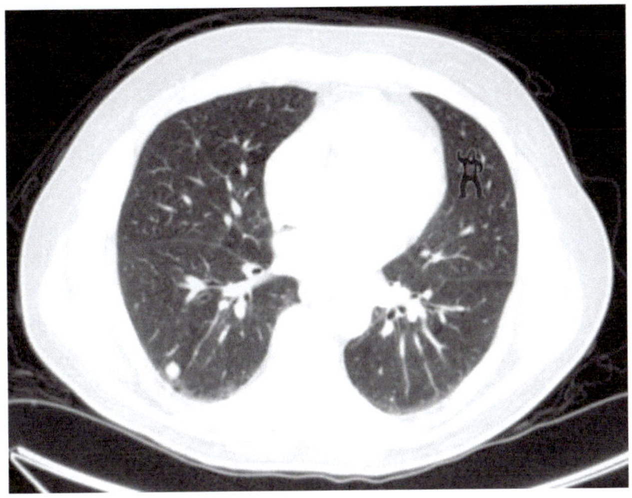

Fig. 5.2 Gorilla in the CT chest. (Reproduced with the permission of Drew T, Võ ML, Wolfe JM. The invisible gorilla strikes again sustained inattentional blindness in expert observers. Reproduced with the permission of Psychological science. 2013 Sep 1;24(9):1848–53 [45])

One way to improve situational awareness, as described by Rhona Flin and Lucy Mitchell in their book *Safer Surgery*, is to find clues within the operating room that can allow you to better anticipate difficult situations. The environmental clues they provide include (1) listening to conversation exchanges between other team members; (2) listening to and understanding changes in patient status; (3) observing changes in other team members' tones of voice, body language, or demeanors; and (4) observing overall changes in the environment [3]. Improvement in situational awareness requires experience and practice. In the invisible gorilla study mentioned above, experts performed better than naïve observers; this was also seen in the basketball experiment, likely because the demand of paying attention to the primary task is less with increased experience, allowing for increased awareness of surrounding activities. The authors point out that expertise in a certain task does not make one immune to the "inherent limitations of human attention and perception." This again highlights the key role that simulation training can play in preparing participants to anticipate and react to unexpected events, thus providing the space to gain experience and awareness, before actual patient interactions take place. One other interesting example highlighting "change blindness" can be found online by conducting a basic Internet search for the phrase "Wiseman Colour Changing Card Trick." In this video, psychologist and magician Richard Wiseman demonstrates a color changing card trick with insight worth watching on video (if one hasn't already) [46]. There are many more examples in the literature of the effects of situational awareness in task performance, and we encourage the reader to not only use the examples listed above but seek out other studies on this topic, which can then be incorporated into simulation training.

Leadership

Leadership within the operating room environment is slightly different from other concepts of leadership with which the reader may be familiar. In this context, leadership is defined as "the provision of direction, assertiveness, and support among members of the team" [47, 48] In this context, the definition of leadership is much more based on the effective role that a leader can play within the surgical team, such that leadership style and team dynamics play a crucial role in the overall success of the leader.

Hu and colleagues studied the impact of leadership style on team behavior in the OR through the scoring of video observations of five surgeons performing complex operations. They correlated the Multifactor Leadership Questionnaire with the Surgical Leadership Inventory to assess leadership behaviors and found that team-oriented (transformational) versus task-focused (transactional) leadership styles were associated with improved team behavior [49]. The study results pointed out that the surgeon with the highest transformational score displayed characteristics consistent with transformational leadership early and throughout the process, engaging all members of the team in a shared mission. They also noted that critical characteristics to improve patient safety, including voicing "constructive change-oriented communication intended to improve a situation," cooperation, and information sharing occurred more often through leaders scoring higher on transformational leadership. Looking closely at these characteristics, we can see that they are the mainframe principles of CRM that we have described. One way that they can be combined with transformational leadership is by connecting communication and assertiveness, teamwork, and information sharing to ultimately result in the most appropriate decision-making strategy.

Considering team preferences for leadership style is also important in implementing the most effective leadership strategy. Kissane-Lee and colleagues compared the experiences and preferences of junior residents in the operating room with surgeon leadership styles and found that trainees preferred explanatory or consultative leadership styles, akin to information sharing and cooperation listed above, but actually encountered authoritative styles in their OR experiences [50]. They pointed out that this disconnect between preference and reality could lead to tension and erosion of team performance and highlighted the importance that awareness of this discrepancy could have on future leadership training.

Effective leadership, in this way, can be seen as a pivotal component to the integration of CRM principles. As was stated in the introductory paragraph, the principles in CRM are interrelated in such a way that when one is addressed and improved, others are also enhanced. By addressing and improving leadership skills, teams can achieve functional and cohesive team dynamics that result in improved patient safety and decreased complications.

Decision Making

Decision making, while an ubiquitous term in CRM literature, is challenging to define and prone to differing views [17, 51, 52]. In addition, there is interplay in healthcare between what some would call "non-technical" decision making (e.g., leadership decisions, teamwork decisions) and "technical decisions" (e.g., which lab tests to send for a complex patient having a medical emergency, whether to perform a complex surgical technique in the setting of unexpected challenging anatomy). Some may even disagree on whether behavioral skills should be labeled as "non-technical." Nevertheless, there is something to be lost by perseverating on these nuances and/or viewing these interrelated aspects in a vacuum. In a study by Phitayakorn et al., the authors sought to determine the relationship between teamwork and communication in the operating room and adherence to patient guidelines in a simulation setting. The study concluded that "separating non-technical and technical skills when teaching OR teamwork is artificial and may even be damaging, because an approach could produce teams with excellent communication skills as they unsuccessfully manage the patient" [53]. For this reason, we adapt from a definition by Flin et al. [3] and define decision making broadly as "a cognitive skill involving multiple interrelated steps." They describe these steps to include the following: (1) recognition that choices between different courses of action are available, (2) perception of different courses of action, (3) evaluation of each course of action in relation to its potential risks and benefits, (4) actual choice, (5) monitoring of the patient's progress in relation to the decision taken (with review and change of plan if appropriate).

In terms of putting this concept of decision-making into the context of anesthesiology and crew/crisis resource management, we mention the example of operating room crisis checklists and emergency manuals, which are cognitive aids that can improve adherence to lifesaving processes of care and overall team performance. The story of these tools is extensive, and we refer the reader to a recent dedicated review article on the topic to learn their history [35]. There is also a dedicated book by leaders in the fields of CRM and anesthesiology, which is the same book for which the definition we used for CRM was referenced [2]. In a multi-center randomized, controlled trial involving both academic and community hospitals, operating room teams were 75% less likely to fail to adhere to critical processes of care when crisis checklists were available during intraoperative emergency scenarios (e.g., cardiac arrest, massive hemorrhage) in a simulated operating room (adjusted relative risk, 0.28; 95% confidence interval, 0.18–0.42; $P < 0.001$). Every team performed better with the crisis checklists available, and 97% of all participants reported that they would want the crisis checklists used if they were a patient undergoing an operation and had the intraoperative emergency being simulated [54]. There have been at least two published case reports involving the use of such cognitive aids to save lives in real operating rooms [55, 56], and there is a growing movement toward determining the best ways to improve clinical implementation [57]. Links to copies of cognitive aids for intraoperative emergencies (including ones that are free to download/customize) can be found at www.projectcheck.org/crisis and www.emergencymanuals.org. These sites also provide materials to aid in effective implementation, which has been shown to be an essential part in improving clinical outcomes from checklist interventions [58].

In the spirit of the saying "an ounce of prevention is worth a pound of cure," we also note that the World Health Organization (WHO) Surgical Safety Checklist is an intraoperative tool that leverages many of the CRM principles discussed above (such as teamwork and communication) toward improving patient outcomes during routine care. It has been shown to reduce morbidity and mortality in a global population [59], with subsequent studies using surgical safety checklists showing improved patient outcomes [60, 61]. One notable study raised the question of surgical safety checklist effectiveness [62], but the responses to this article [63–65] and the article's own editorial [66] noted that the actual use of the checklists in the sites studied was likely lacking and/or reflective of poor implementation.

Lastly, even though this chapter is focused on the intraoperative environment, we would be remiss if we did not mention that there was one notable checklist study that embraced CRM principles toward the reduction of catheter-related bloodstream infections in the ICU [67]. Of note, an anesthesiologist served as the lead author of this study, and readers may take interest, particularly given the role of intensive care for the anesthesiology provider. Given the role of the surgical safety checklist as a valuable tool for enhanced decision making, we provide a link to the WHO Surgical Safety Checklist: http://www.who.int/patientsafety/safesurgery/checklist/en/.

Teamwork

We base our definition of teamwork from the definition of "team" developed by Dr. Eduardo Salas, an organizational psychologist and international expert on simulation and teamwork training. Teamwork is the activity of "a distinguishable set of two or more people who interact, dynamically, interdependently, and adaptively toward a common and valued goal/objective/mission" [68–70]. Salas points out that the members of a team have each been assigned specific roles or functions to perform. A definition of teamwork in the medical literature has added that it is a process that fosters "collaboration, open communication and shared decision-making, and generates value-added patient, organizational and staff outcomes" [71]. The promotion of more effective team functioning, or "teamwork," in healthcare organizations was one of the five principles highlighted by the Institute of Medicine's *To Err Is Human* [72].

In 2009, Mazzoco et al. assessed surgical team behaviors and patient outcomes and found that when certain behaviors were less frequent, patients were more likely to experience major complications or even death. As noted in the literature [5], this is just one of many studies that have associated breakdowns in teamwork and/or communication to operative delays [37], preventable mishaps [9, 73], technical errors [74], clinician testing and stress [75], poorer overall clinical performance [76, 77], and patient morbidity and mortality [78]. Given the fundamental importance of teamwork, it comes as no surprise that teamwork has been linked to patient outcomes and as such plays a critical role within the field of crew/crisis resource management. In the following section, we will discuss the essentials of interprofessional team training and how these principles can be integrated into successful simulation training within diverse teams of medical professionals.

Debriefing and Feedback

We purposefully defer this section to Chap. 4 on *Essentials of Debriefing in Simulation-Based Education*. We merely create this section heading to emphasize that it is too important of a topic to overlook when reviewing the principles of CRM. We strongly encourage the reader to explore the debriefing/feedback chapter, a topic that readily appears in articles in major medical journals, [5, 79] to gather skills and implementation strategies on utilizing debriefing and feedback to simulation sessions and programming within and outside the operating room.

Essentials of Interprofessional Team Training Using Medical Simulation

Based on the knowledge of the above principles, one can use healthcare simulation as a vehicle for multidisciplinary and even interprofessional training of healthcare providers (for example: surgeons, nurses, anesthesiologists, and other operating room staff for intraoperative simulation). Interprofessional training of surgical teams, where participants learn with, from, and about each other, has become increasingly popular, and studies of these efforts have shown evidence toward meaningful feasibility and reductions in surgical mortality [5, 60]. While the above principles of crew/crisis resource management can be used to drive the CRM content of these sessions, we wanted to touch on four essential considerations for interprofessional team training, adapted from the summary curriculum design of a multicenter simulation program for operating room teams (Table 5.4): (1) educational objectives, (2) participant teams, (3) scenarios and course format/length, and (4) scientific measurement (Table 5.4).

Educational Objectives

An important first step in designing interdisciplinary training is the selection of clear and attainable objectives. The body of this chapter contains several principles of CRM to be considered. It is essential that these objectives represent the needs of the different disciplines, and possibly different institutions, involved. One should consider as much relevant multidisciplinary expertise as is available to weigh in on these decisions. Previous work on operating room team training and/or the development of tools for such sessions has included surgeons, anesthesiologists, nurses, operating room directors, biomedical engineers, hospital administrators, risk management, and specialists in simulation, patient safety, education, and cognitive psychology [5, 80]. The developers of the particular curriculum in Table 5.4 chose to focus on three CRM objectives (surgical safety checklists, closed-loop communication, and assertiveness). It is important that those developing their curriculum decide on core objectives that address areas of improvement while also understanding that many of the principles are interrelated (e.g., it is hard to be good at leadership if one is a bad communicator) and allowing other CRM principles to have a presence as the actual sessions are produced and administered.

Table 5.4 Curriculum Design

Objectives
To prepare colleagues from surgery, anesthesia, and nursing to Practice and use operating room surgical safety checklists, including the World Health Organization Surgical Safety Checklist. Consistently close the loop in communication of important information in routine and emergency situations. Speak up readily and effectively with information or concerns.
Participant teams
Active clinical operating room staff, with each team containing at least 1 attending surgeon, one attending anesthesiologist and 1 operating room nurse.
Scenario
Uncontrolled hemorrhage Cardiac arrest of a surgical patient outside of the operating room. Additional case customized to the desires/expertise of the institution (eg, operating room fire, air embolism, etc).
Course format and length
The course must be primarily experiential and of sufficient realism to engage the full operating room team in the learning objectives. The course should include a hands-on practicum and debriefing with minimal didactic (no more than 20% of total time can be didactic). There must be a uniform posttraining course evaluation to be distributed to all participants across all centers. The course be 4–6 h in length.

Source: Arriaga et al. [5]. Used with permission

Participant Teams

With regard to participant teams, we highlight a notion mentioned in the article from which Table 5.4 is based: "Simple retrofitting of a program designed for one clinical domain to an entire operating room team, or design of a program without proper mechanisms to address lost operative time, can lead to significant obstacles to meaningful implementation" [5]. The same multidisciplinary team mentioned above for the creation of curriculum objectives can be integral in this regard. A multidisciplinary panel likely understands the needs of relevant parties and can facilitate ideas on how to incentivize different disciplines to participate relative to resources available. A high-fidelity simulation center containing in-house simulation experts and a repertoire of multidisciplinary and high-technology equipment may be attractive to certain audiences. In-situ *simulation* may also provide advantages, particularly if the simulation center is far away from the primary clinical site and/or represents a hardship for one or more of the disciplines. There can be value in assembling simulation participant teams that commonly work together in real life, but this may not always be feasible. One can also acknowledge that in the reality of many operating rooms, there are often situations where teams that do not commonly work together are assembled.

Scenarios and Course Format/Length

Similar to the above section on debriefing, we purposely defer most of this section to Chap. 3 on *Essentials of*

Scenario Building and Chaps. 10, 11, and 12 on other choices of simulation modalities (e.g., standardized patients, mannequins, virtual simulation, etc.). Nevertheless, regarding multidisciplinary teams, we would like to point out that different audiences may respond to different simulation modalities to foster realism and engagement. These modalities can often be combined for the multidisciplinary participant audience. As noted in the literature, consideration can be given to previously validated surgical props and models [81–83], simulation training sessions that have been successfully used for anesthesiologists [12], and realistic tasks for nursing and other operating room staff [5]. We again emphasize the importance of integrating debriefing into the course format in order to enhance educational value and improve patient care [84–88]. To quote Dr. Jeffrey Cooper, an internationally renowned expert on medical simulation: "It's often said (partly in jest) that simulation is an excuse to do a debriefing" [89]. As the multifaceted needs of an interprofessional team training program are extensive, we point out that there are institutes, such as the Institute for Medical Simulation (http://harvardmedsim.org) [90], that offer simulation instructor "train the trainer" courses for interested parties.

Scientific Measurement

Consider integrating a research component into any simulation programming initiative. Multidisciplinary team training can take substantial effort and is likely to contain findings that would add to generalizable knowledge. Options range from surveys aimed at broad implications [5] and the linkage of medical team training to patient outcomes [60]. There are numerous observation tools of CRM principles that have been validated through studies of observing simulated and/or real intraoperative environments [3], and there are a growing number of studies aimed at evaluating the operating room environment through video observation [91–94]. As an example, the *Observational Teamwork Assessment for Surgery (OTAS)* rates domains such as leadership, communication, and teamwork [95–97]. There are also instruments to measure debriefing [98]. Further, the relationship between cognitive aids designed for crises and their relationship to performance on critical processes of care have also been studied [54]. If one decides to include research within their team training effort, early attention must be given to important steps, including appropriate approval/exemption from an Institutional Review Board and epidemiological/biostatistical concerns, which must be addressed as part of an appropriate study design.

Conclusion

It is our goal that the above sections paint a picture of many of the essential components of CRM and interdisciplinary team training that can be applied to medical simulation sessions. Through a firm understanding of the principles of CRM and their applications both historically and currently, the reader will be able to integrate CRM principles to address issues of patient safety and improved team dynamics. This can lead to the creation of simulation scenarios that train clinicians to avoid pitfalls that have been found to result in human error and adverse patient outcomes. Ultimately, the reader is encouraged to integrate the objectives learned in this chapter to those of other chapters within this book to develop a cohesive simulation setting and program that is adaptable to the needs of their specific teams. The field of anesthesiology has a rich history in the implementation and integration of CRM principles into the healthcare setting. We hope to foster a continued passion and pursuit of practitioners to embrace a cultural atmosphere that continues to advance knowledge and improve patient care.

References

1. Kanki B, Helmreich R, Anca J. Crew resource management. 2nd ed. Amsterdam: Academic Press/Elsevier; 2010.
2. Gaba DM, Fish KJ, Howard SK, Burden A. Crisis management in anesthesiology. Philadelphia: Elsevier Health Sciences; 2014.
3. Mitchell ML, Flin R, editors. Safer surgery: analysing behaviour in the operating theatre. Farnham: Ashgate Publishing, Ltd.; 2012.
4. Salas E, Cannon-Bowers JA. Methods, tools, and strategies for team training. Washington D.C.: American Psychological Association; 1997.
5. Arriaga AF, Gawande AA, Raemer DB, Jones DB, Smink DS, Weinstock P, et al. Pilot testing of a model for insurer-driven, large-scale multicenter simulation training for operating room teams. Ann Surg. 2014;259(3):403–10.
6. Kapur N, Parand A, Soukup T, Reader T, Sevdalis N. Aviation and healthcare: a comparative review with implications for patient safety. JRSM Open. 2016;7(1):2054270415616548.
7. Heinemann GD, Zeiss AM, editors. Team performance in health care: assessment and development. New York: Springer Science & Business Media; 2002.
8. Salas E, Bowers CA, Edens E, editors. Improving teamwork in organizations: applications of resource management training. Boca Raton: CRC Press; 2001.
9. Cooper JB, Newbower RS, Long CD, McPeek B. Preventable anesthesia mishaps: a study of human factors. Anesthesiology. 1978;49:399–406.
10. Gaba DM, Maxwell MS, DeAnda A. Anesthetic mishaps: breaking the chain of accident evolution. Anesthesiology. 1987;66:670–6.
11. Howard SK, Gaba DM, Fish KJ, Yang G, Sarnquist FH. Anesthesia crisis resource management training: teaching anesthesiologists to handle critical incidents. Aviat Space Environ Med. 1992;63:763–70.
12. Holzman RS, Cooper JB, Gaba DM, Philip JH, Small SD, Feinstein D. Anesthesia crisis resource management: real-life simulation training in operating room crises. J Clin Anesth. 1995;7(8):675–87.

13. National Transportation Safety Board (NTSB). Pan American World Airways Flight 736, NTSB number DCA77RA014. 1977. Retrieved 28 Sept 2016, from: http://www.ntsb.gov/_layouts/ntsb.aviation/brief.aspx?ev_id=55835&key=0&queryId=a39.
14. National Transportation Safety Board (NTSB). Special Investigation Report. Runway Incursions At Controlled Airports In The United States, NTSB number SIR-86/01. 1986. Retrieved 28 Sept 2016, from: http://www.ntsb.gov/safety/safety-studies/Documents/SIR8601.pdf.
15. National Transportation Safety Board (NTSB). United Airlines flight 173 accident report, NTSB number AAR-79-07. 1978. Retrieved 28 Sept 2016, from: http://www.ntsb.gov/investigations/AccidentReports/Reports/AAR7907.pdf.
16. Cooper GE, editor. Resource management on the flight deck. National Aeronautics and Space Administration. Moffett Field: Ames Research Center; 1980.
17. Helmreich RL, Merritt AC, Wilhelm JA. The evolution of crew resource management training in commercial aviation. Int J Aviat Psychol. 1999;9(1):19–32.
18. Federal Aviation Administration. Crew resource management training. (Advisory circular no. 120-51E). Washington, D.C.: Author; 2004.
19. National Transportation Safety Board. Aircraft Accident Report: Eastern Air Lines, Inc.; L-1011, N310EA; Miami, Florida; December 29, 1972. Washington, D.C.: National Transportation Safety Board; 1973.
20. Graafland M, Schraagen J, Boermeester M, Bemelman W, Schijven M. Training situational awareness to reduce surgical errors in the operating room. Br J Surg. 2014;102(1):16–23.
21. Ministerio de Transportes Y Comunicaciones. Colision Aeronaves Boeing 747 PH-BUF de K.L.M Y Boeing 747 N 736 PA de Panam en Los Rodeos (Tenerife) el 27 de Marzo de 1.977. Madrid; 1978.
22. Air Line Pilots Association. Human Factors Report on the Tenerife Accident [Internet]. Washington, D.C.; 1979. Available from: http://www.project-tenerife.com/engels/PDF/alpa.pdf.
23. Minehart R, Pian-Smith M, Walzer T, Gardner R, Rudolph J, Simon R, et al. Speaking across the drapes. Simul Healthc. 2012;7(3):166–70.
24. National Transportation Safety Board. Aircraft Accident Report – United Airlines, Inc., McDonnell-Douglas DC-8-61, N8082 U, Portland, Oregon, December 28, 1978. Washington, D.C.: National Transportation Safety Board; 1978.
25. Raemer D, Kolbe M, Minehart R, Rudolph J, Pian-Smith M. Improving anesthesiologists' ability to speak up in the operating room. Acad Med. 2016;91(4):530–9.
26. National Transportation Safety Board. Aircraft Accident Report: Controlled Flight Into Terrain; Korean Air Flight 801; Boeing 747–300, HL7468; Nimitz Hill, Guam; August 6, 1997. Washington, D.C.: National Transportation Safety Board; 2000.
27. Just K, Hubrich S, Schmidtke D, Scheifes A, Gerbershagen M, Wappler F, et al. The effectiveness of an intensive care quick reference checklist manual—a randomized simulation-based trial. J Crit Care. 2015;30(2):255–60.
28. National Transportation Safety Board. Aircraft Accident Report: Loss of Thrust in Both Engines After Encountering a Flock of Birds and Subsequent Ditching on the Hudson River; US Airways Flight 1549; Airbus A320–214, N106US; Weehawken, New Jersey; January 15, 2009. Washington, D.C.: National Transportation Safety Board; 2010.
29. Fernandez Castelao E, Boos M, Ringer C, Eich C, Russo S. Effect of CRM team leader training on team performance and leadership behavior in simulated cardiac arrest scenarios: a prospective, randomized, controlled study. BMC Med Educ. 2015;15:116.
30. Bureau d'Enque^tes et d'Analyses pour la Se'curite' de l'Aviation Civile. Final report on the accident on first June 2009 to the Airbus A330–203 registered F-GZCP operated by Air France, flight AF 447 Rio de Janerio–Paris. https://www.bea.aero/docspa/2009/f-cp090601.en/pdf/f-cp090601.en.pdf. Accessed 20 Sept 2016.
31. Andrew B, Plachta S, Salud L, Pugh C. Development and evaluation of a decision-based simulation for assessment of team skills. Surgery. 2012;152(2):152–7.
32. About the National Transportation Safety Board. Available at: http://www.ntsb.gov/about/. Accessed 28 Sept 2016.
33. Bureau d'Enque^tes et d'Analyses pour la Se'curite' de l'Aviation Civile. Final report on the accident on June 1, 2009, to the Airbus A330–203 registered F-GZCP operated by Air France, Flight AF 447 Rio de Janerio–Paris; Appendix 1. https://www.bea.aero/docspa/2009/f-cp090601.en/pdf/f-cp090601.en.pdf. Accessed 20 Sept 2016.
34. National Transportation Safety Board (NTSB). Amtrak NTSB preliminary report: railroad DCA15MR010. Retrieved 28 Sept 2016, from: http://www.ntsb.gov/investigations/AccidentReports/Reports/DCA15MR010_preliminary.pdf
35. Hepner DL, Arriaga AF, Cooper JB, Goldhaber-Fiebert SN, Gaba DM, Berry WR, et al. Clinical concepts and commentary: operating room crisis checklists and emergency manuals. Anesthesiology. 2017;127:384–92.
36. Flin RH, O'Connor P, Crichton M. Safety at the sharp end: a guide to non-technical skills. Aldershot: Ashgate Publishing, Ltd.; 2008.
37. Lingard L, Espin S, Whyte S, Regehr G, Baker GR, Reznick R, et al. Communication failures in the operating room: an observational classification of recurrent types and effects. Qual Saf Health Care. 2004;13(5):330–4.
38. Vincent C. Patient safety. 2nd ed: Wiley-Blackwell; 2010.
39. Bowers CA, Jentsch F, Salas E, Braun CC. Analyzing communication sequences for team training needs assessment. Hum Factors. 1998;40(4):672–9.
40. Pian-Smith MC, Simon R, Minehart RD, Podraza M, Rudolph J, Walzer T, et al. Teaching residents the two-challenge rule: a simulation-based approach to improve education and patient safety. Simul Healthc. 2008;4(2):84–91.
41. Raemer DB, Kolbe M, Minehart RD, Rudolph JW, Pian-Smith MC. Improving anesthesiologists' ability to speak up in the operating room: a randomized controlled experiment of a simulation-based intervention and a qualitative analysis of hurdles and enablers. Acad Med. 2016;91(4):530–9.
42. Sexton JB, Thomas EJ, Helmreich RL. Error, stress, and teamwork in medicine and aviation: cross sectional surveys. BMJ. 2000;320(7237):745–9.
43. Labor and Delivery: CUS. TeamSTEPPS training video. Available at: http://www.ahrq.gov/teamstepps. Accessed 28 Sept 2016.
44. Simons DJ, Chabris CF. Gorillas in our midst: sustained inattentional blindness for dynamic events. Perception. 1999;28(9):1059–74.
45. Drew T, Võ ML, Wolfe JM. The invisible gorilla strikes again sustained inattentional blindness in expert observers. Psychol Sci. 2013;24(9):1848–53.
46. Martinez-Conde S, Macknik SL. Magic and the brain. Sci Am. 2008;299(6):72–9.
47. OTAS User Training Manual. Available at: https://www.imperial.ac.uk/medicine/. Accessed 28 Sept 2016.
48. Healey AN, Undre S, Vincent CA. Developing observational measures of performance in surgical teams. Qual Saf Health Care. 2004;13(Suppl 1):i33–40.
49. Hu YY, Parker SH, Lipsitz SR, Arriaga AF, Peyre SE, Corso KA, et al. Surgeons' leadership styles and team behavior in the operating room. J Am Coll Surg. 2016;222(1):41–51.
50. Kissane-Lee NA, Yule S, Pozner CN, Smink DS. Attending surgeons' leadership style in the operating room: comparing junior residents' experiences and preferences. J Surg Educ. 2016;73(1):40–4.
51. Pizzi L, Goldfarb NI, Nash DB. Crew resource management and its applications in medicine. In: Making health care safer: a critical analysis of patient safety practices, vol. 44. Rockville: The Agency; 2001. p. 511–9.

52. Zsambok CE. Naturalistic decision making research and improving team decision making. In: Naturalistic decision making. New York: Routledge; 1997. p. 111–20.
53. Phitayakorn R, Minehart RD, Hemingway MW, Pian-Smith MC, Petrusa E. The relationship between intraoperative teamwork and management skills in patient care. Surgery. 2015;158(5):1434–40.
54. Arriaga AF, Bader AM, Wong JM, Lipsitz SR, Berry WR, Ziewacz JE, et al. Simulation-based trial of surgical-crisis checklists. N Engl J Med. 2013;368(3):246–53.
55. Ramirez M, Grantham C. Crisis checklists for the operating room, not with a simulator. J Am Coll Surg. 2012;215(2):302–3.
56. Ranganathan P, Phillips JH, Attaallah AF, Vallejo MC. The use of cognitive aid checklist leading to successful treatment of malignant hyperthermia in an infant undergoing cranioplasty. Anesth Analg. 2014;118(6):1387.
57. Goldhaber-Fiebert SN, Howard SK. Implementing emergency manuals: can cognitive aids help translate best practices for patient care during acute events? Anesth Analg. 2013;117(5):1149–61.
58. Van Klei WA, Hoff RG, Van Aarnhem EE, Simmermacher RK, Regli LP, Kappen TH, et al. Effects of the introduction of the WHO "surgical safety checklist" on in-hospital mortality: a cohort study. Ann Surg. 2012;255(1):44–9.
59. Haynes AB, Weiser TG, Berry WR, Lipsitz SR, Breizat AH, Dellinger EP, et al. A surgical safety checklist to reduce morbidity and mortality in a global population. N Engl J Med. 2009;360(5):491–9.
60. Neily J, Mills PD, Young-Xu Y, Carney BT, West P, Berger DH, et al. Association between implementation of a medical team training program and surgical mortality. JAMA. 2010;304(15):1693–700.
61. de Vries EN, Prins HA, Crolla RM, den Outer AJ, van Andel G, van Helden SH, et al. Effect of a comprehensive surgical safety system on patient outcomes. N Engl J Med. 2010;363(20):1928–37.
62. Urbach DR, Govindarajan A, Saskin R, Wilton AS, Baxter NN. Introduction of surgical safety checklists in Ontario, Canada. N Engl J Med. 2014;370(11):1029–38.
63. Robblee JA. Surgical safety checklists in Ontario, Canada. N Engl J Med. 2014;370(24):2349.
64. Weiser TG, Krummel TM. Surgical safety checklists in Ontario, Canada. N Engl J Med. 2014;370(24):2349.
65. Haynes AB, Berry WR, Gawande AA. Surgical safety checklists in Ontario, Canada. N Engl J Med. 2014;370(24):2350.
66. Leape LL. The checklist conundrum. N Engl J Med. 2014;370(11):1063–4.
67. Pronovost P, Needham D, Berenholtz S, Sinopoli D, Chu H, Cosgrove S, et al. An intervention to decrease catheter-related bloodstream infections in the ICU. N Engl J Med. 2006;355(26):2725–32.
68. Salas E, Dickinson TL, Converse SA, Tannenbaum SI. Toward an understanding of team performance and training. Norwood: Ablex Publishing; 1992.
69. Swezey RW, Salas EE. Teams: their training and performance. Norwood: Ablex Publishing; 1992.
70. Stout RJ, Salas E, Fowlkes JE. Enhancing teamwork in complex environments through team training. Group Dyn Theory Res Pract. 1997;1(2):169.
71. Xyrichis A, Ream E. Teamwork: a concept analysis. J Adv Nurs. 2008;61(2):232–41.
72. Kohn LT, Corrigan JM, Donaldson MS, editors. To err is human: building a safer health system. Washington, D.C.: National Academies Press; 2000.
73. Webb RK, Currie M, Morgan CA, Williamson JA, Mackay P, Russell WJ, et al. The Australian Incident Monitoring Study: an analysis of 2000 incident reports. Anaesth Intensive Care. 1993;21:520–8.
74. Wiegmann DA, ElBardissi AW, Dearani JA, Daly RC, Sundt TM. Disruptions in surgical flow and their relationship to surgical errors: an exploratory investigation. Surgery. 2007;142(5):658–65.
75. Arora S, Hull L, Sevdalis N, Tierney T, Nestel D, Woloshynowych M, et al. Factors compromising safety in surgery: stressful events in the operating room. Am J Surg. 2010;199(1):60–5.
76. Manser T, Harrison TK, Gaba DM, Howard SK. Coordination patterns related to high clinical performance in a simulated anesthetic crisis. Anesth Analg. 2009;108(5):1606–15.
77. Carthey J, de Leval MR, Wright DJ, Farewell VT, Reason JT. Behavioural markers of surgical excellence. Saf Sci. 2003;41(5):409–25.
78. Mazzocco K, Petitti DB, Fong KT, Bonacum D, Brookey J, Graham S, et al. Surgical team behaviors and patient outcomes. Am J Surg. 2009;197(5):678–85.
79. Minehart RD, Rudolph J, Pian-Smith MC, Raemer DB. Improving faculty feedback to resident trainees during a simulated case: a randomized, controlled trial of an educational intervention. Anesthesiology. 2014;120(1):160–71.
80. Ziewacz JE, Arriaga AF, Bader AM, Berry WR, Edmondson L, Wong JM, et al. Crisis checklists for the operating room: development and pilot testing. J Am Coll Surg. 2011;213(2):212–7.
81. Powers KA, Rehrig ST, Irias N, Albano HA, Malinow A, Jones SB, et al. Simulated laparoscopic operating room crisis: an approach to enhance the surgical team performance. Surg Endosc. 2008;22(4):885–900.
82. Berry W, Raemer D. The tumor: a simulator for open surgery. Simul Healthc. 2006;1(2):115.
83. Rehrig ST, Powers K, Jones DB. Integrating simulation in surgery as a teaching tool and credentialing standard. J Gastrointest Surg. 2008;12(2):222–33.
84. Rudolph JW, Simon R, Raemer DB, Eppich WJ. Debriefing as formative assessment: closing performance gaps in medical education. Acad Emerg Med. 2008;15(11):1010–6.
85. Rudolph JW, Simon R, Dufresne RL, Raemer DB. There's no such thing as "nonjudgmental" debriefing: a theory and method for debriefing with good judgment. Simul Healthc. 2006;1(1):49–55.
86. Dismukes RK, Gaba DM, Howard SK. So many roads: facilitated debriefing in healthcare. Simul Healthc. 2006;1(1):23–5.
87. Raemer D, Anderson M, Cheng A, Fanning R, Nadkarni V, Savoldelli G. Research regarding debriefing as part of the learning process. Simul Healthc. 2011;6(7):S52–7.
88. Rudolph JW, Simon R, Rivard P, Dufresne RL, Raemer DB. Debriefing with good judgment: combining rigorous feedback with genuine inquiry. Anesthesiol Clin. 2007;25(2):361–76.
89. JB Cooper. Josiah Macy Jr. website: http://macyfoundation.org/news/entry/simulation-is-for-faculty-development-experience-from-the-center-for-medica. Accessed 28 Sept 16.
90. Center of Medical Simulation. Comprehensive instructor workshop in medical simulation. http://www.harvardmedsim.org/center-for-medical-simulation-ims.php. Accessed 28 Sept 16.
91. Hu YY, Arriaga AF, Roth EM, Peyre SE, Corso KA, Swanson RS, et al. Protecting patients from an unsafe system: the Etiology & Recovery of intra-operative deviations in care. Ann Surg. 2012;256(2):203.
92. Hu YY, Peyre SE, Arriaga AF, Osteen RT, Corso KA, Weiser TG, et al. Postgame analysis: using video-based coaching for continuous professional development. J Am Coll Surg. 2012;214(1):115–24.
93. Hu YY, Peyre SE, Arriaga AF, Roth EM, Corso KA, Greenberg CC. War stories: a qualitative analysis of narrative teaching strategies in the operating room. Am J Surg. 2012;203(1):63–8.
94. Hu YY, Arriaga AF, Peyre SE, Corso KA, Roth EM, Greenberg CC. Deconstructing intraoperative communication failures. J Surg Res. 2012;177(1):37–42.
95. Sevdalis N, Lyons M, Healey AN, Undre S, Darzi A, Vincent CA. Observational teamwork assessment for surgery: construct validation with expert versus novice raters. Ann Surg. 2009;249(6):1047–51.

96. Russ S, Hull L, Rout S, Vincent C, Darzi A, Sevdalis N. Observational teamwork assessment for surgery: feasibility of clinical and nonclinical assessor calibration with short-term training. Ann Surg. 2012;255(4):804–9.
97. Hull L, Arora S, Kassab E, Kneebone R, Sevdalis N. Observational teamwork assessment for surgery: content validation and tool refinement. J Am Coll Surg. 2011;212(2):234–43.
98. Brett-Fleegler M, Rudolph J, Eppich W, Monuteaux M, Fleegler E, Cheng A, et al. Debriefing assessment for simulation in healthcare: development and psychometric properties. Simul Healthc. 2012;7(5):288–94.

Competency Assessment

6

Anjan Shah, Samuel DeMaria, and Andrew Goldberg

Introduction

Competency assessment is a comprehensive and often controversial topic given the challenges inherent to the fair assessment of a practitioner's knowledge, skills, and attributes. Currently, simulation has been identified as a critical educational tool but is increasingly being used for high-stake competency assessments. High-fidelity simulation offers flexibility, realism, and inherent patient safety that makes it ideal for the assessment of undergraduate, graduate, and postgraduate anesthesiology providers, whether in the setting of residency training (or anesthesiology assistant or nurse anesthetist training), Maintenance of Certification in Anesthesiology (MOCA) courses, and even the retraining of physicians (or certified registered nurse anesthetists) seeking reentry to clinical practice [1]. Over the years, significant research and experience have been accumulated on assessment procedures in general, as well as the specifics of simulation-based assessment [2–4]. The goal of this chapter is not only to lay out the importance of assessment to the field of anesthesiology and a framework for how to approach simulation-based assessment but also to understand the complexities that must be overcome when dealing with practitioner assessment.

Competency Assessment

Competency assessment of any practitioner is multifactorial and poses significant challenges with regard to controlling the assessment between individuals. Since there are a wide variety of tools that can be used for assessment purposes (each one with different strengths and weaknesses), reproducibility becomes a central concern. As such, two critically important concepts must be considered when attempting to utilize an assessment tool, namely reliability and validity.

Reliability

In general, reliability refers to the consistency of a measure when utilized under similar conditions. *Test-retest reliability* refers to the degree to which test scores are consistent from one administration event to the next, in which there is a single rater using the same methods and instruments under the same testing conditions. When relating it to assessment in academic performance, it refers to the ability of a method of assessment in consistently producing the scores, when administered multiple times under comparable conditions. This is a critical point to consider if an assessment tool is going to become universal.

Consider an analogy of two people, A and B, throwing darts at a dartboard where different sections have different point values assigned to them. Person A consistently hits the center mark, while Person B consistently hits the bottom right corner of the dart board. Both of these people, undergoing two individual assessments, would be classified as reliable. If these same subjects undergo the same exact assessment several times, but at different times, they each would receive the same exact score as their previous tries if the test had good test-retest reliability (Fig. 6.1).

Validity

Validity refers to the degree of accuracy of what is being assessed. The purpose of validation is to gather evidence that evaluates whether a decision is useful. An analogy to the validity argument is an investigator examining a crime

A. Shah · S. DeMaria (✉)
Department of Anesthesiology, Perioperative and Pain Medicine, Icahn School of Medicine at Mount Sinai, New York, NY, USA
e-mail: Samuel.demaria@mssm.edu

A. Goldberg
Department of Anesthesiology, James J Peters VA Medical Center, New York, NY, USA

B. Mahoney et al. (eds.), *Comprehensive Healthcare Simulation: Anesthesiology*, Comprehensive Healthcare Simulation,
https://doi.org/10.1007/978-3-030-26849-7_6

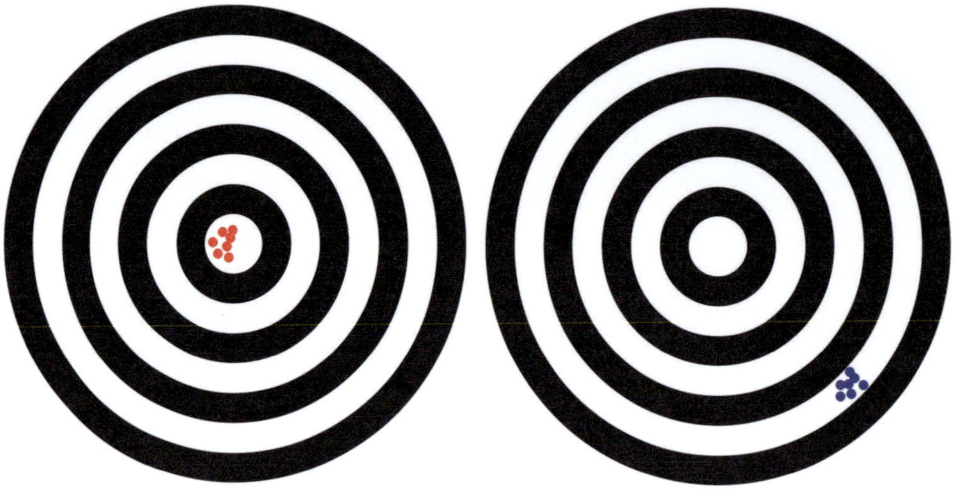

Fig. 6.1 Two individuals, Person A and Person B, throwing darts at separate targets. Both demonstrate high reliability as the results are consistent over seven tries. Accuracy depends on what exactly is being measured. Person A is more accurate than Person B if the center of the target was the goal

scene: the investigator is looking for a wide variety of evidence that may link the defendant to the crime, such as DNA evidence on hair or blood, fingerprints on the weapon used, footage from nearby cameras, eye-witness interviews, interviews with known acquaintances, etc. The prosecuting attorney must then organize all the data collected and make an argument to the jury that the defendant is guilty of the said crime by presenting all the evidence and interpretations of the evidence, in the hopes of persuading the jury into making the wanted decision [5, 6]. Unlike reliability, validity is not a characteristic of the data collected from an assessment but rather a characteristic from the interpretations made from the collected data as representations of the truth. Although the process of building a successful assessment tool is rigorous and involves much more than just optimizing and controlling for reliability and validity, weakness in these two domains will negatively impact the results of an assessment. The use of simulations (including simulators, virtual-reality devices, part-task trainers, and standardized patients) in healthcare education as an assessment tool provides high reliability from the ease of manipulation of physical parameters and delivery of consistent information, as well as providing strong validity evidence by controlling parameters in the weaker inferences in the validity argument (to be explained in greater detail below).

Kane's Validity Framework

According to Kane, when building an assessment tool, the process of validation cannot begin until both the purpose of an assessment and the use of its scores are specified. Once the purpose has been clearly stated, Kane lays out a two-step process to build a validity argument—stating the claims to be made in what he calls the interpretation/use argument (IUA) [7] and then evaluating each of the claims by moving through the four inferences: scoring, generalization, extrapolation, and implication:

1. *Scoring inference*—this relates to an observation about a performance. Evidence accumulated in regard to this inference evaluates whether a standardized protocol was used in establishing scores for the encounter. This includes a set scoring rubric applied correctly, as well as the exam being performed under appropriate and specified conditions.
2. *Generalization inference*—in practicality, there is a finite number of questions or stations that one can make observations on, but in theory, there is an infinite amount. Generalization inference relies on taking the scores from a select sample of items in the assessment(s) and applying them to the bottomless pool in the assessment universe. For qualitative assessments, this includes forming an accurate and descriptive narrative from singular pieces of qualitative data. As Cook et al. mentions, interrater variability for qualitative assessments may be a differing perspective and give alternative insights into a performance rather than an error for numeric scores as with quantitative measures [6, 8, 9]. Evidence gathered under this inference addresses the actual construction of the assessment and assumes that reliability issues of internal consistency were checked.
3. *Extrapolation inference*—the real goal of competence assessments is to be able to predict performance in the real-world clinical setting. Evidence here is used to confirm or refute the relationship between scores on the assessment and the outcomes that stakeholders are interested in.
4. *Decision inference*—evidence gathered here will lead to a final decision regarding the purpose of the assessment. The decision will depend on the stakeholders at play and the assumption that the implications of the said decision (both intended and unintended) were considered.

A Framework for Assessment: Outcomes and Levels of Assessment, Stages of Development, and Context

Once all of these inferences have been considered, the next step in creating a successful assessment is determining the framework in which it will be administered. There are a wide variety of assessment tools available, and they are now generally classified into broad categories (see Table 6.1). It is important to consider several aspects of the evaluation/assessment prior to choosing an appropriate assessment modality. The overall purpose of an assessment should be stated clearly as this provides the context in which the assessment will occur, as well as the stakes of the assessment. In addition, other components to consider in this framework include the specific outcomes to be assessed, the appropriate levels of assessment, and the developmental stage of those who are being assessed.

Outcomes of Assessment

As will be mentioned in greater detail later, in the United States, the Accreditation Council of Graduate Medical Education (ACGME) has listed six core competencies (patient care and procedural skills, medical knowledge, practice-based learning and improvement, interpersonal and communication skills, professionalism, and system-based practice) that a general physician must be competent in by the end of medical education [10]. Specific skills within each competency can be tailored to specific specialties and their needs and challenges. For example, referring to *The Anesthesiology Milestone Project*, one can see specific outcomes expected of anesthesiology residents in each of the six core competency domains, and each one is graded from level 1 to level 5: preanesthetic evaluation, crisis management, management of a critically ill patient in a nonoperative setting, coordination of patient care, team and leadership skills, etc. [11]. The ACGME has also created a list of assessment methods matched to each outcome being assessed within a core competency as a guide to those performing assessments [12]. Consequently, one path to choosing an assessment method would be to clearly identify an outcome to be measured and to match it with an appropriate modality.

Levels of Assessment

There are four levels of assessment in the model first described by George Miller: The first level, *knows*, represents the knowledge base of medical facts and physiology; level 2, *knows how*, is the application of the knowledge in order to make decisions regarding a management plan; the third level, *shows how*, tries to look at how exactly the student would tackle a problem when faced with a patient; the final and fourth level, *does*, is meant to evaluate the learner in an actual clinical practice [13]. The four levels of assessment are also commonly known (and illustrated) as "Miller's Pyramid" (see Fig. 6.2). Once again, specific methods of assessment evaluate the different levels of assessment with varying degrees of efficiency. Therefore, aligning an assessment method to a level on Miller's Pyramid is another way of choosing between different assessment modalities (see Table 6.2).

Stages of Development

The process of learning and education in general is a continuum, a gradual progress that shows improvement within different competencies. Just like the different stages in training for a physician (medical school, internship, residency,

Table 6.1 Categories of assessment methods and specific examples

Assessment methods	Examples
Performance based	Simulation-based assessments
	Objective Structured Clinical Examinations (OSCEs)
	Long and short cases
Written and oral	Multiple-choice questions
	Oral exams
	True/false items
	Matching items
	Long and short essay questions
Clinical observation	360° evaluations/feedback
	Direct observation of procedural skills
	Mini-clinical evaluation exercise
Miscellaneous	Self-assessments
	Peer assessments
	Logbooks
	Patient surveys

Primary focus of the chapter is highlighted in green

fellowship, attending physician), an anesthesiology assistant (anesthesiology assistant students, certified anesthesiology assistants), and a certified registered nurse anesthetist (student registered nurse anesthetist, certified registered nurse anesthetist), subjects in different stages of development learn differently. There are multiple ways to describe the stages of development that a learner is advancing through, and different organizations in various parts of the world use unique models. One approach, the RIME scheme (Reporter, Interpreter, Manager, Educator), was originally designed for internal medicine residency in the United States, and later the Dreyfus brothers created an alternative and original model for skill acquisition for learners in general (novice, competent, proficient, expert, master) that was later summarized by Michael Eraut into the widely accepted stages: novice, advanced beginner, competent, proficient, expert (Fig. 6.3) [14, 15, 16].

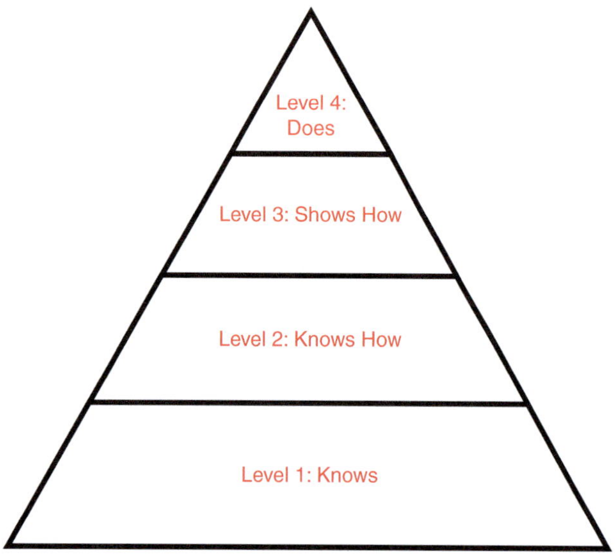

Fig. 6.2 Based on George Miller's Pyramid for levels of assessment [13]

Context

As mentioned previously, the purpose of an assessment is of paramount importance. In the outcome-based educational model, formative feedback (or "assessment *for* learning") is as important as the traditional summative reasons (or "assessment *of* learning"). Moreover, George Miller stated, "Tests of knowledge are surely important, but they are also incomplete tools in this appraisal if we really believe there is more to the practice of medicine than knowing" [13]. Furthermore, different stakeholders may make different decisions based on the same results from rating scales and scores. As such, assessment for its own sake should be avoided, and an a priori justification is crucial to guiding the process and informing the assessment itself.

Rating Instruments and Scoring

There are numerous rating scores and checklist forms validated for use, and they can often be used interchangeably with most methods of assessment. Examples of rating instruments include ANTS (Anesthetists' Non-Technical Skills),

Table 6.2 Aligning the level of assessment with a matching assessment methodology

Level of assessment	Assessment methods	Examples
1 – Knows	Written and oral	Multiple-choice questions
		Oral exams
		True/false items
		Matching items
	Performance based	Simulation-based assessments
2 – Knows How	Written and oral	Oral exams
		Long and short essay questions
	Performance based	Simulation-based assessments
3 – Shows How	Performance based	Simulation-based assessments
		Objective structured clinical examinations
4 – Does	Clinical observation	Direct observation of procedural skills
		360° evaluations/feedback
		Mini-clinical evaluation exercise
	Miscellaneous	Medical record audits
		Peer assessments
		Self-assessments
		Logbooks

Highlighted in green, simulation-based assessments under the category of "Performance based" is primarily used to evaluate level 3 in the "Miller's Pyramid" scheme—"shows how." However, there is also value in using simulations to assess levels 1 and 2 ("Knows" and "Knows How," respectively), as shown in yellow

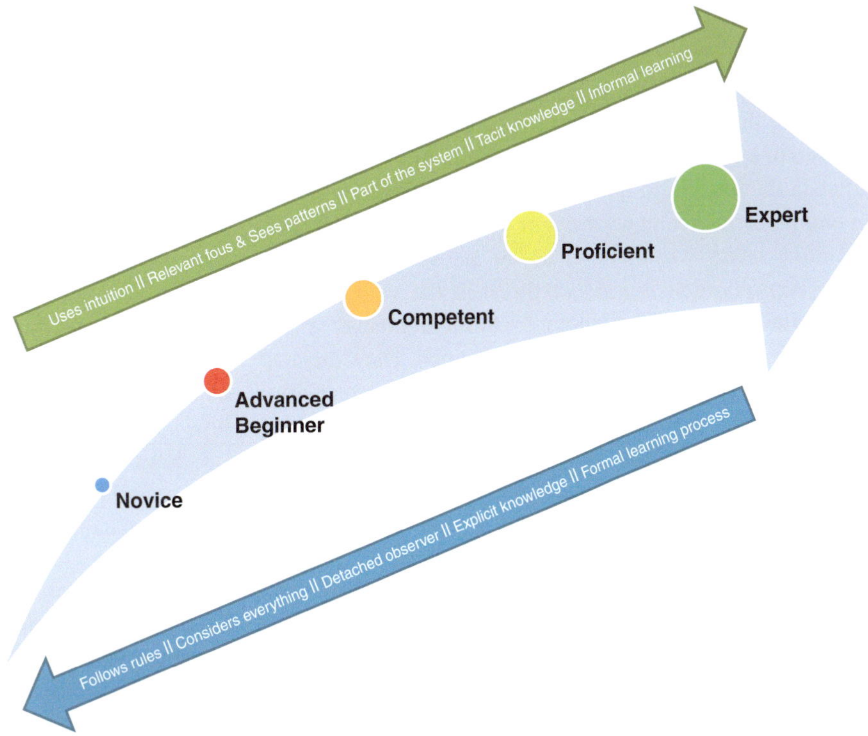

Fig. 6.3 Model of skill acquisition (and the basis of action learners). (Based on the Dreyfus brothers' original model, later summarized by Michael Eraut [15, 16])

NOTSS (Non-Technical Skills for Surgeons), and RIME (Reporter, Interpreter, Manager, Educator), to name a few. Rating instruments undergo demanding procedures during development, and those developed are said to be "validated." However, it is important to note that the context of an assessment is extremely important in the validation process and that adjustments must be made when using previously developed rating instruments (even if the outcomes of a competency being measured are similar) when used under different circumstances.

Competency Assessment of Practitioners Using Simulation

When assessing competence in a clinical setting, there is a layer of variance in reliability that cannot normally be controlled, and this is largely due to the factors introduced by the patient being studied (or the specific physiological changes present from certain diseases) or the clinical task at hand. Abrahamson and Barrows had the foresight to recognize these difficulties and created what is now recognized as the standardized patient (SP), one of the first true simulation modalities used for assessment (see also Chap. 10). For decades, SPs have been recognized as a means of delivering history and physical findings consistently and have proven key to simulation-based assessments [17]. In addition to SPs, Abrahamson created Sim One, the first computer-enhanced mannequin that was used to train anesthesiology residents in endotracheal intubation (see also Chaps. 1, 11, and 12). He showed that residents achieved a higher level of proficiency with intubation in overall fewer days in training, as well as with fewer attempts within the operating room, remarking that this leads to increased patient safety [18]. Over the years, technological advances in computer-enhanced mannequins allow manipulation of multiple physiologic parameters so that anesthesiology trainees (as well as members of other specialties) can become acquainted with the scenarios most commonly encountered within the operating room, as well as introduced to the rare scenarios with potential for major morbidity and mortality, all while in a controlled environment. The ability to reproduce the same parameters, accurately, across multiple administrations of the assessment to different groups of subjects is a great strength of using simulators in assessments. However, simulation adds a different layer to the already complex process of competency assessment, through separate challenges regarding validity and fidelity of the simulated environment.

For an assessment being performed for a specific purpose, it is important to note that the individual properties of various assessment methods will determine in part which components of the validity argument are the weakest. As Kane states, "Validity evidence is most effective when it addresses the weakest parts of the interpretive argument … The most questionable assumptions deserve the most attention" [19]. In regard to observational methods for conducting assessments, including the use of simulated environments, the *generalization* component of the validity argument is often questioned, due to construct underrepresentation, when it is believed that a single encounter in the test world is not generalizable to the real world [20]. However, this threat can be overcome by increasing the volume of observations in one assessment. For example, increasing the number of different cases that the subject is exposed to and assessed on, a better prediction can be made between the test world and the real world regarding behavior and performance in a variety of clinical encounters [20].

Unlike using written tests as an assessment modality, where *extrapolation* is a major threat to the validity argument, simulations add strength to this component of the validity argument via realism of the scenarios. The simulated environment is one that attempts to reproduce an actual clinical environment that the subjects will encounter in practice, specifically the conditions that anesthesiology residents and attending residents experience in the perioperative care of their patients. *Fidelity* is the degree of exactness to which this simulated environment parallels real-world circumstances. Certain aspects that contribute to increased or high-fidelity simulations are as follows: (1) physical appearance of mannequins tailored to specific scenarios; (2) extra support staff playing the roles of surgeons, nurses, technicians in and around the operating room environment; (3) presence of appropriate equipment to simulate an operating room, such as anesthesia machine, operating table, surgical equipment, proper draping, IV poles, etc. In a simulation lab, subjects are expected to interact with the computer-enhanced mannequin and with the other support staff as they normally would if they were a real patient or real interdepartmental colleagues.

Several simulators have been developed and are used to aid in the learning of specific technical skills by a trainee in anesthesiology. Examples of these part-task trainers include head mannequins for direct laryngoscopy, virtual reality (VR) simulators for fiberoptic bronchoscopy, or surgical trainers. With each of these devices, a singular technical skill was shown to be more easily acquired when compared to groups that did not use the devices [18, 21]. However, the critical piece missing from these devices that are high in engineering fidelity is the interplay of psychological fidelity, which deals with the actual skills and behaviors required in real clinical situations [22]. The ability to create an environment rich in both engineering fidelity and psychological fidelity is invaluable as it allows the assessor to witness and grade nontechnical skills, such as communication, as well as technical skills in a fluid and busy environment.

Regardless of the level of anesthesiology practitioners, it is important to assess how their technical and nontechnical skills are affected or change in an environment filled with various distractors. Imagine an operating room environment where the surgeon is placing pressure to get the operation started and upon induction, the patient rapidly desaturates and all eyes are on the anesthesiology provider who will make attempts to secure the airway—one can simulate this and even more complex scenarios in the simulation lab. In fact, it has been shown that having a simulated environment that triggers extreme emotional responses within the subjects can increase future performance [23].

Often the underlying assumption is that the closer the simulation is to the real-life environment, the better the assessment of performance will be in predicting clinical behaviors. However, as one can imagine a plastic mannequin, even the most advanced model, certainly has limitations. Furthermore, other aspects of the simulated environment can distract the subject, creating "simulation artifact" and can interfere with the assessment of performance. Therefore, creating too rigid of a scenario may not necessarily be optimal depending on how a participant interacts in the simulated environment, and "sticking to a script" may also negate a scenario's validity with regard to generalization into real-world clinical practice (see also Chap. 3).

The Role of Simulations in Competency Assessment

Using the framework outlined above for assessment, we will now focus on specific simulations (including SPs, computer-enhanced mannequins, virtual reality simulators) and their current and evolving role in assessment in medical education, specifically as they relate to the specialty of anesthesiology. To be sure, individuals and practitioners in different stages of training learn differently, necessitating distinct assessment programs for each level, including undergraduate medical education, anesthesiology resident training, certification or continuing education of attending anesthesiologists, and even reentry of attending anesthesiologists. In addition, there are similar programs targeting anesthesia assistants, student registered nurse anesthetists, certified registered nurse anesthetists, and reentry of certified registered nurse anesthetists into practice.

Undergraduate Trainees in Anesthesiology

We have witnessed the national impact of simulations upon medical education with the implementation of Step 2 Clinical Skills (Step 2 CS) portion of the United States Medical Licensing Examination (USMLE). This simulation exam is for summative purposes and consists of multiple stations that assess students' ability to perform a history and physical examination upon SPs, who provide highly reliable and accurate histories for specific disease processes, as well as objective physical exam findings [24]. SPs provide a score to each student using standardized checklists, and this provides input in a high-stake decision of whether the medical students will "pass" or "fail" and whether they may move on to the next phase of medical education in residency. Once this Step 2 CS component of the USMLE was announced, medical schools around the United States began the development of programs with the training of SPs to simulate this very exam and to facilitate the teaching and assessment of the clinical skills, including history taking, performing physical examinations, and creating differential diagnoses.

As mentioned previously, nearly all medical schools now employ a program to help prepare the students for various clerkships and for the Step 2 CS exam by means of the SP. These same SPs can be used to help foster a preoperative history and physical examination to help prepare for a clerkship in anesthesiology. For centers that have head mannequins and part-task trainers, holding workshops for basic yet vital technical skills such as bag-mask ventilation and intravenous line placement will aide these students over various clerkships and residencies regardless of specialty. More advanced workshops requiring more sophisticated simulators for endotracheal intubation, advanced cardiac life support (ACLS), central line placement, neuraxial/regional anesthesia for these medical students can also promote interest in the field of anesthesiology. One program has developed a six-week externship for third-year medical students, which includes didactics and procedural and simulation education, where they had a statistically significant increase in applications for the field of anesthesiology by the program's completion [25]. As the medical students are progressing through the anesthesiology clerkship, the use of periodic high-fidelity simulation scenarios as a means of assessment can help gauge student interest, as well as student adherence to readings and to establish if they are meeting the various stated goals and objectives. In addition, varying proportions of medical students who pass through an anesthesiology clerkship and who have interest in applying for a residency inevitably speak with the program director in anesthesiology at the host institution. The summative and formative feedback from various simulation assessments, in addition to the more basic and general exam scores from USMLE Steps 1 and 2, can help program directors better direct the applicants.

In addition to the increased use of simulation in medical school and specifically the potential benefits of teaching by simulation during anesthesiology clerkships, schools for student registered nurse anesthetists (SRNAs) have also found value in incorporating simulation within the curriculum. The importance of nontechnical skills (NTS) on anesthetist performance and the resultant excellence in care and patient safety outcomes has been reviewed and validated [26, 27]. The previously mentioned ANTS rating score has been used during simulations to assess these very skills in new trainees and practicing anesthesiologists. However, there has been little incorporation of simulation into the SRNA curriculum in the United States. Among various international institutions, there has recently been incorporation of simulation into SRNA curriculum where they have also created and validated modified rating instruments (NANTS-no and N-ANTS) suited for their specific assessments [28, 29]. In the United States, a program for SRNAs has moved toward the development and incorporation of an Objective Structured Clinical Examination (OSCE) for summative assessment via simulation for first-year SRNAs to ensure competence prior to entering their clinical year [30]. A follow-up study by Wunder was conducted to see the effect of a 3-hour intervention on first-year SRNAs on their NTS; results showed a statistically significant increase in post-test scores as measured by six high-fidelity scenarios simulating crisis [31].

Anesthesiology Residents

In respect of outcomes and the ACGME Toolbox, experts have placed simulations as a preferred or "most desirable" modality to evaluate clinical skills, knowledge, and attitudes in areas involving patient care and procedural proficiency, as well as interpersonal and communication skills. Similarly, when thinking about levels of assessment in "Miller's Pyramid" model, simulations tend to emphasize the *shows how* level, in which anesthesiologists in training can show how they would perform a skill, whether it be technical or nontechnical.

Key to simulation-based assessment for anesthesiology residents is the ability to provide fidelity of a very complex environment with varying degrees of workload, time pressure, and nontechnical challenges. Most importantly, it adds to patient safety by having new residents in anesthesiology learn in, and periodically be assessed in, a controlled, high-fidelity environment.

Anesthesiology as a specialty assumes proficiency in numerous technical and nontechnical skills, in addition to a broad knowledge base regarding human physiology and pharmacology; these include airway management (whether basic bag-mask ventilation or direct laryngoscopy and fiber-optic bronchoscopy skills), ACLS, central-line placement, performing neuraxial blocks and peripheral nerve blocks, team leadership skills, interpersonal and communication skills, and overarching crisis resource management skills, to name a few essential components. It is important to assess these skills as many of them deal with emergency situations in which a potential outcome is the death of the patient being cared for if not performed properly and in a timely manner. Current restrictions on duty hours imposed by the ACGME for anesthesiology residents and having a minimum of eight consecutive hours off between shifts [32], along with a finite amount of operating room cases with technical and nontechnical skills needing to be deployed, are some limitations that exist when learning and practicing said tasks. Here again, we suggest the use of simulation for the training and assessment of anesthesiology practitioners to increase their efficiency, proficiency, and ultimately patient safety.

Several studies have utilized simulation-based assessment for anesthesiology residents, where the instruments used were to assess explicit procedural skills and those of communication and collaboration, with the majority of the simulation studies devoid of evidence to support the validity of the performance measures [33–39]. The authors of one paper created tested a behaviorally anchored rating scale used during a simulation-based assessment to help identify critical gaps in anesthesia performance and to increase patient safety [40]. Two trained faculty (blinded to outside anesthesiology trainee program and level of training) applied the behaviorally anchored scale in a multiscenario setting and used surveys completed by the residents, fellows, facilitators, and raters to gain feedback on the overall assessment system. The results showed evidence that supported the reliability and validity of the assessment scores that included high generalizability, and the feedback from the surveys illustrated that the multiscenario simulation-based assessment was "useful, realistic, and representative of critical skills required for safe practice" [40].

Many anesthesiology residency programs that have a simulation center or program in place are incorporating its use and have integrated it into the standard training curriculum. It is particularly important to give the Clinical Anesthesia Level 1 (CA-1) residents this exposure early on in their training so that any gaps in knowledge and skills identified from the formative assessment can be used to further tailor and stimulate growth within those residents. Some critics have stated that the outcomes from a simulation scenario may impact the scoring and validity as some learners may become emotionally invested in negative outcomes and potentially employ avoidance behaviors when similar situations arise in the future (whether in more simulated environments or clinical practice). However, in a particularly rare but critical case scenario of pipeline contamination of oxygen supply during a simulated intraoperative environment, Goldberg et al. demonstrated that a negative outcome to the patient during a simulated independent practice (one where the facilitator is hands off and is simply there to drive the scenario and watch it unfold) led to better retention of clinical skills upon retesting the scenario 6 months later as compared to those who performed in a simulated supervised practice (one where an attending intervened to "save" the patient) [41]. In addition, simulation-based assessments can be performed that are targeted to more specific and advanced areas within the specialty of anesthesiology, to continue the educational growth of the anesthesiology residents on specific rotations during residency.

Regardless of the stage of development of the learner, one can tailor a simulated environment to assess competencies, as well as constructive data in a formative assessment. For example, to assess specific skills in a novice anesthesiology resident, one might separate them into individual components, such as preanesthetic evaluation, airway intubation, and hemodynamic management intraoperatively. A resident in the advanced or expert stage of development may get all the same components tested but in a more intricate environment that involves an acutely decompensating patient, which requires multitasking.

Practicing Anesthesiologists

Whether the assessment being performed is considered high stakes or low stakes, whether it is for summative (assessment *of* learning) or formative (assessment *for* learning) purposes, the results from one individual modality alone never solely determine the outcome. It is important to note George Miller's words in that "…no single assessment method can provide all the data required for judgement of anything so complex as the delivery of professional services by a successful physician" [13]. Rather, we make a strong case to use simulation as another assessment modality, an extra tool to assist in gathering the evidence to lead to the appropriate decision.

To work as a trainee or faculty within the hospital setting, these practitioners (especially those within the department of anesthesiology) are required to have active Basic Life Support (BLS) and ACLS certification. Currently, all American Heart Association (AHA) courses for the certification of BLS and ACLS involve the use of simulations, including part-task training for evaluating chest compressions and airway management skills on mannequins, as well as high-fidelity scenarios for mega-codes. In fact, studies have demonstrated an increased retention of skills and knowledge of ACLS when using full-scale, high-fidelity environments as compared to the standard part-task mannequins of the past [42–45].

Another clear example of utilizing simulations for high-stake situations deals with the evolving nature of the certification process of anesthesiologists after the completion of residency. The traditional exam consisted of two parts: an advanced written exam portion and an oral exam portion. Now, physicians must take three different assessments of different modalities: a written exam and what is now known as the "APPLIED" exam, which consists of the traditional oral exam, as well as a third portion that follows the OSCE format. The OSCE started in March of 2018, and the goal with this addition has been to "assess two domains that may be difficult to evaluate in written or oral exams—communication and professionalism and technical skills related to patient care" [46]. The nontechnical skills regarding communication and professionalism include informed consent, discussing various treatment options, working through periprocedural complications, navigating ethical issues, communication with other professionals, practice-based learning and improvement; the technical skills being assessed include the interpretation of a variety of simulated monitors, interpretation of various views of echocardiography, and application of ultrasonography [47]. It seems that preparation for this high-stake summative exam, which now includes a larger portion of simulations via both simulators and SPs, will best be achieved by the increased, periodic use of simulations by individual institutions that cover the various aspects of the examination.

Maintenance of Certification

Nowadays, the initial certification upon passing the high-stake examinations and becoming a new anesthesiology attending is time limited. This means that anesthesiology practitioners must partake in periodic evaluations to demonstrate continued and up-to-date knowledge in the field in order to become recertified. This process is known as the Maintenance of Certification in Anesthesiology (MOCA). This recertification process currently consists of multiple components, and traditionally, part 4 of the MOCA consisted of a simulation course at a center endorsed by the American Society of Anesthesiologists (ASA). With the evolution of times, this last portion of the MOCA now includes a wide variety of activities, including being an institutional/departmental leader of a quality improvement project, clinical pathway development leader, or self-directed case discussion/presentation of Mortality & Morbidity (M&M) case, to name a few [48]. However, undergoing the simulation course will likely remain a popular choice for those seeking recertification because "simulation experiences stimulate active learning and motivate personal and collaborative practice improvement changes" [48]. Furthermore, the simulation course offers the most points per hour and is beneficial in terms of time commitment. A study looking at practice improvement plans over a period of 3 years after anesthesiologists participated in MOCA part IV simulation course demonstrated that 94% of these practitioners successfully applied some or all of their planned improvements in practice [49].

There exists a minimum of certain requirements for the MOCA courses imposed by the ASA, such as duration of the course, content, and ratio of faculty to attendees, but the specifics of the content and structure/organization of the MOCA courses are left up to the discretion of the endorsed simulation center. One course design is described by the Mount Sinai Human Emulation, Education and Evaluation for Patient Safety and Professional Study (HELPS) Center. They developed a course using a variety of educational formats, which included traditional lectures on topics such as airway management, small group activities on part-task training mannequins and virtual-reality simulators to break the ice among the attendees, team-building exercises, and large "grand simulation" scenarios that ties everything together in high-fidelity simulations followed by debriefing [50].

Physician Reentry

In addition to simulations being integrated into the curriculum during anesthesiology residency, they are also being used for the purpose of retraining anesthesiology practitioners from returning to practice after a leave of absence. Relative physician shortages through a mismatch of supply and/or demand are a reality in modern medicine and can be attributed to a multitude of factors, both personal and economic [51, 52]. Although there is no standardized curriculum for reentry program and therefore allows flexibility for customization to the individual, a lot of the programs provide opportunities of observership that may assess the *knows* and *knows how* levels but not much more. The effectiveness of simulation-based assessment has been demonstrated for physician reentry across a variety of fields [53–56]. However, the use of a high-fidelity and high-stake simulation-based assessment "to assess the individual practitioner's deficits and provide a means to tailor the educational program to fill skills and knowledge gaps without risk of patient harm" is a unique method and consists of a two-part process: (1) a two-day assessment involving two standardized written tests (Anesthesiology Knowledge Test and AHA ACLS), as well as several repetitive simulations of varying complexities and covering various concepts (common and rare but critical scenarios) that are scored using a global rating Likert scale 1 to 5; (2) retraining phase that consists daily simulations covering distinct learning objectives over a variable and flexible 1- to 6-week duration, as well as operating room observation with one simulation faculty member [1, 57]. A case series that was published by DeMaria et al. demonstrated the success of the program with 73% of participants having successfully reentered into active practice for at least 1 year [57].

Rating Instruments in Simulation-Based Assessment

We have discussed the general criteria for good assessment, briefly mentioned different modalities of assessment, and then focused on the use of simulation for competency assessment, with examples specific to the specialty of anesthesiology. The assessment is not complete without a composite score that can be used to make a decision about the learners. As stated earlier, there are a host of global rating scales and various checklists already present, and it is beyond the scope of this chapter to list and analyze each one but rather to give a comparison. There was a systematic review performed of simulation-based assessments, in which the authors reviewed the evidence of the checklists and global rating scales used; the results from their study showed that the global-rating scale (GRS) to checklist correlation was 0.76, a similar interrater reliability between the two methods; and GRS had higher inter-item and interstation reliabilities than checklists [58]. So checklists are certainly a good alternative to GRS, but if a scenario has multiple tasks being measured, a separate checklist needs to be developed and used for each task, whereas the GRS can be used across several tasks.

Conclusion

Using simulation as an educational modality is gaining traction in the medical field, and their use in competency assessment is growing with it. Using the framework described as applied to simulation-based assessments, the purpose of the assessment to be performed must clearly be stated. In regard specific outcome to be assessed and the level of assessment to be evaluated, simulations are known to be the strongest in the clinical skills and interpersonal and communication skill areas and *shows how* level; however, the complexity of the scenario and questions asked within the scenario or in the debrief can elucidate and assess other aspects and levels of assessment. Simulation-based assessments (ranging from the use of SPs to computer-enhanced mannequins) are invaluable in the field of anesthesiology, where patient safety is addressed daily through invasive procedures, maintaining vigilance for the common and rare yet potentially fatal scenarios, along with knowledge and implementation of ACLS. This method of assessment of competencies in anesthesiology residents ensures little to no harm for patients while allowing for high reliability, as well as strengthening of the weaker components of the validity argument (generalization and extrapolation inferences) by manipulation of variables and organizing and conducting assessments with the appropriate level of fidelity. The use of simulation by the department of anesthesiology at individual teaching institutions as a method of teaching and assessing anesthesiology practitioners for both technical and nontechnical skills throughout the stages of training, and for new trainees and physicians seeking reentry into clinical practice, is all encouraged as the formative feedback will prove invaluable to both the assessor and those being assessed. Especially now with the movement by the American Board of Anesthesiology in incorporating simulations to provide summative feedback in the high-stake initial certification process, along with the ongoing MOCA requirements, anesthesiology practitioners should be familiarized with the simulated environments in all the components that will be tested.

References

1. Goldberg A, et al. High-stakes simulation-based assessment for retraining and returning physicians to practice. Int Anesthesiol Clin. 2015;53(4):70–80.
2. McGaghie WC, et al. A critical review of simulation-based medical education research: 2003–2009. Med Educ. 2010;44(1):50–63.
3. Issenberg SB, et al. Features and uses of high-fidelity medical simulations that lead to effective learning: a BEME systematic review. Med Teach. 2005;27(1):10–28.
4. Weller JM, et al. Psychometric characteristics of simulation-based assessment in anaesthesia and accuracy of self-assessed scores. Anaesthesia. 2005;60(3):245–50.
5. Cook DA. When I say... validity. Med Educ. 2014;48(10):948–9.
6. Cook DA, et al. A contemporary approach to validity arguments: a practical guide to Kane's framework. Med Educ. 2015;49(6):560–75.
7. Kane MT. Validating the interpretations and uses of test scores. J Educ Meas. 2013;50(1):1–73.
8. Gingerich A, Regehr G, Eva KW. Rater-based assessments as social judgments: rethinking the etiology of rater errors. Acad Med. 2011;86(10 Suppl):S1–7.
9. Yeates P, et al. Seeing the same thing differently: mechanisms that contribute to assessor differences in directly-observed performance assessments. Adv Health Sci Educ Theory Pract. 2013;18(3):325–41.
10. Accreditation Council for Graduate Medical Education. Next Accreditation System (NAS) and Milestones – a resident perspective. 2014 [cited 2016 09/25]. Available from: http://www.acgme.org/portals/0/pdfs/resident-services/9nasresidentsmay2014.pdf.
11. The Accreditation Council for Graduate Medical Education and The American Board of Anesthesiology. The Anesthesiology Milestone Project. 2015 [cited 2016 09/20]. Available from: https://www.acgme.org/Portals/0/PDFs/Milestones/AnesthesiologyMilestones.pdf.
12. Accreditation Council for Graduate Medical Education and The American Board of Medical Specialties. ACGME competencies: suggested best methods for evaluation (Toolbox of assessment methods). 2000 [cited 2016 09/26]. Available from: https://www.partners.org/Assets/Documents/Graduate-Medical-Education/ToolTable.pdf.
13. Miller GE. The assessment of clinical skills/competence/performance. Acad Med. 1990;65(9 Suppl):S63–7.
14. Pangaro L. A new vocabulary and other innovations for improving descriptive in-training evaluations. Acad Med. 1999;74(11):1203–7.
15. Dreyfus, S.E. A five-stage model of the mental activities involved in directed skill acquisition. 1980 [cited 2016 09/28]. Monograph available online. Available from: http://www.dtic.mil/cgi-bin/GetTRDoc?AD=ADA084551&Location=U2&doc=GetTRDoc.pdf.
16. Eraut M. Developing professional knowledge and competence. London: RoutledgeFalmer; 1994. p. 124.
17. Barrows HS, Abrahamson S. The programmed patient: a technique for appraising student performance in clinical neurology. J Med Educ. 1964;39:802–5.
18. Abrahamson S, Denson JS, Wolf RM. Effectiveness of a simulator in training anesthesiology residents. J Med Educ. 1969;44(6):515–9.
19. Kane MT. An argument-based approach to validity. Psychol Bull. 1992;112(3):527–35.
20. Downing SM, Haladyna TM. Validity and its threats. In: Downing SM, Yudkowsky R, editors. Assessment in health professions education. New York: Routledge; 2009. p. 21–56.
21. Goldmann K, Steinfeldt T. Acquisition of basic fiberoptic intubation skills with a virtual reality airway simulator. J Clin Anesth. 2006;18(3):173–8.
22. Maran NJ, Glavin RJ. Low- to high-fidelity simulation – a continuum of medical education? Med Educ. 2003;37(Suppl 1):22–8.

23. Demaria S Jr, et al. Adding emotional stressors to training in simulated cardiopulmonary arrest enhances participant performance. Med Educ. 2010;44(10):1006–15.
24. USMLE. Bulletin of Information. 2016 [cited 2016 09/30]. Available from: http://www.usmle.org/pdfs/bulletin/2016bulletin.pdf.
25. Baker KS, Cormican D, Seidman PA. Summer anesthesiology externship: demonstrating the ability of early clinical involvement to educate and increase specialty interest. J Educ Perioper Med. 2012;14(4):E063.
26. Fletcher GC, et al. The role of non-technical skills in anaesthesia: a review of current literature. Br J Anaesth. 2002;88(3):418–29.
27. Glavin RJ. Excellence in anesthesiology: the role of nontechnical skills. Anesthesiology. 2009;110(2):201–3.
28. Flynn FM, Sandaker K, Ballangrud R. Aiming for excellence – a simulation-based study on adapting and testing an instrument for developing non-technical skills in Norwegian student nurse anaesthetists. Nurse Educ Pract. 2016;22:37–46.
29. Lyk-Jensen HT, et al. Assessing nurse anaesthetists' non-technical skills in the operating room. Acta Anaesthesiol Scand. 2014;58(7):794–801.
30. Wunder LL, et al. Objective structured clinical examination as an educational initiative for summative simulation competency evaluation of first-year student registered nurse anesthetists' clinical skills. AANA J. 2014;82(6):419–25.
31. Wunder LL. Effect of a nontechnical skills intervention on first-year student registered nurse anesthetists' skills during crisis simulation. AANA J. 2016;84(1):46–51.
32. Accreditation Council for Graduate Medical Education. Specialty-specific Duty Hour Definitions. 2012 [cited 2016 09/29]. Available from: http://www.acgme.org/Portals/0/PDFs/DH_Definitions.pdf.
33. Mudumbai SC, et al. External validation of simulation-based assessments with other performance measures of third-year anesthesiology residents. Simul Healthc. 2012;7(2):73–80.
34. Berkenstadt H, et al. Deficits in the provision of cardiopulmonary resuscitation during simulated obstetric crises: results from the Israeli Board of Anesthesiologists. Anesth Analg. 2012;115(5):1122–6.
35. Ben-Menachem E, et al. Objective structured clinical examination-based assessment of regional anesthesia skills: the Israeli National Board Examination in anesthesiology experience. Anesth Analg. 2011;112(1):242–5.
36. Flin R, et al. Anaesthetists' non-technical skills. Br J Anaesth. 2010;105(1):38–44.
37. Fehr JJ, et al. Simulation-based assessment of pediatric anesthesia skills. Anesthesiology. 2011;115(6):1308–15.
38. Blum RH, et al. A method for measuring the effectiveness of simulation-based team training for improving communication skills. Anesth Analg. 2005;100(5):1375–80, table of contents
39. Malec JF, et al. The mayo high performance teamwork scale: reliability and validity for evaluating key crew resource management skills. Simul Healthc. 2007;2(1):4–10.
40. Blum RH, et al. Simulation-based assessment to identify critical gaps in safe anesthesia resident performance. Anesthesiology. 2014;120(1):129–41.
41. Goldberg A, et al. Learning through simulated independent practice leads to better future performance in a simulated crisis than learning through simulated supervised practice. Br J Anaesth. 2015;114(5):794–800.
42. Wayne DB, et al. A longitudinal study of internal medicine residents' retention of advanced cardiac life support skills. Acad Med. 2006;81(10 Suppl):S9–S12.
43. Wayne DB, et al. Mastery learning of advanced cardiac life support skills by internal medicine residents using simulation technology and deliberate practice. J Gen Intern Med. 2006;21(3):251–6.
44. Wayne DB, et al. Simulation-based education improves quality of care during cardiac arrest team responses at an academic teaching hospital: a case-control study. Chest. 2008;133(1):56–61.
45. Rodgers DL, Securro S Jr, Pauley RD. The effect of high-fidelity simulation on educational outcomes in an advanced cardiovascular life support course. Simul Healthc. 2009;4(4):200–6.
46. The American Board of Anesthesiology. The American Board of Anesthesiology: APPLIED (Staged Exams). 2016 [cited 2016 09/30]. Available from: http://www.theaba.org/Exams/APPLIED-(Staged-Exam)/About-APPLIED-(Staged-Exam).
47. The American Board of Anesthesiology. Applied Examination. [cited 2016 12/13/2016]. Available from: http://www.theaba.org/PDFs/APPLIED-Exam/APPLIED-OSCE-ContentOutline.
48. The American Board of Anesthesiology. MOCA Part 4 Requirements. [cited 2016]. Available from: http://www.theaba.org/PDFs/MOCA/MOCA-2-0-Part-4-Requirements.
49. Steadman RH, et al. Practice improvements based on participation in simulation for the maintenance of certification in anesthesiology program. Anesthesiology. 2015;122(5):1154–69.
50. Levine AI, et al. Simulation-based Maintenance of Certification in Anesthesiology (MOCA) course optimization: use of multi-modality educational activities. J Clin Anesth. 2012;24(1):68–74.
51. Grace ES, et al. Physicians reentering clinical practice: characteristics and clinical abilities. J Contin Educ Heal Prof. 2011;31(1):49–55.
52. Jewett EA, Brotherton SE, Ruch-Ross H. A national survey of 'inactive' physicians in the United States of America: enticements to reentry. Hum Resour Health. 2011;9:7.
53. Gallagher CJ, Tan JM. The current status of simulation in the maintenance of certification in anesthesia. Int Anesthesiol Clin. 2010;48(3):83–99.
54. DeMaria S Jr, Levine AI, Bryson EO. The use of multi-modality simulation in the retraining of the physician for medical licensure. J Clin Anesth. 2010;22(4):294–9.
55. Levine AI, et al. Role of simulation in U.S. physician licensure and certification. Mt Sinai J Med. 2012;79(1):140–53.
56. Steadman RH, Huang YM. Simulation for quality assurance in training, credentialing and maintenance of certification. Best Pract Res Clin Anaesthesiol. 2012;26(1):3–15.
57. DeMaria S Jr, et al. Simulation-based assessment and retraining for the anesthesiologist seeking reentry to clinical practice: a case series. Anesthesiology. 2013;119(1):206–17.
58. Ilgen JS, et al. A systematic review of validity evidence for checklists versus global rating scales in simulation-based assessment. Med Educ. 2015;49(2):161–73.

7 Role of Simulation in Healthcare Quality Assurance

Oren T. Guttman, Kristina L. Goff, and Scott C. Watkins

Introduction

What Is Quality?

> Every system is perfectly designed to get the results it gets. [6]
> – Dr. Paul Batalden

Healthcare systems are very complex. Contributing factors include the integration of multisystem teams, constantly changing technology, and a dizzying amount of new medical knowledge that must be rapidly assimilated in the face of ever-increasing production pressure. Regulatory and cost constraints add layers of complexity to the healthcare system that may actually harm the very patients it is trying to serve.

In 2015, it was estimated that hospital care harms and/or kills approximately 250,000 people annually in the US and the number of preventable harm events is likely much higher [1]. This places harm from healthcare as the third leading cause of death, exceeded only by heart disease (#1) and cancer (#2) [7]. In 2000, the Institute of Medicine (IOM) began a national campaign to remedy this situation. In its landmark publication, *To Err Is Human*, the IOM defined "Quality" in healthcare as *the degree to which health services for individuals and populations increase the likelihood of desired health outcomes and are consistent with current professional knowledge* [8].

Since then, many lessons have been translated from the world of manufacturing, aviation, and other highly reliable industries to improve "Quality" in healthcare [9]. We can differentiate "Quality" into two identifiable applications, namely quality assurance (QA) and quality improvement (process improvement) (QI), whose definitions are as follows [10]:

- *Quality assurance* is everything (policies/processes/procedures/practices) that enables an organization to "control" its ability to meet current requirements (regulations, standards, etc.)
- *Quality improvement*—synonymous to process improvement—is everything that focuses on improving processes, incrementally and continuously, to consistently meet desired standards.

While there is not a universal agreement on these definitions, they enable us to focus and study our efforts aimed at the current state and differentiate these efforts from those aimed at bringing the system to a future state.

Simulation and Healthcare Quality

Simulation is an educational technique that replaces or amplifies real experiences with guided experiences in order to *create a situation or environment to allow persons to experience a representation of a real event for the purpose of practice, learning, evaluation, testing, or to gain understanding of systems or human actions* [3]. This immersive learning strategy has particular relevance in high-stake industries. Threats to safety in healthcare include challenges from a constant influx of trainees, high rates of staff turnover, and the need for continuing medical education to maintain skills [5]. Simulation offers healthcare a multidimensional tool that aims to improve the quality and safety of patient care.

O. T. Guttman
Department of Anesthesiology, Health System Vice President For High Reliability and Patient Safety, Jefferson Health, Philadelphia, PA, USA

K. L. Goff
Department of Anesthesiology and Pain Management, University of Texas Southwestern Medical Center, Dallas, TX, USA

S. C. Watkins (✉)
Department of Anesthesiology and Critical Care Medicine, Johns Hopkins University School of Medicine, Johns Hopkins All Children's Hospital, Saint Petersburg, FL, USA
e-mail: scott.watkins@jhmi.edu

B. Mahoney et al. (eds.), *Comprehensive Healthcare Simulation: Anesthesiology*, Comprehensive Healthcare Simulation,
https://doi.org/10.1007/978-3-030-26849-7_7

This chapter will highlight specific examples of how simulation can help improve quality in healthcare, with initiatives categorized as either quality assurance or quality improvement.

Screen-Based Simulation

Screen-based simulation (SBS) in healthcare is defined as *digital technology used to represent patients, populations, or other healthcare encounters on a computer screen or other screen-based device with the use of virtual patients or virtual worlds* [11] in order to engage a learner in the acquisition of knowledge, application of knowledge (sense making), and problem solving (critical thinking). SBS has been shown to be an effective method for teaching resuscitation guidelines [12] and a better method to teach procedural knowledge over traditional classroom settings [13]. It is considered to be superior to traditional learning methods (lecture, handouts) in teaching medical staff how to handle medical emergencies [14] and has also been shown to improve the retention of medical guidelines compared with other standard methods of knowledge acquisition, such as simply reading text [15].

A virtual reality simulator is a form of SBS where participants are immersed in a three-dimensional world "screen" performing a simulated task while wearing a head-mounted display (HMD) or looking at a large-scale display. This modality has played an active role in procedural skill acquisition [16, 17], verification [18], and novice versus expert differentiation [19]. In fields that utilize endoscopy, this learning modality has been endorsed as a tool to ensure quality assurance [20, 21].

SBS has been utilized as a tool for improving surgical patient safety by educating perioperative healthcare personnel on the fundamentals of electrosurgical safety (FUSE) [22], for informing surgeons on the effects of distractions on their cognitive load, their metacognition, and surgical performance [23].

SBS is likely to be useful for optimizing the experience and safety of patients in the ambulatory care setting. For example, SBS modules could be used to enable assessment and feedback to clinicians about underlying cognitive biases affecting diagnostic skills. Nursing staff could utilize modules focused on their ability to correctly apply delegated medical orders to online patient portals in which patients ask medical questions and seek medical consultation (i.e., mychart, myhealth). Medical assistants and nonclinical staff could engage in modules that simulate patient phone inquiries and front-desk complaints and inform their ability to manage staffing challenges, engage in conflict resolution, and respond to production pressure challenges.

Onboarding, Patient Experience, and Simulation

Validating House Staff Competency

In healthcare, a rapid workforce turnover rate (~19% [24]) threatens the reliable delivery of safe care. Organizations require an ability to effectively and efficiently onboard staff to new processes, policies, and procedures and to identify and correct knowledge gaps in new employees. Simulation is a tool that has been used effectively in this context, reducing both the time and cost of new employee orientation in healthcare [25].

A simulation-based orientation for new nurses utilizing standardized patient actors has been shown to significantly improve knowledge acquisition, provide self-confidence in skills, and diminish workplace performance anxiety when compared with traditional non-simulation-based orientations [26]. Otolaryngology residents demonstrated improved self-confidence for up to 6 months after a one-day hybrid boot camp using medium and high fidelity mannequins to practice both technical skills (mask ventilation, intubation, flexible laryngoscopy, microlaryngoscopy/bronchoscopy, epistaxis control, and cricothyroidotomy) and adaptive skills (triaging and team leadership). The residents' improved confidence was significant for all skills, and the majority of participants felt that the intervention was useful in developing their knowledge, technical skills, and self-confidence and improving their self-assessment of clinical performance [27].

The ability of healthcare professionals to function as a team is critical to effective patient care. Effective teamwork is dependent on trust, and establishing trust within teams can be developed and augmented through interprofessional training and orientation. Interprofessional orientation, focusing on exposing the shared vulnerability of clinicians caring for patients, may serve to break down barriers of communication between providers and build teamwork from the start. Clinicians at Mayo utilized a simulation training session focused on communication, collaboration, and healthcare roles and responsibilities, followed by facilitated reflection with positive staff feedback [28]. Specifically, the Mayo study participants reported that "their communication had improved with other health disciplines" and that "they were more likely to call other health professions when needed to provide optimal patient care", both are behaviors that are critical to patient care. There is evidence that onboarding using simulation plays an important role in employee retention. In a study involving new graduate nurses, a 12-week simulation onboarding program that focused on critical clinical competencies led to an almost 90% retention of the first group of new graduate nurses and enhanced organizational integration [29].

Critical Patient Safety Language

The ability to speak up when one has a concern about a patient's safety is critical to preventing harm to patients. Sadly, one study showed that 53% of professionals (*n*: 192,462) are afraid to "speak up" despite feeling that something does not seem right [30]. The literature is mixed on whether simulation can affect clinician's ability to speak up, demonstrating a positive impact on residents [31] but no impact on getting nontrainee staff to change behavior [32]. Another component of critical patient safety language is conflict resolution. Poor conflict resolution among healthcare providers is a poor prognostic indicator for patient outcomes. If conflict is not managed appropriately, it can lead to burnout and loss of employee morale and negatively impact patient safety culture. One group has successfully utilized standardized patient instructor training to ready their student learners to prepare for peer-to-peer conflict situations. They found that the learners self-reported a high level of satisfaction for skill training. However, the program's value and applicability appeared to have been limited over time [33].

Giving bad news to patients is a difficult task, which continues to be a challenge for providers [34]. One approach, utilizing a four-day workshop with standardized patients, has been successfully leveraged to improve oncology fellows' ability to deliver bad news to patients about their new diagnosis [35]. Another approach using standardized patient (SP) simulation training with reflective practice (debriefing) was superior to lecture in enabling obstetric residents to break bad news to patients [36]. Surgical residents benefit from SP simulation with scenarios focused on breaking bad news to patients, such as disclosing a medical error, obtaining informed consent, or discussing unexpected events [37].

In Situ Simulation (ISS), Teamwork, and Resuscitation

ISS has been shown to improve teamwork on patient care units [38, 39]. In a large, multicenter, long-term study of perinatal care, authors studied 342,754 birth events across 14 widely distributed hospitals over a seven-year time frame. The study included both employed physicians and private hospital staff and found that only ISS and didactic team training independently achieved statistical significance, resulting in a 14% reduction in the Perinatal Adverse Outcome Index [40]. In a two-year study in the setting of cardiac arrest, ISS improved nursing staff response times for calling for help by 12% and reduced the time elapsed before initiating compressions and to initial defibrillation by 52% and 37%, respectively [41]. ISS improved both teamwork and clinical performance of multidisciplinary trauma teams, increasing the frequency of near-perfect task completion to 76% and reducing overall emergency room resuscitation time by 16% [42]. Finally, ISS improved code response time for a pediatric code blue team that services two adjoining hospitals, decreasing the response time for secondary providers coming from the second hospital from 29 to 7 min, decreasing time to CPR initiation from 90 to 15 seconds, and decreasing time to vascular access from 15 to 3 min [43].

In Situ Simulation (ISS) and High Acuity, Low Frequency Events

Healthcare struggles to prepare its staff to successfully manage high-acuity, low-frequency events. These events frequently involve multiple service lines, multifaceted technology, and clinically challenging situations of various diagnostic and therapeutic complexity. One example is when hospital staff is tasked with caring of a patient with a rare and high-risk pathogen (e.g., Ebola). The staff must manage a complex series of tasks, including containing the spread of the pathogen in the hospital, avoiding occupational injury, and assuaging an overactive media/public outcry. ISS has been effectively used to prepare for these situations, with one group utilizing a hybrid simulation model with a projected virtual reality environment for Ebola training, enabling staff to train in various tasks required for Ebola readiness (personal protective equipment (PPE) usage, IV placement, blood draws, and other patient care tasks) [44].

ISS and Latent Safety Threats (LST)

In the context of high-acuity, low-frequency events, ISS is a useful tool for exposing errors, performance gaps, and mistakes that personnel make in these stressful situations [45]. Furthermore, ISS has been leveraged as a tool for *prospectively* improving patient safety by exposing latent safety threats in a healthcare ecosystem [4]. In one study of over 90 unannounced in situ simulations conducted over 12 months, a total of 73 latent system threats (LST) were exposed, resulting in a rate of one LST for every 1.2 simulations performed [46]. In another study, 64 scheduled in situ simulations over a 21-month period produced 134 latent safety threats that were corrected before harm could reach patients [47]. ISS is superior to simulation-center-based simulation programs for the identification of LSTs [48].

ISS and Guideline Adherence

Adherence to best practice guidelines in critical patient situations has been shown to improve outcomes in cardiac arrest [49] and sepsis [50]. Despite the many dollars and hours spent on the certification of resuscitation skills, the application of these guidelines quickly fade after initial education [51]. The literature suggests that both medical and surgical patients are often not adequately resuscitated, necessitating continued maintenance of this skill set [52]. Finally, ISS has a special role in assessing guideline adherence of staff at the sharp end of care. An ISS study done in the emergency department showed marked variability in adherence to sepsis guidelines among providers and opportunities for focused improvements [53].

ISS and Operational Readiness

ISS has been shown to be a useful tool to achieve operational readiness in new areas of hospitals. In one study, four shifts of ISS were performed to assess critical services of a new free-standing emergency room. The simulation focused on patient flow, the physical design and layout of corridors and the triage area, and the community access points (entry and exit). Staff skills such as the ability to give bad news to patients, and to escalate care were assessed by ISS [54].

In Situ Simulation-Based FMECA and Latent Safety Threats

A robust method for exposing latent safety threats in a system is to conduct in situ simulations followed by a failure modes effects criticality analysis (FMECA). In this paradigm, one takes each failure mode exposed in the simulation, during the debriefing, and from video analysis and applies a series of questions to each of the failure modes. Multiple causes for each failure mode are identified and then systematically ranked with a risk priority number (RPN). The RPN is derived for each cause of failure by multiplying the probability of occurrence for a specific cause of failure (occurrence score), by the impact on the patient's health if the cause were to occur (severity score), by the system's current (not future) ability to detect this specific cause of failure should it occur (detection score). The RPN numbers allow for streamlined action planning to improve system safety by prioritizing scarce resources to correct the most critical gaps [55]. In one study, the authors conducted ten in situ simulations on a labor and delivery unit, identifying ten causes of failure with RPN scores ranging from 40 to 720, which led to rapid cycle quality improvements that included policy changes, process improvement, and staff education [56].

Simulation and Accreditation

Accreditation can be defined as a formal process conducted by an external body, e.g., The Joint Commission, for determining if a healthcare organization meets predetermined standards for quality of care [57]. Unlike certification, which focuses on both organizational and individual level competencies, accreditation focuses exclusively on quality at the level of systems and microsystems within healthcare organizations [2]. While often undervalued by clinicians, numerous studies have demonstrated improved clinical outcomes delivered by accredited systems compared to nonaccredited systems, particularly in the management of acute myocardial infarction, trauma care, and ambulatory surgical care [58]. Accrediting bodies often require systems and microsystems to demonstrate competency in processes of care for managing rare and uncommon events. A system capable of effectively managing a "worst case scenario" is assumed to have the structures and processes in place to manage routine care. The American Association for Accreditation of Ambulatory Surgery Facilities mandates that accredited facilities have numerous emergency protocols in place, including protocols for security emergencies, e.g., active shooter, fires and fire drills, malignant hyperthermia (MH), cardiopulmonary resuscitation (CPR), situations in which clinician(s) become incapacitated, power failure, and emergency evacuation, e.g., natural disaster [59]. It is the expectation of accrediting bodies that these protocols be maintained in writing, that the staff possesses working knowledge of the protocols and that the staff is able to implement the protocols if asked, i.e., during an inspection by the accrediting body. To meet these requirements, many organizations turn to simulation to maintain and demonstrate staff competency to accrediting bodies. In situ simulations (ISS) are excellent methods for ensuring that systems are prepared to manage specific situations, e.g., cardiopulmonary resuscitation, and to uncover deficiencies in system processes, e.g., staff unable to use or locate resuscitation carts. Many organizations, including the authors', use ISS periodically to train and test their system's response to fires, MH, evacuation for natural disaster and, sadly, active shooter. One author's (SCW) institution has used ISS to prepare and maintain accreditation as a pediatric level one-trauma center and as a pediatric liver transplantation program. In both cases, multi- and interdisciplinary simulations were invaluable in developing core processes and organizational structure and to prospectively identify system and microsystem gaps. The quality of healthcare systems is increasingly being defined by external indicators, which strive for reduced variability and the demonstration of reliability and resiliency. Simulation is well suited to aid systems in their pursuit of quality, reliability, and resiliency.

Assessing Competence Using Simulation Technology

As medical education has evolved over the past 20 years, we have seen an increased focus on outcome-based education. In 2012, an evaluative tool, the Milestones by the Accreditation Council for Graduate Medical Education (ACGME), was developed to ensure comprehensive assessment of our medical trainees in six core areas of competency [60]. Milestones not only play a role in the assessment of individual residents, but their effective implementation is now also a critical component in program accreditation.

Developing and assessing competency are increasingly challenging as the practice of medicine becomes more complex. New techniques and technologies used for nuanced diagnosis and treatment demand a more complicated skill set. Simultaneously, work-hour restrictions limit the time that residents are permitted to spend practicing and demonstrating their abilities. The transition from novice to expert requires a progression in knowledge and skills described in Miller's pyramid as a continuum from knowing to knowing how to showing how, and ultimately to independently doing [61]. As previously discussed, the Institute of Medicine and other professional societies have begun taking a much closer look at medical errors and patient safety over the past two decades, pushing the "see one, do one, teach one" tradition into the past and placing greater importance on our ability to ensure competence among trainees. Although necessary, this paradigm shift has resulted in decreased opportunities for trainees to practice clinical skills, further complicating the process of medical education.

Simulation, as previously discussed, can offer an excellent alternative to traditional teaching methods. Simulation technology also provides a new platform to evaluate competency across a wide-ranging array of skills and situations, with many benefits over "real life" procedural skill assessment. Simulation-based evaluations allow for a more reliable and reproducible exam and avoid the possibility of inadvertent patient harm by utilizing a risk-free environment [62]. The ACGME specifically recommends the use of simulation-based assessment in the evaluation of competencies in patient care, medical knowledge, and interpersonal communication [63]. This recommendation has been echoed by the American Thoracic Society Skills-Based Work Group, which advocates for the use of simulation in teaching and assessing procedural skills, including point-of-care ultrasound (especially echocardiography, thoracentesis, and vascular access), and airway management and bronchoscopy [64]. The legitimacy of simulation-based competency assessments in the healthcare setting has been verified in several studies over the past decade [65–67].

It has been well demonstrated that the evaluation of simulation performance can reliably distinguish between healthcare providers with different levels of experience [65, 68]. A number of validated instruments have been developed to help guide the evaluation process. Many of these are being incorporated into simulation-based education in nursing, undergraduate courses, and graduate medical training [69]. These tools focus on establishing competency by both objective (e.g., duration of task performance, technical error rates) and subjective (e.g., summative assessment given by preceptor) criteria.

Simulation modalities used to assess competence exist in a number of forms. The most basic form is the part-task trainer. Partial task trainers are reproductions of various body parts that are used as passive simulation elements. Partial task trainers are particularly useful in evaluating a trainee's ability to perform common procedures. For example, partial task trainers are available to allow trainees to demonstrate tracheal intubation, the placement of central venous catheters, laparoscopy, and lumbar puncture. This may be helpful in decreasing complications, especially with procedures with high complication rates, and permits the assessment of skills in a controlled environment without harm to real patients. For example, a number of studies have evaluated the use of simulation in teaching and assessing the placement of central venous catheters. A review of these studies indicates that trainees who learn using simulation have significantly improved learner outcomes, including better performance on simulators and increased confidence. This also translates to an improvement in patient outcomes, with fewer needle passes and a decreased rate of pneumothorax observed in procedures performed by trainees who had undergone simulation-based training [70]. Partial task trainers may also be useful in demonstrating and assessing more difficult skill sets and less commonly practiced procedures, although in these situations, more sophisticated simulation modalities may be preferable.

Simulation and Certification

Given the efficacy of simulation-based assessment in establishing competency, it is now being used in various certification processes required of healthcare providers. Simulation is ideal for high-stake certification examinations because of its reliability and reproducibility and has been a key component of many standardized competency assessments for years. For example, basic life support (BLS) and advanced cardiac life support (ACLS) certification training from the American Heart Association utilizes computer-based simulations to teach and test BLS/ACLS content via a series of online courses. This is followed by a hands-on skill assessment, using either partial task trainers or computer-enhanced mannequins, in addition to the standard written examination [71]. The application of simulation technology in the certification of healthcare workers continues to broaden as the field of medicine becomes more complex and subspecialized.

A number of certification programs employing simulation exist within surgical specialties. The Fundamentals of Laparoscopic Surgery (FLS) program was originally developed by the Society of American Gastrointestinal and Endoscopic Surgeons (SAGES) as a means of training and assessing both knowledge and technical skills in laparoscopy. This program has been studied extensively, with strong correlation between performances during the FLS simulations and in the operating room, and now represents a critical aspect of general surgical training [72]. A similar curriculum, known as the Fundaments of Endoscopic Surgery (FES), has been developed by SAGES to offer certification in endoscopy [73]. Simulation plays a particularly important role in the emerging field of robotic surgery. The wide application of robotic surgery across multiple surgical subspecialties and the variability in exposure during residency training has created a dilemma in ensuring operator competency. While formal certification in robotic surgery is not universally required to obtain credentialing at present, participation in the Fundamentals of Robotic Surgery (FRS) program for certification—a course that combines didactics with virtual-reality-based simulation to establish both technical proficiency and necessary team training skills—is quickly becoming standard for surgeons who wish to practice robotic surgery. This course was developed as the result of several consensus conferences attended by 14 surgical subspecialty societies and represents the first effort to standardize curriculum required for training in robotic surgery [74].

Many medical subspecialty societies have mandated some of these simulation-based certification programs and others for trainees prior to independent practice. For example, in 2009, the American Board of Surgeons announced that all graduating surgical residents must first complete the Fundamentals of Laparoscopic Surgery (FLS) certification in order to be considered eligible to take their board certification examination [65]. Objective Structured Clinical Examinations (OSCEs) are interactive examinations that employ simulators and standardized patients to test healthcare providers' diagnostic and procedural skills, as well as communication and professionalism, across a wide range of clinical scenarios. OSCEs have played an important role in medical school education since the 1970s. These exams offer improved reliability and validity in assessing competency, as opposed to standard bedside clinical skill examination. For over 10 years, medical students in the United States have been required to pass an OSCE administered as part of the United States Medical Licensing Examination Step 2 Clinical Skills Exam prior to graduation. Now OSCEs are being used with increasing frequency as part of the board certification process for medical subspecialties as well. In Canada, the Royal College of Physicians and Surgeons includes a cardiopulmonary and a cardiac audiovisual simulator as part of its OSCE for Internal Medicine Specialty Certification [75]. The American Board of Anesthesiologists added an OSCE to the traditional oral examination required for board certification in 2018. Simulation-based technology plays an especially prominent role in this exam as examinees are expected to demonstrate ultrasound use and regional anesthetic techniques, interpret a variety of simulated monitors, and analyze echocardiograms [76].

The role of simulation is also expanding in Maintenance of Certification (MOC) programs offered by a number of subspecialty boards, including the American Board of Internal Medicine (ABIM) and the American Board of Anesthesiology (ABA). The ABIM offers a high-fidelity simulation as part of the self-assessment of knowledge component of MOC for interventional cardiologists. A number of other internal medicine subspecialties are considering the addition of similar tools. The ABA was the first specialty board to require an immersive simulation-based course as part of its MOC curriculum [77]. Although no longer required for MOC, courses continue to be offered at a growing number of simulation centers across the country, incorporating high-fidelity computer-enhanced mannequins and virtual reality simulators to reinforce both technical skills and team training, often with a heavy emphasis on crisis resource management practices.

Conclusion

The use of simulation as a means of establishing competency and testing for certification is an area with tremendous potential for growth. In the last 10 years, there has been a dramatic increase in the use of simulation in this capacity, but it is still far from mainstream. As technology becomes more complex, and scrutiny on patient safety and quality assurance intensifies, simulation-based assessments may well become the most adaptive and comprehensive means of evaluating both trainees and experts to ensure the safe and appropriate practice of medicine.

References

1. James JT. A new, evidence-based estimate of patient harms associated with hospital care. J Patient Saf. 2013;9(3):122–8.
2. Makary MA, et al. Medical error—the third leading cause of death in the US. BMJ. 2016;353:i2139.
3. Healthcare Simulation Dictionary. 1st ed. 2016. p. 33. www.ssih.org/dictionary.
4. Deutsch ES, et al. Leveraging health care simulation technology for human factors research: closing the gap between lab and bedside. Hum Factors. 2016;58(7):1082–95.
5. IOM. Redesigning continuing education in the health professions. Washington, D.C.: The National Academies Press; 2010.

6. Said by Paul Batalden, quoted in article by Kimberly Mitchell, Like Magic? (Every system is perfectly designed…"), Friday August 21, 2015. www.Ihi.org.
7. Makary MA, Daniel M. Medical error-the third leading cause of death in the US. BMJ. 2016;353:i2139.
8. Institute of Medicine (IOM). In: Kohn LT, Corrigan JM, Donaldson MS, editors. *To Err is Human*: building a safer health system. Washington, D.C: National Academy Press; 2000.
9. Crosby PB. Quality is free. New York: McGraw-Hill; 1979.
10. Duffy GL. The ASQ quality improvement pocket guide: basic history, concepts, tools, and relationships. Milwaukee, Wisconsin: ASQ Quality Press; 2013. p. 62–5.
11. Chang TP, Gerard J, Pusic MV. Screen-based simulation, virtual reality, and haptic simulators. In: Comprehensive healthcare simulation: pediatrics. Cham: Springer; 2016. p. 105–114.
12. Schwid H, Rooke G, Alec MD, et al. Use of a computerized advanced cardiac life support simulator improves retention of advanced cardiac life support guidelines better than a textbook review. Crit Care Med. 1999;27(4):821–4.
13. Tan GM, Ti LK, Tan K, Lee T. A comparison of screen-based simulation and conventional lectures for undergraduate teaching of crisis management. Anaesth Intensive Care. 2008;36(4):565–9.
14. Schwid HA, Rooke GA, Michalowski P, et al. Screen-based anesthesia simulation with debriefing improves performance in a mannequin-based anesthesia simulator. J Teach Learn Med. 2001;13(2):92–6.
15. Schwid HA, Rooke GA, Ross BK, Sivarajan M. Use of computerized advanced cardiac life support simulator improves retention of advanced cardiac life support guidelines better than a textbook review. Crit Care Med 1999;27:821–824.
16. McClusky DA, Gallagher AG, Ritter EM, et al. Virtual reality training improves junior residents' operating room performance: results of a prospective, randomized, double-blinded study of the complete laparoscopic cholecystectomy. J Am Coll Surg. 2004;199:73–8.
17. Aggarwal R, Grantcharov T, Moorthy K, et al. A competency-based virtual reality training curriculum for the acquisition of laparoscopic psychomotor skill. Am J Surg. 2006;191(1):128–33.
18. Neis F, Brucker S, Henes M, et al. Evaluation of the HystSim™-virtual reality trainer: an essential additional tool to train hysteroscopic skills outside the operation theater. Surg Endosc. 2016;30(11):4954–61. Epub 2016 Mar 9
19. Mohtashami F, Dadelszen P, Allaire C, et al. A surgical virtual reality simulator distinguishes between expert gynecologic laparoscopic surgeons and perinatologists. JSLS. 2011;15(3):365–72.
20. Cohen AR, Lohani S, Manjila S, Natsupakpong S, et al. Virtual reality simulation: basic concepts and use in endoscopic neurosurgery training. Childs Nerv Syst. 2013;29(8):1235–44.
21. Haycock A, Koch A, Familiari P, et al. Training and transfer of colonoscopy skills: a multinational, randomized, blinded, controlled trial of simulator versus bedside training. Gastrointest Endosc. 2010;71(2):298–307.
22. Olasky J, Sankaranarayanan G, Seymour N, et al. Identifying opportunities for virtual reality simulation in surgical education: a review of the proceedings from the Innovation, Design, and Emerging Alliances in Surgery (IDEAS) conference: VR surgery. Surg Innov. 2015;22(5):514–21.
23. Weigl M, Stefan P, Abhari K. Intra-operative disruptions, surgeon's mental workload, and technical performance in a full-scale simulated procedure. Surg Endosc. 2016;30(2):559–66.
24. http://www.compdatasurveys.com/2015/09/17/rising-turnover-rates-in-healthcare-and-how-employers-are-recruiting-to-fill-openings-2/.
25. Zigmont JJ, Wade A, Edwards T, Hayes K, Mitchell J, Oocumma N. Utilization of experiential learning, the learning outcomes model reduces RN orientation time by more than 35%. Clin Simul Nurs. 2015;11:79–94.
26. Dearmon V, Graves RJ, Hayden S, et al. Effectiveness of simulation-based orientation of baccalaureate nursing students preparing for their first clinical experience. J Nurs Educ. 2013;52(1):29–38.
27. Malekzadeh S, Malloy KM, Chu EE, et al. ORL emergencies boot camp: using simulation to onboard residents. Laryngoscope. 2011;121(10):2114–21.
28. Will KK, Stepanek J, Brewer KK, et al. Interprofessional orientation for health professionals utilizing simulated learning: findings from a pilot study. J Interprof Care. 2016;30(2):254–6.
29. Fey MK, Miltner RS. A competency-based orientation program for new graduate nurses. J Nurs Adm. 2000;30(3):126–32.
30. John Ovretveit. Achieving "value improvements" changes which improve quality and save money. The International Society for Quality in Health Care (ISQua). http://www.isqua.org/docs/geneva-2012-docs/john-ovretveit.pdf?sfvrsn=0.
31. Pian-Smith MC, Simon R, Minehart RD, et al. Teaching residents the two-challenge rule: a simulation-based approach to improve education and patient safety. Simul Healthc. 2009;4(2):84–91.
32. Raemer DB, Kolbe M, Minehart RD, Rudolph JW, Pian-Smith MC. Improving anesthesiologists' ability to speak up in the operating room: a randomized controlled experiment of a simulation-based intervention and a qualitative analysis of hurdles and enablers. Acad Med. 2016;91(4):530–9.
33. Beattie BE, Kinney J, Fitzgerald M, et al. Dental and dental hygiene students' perceptions of a standardized patient instructor conflict resolution program. J Dent Educ. 2014;78(10):1397–404.
34. Foley KM, Gelband H. Improving palliative care for cancer: summary and recommendations. Washington, D.C.: Institute of Medicine and National Academy Press; 2001.
35. Back A, Arnold R, Baile W, et al. Efficacy of communication skills training for giving bad news and discussing transitions to palliative care. Arch Intern Med. 2007;167:453–60.
36. Karkowsky CE, Landsberger EJ, Bernstein PS, et al. Breaking bad news in obstetrics: a randomized trial of simulation followed by debriefing or lecture. J Matern Fetal Neonatal Med. 2016;29(22):3717–23.
37. Lamba S, Tyrie LS, Bryczkowski S, Nagurka R. Teaching surgery residents the skills to communicate difficult news to patient and family members: a literature review. J Palliat Med. 2016;19(1):101–7.
38. Jewll K, McGiffert L. "To err is human—to delay is deadly" consumers union. 2009. Available at: http://www.safepatientproject.org/pdf/safepatientproject.org-to_delay_is_deadly-2009_05.pdf.
39. Weaver SJ, Salas E, Lyons R, et al. Simulation-based team training at the sharp end: a qualitative study of simulation-based team training design, implementation, and evaluation in healthcare. J Emerg Trauma Shock. 2010;3:369–77.
40. Riley W, Begun JW, Meredith L, et al. Integrated approach to reduce perinatal adverse events: standardized processes, interdisciplinary teamwork training, and performance feedback. Health Serv Res. 2016;51:2431.
41. Herbers MD, Heaser JA. Implementing an in situ mock code quality improvement program. Am J Crit Care. 2016;25(5):393–9.
42. Steinemann S, Berg B, Skinner A, et al. In situ, multidisciplinary, simulation-based teamwork training improves early trauma care. J Surg Educ. 2011;68(6):472–7.
43. Yager P, Collins C, Blais C, et al. Quality improvement utilizing in-situ simulation for a dual-hospital pediatric code response team. Int J Pediatr Otorhinolaryngol. 2016;88:42–6. Epub 2016 Jun 7
44. Ragazzoni L, Ingrassia PL, Echeverri L, et al. Virtual reality simulation training for Ebola deployment. Disaster Med Public Health Prep. 2015;9(5):543Y6.
45. Rosen MA, Hunt EA, Pronovost PJ, et al. In situ simulation in continuing education for the health care professions: a systematic review. J Contin Educ Health Prof. 2012;32:243–54.
46. Patterson MD, Geis GL, Falcone RA, LeMaster T. In situ simulation: detection of safety threats and teamwork training in a high risk

emergency department. BMJ Qual Saf. 2013;22(6):468–77. https://doi.org/10.1136/bmjqs-2012-000942.
47. Wheeler DS, Geis G, Mack EH, LeMaster T, Patterson MD. High-reliability emergency response teams in the hospital: improving quality and safety using in situ simulation training. BMJ Qual Saf. 2013;22(6):507–14. https://doi.org/10.1136/bmjqs-2012-000931. Epub 2013 Mar 1.
48. Wetzel EA, Lang TR, Pendergrass TL, Taylor RG, Geis GL. Identification of latent safety threats using high-fidelity simulation-based training with multidisciplinary neonatology teams. Jt Comm J Qual Patient Saf. 2013;39(6):268–73.
49. McEvoy MD, Field LC, Moore HE, et al. The effect of adherence to ACLS protocols on survival of event in the setting of in-hospital cardiac arrest. Resuscitation. 2014;85(1):82–7.
50. Paul R, Neuman MI, Monuteaux MC, Melendez E. Adherence to PALS sepsis guidelines and hospital length of stay. Pediatrics. 2012;130:e273–80.
51. Smith KK, Gilcreast D, Pierce K. Evaluation of staff's retention of ACLS and BLS skills. Resuscitation. 2008;78(1):59–65. [PubMed: 18406037]
52. Chan PS, Nichol G, Krumholz HM, Spertus JA, Nallamothu BK. American Heart Association National Registry of cardiopulmonary resuscitation I. hospital variation in time to defibrillation after in-hospital cardiac arrest. Arch Intern Med. 2009;169(14):1265–73. [PubMed: 19636027]
53. Kessler DO, Walsh B, Whitfill T, et al. Disparities in adherence to pediatric sepsis guidelines across a spectrum of emergency departments: a multicenter, cross-sectional observational in situ simulation study. Emerg Med. 2016;50(3):403–15.e1-3.
54. Kerner RL Jr, Gallo K, Cassara M, et al. Simulation for operational readiness in a new freestanding emergency department: strategy and tactics. Simul Healthc. 2016;11(5):345–56.
55. DeRosier J, Stalhandske E, Bagian JP, et al. Using health care failure mode and effect analysis: the VA national center for patient safety's prospective risk analysis system. Jt Comm J Qual Improv. 2002;28:248–67.
56. Davis S, Riley W, Gurses AP, Miller K, Hansen H. Failure modes and effects analysis based on in situ simulations: a methodology to improve understanding of risks and failures. In: Henriksen K, Battles JB, Keyes MA, Grady ML, editors. Source advances in patient safety: new directions and alternative approaches, Performance and tools, vol. 3. Rockville: Agency for Healthcare Research and Quality; 2008.
57. Viswanathan HN, Salmon JW. Accrediting organizations and quality improvement. Am J Manag Care. 2000;6(10):1117–30.
58. Alkhenizan A, Shaw C. Impact of accreditation on the quality of healthcare services: a systematic review of the literature. Ann Saudi Med. 2011;31(4):407–16.
59. Regular standards and checklist for accreditation of ambulatory surgery facilities. In: American Association for Accreditation of ambulatory surgery facilities I, ed. Version 144, Gurnee; 2016.
60. www.acgme.org/what-we-do/accreditation/milestones/overview.
61. Miller GE. The assessment of clinical skills/competence/performance. Acad Med. 1990;65(Suppl):S63–7.
62. Scalese RJ, Obeso VT, Barry Issenberg S. Simulation technology for skills training and competency assessment in medical education. J Gen Intern Med. 2008;23(Suppl 1):46–9. *PMC*. Web. 11 Nov. 2016
63. https://www.acgme.org/Portals/0/MilestonesGuidebook.pdf?ver=2016-05-31-113245-103.
64. McSparron JI, et al. Simulation for skills-based education in pulmonary and critical care medicine. Ann Am Thorac Soc. 2015;12(4):579–86.
65. Devitt JH, et al. The validity of performance assessments using simulation. Anesthesiology. 2001;95(1):36–42.
66. Sidi A, et al. Simulation-based assessment to evaluate cognitive performance in an anesthesiology residency program. J Grad Med Educ. 2014;6(1):85–92.
67. Michelson J, et al. Competency assessment in simulation-based procedural education. Am J Surg. 2008;196(4):609–15.
68. Adrales GL, et al. A valid method of laparoscopic simulation training and competence assessment. J Surg Res. 2003;114(2):156–62.
69. Fried GM. FLS assessment of competency using simulated laparoscopic tasks. J Gastrointest Surg. 2008;12:210–2.
70. Ma IW, et al. Use of simulation-based education to improve outcomes of central venous cathetrization: a systematic review and meta-analysis. Acad Med. 2011;86(9):1137–47.
71. https://www.onlineaha.org/course_format.
72. Hafford ML, Van Sickle KR, Willis RE, et al. Ensuring competency: are fundamentals of laparoscopic surgery training and certification necessary for practicing surgeons and operating room personnel? Surg Endosc. 2013;27:118.
73. http://www.fesprogram.org/.
74. Smith R, et al. Fundamentals of robotic surgery: a course of basic robotic surgery skills based upon a 14-society consensus template of outcome measures and curriculum development. Int J Med Robotics Comput Assist Surg. 2014;10:379–284.
75. Royal College of Physicians and Surgeons of Canada Format of the comprehensive objective examination in internal medicine. http://www.royalcollege.ca/cs/groups/public/documents/document/y2vk/mday/~edisp/tztest3rcpsced002085.pdf.
76. American Board of Anesthesiology. Applied examination objective structure clinical examination content outline. http://www.theaba.org/PDFs/APPLIED-Exam/APPLIED-OSCE-ContentOutline.
77. Ross BK, Metzner J. Simulation for maintenance of certification. Surg Clin N Am. 2015;95(4):893–905.

Licensure and Certification

8

Jonathan Lipps

Introduction

Similar to any high-stake industry in which human welfare is at risk, healthcare, and anesthesiology in particular, must ensure that its practitioners achieve and maintain competence. Multiple stakeholders—patients, society at large, insurance companies, hospital and health care systems, and professional societies—all demand high-quality, cost-effective patient care. Concomitant with the rise of simulation as a teaching modality in healthcare has been its application as a tool for assessment. Many of the qualities that make simulation an effective teaching tool also make it useful for assessment for licensure and certification: recreation of a realistic clinical environment, standardization, and reproducibility without exposing patients to harm [1]. While simulation-based assessment for the trainee is often formative or designed for providing feedback and performance improvement, summative, high-stake assessment of competence is also utilized as a standard for licensure and certification. As advances in simulation-based technology have allowed for increasingly realistic recreations of the clinical environment, licensing and certifying bodies have gained confidence in its utility and validity as a tool for the assessment of clinical proficiency. Miller's model of clinical competence describing a pyramid of four levels of competence in which the base, "knows," precedes "knows how," followed by "shows how," and finally "does," is often cited in support of the benefits of simulation for healthcare education and assessment [2]. Unlike traditional measures of assessment (written and oral examinations) in which examinees demonstrate that they "know how," by placing them in a simulated clinical environment, they can perform under direct observation or, in the phrasing of Miller's model, "show how." Currently, simulation is being used to assess for competence at all levels of healthcare education. As such, the current anesthesiologist in training is guaranteed to encounter simulation-based assessment at many points along their career. Given anesthesiologists' role as pioneers in the use of simulation as a tool for instruction, leaders in the field are in the midst of a period of rapid innovation as simulation-based assessments are being introduced to measure proficiency throughout anesthesiology training and practice. In this chapter, we review the current uses and evidence for simulation as an assessment tool for licensure and certification for undergraduate, graduate, and postgraduate medical professionals in the field of anesthesiology. We will explore current practice in the United States in addition to practice outside of the U.S. At the conclusion, we will briefly glimpse at the potential future for simulation-based certification based on the current trajectory.

Licensure

The most widely recognized current example of simulation-based credentialing is its use as a component of the United States Medical Licensing Exam (USMLE). Since 2004, completion of the USMLE Step 2 Clinical Skills (CS) exam has been a requirement for gaining licensure to practice medicine in the US. The purpose of the exam is to evaluate students in the areas of communication and interpersonal skills, spoken English proficiency, and data gathering/interpretation—topics difficult to assess through written testing alone. The first iteration was introduced in 1998 by the Education Commission for Foreign Medical Graduates for non-US physicians before entering practice and consisted of a series of standardized patient interactions [3]. The National Board of Medical Examiners (NBME) introduced a similar exam in the form of the Step 2 CS in 2004 due to increased reports of malpractice, medical errors, and decreased patient satisfaction. The current form of the Step 2 CS consists of 12 15-minute standardized patient encounters divided over the course of an eight-hour day. Most of the encounters

J. Lipps (✉)
Department of Anesthesiology, The Ohio State University Wexner Medical Center, Columbus, OH, USA
e-mail: jonathan.lipps@osumc.edu

B. Mahoney et al. (eds.), *Comprehensive Healthcare Simulation: Anesthesiology*, Comprehensive Healthcare Simulation,
https://doi.org/10.1007/978-3-030-26849-7_8

involve face-to-face interaction with a standardized patient actor, although some may be telephone based. In addition to testing nontechnical communication skills, encounters are scripted in order that tasks such as physical examination skills, note writing, and imaging interpretation can be evaluated. The examination is comprised of three separate subcomponents, which all must be passed: Communication and Interpersonal Skills (CIS), Spoken English Proficiency (SEP), and Integrated Clinical Encounter (ICE). [4] A prototype of the exam was found to correlate significantly with intern performance, as measured by residency directors' ratings and was a better predictor than the multiple-choice Step 1 and Step 2 exams [5].

As with other mandatory simulation-based examinations, the Step 2 CS is not without controversy [6]. Alvin identifies "convenience, cost, and value" as being in question for an examination requiring heavy manpower for its administration, leading to its limited availability at only a handful of sites nationally. This can be a challenge for U.S. medical students, many of whom already carry significant student loan debt and must pay a $1290 examination cost (as of 2019), which does not include the cost of travel, while simultaneously balancing medical school requirements and residency interviews. Furthermore, the utility or "value" of the exam is not without criticism, given its pass/fail nature and the fact that no formative feedback is provided to the examinee. Many students with marginal performance could potentially make use of a detailed performance report in order to focus their efforts on improving clinical performance. Furthermore, data suggest that results from this component of the USMLE is not particularly useful to residency programs seeking data on preparedness for residency training. In the 2012–2013 year, 98% of 20,201 US medical students taking Step 2 CS for the first time achieved a result of "pass." Eighty percent of those having previously failed taking the exam also achieved a result of "pass." Such a large proportion of students receiving the same result for an exam yields little utility for the stratification of ability. Another study showed a positive but only modest correlation between performance on the Step 2 CS and performance ratings provided by residency program directors based on students' first year of residency training [7]. Despite this criticism, the Step 2 CS continues to be a requirement for all graduating medical students and as a result serves as a factor in medical schools' curriculum development. Simulation is now nearly ubiquitous as a component of clinical curriculum in U.S. medical schools and often consists of objective structured clinical exams (OSCEs) that are created to mimic those standardized patient (SP) encounters seen in the Step 2 CS exam [8].

The final stage in the series of U.S. medical licensing examinations, the USMLE Step 3, though quite different from the USMLE Step 2 in content and format, contains portions involving simulation-based assessment. As a prerequisite to taking the exam, examinees must have an undergraduate medical degree and therefore often sit for the examination early in residency training. The exam consists of two sections occurring on consecutive days: Fundamentals of Independent Practice, a multiple-choice format assessment of clinical knowledge, and Advanced Clinical Medicine, which involves the application of medical knowledge in the clinical setting. This latter portion is comprised of multiple-choice items, as well as 13 computer-based case simulations (CCS) that employ Primum® software and are entirely virtual and screen based [9]. In each scenario, the examinee is provided with a virtual patient vignette and an accompanying explanation of the purpose of the encounter, which can take place in the inpatient or outpatient setting. The examinee must initiate patient care actions such as physical examination, diagnostic testing, procedural intervention, or medication administration through free texting within the software. Results of each action are revealed when the examinee advances the scenario through "advancing the clock," and each scenario ends after either a maximum allotted time has been utilized or after the objectives of the scenario are achieved. The virtual, screen-based scenarios presented in the USMLE Step 2 allow for the assessment of patient care over time and location free of the constraints imposed by standard patient-based scenarios. For example, follow-up over extended periods (weeks to months) is possible, as is interaction with a single patient over a variety of settings, such as in a clinic, emergency department, or nursing home. While there is a seven-minute tutorial built into the start of the examination, the USMLE encourages examinees to practice and become familiar with the Primum® software in advance. Unlike the USMLE Step 2 CS standard patient encounters, this format does not allow for the assessment of interpersonal communication, professionalism, and physical exam skills. Through the use of standard patient and screen-based simulation, the USMLE Step 2 CS and Step 3 CCS provide complementary assessments of examinees and demonstrate the benefits and limitations of two very different simulation assessment modalities.

Specialty Certification

Despite the widespread use of simulation-based assessment in the United States for medical licensure during the early twenty-first century, its use in specialty board certification is relatively new. The American Board of Family Medicine and the American Board of Surgery have required simulation-based assessments for primary certification since 2004 and 2009, respectively [10]. The American Board of Anesthesiology (ABA), traditionally having assessed clinical application of medical knowledge through case-based oral examination, began the implementation of simulation-based OSCEs as a part of the Applied Examination in 2018. Prior to this time, the only mandated simulation requirement for anesthesiology trainees consisted of at least one simulated experience per year, a mandate put forth by the Accreditation Council for Graduate Medical Education (ACGME) [11]. Although the addition of the OSCE to the applied exam represents a dramatic change in board certification of anesthesiologists in the United States, precedent exists internationally, most notably in Israel, the UK and Canada, all of which have credentialing bodies that incorporate simulation-based assessments into their primary certification process. The Israeli OSCE was first introduced for primary certification by the Israeli Board of Anesthesiology in 2003 [12]. The creation of the examination relied upon national consensus using a modified Delphi technique to ensure content and face validity. The OSCE in its current form consists of five stations covering the domains of trauma management, resuscitation, operating room crisis management, mechanical ventilation, and regional anesthesia (Table 8.1). During each 15-minute OSCE, examiners assess participants utilizing both a technical skill checklist and a nontechnical skill scale. The technical checklist consists of critical actions that are identified as performed or not performed. The exam employs a variety of simulation modalities, including standardized patients, mannequin-based simulation, and partial task trainers. The Israeli OSCE is innovative in its assessment of competency in regional anesthetic technique, requiring that participants position a standardized patient, identify relevant anatomy and landmarks, position a block needle (without insertion), and explain the choice of local anesthetic, expected duration of action, and possible complications to a facilitator. Through this original approach, the examination combines elements of a traditional oral examination with a simulation-based component [13]. An analysis of OSCE validity yielded good interrater reliability; however, correlation of OSCE performance with that of the traditional oral exam was poor. This is a not entirely unexpected result, which may suggest that the OSCE assesses competence in areas previously not testable through other modalities.

The Royal College of Anaesthetists (UK) has also implemented an OSCE-based assessment as a requirement for primary certification. This pass/fail exam consists of 18 stations overlapping many of the topics found in the Israeli OSCE with additional stations dedicated to the assessment of communication skills, history taking, the understanding of anatomic relationships, and imaging interpretation. The exam is unique in that the participants may also be asked to perform a safety check on common anesthesia equipment and assess for faults [14]. In recognition of the utility of the Israeli and UK simulation-based requirements for certification, along with a growing confidence in the fidelity and validity of simulation-based assessment, other countries are also turning to simulation-based components to enhance their certification processes. While it does not employ the OSCE-based format listed above, since 2010 the Royal College of Physicians and Surgeons of Canada (RCPSC) has incorporated what it refers to as "enhanced reality" into its oral examination for certification. This includes a screen-based display of changing vital signs, laboratory data, and diagnostic imaging provided to the examinee. While this format does allow the examinee to engage in the content in a visual manner, it does not meet the standard of allowing the examinee to "show how" in the language of Miller's pyramid model of clinical competence [15]. This approach has been described as "simulation-assisted" in that it utilizes multimedia features common to simulation-based activities while excluding the kinesthetic aspects of simulation-based learning or assessment.

Table 8.1 Israeli OSCE content

Module	Content	Simulation modality
Trauma	Principles of ATLS	High fidelity
Resuscitation	Principles of ACLS	High fidelity
OR crisis management	Management of hemodynamic changes	High fidelity
Mechanical ventilation	Lung compliance, ventilator settings, blood gas interpretation	Task trainer, low fidelity
Regional anesthesia	Surface anatomy, needle placement, complications	Task trainer, standardized patient

More recently, the ABA has sought to transform board certification for U.S. anesthesiologists through the modification of its staged series of examination for certification culminating in the Applied Examination. This most recent iteration of the final staged examination in the certification process to be introduced in 2018 includes both the traditional oral examination and an OSCE component somewhat similar to that offered in Israel and the UK and consists of seven encounters, each of which are eight minutes in duration [16]. This OSCE component was created to allow candidates to demonstrate nontechnical skills in competencies otherwise difficult to assess through traditional oral and written examinations in order that Miller's "shows how" and "does" levels of medical competence can be assessed [17].

The ABA Applied Examination OSCE component will utilize standardized patients, simulated anesthesia monitors, and simulated echocardiographic examinations to assess proficiency in a variety of competency domains (Table 8.2) [18].

While the OSCE portion of the Applied Examination aims to assess proficiency in some technical and nontechnical clinical skills, a practicing anesthesiologist must be able to function effectively in a stressful and dynamic operating room setting. At present there is no plan for the inclusion of high-fidelity simulation (HFS), which can recreate a realistic clinical scenario through the use of mannequin-based human patient simulation in any portion of the ABA certification process. Most of the interactions on

Table 8.2 ABA OSCE content

Skill to be tested	Core competency	Type of simulation
Informed consent	Interpersonal and communication skills, patient care	Standardized patient
Treatment options	Interpersonal and communication skills, patient care	Standardized patient
Periprocedural complications	Interpersonal and communication skills, patient care	Standardized patient
Ethical issues	Interpersonal and communication skills, professionalism	Standardized patient
Communication with other professionals	Interpersonal and communication skills	Standardized patient
Practice-based learning and improvement	Practice-based learning and improvement	Standardized patient
Interpretation of monitors	Patient care	Computer-based
Interpretation of echocardiograms	Patient care	Computer-based
Application of ultrasonography	Patient care	Task trainer

Table 8.3 Effective Management of Anaesthetic Crises (EMAC) course content

Module	Content	Simulation modality
Human performance	Human factors, systems approach to patient safety	Discussion, video review, games, HFS
Airway emergencies	Non-invasive airway, surgical airway, planning for difficult airway	Video review, task trainer, HFS
Anesthetic emergencies	Emergencies related to drugs or equipment, strategies for diagnosis and management	HFS followed by video-assisted debrief
Cardiovascular emergencies	ACLS, emergency vascular access	Case-based discussion, HFS
Trauma management	Primary and secondary survey, patient transfer, c-spine injury, head trauma, chest trauma	HFS – complex, multitrauma scenario

the seven-station circuit will take place in a preoperative or postoperative environment. Outside of a realistic recreation of the anesthesiologist's clinical operating room environment, the assessment of many technical and nontechnical skills is somewhat limited. Arguably, an anesthesiologist's proficiency in skills, such as situational awareness, effective communication, resource utilization, and timely clinical decision making based on changing information, can mean the difference between life and death for patients within the context of a high-stress, dynamic operative environment. While the traditional oral examination for ABA certification allows candidates to display the application of medical knowledge to clinical decisions, they respond to verbal information and provide a verbal response. This certainly loses a high degree of fidelity in comparison with the clinical situation under discussion, which may involve a pulse-oximeter alarm that indicates impending hypoxia prior to the application of the difficult airway algorithm. This loss of fidelity creates a gap between a candidate demonstrating that he or she "knows how," as opposed to the ability to "show how," and depriving the examiners of the ability to assess a great degree of clinical competence. A simulation-based assessment tool capable of assessing the higher levels of Miller's pyramid of competency would certainly provide a tool valued by examinees, certifying bodies, and society at large.

The Australian and New Zealand College of Anesthetists (ANZCA) is one of the first certifying bodies to attempt to apply the potential of HFS to address some of the gaps in the traditional certification process [19]. Since 2002, the College has required its trainees to undergo a simulation-based Effective Management of Anaesthetic Crises (EMAC) course. The two-and-a-half-day course offered in Australia, New Zealand, and Hong Kong consists of five modules consisting of human factors, airway management, cardiovascular emergencies, anesthetic emergencies, and trauma management [19, 20] (Table 8.3). The EMAC course is taught in groups of 12 and utilizes high-fidelity, mannequin-based simulation. Many of the principles taught in this course are based on the anesthesia crisis resource management first described by Gaba and colleagues almost two decades ago [21]. Although participation is compulsory, unlike the summative Israeli and UK OSCE component for certification, assessment is formative, and as such the EMAC is not considered a high-stake assessment. Given the nature of the EMAC, the ANZCA is able to provide exposure and assessment for rare and critical scenarios, an established benefit of HFS.

Maintenance of Certification

In parallel with the recognition by certifying bodies of a need to establish standards for quality in newly trained physicians, there has been an effort to provide meaningful continuing medical education (CME) experiences to ensure continued competency among practicing physicians. The constantly evolving nature of medicine requires physicians to maintain a commitment to lifelong learning as advances in clinical knowledge and management accumulate in their respective fields. As a result, the American Board of Medical Specialties (ABMS) committed member boards to developing Maintenance of Certification (MOC) programs in order that the public could have confidence that physicians were dedicated to the highest standards of patient safety and quality care [22]. In 2004, Maintenance of Certification in Anesthesiology (MOCA) was launched and has evolved over the last decade to its current four-part iteration: Part I: Professionalism and Professional Standing; Part II: Lifelong Learning and Self-Assessment; Part III: Assessment of Knowledge, Judgment; and Part IV: Skills, and Improvements in Medical Practice [23]. The MOCA Part IV requirements can be fulfilled through participation in a simulation-based experience provided by a simulation center endorsed by the American Society of Anesthesiologists (ASA). The ABA was the first of the ABMS boards to include a simulation-based component as a part of its MOC program and in 2010 made this component a requirement of all diplomates [24]. This requirement was subsequently removed in the newest iteration, MOCA 2.0 in 2015 as other options for fulfilling the MOCA Part IV requirement were introduced [23]. Despite the removal of a mandate, the simulation course remains a popular option for anesthesiologists seeking to meet the MOCA Part IV requirements. Much like the ANZCA EMAC, the MOCA simulation course offered at almost 50 American Society of Anesthesiologists (ASA) Simulation Education Network (SEN)-endorsed centers consists largely of high-fidelity, mannequin-based simulation experiences in which elements of intraoperative crisis management are addressed with a high instructor to participant ratio. Unlike the EMAC, a MOCA Part IV simulation course occurs over 6–8 hours during a single day. While each ASA simulation center is granted great leeway in the development of the MOCA course it provides, certain elements are mandated by the ABA: active participation in realistic simulated scenarios followed by postscenario peer debriefing with an emphasis on teamwork and communication, an instructor-to-student ratio of no less than 1 to 5, an opportunity for all participants to be in the "hot seat" role, as the anesthesiologist in charge. While some simulation scenarios will involve hemodynamic disturbances and hypoxemia, scenario content can differ between institutions despite some efforts at standardization [25]. Given the rigorous accreditation process for endorsed centers, by the ASA Simulation Editorial Board, the format, scenario content, and debriefing techniques of each course bear some similarities. Centers may utilize didactic content in varying degrees as a component of postscenario debriefing or introduce partial task trainers to supplement the high-fidelity mannequin-based scenarios. Courses are not pass/fail, no formal evaluation occurs, and participant performance is in no way shared with the ABA. All feedback and assessment are formative and occurs through the facilitated postscenario debriefing process [26]. Video recordings of the sessions may be used to aid in postscenario debriefing but are not used in the creation of any summative report of the participant's performance.

Given that MOCA Part IV activities are meant to produce reflection on practice and practice improvement, immediately following participation in a course, each participant must submit three practice improvement plans to the ABA inspired by their simulation experience. Ninety days later, participants are required to submit an additional report on the status of their implementation to receive full credit for the Part IV component of MOCA. Based on a recent analysis, within 3 months after their simulation experience, over 90% of participants reported having implemented at least one of their proposed improvement plans, most of which fell within three broad categories: system-based practice, teamwork or CRM, and knowledge [27].

In the initial years after the simulation course was introduced as a requirement for MOCA Part IV, feedback was overwhelmingly positive. In a study of the initial 583 diplomates to undergo the course, 99% agreed or strongly agreed with the statement that "course content was relevant to my practice," 94% agreed with the statement that it would "change my practice," and all reported it as a positive experience [24]. Nonetheless, the requirement that all ABA diplomates participate in a MOCA simulation course during each ten-year reaccreditation cycle was not without controversy. At the fore of arguments critical of MOCA simulation lies cost in time and money. The resources required to design and host a six- to eight-hour course are not insignificant, and while it will vary by institution, the cost to register for the course is no less than $1500 per participant. These courses are only offered at a geographically limited number of ASA-endorsed centers leading to potentially substantial travel and lodging expenses for participants [28]. In 2015, based on member feedback, the ABA amended the MOCA Part IV requirements such that simulation became an option among many for fulfilling MOCA Part IV. Despite these changes, simulation remains popular, in part due to its being encouraged by the ABA as the most efficient method for completing MOCA Part IV every 5 years. Participants are awarded 3 credit points for every hour of attendance compared with self-reported documentation of quality improvement initiatives, which are awarded only 1 credit point for each hour of work.

Most recently, the ASA has supported an initiative to introduce screen-based simulation for MOCA Part IV credit. Module 1 of the ASA SimSTAT, or Screen-Based Technology for Advanced Training, was released in July 2017. The program was developed through cooperation with CAE Healthcare and several anesthesiologist consultants recognized as experts in simulation-based education [29]. With the purchase of SimSTAT software, users can access content consisting of scenarios within a virtual operating room (OR) through their personal computer. Taking the role of the primary anesthesiologist, the user will interact with his or her environment by communicating with other providers, administering medications, and using standard anesthesia-related equipment to solve and treat a diagnostic challenge. On-screen monitors will display dynamic changes in the patient's vital signs based on the progression of the scenario and actions taken by the user. At present, five listed modules have been produced involving trauma, appendectomy, robotic surgery, PACU, and labor and delivery. Unlike day-long MOCA courses at ASA-endorsed simulation centers, this format allows for self-directed learning at the user's own pace and convenience and is paired with after-course educational modules produced by Dr. Larry Chu through the Stanford Medicine Anesthesia Informatics and Media (AIM) Lab. Scenarios can be repeated in order to explore the effects of alternative user actions on scenario outcome. While many of the topics well addressed through postscenario small group debriefing such as CRM principles like effective communication, leadership, and role clarity may be less effectively reinforced with a screen-based modality, for other objectives such as medical decision making, interpretation of monitors, and mobilization of resources, the virtual OR may prove to be equally effective. On the other hand, the convenience of an on-demand style software-based program may make screen-based simulation an attractive option for obtaining CME or MOCA credit. SimSTAT is unlikely to replace the demand for live simulation courses for the maintenance of certification but may provide an alternative for those with geographic or other limitations in accessing an ASA-endorsed simulation course.

Conclusion

The demand by our public, health care system, and professional societies for ensuring practitioner competence has led licensing and certifying bodies to seek more effective assessment methods for licensure, primary certification, and continuing certification. The use of simulation technology in healthcare, long valued for its ability to provide repeatable, realistic experiences within a safe environment, has provided multiple tools to meet this demand and is now encountered at the undergraduate, graduate, and postgraduate levels. As an undergraduate medical student, prospective anesthesia trainees encounter simulation-based assessment during the USMLE STEP2 CS, which makes use of OSCE-based simulations and standardized patient encounters, as well as USMLE STEP 3, which incorporates screen-based simulated clinical scenarios. Following residency training, simulation-based assessment is again encountered in the form of the ABA Applied Exam OSCE component, which will test candidates' competence in both technical and non-technical skills. Following initial certification new requirements for maintenance of certification in anesthesiology incorporate mannequin-based, high-fidelity simulation. Immersive screen-based simulation is available as well for those seeking CME and MOCA credit, though this software is likely to change considerably as this technology advances. This trend of increasing utilization of simulation-based technology in summative assessment shows little sign of slowing and creates opportunities for a profession that has always found itself at the forefront of simulation-based education and assessment.

References

1. Banerjee AA. Using simulation for primary certification. Int Anesthesiol Clin. 2015;53:42. Lippincott Williams and Wilkins.
2. Miller GEG. The assessment of clinical skills/competence/performance. Acad Med. 1990;65:S63. Hanley Belfus.
3. AIA L. Standardized patients: the "other" simulation. J Crit Care. 2008;23(2):179.
4. Step 2 Clinical Skills (CS) Content Description and General Information. [Internet] National Board of Medical Examiners and Federation of State Medical Boards of the United States, Inc [updated 2017 May; cited 2017 June 1]. Available from: http://www.usmle.org/pdfs/step-2-cs/cs-info-manual.pdf.
5. Taylor MLM. The relationship between the National Board of Medical Examiners' prototype of the Step 2 clinical skills exam and interns' performance in the six core ACGME competencies. Acad Med. 2005;80(5):496.
6. Alvin MDM. The USMLE Step 2 CS: time for a change. Med Teach. 2016;38(8):854.
7. Winward MLM. The relationship between communication scores from the USMLE step 2 clinical skills examination and communication ratings for first-year internal medicine residents. Acad Med. 2013;88(5):693.
8. Medical simulation in medical education: results of a AAMC survey. [Internet] Association of American Medical Colleges. Washington D.C. 2011. [cited Sept 29]. Available from: https://www.aamc.org/download/259760/data.
9. Step 3 Content Description and General Information. [Internet] National Board of Medical Examinders and Federation of State Medical Boards of the United States, Inc [updated 2016 November; Cited 2017 June 1] Available from.: http://www.usmle.org/pdfs/step-3/2015content_Step3.pdf
10. Levine AI, Schwartz AD, Bryson EO, DeMaria S. Role of simulation in US Physician Licensure and Certification. Mt Sinai J Med. 2012;79:140–53.
11. Steadman RH, Huang YM. Simulation for quality assurance in training, credentialing and maintenance of certification. Best Pract Res Clin Anaesthesiol. 2012;26:3–15.
12. Berkenstadt H, Ziv A, Gafni N, et al. Incorporating simulation-based objective structured clinical examination into the Israeli National Board Examination in anesthesiology. Anesth Analg. 2006;102:853–8.
13. Ben-Menachem EE. Objective structured clinical examination-based assessment of regional anesthesia skills: the Israeli National Board Examination in anesthesiology experience. Anesth Analg. 2011;112:242. Williams & Wilkins.
14. The Royal College of Anaesthetists Examination Overview [Internet]. Accessed June 1. Available from: http://www.rcoa.ac.uk/examinations/primary-frca-osce-soe. http://www.rcoa.ac.uk/node/293.
15. Blew PP. The evolving Royal College examination in anesthesiology. Can J Anesthesia. 2010;57:804. Canadian Anaesthetists' Society.
16. ABA Staged Exam Policy Book [Internet]. American Board of Anesthesiology [updated 2017 February; cited 2017 June 1]. Available from: http://www.theaba.org/PDFs/BOI/StagedExaminations-BOI.

17. Rathmell JPJ. Objective structured clinical examination and board certification in anesthesiology. Anesthesiology (Philadelphia). 2014;120:4. American Society of Anesthesiologists.
18. ABA Applied Examination Objective Structured Clinical Examination Content Outline [Internet] cited June 1 2017. Available from: http://www.theaba.org/PDFs/APPLIED-Exam/APPLIED-OSCE-ContentOutline.
19. Weller J. Effective management of anaesthetic crises: development and evaluation of a college-accredited simulation-based course for anaesthesia education in Australia and New Zealand. Simulation in healthcare: journal of the Society for Medical Simulation. 2006;1:209. Lippincott Williams and Wikins.
20. Effective Management of Anaesthetic Crises Course Handbook. [Internet]. Austraian and New Zealand College of Anaesthetists [updated 2017 February; cited 2017 June 1]. Available from: http://www.anzca.edu.au/documents/eu-emac-course-handbook-20170216-v1-0.pdf.
21. Gaba D, Fish K, Howard S. Crisis management in anesthesiology. 1st ed. London: Churchill Livingston; 1994. p. 290.
22. Miller SHS. American Board of Medical Specialties and repositioning for excellence in lifelong learning: maintenance of certification. J Contin Educ Health Prof. 2005;25:15. John Wiley & Sons Inc.
23. About MOCA 2.0 [Internet]. The American Board of Anesthesiology [cited 2017 June 1]. Available from: http://www.theaba.org/MOCA/About-MOCA-2-0.
24. McIvor WW. Simulation for maintenance of certification in anesthesiology: the first two years. J Contin Educ Health Prof. 2012;32:236. John Wiley & Sons Inc.
25. McIvor WR. A taxonomy of delivery and documentation deviations during delivery of high-fidelity simulations. Simul Healthc. 2017;12(1):1. (1559–2332).
26. Weinger MBM. Misconceptions surrounding the maintenance of certification in anesthesiology simulation course. Anesthesiology (Philadelphia). 2014;121:655. American Society of Anesthesiologists.
27. Steadman RHR. Practice improvements based on participation in simulation for the maintenance of certification in anesthesiology program. Anesthesiology (Philadelphia). 2015;122:1154. American Society of Anesthesiologists.
28. Endorsed Simulation Centers [Internet]. American Society of Anesthesiologists [cited 2017 June 1]. Available from: https://education.asahq.org/totara/asa/core/drupal.php?name=sim-endorsed.
29. Anesthesia SimSTAT [internet]. American Society of Anesthesiologists [cited 2017 June 1]. Available from: https://www.asahq.org/education/simulation-education/anesthesia-simstat.

Leadership and Endorsement

9

Amanda Burden

Introduction

Simulation Leadership: Anesthesiology at the Forefront

Anesthesiologists led efforts to create and expand simulation-based medical education beginning as early as the 1920s (Table 9.1). Their goal in these efforts was improving patient safety. Interest in this educational methodology has exploded during the past decade. More medical schools and hospitals are building simulation programs, and credentialing bodies are beginning to require the addition of simulation to both educational and certification processes. The leadership of anesthesiologists in simulation continues to be a critical force.

Table 9.1 Anesthesiology leaders in simulation

1920s	Lundy	Created laboratory environment to teach physicians practice of regional techniques and to deal with patient challenges in operating room environment
1960s	Safar, Lund	Created process for CPR and forced ventilation; CPR mannequin
1960s	Denson	Created Sim one, first physiologically realistic mannequin
1970s	Cooper	Identified human factor errors in anesthesia incidents; work led to founding of APSF
1980s	Gaba	Created anesthesia crisis resource management; created simulator and realistic simulated environment
1980s	Good, Gravenstein	Created computerized simulator: Gainesville anesthesia simulator

This table highlights the patient safety contributions in anesthesiology leading to the introduction and advancement of simulation [1–4]

Anesthesiologists were the first to develop simulation technology and incorporate simulation into medical education. The earliest record of the use of simulation to educate physicians can be traced to the "anatomy laboratory" that was created by John Lundy, MD. Dr. Lundy, head of anesthesia for the Mayo Clinic in the 1920s, first developed a program to educate surgical fellows in anatomy in an effort to improve their performance of regional anesthesia and as part of an effort to interest them and other physicians in the emerging field of anesthesiology. He created the anatomy laboratory, which consisted of cadavers, so these residents would be able to practice procedures. Initially, surgical residents primarily used this clinic, but it ultimately became a multidisciplinary laboratory [1, 2].

The anatomy laboratory grew at a rapid pace. Dr. Lundy observed that surgical fellows who studied in his laboratory before assisting with patients in the OR were better able to understand the anatomy and regional anesthesia techniques on real patients than those who had not [2, 3]. Dr. Lundy also developed a simulation program that recreated the OR environment so residents could learn how to perform procedures under conditions similar to those in the operating room (OR). This allowed the surgical fellows to practice procedures, learn anatomy, and receive feedback about their performance, which was not possible in the OR [3].

Leadership in Patient Safety

Two mannequin simulators were developed in the 1980s. Developed independently, both were inspired by the research of Jeffrey Cooper, PhD, and his colleagues into error and human factors. Dr. Cooper's research was among the influences leading to the formation of the Anesthesia Patient Safety Foundation (APSF), which was an early funder for simulation research [4–6]. With funding from APSF, David Gaba, MD, and colleagues at Stanford and the Veterans' Affairs Palo Alto Health Care System developed the prototype of a mannequin

A. Burden (✉)
Department of Anesthesiology, Clinical Skills and Simulation, Cooper Medical School of Rowan University, Cooper University Hospital, Camden, NJ, USA
e-mail: burdena@rowan.edu

B. Mahoney et al. (eds.), *Comprehensive Healthcare Simulation: Anesthesiology*, Comprehensive Healthcare Simulation,
https://doi.org/10.1007/978-3-030-26849-7_9

simulator. This new mannequin was able to exhibit vital signs that could be manipulated to simulate critical events. It was housed in a real OR and was surrounded by actual equipment, which created a highly realistic simulation environment to investigate human performance in anesthesiology [7–9]. While performing cardiopulmonary bypass experiments involving animals, Dr. Gaba investigated decision making during patient emergencies [7, 8]. He adapted "crew resource management," an approach to team training used in aviation, to the anesthesia environment, and called it Anesthesia Crisis Resource Management (ACRM) [7, 8]. The course, which is discussed more fully in Chap. 5, concentrates on basic principles of crisis management, which include leadership, teamwork, distribution of workload, communication, use of all available information and resources, and constant re-evaluation of the clinical situation. Dr. Gaba's group used simulation to present and teach ACRM to anesthesiologists and explored clinicians' actions and decision-making in dynamic environments [7, 8].

At the same time Dr. Gaba and his colleagues were working on ACRM, a multidisciplinary team at the University of Florida also received funding from the APSF to develop a simulation program. This effort arose from an interest in improving the clinical skills of anesthesia residents. Led by anesthesiologists Michael Good, MD, and J.S. Gravenstein, MD, the project spawned the Gainesville Anesthesia Simulator, or GAS [10]. (The history of simulation is further described in detail in Chap. 1.)

The American Society of Anesthesiologists

In 2004, the American Society of Anesthesiologists (ASA) appointed a Workgroup on Simulation Education in an effort to identify programs that would appeal to its membership for continuing medical education for attending physician anesthesiologists. Their goal was to organize national network simulation programs. In 2006, the workgroup drafted a white paper, "ASA Approval of Anesthesiology Simulation Programs." Concurrently, the workgroup conducted a survey of ASA members, which revealed that the majority (81%) of the 1350 ASA member respondents had an interest in simulation-based continuing medical education (CME), with a similar percentage (77%) indicating they felt simulation-based CME offered benefits superior to those offered by traditional, lecture-based CME. ASA members identified that features of simulation-based training that were meaningful were a realistic mannequin (77%), a high instructor-to-student ratio (76%), and a realistic simulation of the environment (69%). Videotaping of performance (51%) and multidisciplinary training (50%) were less frequently identified as important elements of simulation-based CME. Additionally, 71% sought an assessment of their performance [11]. Also in 2006, the ASA Committee on Simulation Education was formed to foster access to high-quality simulation-based education for ASA members. The committee developed endorsement criteria for simulation programs, which led to the creation of the Simulation Education Network (SEN). The committee also developed guidelines for the courses, and simulation became an approved component of the Part IV Maintenance of Certification in Anesthesiology (MOCA®) requirement in 2010 [11].

Program Requirements for SEN Membership

The ASA Committee on Simulation Education, which ultimately became the ASA Editorial Board for Simulation-Based Training (SEB), established the required components of a simulation program and created an application process (see Table 9.1). Essential elements of every simulation program include [1] a program director, [2] simulation instructors, [3] content experts, [4] courses, and [5] course directors. Programs are defined by the courses they offer; each program must have a program director with the authority to lead a simulation program by virtue of his or her knowledge of simulation-based instruction, as well as simulation instructors who are also skilled in simulation-based instruction [12]. Additional program requirements closely follow those identified by Issenberg and McGaghie in their comprehensive review of simulation programs (see Table 9.2) [13, 14]. These criteria listed below are intended to provide the minimal requirements for program approval and to encourage programs to continually review and improve their offerings and faculty (see Table 9.3).

Mission Statement The SEB is interested in the program's mission statement and how that informs their course offerings and organization.

Table 9.2 Features of simulation that contribute to effective learning

Features
Feedback: MOST important, provides opportunity for reflection and practice improvement
Repetitive practice with the use of feedback to allow for deliberate practice
Varying degrees of difficulty needed to allow the learner to progress
Multiple learning strategies should be employed
Clinical variation should be appropriate and relevant to participants' practice
Faculty should be able to control the environment
Opportunities for individualized learning should exist
Programs and courses should have defined outcomes and benchmarks
The simulated environment should be realistic
Simulation program should be integrated into a curriculum

This table lists features of simulation programs that provide an effective learning program for participants. Adapted from Issenberg and McGaghie [13]

Table 9.3 Essential elements for American Society of Anesthesiologists (ASA) Simulation Education Network (SEN)

Program overview	Programs should detail their mission statement and overall program goals
Educational programs	Endorsed programs must have robust educational offerings for anesthesiology students, residents, and attending physicians
Scenario	Scenario must be appropriate and relevant for attending physician-level education
Curriculum development	Programs must have a standard process for developing courses and curricula
Instructor and faculty development	Programs must have ongoing faculty development programs for instructors
Leadership	Program director must have appropriate education in use of simulation, institutional support, and time to dedicate to program
Facility and equipment	Infrastructure must be appropriate to support CME offerings
Policies and procedures	Program must address issues of confidentiality and performance anxiety and must continually evaluate and seek to improve its offerings

This table lists the eight application components to become an ASA-endorsed simulation program. Adapted from the ASA website [12]

Educational Offerings The SEB is particularly interested in courses that SEN programs provide, especially the educational objectives and learner populations served.

Curriculum Development Process The program should describe its curriculum development process. This should include information about needs assessment for different learner groups, learning objective development, and the evaluation process used to assure continual improvement.

Scenario A sample scenario must be provided using a standard process like the Duke Scenario Development Template. The scenario presented must be appropriate for and relevant to the practice of attending physicians [15].

Instructor Development The program should have a process for developing, evaluating, and providing credentials for its instructors. This faculty development process should address opportunities for instructors to receive constructive feedback about their performance and opportunities for education and to demonstrate their improvement. Instructors should be evaluated on their ability to educate using simulation, their understanding of and education in simulation and medical education principles, and their expertise in the subject matter for the simulation courses. At least one instructor in each course must be an ABA diplomate enrolled in MOCA.

Program Leadership The program leader is responsible for the ongoing conduct and quality of the simulation program. This individual should have an appropriate educational background and support from the leadership of the institution. She or he must also have appropriate nonclinical time to administer the program and develop the courses.

CME Credit The program should have a track record in providing education for attending physicians and should be able to provide CME credit for the MOCA simulation courses.

Assessing Course Effectiveness An ongoing and reliable process to evaluate course offerings and programming is essential for any simulation program. The program should have a reliable process for participants to evaluate the courses and instructors and should also conduct rigorous self-evaluation. The applicant must document the process for addressing unsatisfactory evaluations and for improving its programs and developing faculty.

Facilities and Technology The program should have the facilities and educational technology needed to conduct simulation courses for attending physicians. The space and equipment should be fully described in the application. The program must also describe how the facilities and equipment are maintained.

Policies and Procedures Policies and procedures are critically important; especially regarding confidentiality and resolving performance anxiety among the participants. The program should have established written policies and procedures regarding these issues as well as the conduct of their courses, mechanisms to assure quality instruction, and issues involving cancellations and refunds.

The American Board of Anesthesiology (ABA)

The ABA initially proposed simulation as a mechanism for practice improvement in January 2010.[11,16] Simulation courses were chosen for these programs for several reasons: (1) its ability to engage and stimulate participants made it likely that improved self-assessment and self-identification of gaps in their practice would result from these programs; (2) simulation can allow clinicians to practice managing critical events that are life-threatening but rarely occur; (3) anesthesiologists can practice leading the team during management of these crisis situations. The simulation courses consist of a one-day simulation course at one of the ASA-endorsed simulation centers. Typically, four to six anesthesiologists participate in these courses; each anesthesiologist acts as the leader in a scenario and manages the patient's care. The MOCA simulation courses (course) address both medical and technical skills required to manage acute perioperative challenges as well as the nontechnical skills of making decisions in dynamic environments and team management. The sessions are debriefed, and participants reflect on their own performances after each simulation scenario, identifying areas in their practice that could be improved. The practice improvements are submitted to ASA. Several weeks later, ASA contacts the participants to identify whether they were able to implement any of the proposed changes or, if not, what barriers were encountered that prevented changes. MOCA simulation is not a test, but is a personal practice assessment and improvement activity [11, 16, 17].

The initial experience with the MOCA simulation activity has been extremely positive. In follow-up surveys, 95% of participants reported that they would recommend simulation to their colleagues, and 98% felt the course was relevant to their practice. Course participants have identified relevance as the most important element of the program. Follow-up surveys identified that 95% of participants had successfully completed changes in their practice based on what they identified during the course [16].

For many of the participants, the nature and impact of these improvements have been impressive. Recently, the follow-up results for more than 1800 self-identified practice improvement plans were reviewed; many compelling, impactful plans were completed, and often the participants overcame barriers and exceeded the scope of the original plan. Examples include plans demonstrating direct benefits for patients related to improving teamwork and communication skills. Other examples of compelling plans include the widespread dissemination of management guidelines (emergency manuals) across departments and across a hospital network. Interprofessional collaboration was remarkable in many instances. Additionally, a participant reported that he used intraosseous insertion techniques he learned during a MOCA simulation course to save a patient's life [17, 18].

Advantages to SEN Membership

Collaboration is the hallmark of the SEN, it is a network of leaders in anesthesiology and in simulation education and their programs. It provides resources to its members, which include a library of scenarios and other shared content. It also provides opportunities for faculty and curricula development, for participating in additional simulation programming, and for networking. Faculty in endorsed programs are expected to participate in the ongoing development and improvement of the educational offerings available to ASA members. Endorsed programs also receive ongoing evaluation data that allows them to gauge participant reaction to their programs and courses.

The advantages to participants in ASA's simulation-based CME courses include experiential training from peer-reviewed programs, an opportunity to improve their knowledge and patient safety through teamwork and critical event training, and a chance to reflect on management of challenging situations in a confidential setting. In addition to CME credit, participants in MOCA simulation courses will be able to receive credit from the ABA toward MOCA.

Medical Malpractice

The use of simulation continues to impact medical malpractice insurance for anesthesiologists. The Risk Management Foundation of the Harvard Medical Institutions Incorporated is 1 of the organizations that combined to form CRICO. The website explanation for them is: rmf.harvard.edu/about-crico - I think the way it is written is OK and is how it has been referenced by them, but wanted to send you this information so you can decide (CRICO) is a patient safety and medical malpractice company that is owned by and serves the Harvard medical community. In 2001, the CRICO Risk Management Foundation began offering insurance premium incentives for anesthesiologists who participated in simulation-based crisis resource management [19, 20]. After several years of simulation courses, CRICO analyzed malpractice claims and concluded that the program had reduced the number and cost of malpractice claims. The company subsequently increased the amount of premium incentives for anesthesiologists who participated in these courses. The benefit was large enough that CRICO worked with the simulation experts to create similar programs in other specialties and a team training program for operating room teams [20]. Other malpractice insurance companies have now made this type of training a component of a group of patient safety provisions that can lead to a reduction in premiums [20, 21].

Simulation and Quality Assurance

As the literature indicates, more evidence linking simulation to direct patient benefits, hospitals and other institutions may mandate simulation as a quality assurance tool [22, 23]. Legislative initiatives such as the Enhancing SIMULATION (Safety in Medicine Utilizing Leading Advanced Simulation Technologies to Improve Outcomes Now) Act, first introduced in the United States Congress in 2007, and again in 2009, have increased awareness among elected officials about this educational method. These efforts, along with increasing research and discussion in the academic literature, have resulted in additional federal funds to encourage further research for simulation as a patient safety tool. The Agency for Healthcare Research and Quality (AHRQ),

Anesthesia Patient Safety Foundation (APSF), Foundation for Anesthesia Education and Research (FAER), and many other specialty societies have allocated funds for simulation research. Furthermore, consensus meetings with simulation experts have generated many questions for collaborative research [24].

As interest in simulation has grown, considerable resources have been dedicated to simulation-based training centers. In addition to the ASA and ABA efforts described earlier, other clinical specialty societies have also established standing committees to endorse simulation education programs. The American College of Surgeons (ACS) created a consortium of ACS-accredited Education Institutes (AEI). These programs offer "global opportunities for collaboration, research, and access to resources" designed to enhance patient safety through simulation. A full description of their application process and programs can be found on the ACS website [25]. The interprofessional society, the Society for Simulation in Healthcare (SSH) whose mission is to "facilitate excellence in healthcare education, practice and research through simulation," also offers accreditation as a quality control for simulation training and research [26].

Justification for Simulation Accreditation

Simulation has been repeatedly identified as a means to address issues of patient safety and practice improvement for attending physicians and residents in all specialties [7, 27, 28]. The ASA Simulation Editorial Board has maintained improving practice and patient safety at the core of its establishment of an educational network of simulation programs. The opportunity for collaboration among simulation programs and faculty represents a unique opportunity to advance patient safety by identifying challenges faced by anesthesiologists and helping to address those issues.

Conclusion

The public demands that physicians maintain their skills, but traditional CME activities are not frequently associated with a change in practice [29]. Substantiation of learning to clinical environments such as that shown in simulation programs has rarely been shown for other educational modalities or CME program [12, 30].

Our specialty has a long tradition of expecting excellence in practice and continued training among our members. We also have a long tradition of advocating for our patients and their safety – anesthesiologists were the first to do that, even in the face of opposition, and long before it was popular. Anesthesiologists have contributed many innovative therapies to the medical community and to patient care that are used each day to make patient care safer. Simulation is only one of these many tools. It is a willingness to do what is right when it is not popular, when it is difficult, and when it requires real effort from each of us that demonstrates the leadership of anesthesiologists. This is what our patients and their families expect of us.

References

1. Lundy JS. Anatomy Service Report, February 14, 1929. In the Collected Papers of John S. Lundy, Mayo Foundation Archive, Rochester; 1929.
2. Ellis TA 2nd, Bacon DR. The anatomy laboratory: a concept ahead of its time. Mayo Clin Proc. 2003;78(2):250–1.
3. Lundy JS. Twenty-one months' experience in operating a dissecting room under the Mayo Foundation. In the Collected Papers of John S. Lundy, Mayo Foundation Archive, Rochester; July 12, 1927.
4. Cooper JB, Taqueti VR. A brief history of the development of mannequin simulators for clinical education and training. Qual Saf Health Care. 2004;13(Suppl 1):i11–8.
5. Cooper JB, Newbower RS, Long CD, et al. Preventable anesthesia mishaps: a study of human factors. Anesthesiology. 1978;49(6):399–406.
6. Anesthesia Patient Safety Foundation. www.apsf.org. Accessed 8 Sept 2016.
7. Gaba DM, Howard SK, Fish K, Smith BE, Sowb YA. Simulation-based training in anesthesia crisis resource management (ACRM): a decade of experience. Simul Gaming. 2001;32(2):175–93.
8. Howard SK, Gaba DM, Fish KJ, Yang G, Sarnquist FH. Anesthesia crisis resource management training: teaching anesthesiologists to handle critical incidents. Aviat Space Environ Med. 1992;63(9):763–70.
9. Holzman RS, Cooper JB, Gaba DM, Philip JH, Small SD, Feinstein D. Anesthesia crisis resource management: real-life simulation training in operating room crises. J Clin Anesth. 1995;7(8):675–87.
10. Good M, Lampotang S, Gibby G. Critical events simulation for training in anesthesiology. J Clin Monit Comput. 1988;4:140.
11. Steadman RH, Berry AJ, Coursin DB, Andrews JJ. Simulation and MOCA®: ASA and ABA perspective, after the first three years. ASA Newsl. 2013;77(8):30–2.
12. American Society of Anesthesiologists Simulation Education. https://education.asahq.org/totara/asa/core/drupal.php?name=sim-endorsed. Accessed 11 Sept 2016.
13. Issenberg SB, McGaghie WC, Petrusa ER, Lee Gordon D, Scalese RJ. Features and uses of high-fidelity medical simulations that lead to effective learning: a BEME systematic review. Med Teach. 2005;27(1):10–28.
14. McGaghie WC, Issenberg SB, Petrusa ER, Scalese RJ. Effect of practice on standardized learning outcomes in simulation-based medical education. Med Educ. 2006;40(8):792–7.
15. Duke University Template for Case-Based Scenarios. http://anesthesiology.duke.edu/?page_id=825706. Accessed 11 Sept 2016.
16. McIvor W, Burden A, Weinger MB, Steadman R. Simulation for maintenance of certification in anesthesiology: the first two years. J Contin Educ Health Prof. 2012;32:236–42.
17. Steadman RH, Burden AR, Huang YM, Gaba DM, Cooper JB. Practice improvements based on participation in simulation for the maintenance of certification in anesthesiology program. Anesthesiology. 2015;122(5):1154–69.
18. Anson JA. MOCA saves a life [letter]. ASA Newsl. 2013;77(1):47.
19. Hanscom R. Medical simulation from an insurer's perspective. Acad Emerg Med. 2008;15:984–7.

20. CRICO/RMF. Clinician resources: team training https://www.rmf.harvard.edu/Clinician-Resources/Article/2014/OR-Team-Training-Incentive Accessed 24 Aug 2016.
21. The Doctors Company Resources. http://www.thedoctors.com. Accessed 24 Aug 2016.
22. Geis GL, Pio B, Pendergrass TL, et al. Simulation to assess the safety of new healthcare teams and new facilities. Simul Healthc. 2011;6(3):125–33.
23. Hamman WR, Beaudin-Seiler BM, Beaubien JM, et al. Using simulation to identify and resolve threats to patient safety. Am J Manag Care. 2010;16(6):e145–50.
24. Dieckmann P, Phero JC, Issenberg SB, et al. The first research consensus summit of the Society for Simulation in healthcare: conduction and a synthesis of the results. Simul Healthc. 2011;6(6 Suppl):S1–9.
25. American College of Surgeons, Division of Education Accredited Education Institutes, Enhancing Patient safety Through Simulation. Accessed 21 Sept 2016. http://www.facs.org/education/accreditationprogram/requirements.html.
26. Society for Simulation in Healthcare Council for Accreditation of Healthcare Simulation Programs Informational Guide for the Accreditation Process from the SSH Council for Accreditation of Healthcare Simulation Programs. Accessed 21 Sept 2016. http://ssih.org/cats-accreditation.
27. Institute of Medicine. Crossing the quality chasm: a new health delivery system for the 21st century. Washington, D.C.: National Academy Press; 2001.
28. ACGME. Simulation: new revision to program requirements. RRC News Anesthesiology. March 2011; Sect. 1–6. http://www.acgme.org/Portals/0/PFAssets/PublicationsNewsletters/Anesthesiology_Newsletter_Mar11.pdf
29. Davis D, O'Brien MA, Freemantle N, et al. Impact of formal continuing medical education: do conferences, workshops, rounds, and other traditional continuing education activities change physician behavior or health care outcomes? JAMA. 1999;282(9):867–74.
30. Steadman RH. Improving on reality: can simulation facilitate practice change? Anesthesiology. 2010;112(4):775–6.

Part II

Simulation Modalities and Technologies

Standardized Patients

10

Roxane Gardner

Introduction

Brief History of Standardized Patients in Healthcare Education and Assessment

The history of using standardized patients as a technique for healthcare simulation-based education is rich, and their use has generated revolutionary changes in training and assessment of healthcare professionals. A number of key individuals and events that have contributed greatly to the field of standardized patients will be highlighted in this section. First and foremost are Dr. Howard Barrows and Professor Stephen Abrahamson at the University of Southern California School of Medicine, Los Angeles, who were concerned about ensuring consistency in testing the clinical skills of medical students. They reported in 1964 their novel assessment technique described as the "programmed patient" [1]. The programmed patient involved training a professional model with acting ability to simulate a patient's signs and symptoms for assessing medical students during their clinical clerkships. This technique involved "training a professional model-actress to simulate a neurological disorder," having students complete a neurological workup and write-up of their encounter, and having the simulated patient provide each student written feedback on their clinical performance. Thereafter, the faculty reviewed the write-ups and corresponding simulated patient's feedback reports with each student. Barrows and Abrahamson concluded their technique avoided problems using observers, guaranteed that the patient and medical circumstances would be constant for all examinees, and allowed faculty to determine how best to modify the curriculum by learning from their students' missteps. Barrows later defined a "simulated patient" as a person trained to perform as a patient who gives a history and simulates clinical findings of a disease or illness [2].

In 1970, Dr. Ray Helfer, from the University of Colorado Medical Center in Denver, described his use of "programmed mothers," women trained to portray mothers of a seriously ill child with underlying psychosocial issues, in effort to standardize assessment of medical students' interviewing skills. He looked to compare differences between cohorts of beginner and advanced medical student [3]. Dr. Paula Stillman, together with her colleagues, capitalized on Helfer's work by training and rehearsing two non-physician actual mothers to consistently give a history of a child's illness [4]. These "patient simulators" were then trained to score the content and process of a medical student's interviewing skills and give them immediate post-interview evaluative feedback. In this way, trained mothers were used as teachers and evaluators of medical students. Stillman and colleagues later used the term "patient instructor" (PI) for describing a non-physician, simulated patient who serves in multiple roles as patient, teacher, and evaluator [5, 6].

In 1985, Norman and colleagues used the term "standardized patient" (SP) to "…include both healthy individuals and patients with chronic, stable physical findings who have been trained to present a clinical problem repeatedly and consistently" [7]. However, Barrows viewed SP as an umbrella term for both a simulated patient and actual patient who had been trained to present the illness in a standardized way [8]. Furthermore, a standardized patient was one who had been carefully coached to simulate an actual patient so accurately that a skilled clinician could not detect the simulation. According to Barrows, the SP "represent[ed] the gestalt of the patient being simulated; not just the history but the body language, the physical findings, and the emotional and personality characteristics as well" [9]. Collins and Harden further broadened the definition of SP in 1998 to include

R. Gardner (✉)
Department of Obstetrics & Gynecology, Brigham and Women's Hospital, Boston, MA, USA

Harvard Medical School, Boston, MA, USA

Department of Anesthesia, Critical Care and Pain Medicine, Massachusetts General Hospital, Boston, MA, USA

Center for Medical Simulation, Boston, MA, USA
e-mail: RGARDNER1@PARTNERS.ORG; rgardner1@bwh.harvard.edu

B. Mahoney et al. (eds.), *Comprehensive Healthcare Simulation: Anesthesiology*, Comprehensive Healthcare Simulation,
https://doi.org/10.1007/978-3-030-26849-7_10

a person with or without actual disease who is trained to consistently portray a medical condition [10]. They viewed standardized patients as being on *a continuum*, ranging from real patients with no training (who portrayed themselves and their medical condition) to simulated patients who were extensively trained and rehearsed to portray a medical condition. They deemed standardization was easier to achieve with a simulated patient who was extensively trained and rehearsed. Churchouse and McCafferty later articulated their distinctions between these terms in 2012, with simulated patient (SiP) being a normal layperson or actor who must be trained and coached carefully to play a patient or directed to take a role in a simulation and standardized patient (SP) being a real patient or a person with or without actual disease who portrays themselves consistently in a healthcare learning activity and may be trained to give feedback as required [11]. Beigzadeh and colleagues' more recent review of the literature for exact definitions of these two terms concurs with that of Churchouse and McCafferty [12]. Despite such distinctions, the terms "simulated patient" and "standardized patient" are often used interchangeably. However, clarity about the differences is relevant to their training, performance, and management as well as in research-related activities [12].

Standardized patients (SPs), whether real or simulated, have become an integral part of a medical school's curriculum for consistently and realistically portraying a patient case for training students, for assessing their competency, and as part of the licensure process for practicing medicine [13–15]. Harden and colleagues first reported on the objective structured clinical exam (OSCE) in 1975, a standardized assessment technique that included simulated patients who were doctors posing as patients [16]. Similar to today's version, the OSCE consisted of multiple stations around which learners or examinees rotate and perform clinical or procedural tasks. Adoption and spread of the OSCE assessment technique coupled with the need to provide consistent teaching and learning experiences in undergraduate and postgraduate clinical education facilitated growth in the use of SP methodologies [14, 17]. Dr. Stillman worked closely with Dr. David Swanson to develop a program using standardized patients for teaching and assessing third-year medical students on how to obtain medical histories and how to interact with ambulatory patients with common problems [18]. Stillman, Swanson, and others were subsequently instrumental in advancing the use of SPs and OSCE format for assessing medical students and for residents on a regional basis, specifically New England [19, 20]. In 1993, Anderson, Stillman, and Wang surveyed medical schools in the United States and Canada to determine how SPs were being used for education and evaluation of clinical skills [21]. They reported that 138 of 142 (97%) schools responded; and 111 of 138 (80%) respondents reported using SPs, corresponding to 17 more schools than in a similar survey in 1989. Compared to results of the prior survey, the 1993 survey respondents reported greater use of SPs in teaching and evaluating interview and history-taking skills of medical students and broader application of SPs in the process of physical examination beyond the male and female genital area. Lane and Rollins reviewed the literature up to 2005 for use of simulated patients and role-play in communication skills training and found them to be used worldwide [22]. Currently, SP methodologies are employed worldwide across the spectrum of health professions training and assessment programs, including ones in anesthesiology as discussed later in this chapter [14, 15, 23].

A number of national and international organizations, agencies, and societies have also contributed greatly to the history, research, and support of SP methodologies. A comprehensive history of their contributions is beyond the scope of this chapter; however, several key events will be highlighted. During the 1980s, the Josiah Macy Jr. Foundation strongly supported the development of clinical practice exams that incorporated standardized patients and provided six grants to support medical schools in developing clinical skills assessment centers where SPs would be used in evaluating students [8, 21]. Around this same time, under the leadership of Dr. Stillman, the Association of the American Medical Colleges created a Special Interest Group on Standardized Patients (AAMC SIG SPs) to unify and facilitate collaboration among those interested in this field [8]. The AAMC subsequently convened a Consensus Conference on the Use of Standardized Patients in the Teaching and Evaluation of Clinical Skills in 1992 [24]. The aims of this conference were to gather ideas and understand issues of concern and areas of agreement and differing points of view in the application of standardized patient methodologies in medical teaching, learning, and assessment.

The Medical Council of Canada (MCC) and the General Medical Council of the United Kingdom (GMC UK) contributed greatly to the history of SPs and OSCEs. In 1992, MCC was the first agency to pioneer their use in the qualification process for obtaining a license to practice medicine in Canada [25, 26]. The GMC UK has included SP-based assessments in their Professional Linguistics and Assessment Board (PLAB) since 1998 [27, 28]. Similar efforts to incorporate SPs in the process of certifying foreign medical graduates to enter graduate medical education programs had begun in the late 1980s in the United States of America (USA) [29]. Inclusion of SPs within the Educational Commission on Foreign Medical Graduates (ECFMG) clinical skills assessment (CSA) methods became official on an international basis by 1998 [30]. The ECFMG CSA was later replaced in 2004 with the United States Medical Licensing Exam (USMLE) Step 2, which included assessment of clinical skills (CS) with SPs in an OSCE format. Since then, graduates of international medical schools are required to take and pass the USMLE Step 2 CS to qualify for a medical license to practice in the USA [31]. Likewise, the National Board of Osteopathic Medical Examiners (NBOME) incorporated SP-based clinical skills assessment for licensure of osteopathic physicians in the USA. The launch of the Comprehensive Osteopathic Medical Licensing Examination Level 2-Performance Evaluation (COMLEX-USA Level 2-PE) took place in 2004. Boulet and colleagues described the advent of SP-based examinations for certification and licensure in medicine as a "monumental achievement" [31].

The Association for Medical Education in Europe (AMEE) and the Association of Standardized Patient Educators (ASPE) have manifested ongoing support and continued efforts to advance the field of SP-based education and assessment. The AMEE was formed in the 1970s with the support of the World Health Organization (WHO). Their aim, as an international association of medical educators from 31 countries, was to encourage communication and collaboration between them. The AMEE has cultivated an international reputation for promoting appreciation and improving education and research in SP and OSCE methodologies and has published numerous guides on various aspects of this topic [8, 10, 14, 32–37]. Likewise, ASPE has garnered an international reputation for promoting best practices in SP methodology and advancing application in the use of this technique for teaching, assessment, and research. ASPE originated from the membership of the AAMC SIG SPs, launching in 2001 as a professional society for health profession educators involved with SP methodologies to organize, share their ideas, and compare and disseminate best practices [38, 39]. Members of ASPE collaborated in the early 2000s to develop a survey aimed at identifying how various programs were approaching SP development and assuring quality in their performance [40]. Four countries with SP programs (Scotland, Ireland, Netherlands, and Belgium) were selected as representing the European experience. Cantillon and colleagues found, of the 22 medical schools surveyed, 19 (86%) responded; and most of these programs reported they employed amateur actors or had volunteer patients serve as SPs. Most viewed SP programs as expensive, yet there seemed to be nil sharing of resources between different centers in the same country; and there was no consistency in assuring quality in SP performance. However, they found respondents were very interested in establishing an SP education networking organization in Europe. These findings resulted in a formal 5-year agreement between AMEE and ASPE to hold a daylong preconference for SP teachers at the annual AMEE meetings as a way to facilitate collaboration and sharing of ideas and resources.

In the field of anesthesiology, the Royal College of Anaesthetists introduced SP-OSCEs into postgraduate examinations in 1994 [41] and examination procedures for obtaining fellowship status in the Royal College of Anaesthetists by 1997 [42, 43]. Ziv et al. reported in 2007 on endeavors undertaken since 2003 to incorporate simulation and SP-OSCE methodologies into the Tel Aviv University Sackler School of Medicine's admissions selection process and into the high-stakes Israeli national board examination in anesthesiology [30]. Such undertakings by Ziv et al. triggered systematic evaluation and modification of residency curricula for training and assessment of clinical skills. The Australian and New Zealand College of Anesthetists (ANZCA) also undertook similar efforts as they incorporated SP-OSCEs into the final exam required for completion of residency training [44, 45].

The history would be incomplete without highlighting the influential prowess of the Accreditation Council for Graduate Medical Education (ACGME) and the American Board of Medical Specialties (ABMS) in their endorsement of SP-based and OSCE format assessments for use in residency training programs. ACGME, established in 1981, collaborated with ABMS in the 1990s to identify general competencies applicable across graduate medical education programs and focus attention on educational outcomes with respect to decisions involving accreditation [46, 47]. Beginning in 1998 and known as "The Outcomes Project", the competencies were categorized and finalized into six domains (patient care, medical knowledge, practice-based learning and improvement, interpersonal and communication skills, professionalism, and systems-based practice) by the following year. ACGME and ABMS next created the first version of a "Toolbox of Assessment Methods." Released for distribution in 2000, the toolbox supported SP-based OSCE assessment methods as reliable, valid, and fair, especially for assessing domains of communication, professionalism, and systems-based practice [46, 48]. ACGME mandated that all residents be taught and assessed in the six general competency domains as of 2002 [46, 47, 49]. However, Tetzlaff noted in 2007 that, even though leaders in the specialty of anesthesiology had responded positively to The Outcomes Project, it took several years for the society to work toward compliance [50]. ACGME transitioned from The Outcomes Project to "Next Accreditation System" between 2013 and 2014, which led to the requirement that anesthesiology residency programs evaluate residents on 25 specific, defined competency milestones [51, 52]. Furthermore, the American Board of Anesthesia (ABA) introduced a "Staged Exam" system that would be applicable to all residents entering training programs as of 2012. This system expanded the board certification exams from an oral exam format to include a series of OSCE stations, some of which would utilize SPs. As a result of these changes, Isaak et al. designed a training program that included twice yearly and standardized OSCE assessment of their anesthesia residents' milestone competencies, experiences that would help them prepare for high-stakes OSCE examinations they would encounter in the process of their board certification [52].

Evidence Associated with Use of Standardized Patients

A wealth of evidence has accumulated since the early days of Barrows and Stillman substantiating the reliability and effectiveness of SP methodologies in clinical skills training, assessments, and high-stakes examinations [8–15, 23, 25–31, 37, 53–67]. Despite the high regard for SP-based teaching, learning, and assessment, efforts to strengthen the evidence-based support for its use are ongoing as evidenced by the following key articles. In their 1990 "state-of-the-art" article, van der Vleuten and Swanson reviewed and analyzed the psychometric properties of SP-based assessments in published and some unpublished large-scale studies [53]. They examined studies for reliability of SP-based scores and pass-fail decisions and for validity of SP-based test score interpretation and the educational impact of such scores. They found inter-rater reliability of SP-based scores varied from 0.42 to 0.93, with the majority (13 of 15) having a Cohen's kappa indicating at least "substantial agreement" (Cohen's kappa >0.60) among the raters. Variation in examinee performance from station to station was identified as the major source of measurement error; therefore, van der Vleuten and Swanson recommended SP tests which include a large number of stations to obtain stable, reproducible assessments of clinical skills. Although disagreement between raters about observed performance and differences between SPs playing the same role can each contribute to measurement error, van der Vleuten and Swanson advised random assignment of examinees to raters and SPs to minimize such effect. While they deemed the results of the validation studies generally favorable, they recommended future research on the impact of scoring procedures; the effects of rater and SP bias; effect of station format and timing; and examinee perception of tasks they are asked to perform. Finally, van der Vleuten and Swanson found little attention had been paid to better understand the educational impact of SP tests on examinees or on the SPs themselves. They recommended future research target all of these topics because of continued growth in SP-based assessments despite their high costs and gaps in fully understanding their psychometric properties and educational impact.

A major aim in performance assessment is to minimize measurement error, an imperative in high-stakes testing [59]. Boulet et al. in 2003 conducted a detailed analysis of ECFMG CSA scores obtained from over 7000 examinees in 2001 and offered several strategies for assuring quality and validity of scores obtained in SP-based performance assessments. They recommended both qualitative and quantitative measures to address two major sources of error, those due to exam content or task sampling and those due to scoring inconsistencies, so that scores obtained were accurate and kept "reasonably free from error." Such measures included a) ensuring case development be informed by knowledgeable, expert professionals; b) standardized procedures for training SPs in their portrayal of a case, the SPs' use of scoring rubrics, and systematic provision of feedback to SPs about their performance; c) using standardized, validated scoring rubrics and checklists; d) employing standardized procedures for administering examinations; and e) stringent monitoring of SP and case performance to identify deficiencies and adjust accordingly. Furthermore, they advised application of generalizability theory as a statistical technique for investigating adequacy of case development and analyzing scoring inconsistencies. Generalizability theory (G theory) allows investigators to estimate multiple sources of error simultaneously and examine the interaction effects across the sources of error; and it can be used to provide alternative strategies for improving dependability of the measures [68]. It is noteworthy that van der Vleuten and Swanson had also recommend the use of G theory for analyzing and reporting results of psychometric analysis of SP-based tests precisely because SP methodologies are subject to multiple sources of error [53]. The recommendations of Boulet et al. in 2003 underscore the significance of those made previously by van der Vleuten and Barrows in 1990.

In their 2009 guide on the use of SPs in training healthcare professionals, Cleland, Abe, and Rethans expressed concern that randomized controlled trials had not yet been conducted comparing SP performance against real patients or role-playing with colleagues [14]. They advocated for conducting robust, well-designed studies on the use of SPs and their impact on teaching and learning on the learners and the SPs themselves; greater use of validated data collection tools and metrics; and researchers to provide detailed information about exactly what training SPs receive prior to their use. In the same year, May, Park, and Lee published their findings of a 10-year review of the literature on the value of using SPs in teaching and learning [15]. They confined their search to English-language articles published between January 1996 and December 2005 and identified 69 articles. Studies identified for inclusion were evaluated with a modified version of Freeth's model of educational outcomes evaluation (a modification of Kirkpatrick's 4 level model of education evaluation). Most studies (59%) reported on satisfaction, changes in knowledge (62.3%), or changes in skills (62.3%), outcomes corresponding to Kirkpatrick levels 1 and 2. Only 6% of studies reported on behavioral change (Kirkpatrick level 3); none reported outcomes related to organization change or change in patient health and well-being (Kirkpatrick level 4). May, Park, and Lee deemed that, although SPs have value and are commonly used on a widespread basis across the fields of health professions education, most of the studies they reviewed had weak research design. They, like Cleland, Abe, and Rethans, urged more rigorous research methodology be employed in future studies to strengthen the evidence for use of SPs in healthcare education.

Baig and colleagues were also concerned about the impact of SPs on reliability of OSCE assessments [66]. They examined the accuracy of SP portrayal of a case, including concordance of appearance and symptom complex and portrayal of the same case by different SPs. They video recorded four of ten OSCE stations, wherein four different SPs were trained per case. Two physicians were trained to use station-specific rating instruments designed according to each specific station's guidelines. Reliability of the rater scores ranged from Cronbach's alpha of 0.47 to 0.74, with most of the differences attributed to lack of consistency in facial expressions portrayed by the 4 SPs trained for their stations. Consequently, they advocated on behalf of more rigorous training and constant monitoring of SPs for quality assurance to ensure examinee scores accurately reflect examinee skills and measurement error is kept to a minimum.

Keifenheim, Teufel, and Ip et al. conducted a systematic literature review of the quality of educational interventions used to teach history-taking skills and published their findings in 2015 [67]. They searched the literature from January 1990 to June 2014 for articles on history-taking for medical students, yielding 1254 potentially relevant ones of which 23 were included for in-depth analysis. They evaluated study quality using the Medical Education Research Study Quality Instrument (MERSQI), a 10-item education research studies evaluation tool that was designed and validated by Reed, Cook, and Beckman et al. in 2007 [69]. The maximum possible MERSQI score is 18, ranging from 5 to 18. According to Keifenheim and colleagues, the mean MERSQI score for the 23 studies they reviewed was 10.4 with scores ranging from 6.5 to 14. Ten of the 23 studies involved SPs, the majority of which achieved MERSQI scores of 9 or greater. Keifenheim's team expressed support for the use of SP-based tests, especially those using an OSCE format, and regarded such as "gold standard in assessing history-taking skills." However, they encouraged employing more rigorous research methodologies, especially when comparing educational approaches for superiority in outcomes.

Based on the studies highlighted, there is a clarion call to strengthen the evidence-based support for the use of SP-based methodologies. Indeed, researchers and educators have an ethical and education science imperative to devise more rigorous training and monitoring of programs for quality assurance involving SPs and to use more robust research methods in the design and evaluation of such projects and programs.

Examples of SP Use in Anesthesiology and the Surgical Disciplines

In 2005, Dr. Elizabeth Sinz strongly advocated for utilizing simulation-based methodologies in anesthesiology training programs and specifically the cardiac, thoracic, and vascular subspecialties [70]. Whether used in clinical encounters or OSCEs or incorporated into scenarios involving mannequin-based simulation or "hybrid simulation" (combining an SP with a part-task trainer for training), Sinz expressed high regard for SPs and considered them as the "highest fidelity simulator." She deemed SP methodology extremely useful in training for difficult conversations such as delivering bad news or disclosing medical error, managing family interactions, or conducting family meetings. Similarly, Lake supported the use of SPs for teaching in cardiovascular and vascular anesthesiology [71].

Drs. Levine and Swartz regarded SP-based education in the field of anesthesia as "an ideal format" for teaching, learning, and evaluating critical skills of communication with interprofessional colleagues, patients, and their families, professionalism, and empathy toward trainees [48]. Even though for decades the field of anesthesiology had championed simulation-based education, Levine and Swartz acknowledged in 2008 that SP methodologies had been underutilized in the training of anesthesiologists. They described two SP-based cases that exemplified how clinical skills of anesthesiologists can be trained and assessed. Case 1 involved a woman with undiagnosed bleeding disorder who is about to have an elective surgery. The anesthesiology trainee is expected to (1) conduct the preoperative anesthesia history and physical examination and uncover the potential of coagulopathy; (2) develop an appropriate plan, including whether to delay or cancel the surgery; and (3) discuss the plan with both the patient and surgeon. In this case, both the SP and the standardized surgeon roles should be well scripted for consistency across all trainee assessment experiences. Case 2 involves incorrect, inadvertent administration of a medication that triggered myocardial ischemia and congestive heart failure during induction of general anesthesia in a patient undergoing elective surgery. Depending on their level of training, the trainee(s) could be asked to conduct a difficult conversation with the standardized surgeon or with the SP's "standardized family" or both. Levine and Swartz offered numerous suggestions for which SPs could be used in the process of training and assessment, ranging from conducting difficult conversations or managing difficult interactions with interprofessional colleagues, patients, or families; obtaining consent or managing refusal of consent; explaining procedures to patients; managing a patient's expectations that may be potentially unreasonable; or dealing with colleagues with whose care the trainee disagrees. They concluded only one's imagination limited the incorporation of SPs into anesthesia training.

Kneebone, Nestel, and Wetzel et al. of the Imperial College of London cogently argued for broader use of SPs within simulations and combining SPs with part-task trainers (hybrid simulators) to achieve "patient-focused simulation (PFS)" as a means to encourage buy-in by clinician participants [72]. They describe how they incorporated SPs into low-, mid-, and high-complexity clinical procedures for teaching and learning. In particular, they developed a PFS carotid endarterectomy (CEA) simulation for training a full surgical team and conducted a multifaceted performance assessment of the surgeon's technical and nontechnical skills. They found the PFS CEA simulation to be feasible and perceived by participants as having a high degree of realism.

A unique application of SP methodology, published in 2008, was the development and evaluation of a "simulated anesthetist" (SA) training program for actors [73]. Nestel, Black, and Kneebone et al. assessed the feasibility of using actor-anesthetists as a way to solve the problem of not having a real anesthetist available to participate in CEA simulations due to last-minute schedule changes. Three actors were recruited from their SP program and, using a variety of educational techniques, trained them to portray authentic anesthetist behaviors. Such techniques included use of written materials, direct observations of anesthetists, role-play with feedback by simulation faculty and by real surgeons; direct audio support during the simulation; and notes written by the SAs on their experiences and reflections immediately after each simulation. Intensive focus group interviews of the three SAs were also conducted after completion of the pilot series of CEA simulations. The SAs participated in a total of 34 CEA scenarios involving 17 surgeons ranging from junior doctor to expert consultant. Nestel et al. found that SAs regarded the program as valuable and came to feel confident in their performance in spite of initial anxieties. At the conclusion of each simulation, surgeons rated the authenticity of the anesthetist (SA) on a scale of 0–10, with scores ranging from 2 to 10 and a mean of 8.1. High-level ratings were supported by positive comments obtained in post-simulation interviews with the surgeons. However, the consultant surgeons were more likely than novices to be critical about the SA performance after learning their anesthetist was actually an actor. This suggested something about perceived credibility that is worth considering, as there may be some risk in using standardized providers and revealing their actual backgrounds are not what they portrayed. A major advantage of this SA program was fewer cancellations of scheduled simulation sessions. Nestel et al. postulated that simulation of other professionals could remedy the problem of cancellation of scheduled training when clinicians are pulled to provide patient care. Nestel et al. noted their study was limited by not directly involving anesthetists in training the SAs beyond reviewing written materials and permitting themselves to be observed by SAs. However, they felt SAs were trained to be authentic from the surgeon's perspective, but not the anesthetist, a provocative notion since they didn't know if or to what degree such differences in perspectives existed a priori. This presents an interesting topic for future research.

The team of Hoelzer, Moeschler, and Seamans published their work in 2015 on using SPs for teaching pain medicine fellows, which provided example templates and case-related storylines involving a patient undergoing a stellate ganglion block under fluoroscopic guidance that became a total spinal [74]. The pain fellow managing the case must have initiated resuscitative procedures, stabilized the patient, and then conversed with a family member (SP) about the complication and updated them on the patient's status. Hoelzer's team developed and integrated this simulation into their Pain Medicine Fellowship curriculum as one way to evaluate ACGME core competencies of professionalism and communication and to provide opportunities for pain medicine fellows to participate in difficult patient interactions. They also suggested possible SP-based scenarios to consider for an anesthesiology residency curriculum such as disclosing wrong-sided procedure or procedural complication with a patient or family member(s), obtaining consent, discussing unexpected findings or end-of-life issues with patients, and using a medical interpreter.

Within the confines of this chapter, it is not possible to provide a comprehensive guide for developing, implementing, and monitoring an SP-based educational program for anesthesiologists. However, several more recently published articles serve as excellent resources [14, 48, 74]. Cantrell and Deloney offer additional general suggestions and issues to consider when integrating SPs into healthcare simulations [75]. A complementary article by Motola, Devine, and Chung et al. provides a practical, evidence-based general guide for introducing simulation in healthcare education that is applicable to implementing SP-based programs [8d]. Additional excellent resources can be found on ASPE's website, www.aspeducators.org, and in Nestel and Bearman's textbook on simulated patient methodology [76].

Future Directions for SP and Virtual Patient Use in Anesthesiology

A wealth of knowledge about SP methodologies has accumulated over the past five decades since Barrows and Abrahamson first reported on their novel assessment technique. Moreover, since the 1990s, there has been steady growth in the use of SPs by anesthesiology residency programs, societies, and professional organizations for training and assessment. In view of this, the future looks bright for SP methodologies becoming systematically incorporated within anesthesiology training and assessment programs on a worldwide basis. Not only has portrayal of patients been standardized; standardized portrayals have broadened to include family members and even healthcare providers, such the "standardized anesthesiologist" described by Nestel et al. [73]. Such portrayals will likely expand to include other disciplines and professions over time.

In addition to use of SPs, efforts have been undertaken to develop virtual patients (VPs), computerized versions of a standardized patient. Such technique was first described in 1971 by Harless, Drennon, and Marxer et al. [77]. Harless et al. developed a "computer-aided simulation of a clinical encounter," also known as CASE. CASE was used to provide an interactive simulated clinical encounter and simulated patient management for trainees. The computer acts as the simulated (and standardized) patient. This technique offers the possibility of longitudinal care that can be condensed over the length of the trainee's rotation or expanded to encompass the trainee's entire academic experience. Results from a survey of their use at medical schools in the USA and Canada were reported in 2007 by Huang, Reynolds, and Candler [78]. They surveyed 142 schools, of which 108 responded, and found that 26 were using virtual patients in their curriculum. They created the first formal inventory about information on use of virtual patients at medical schools in North America, including technical requirements; program, case, and production characteristics; and willingness to share their programs. While they confirmed that virtual patients were well received and facilitated cognitive and behavioral skill acquisition, they found that widespread integration into medical education curricula was lacking. Ellaway, Poulton, and Fors et al. advocated for a commons model to support collaboration and sharing among healthcare education communities about VP methodologies, including the costs of VP case design, implementation, assessment, and research [79]. In 2009, Cook and Triola published their review of the literature on virtual patients and noted that use of computer-based instruction was associated with improved learning over no intervention [80]. They found little difference in the information elicited or number of correct diagnoses obtained when using VPs compared to SPs; however, VPs were treated less warmly and empathically than SPs. They also reported that the research on best practices for VP methodologies was "currently virtually nonexistent." That said, VPs have come to be used in Hong Kong undergraduate anesthesiology and acute pain management coursework [81–83]. Leung, Critchley, Yung, and Kumta undertook efforts to evaluate final-year medical students at Chinese University Hong Kong (CUHK) while rotating in their 2-week anesthesia course using a new longitudinal VP storyline (SL) learning system compared to their Formative Assessment Case Studies (FACS) VP system [84]. They found students using the FACS VP system to learn about acute pain management obtained better scores in their examinations (multiple choice and essays) compared to those using the longitudinal VP SL system. While they could not judge the education role and benefits of using the VP SL, they noted that it used a more English narrative style and provided less interactivity for the learners who were more likely to know English as a second language. Such factors are worthy of consideration when designing and implementing VP learning systems.

In 2014, Schwid and Souter described their decades of experience with using VPs for training first-year anesthesia residents [85]. First used in 1989, completion of a series of VP simulator scenarios was required of all first-year residents as of 1991. Schwid and Souter conducted a survey to evaluate resident perception and use of the VP system and conducted a cost analysis of implementing such curriculum over a 20-year time period [86]. They found that of the 404 residents, 252 (62%) completed the surveys and 97% deemed the VP curriculum as worthwhile; 88% rated it as realistic and 97% felt better prepared to handle anesthesia-related critical events. They estimated cost of their software and faculty time implementing the VP curriculum over 20 years averaged out to about USD $16.00 per hour. Based on their experiences, they concluded that the VP learning system was easy to incorporate into their residency training program, their anesthesiology residents felt better prepared to manage critical events, and the VP system was a low-cost training modality, serving as a cost-effective way to supplement use of mannequin-based simulation training. The use of VPs provides a viable, relatively low-cost solution to reducing the length of time in skill acquisition and competency assessment in the face of time constraints in work hours and financial resources.

Conclusion

When looking to the future, it's important for healthcare educators to gain a better understanding of how to best utilize SP, VP, and mannequin-based methodologies, either independently or in some combination thereof, for learning and assessment of trainees. The need is great for strengthening the evidence-based support for using such methodologies. Indeed, researchers and educators have an ethical and education science imperative to devise more rigorous training and monitoring of programs for quality assurance involving SPs, VPs, and mannequin-patients and to use more robust research methods in the design and evaluation of such projects and programs.

References

1. Barrows HS, Abrahamson S. The programmed patient: a technique for appraising student performance in clinical neurology. J Med Educ. 1964;39:802–5.
2. Barrows HS. Simulated patients in medical teaching. Can Med Assoc J. 1968;98:674–6.
3. Helfer RE. An objective comparison of the pediatric interviewing skills of freshman and senior medical students. Pediatrics. 1970;45(4):623–7.
4. Stillman PL, Sabers DL, Redfield DL. The use of paraprofessionals to teach interviewing skills. Pediatrics. 1976;57(5):769–74.
5. Stillman PL, Ruggill JS, Rutala PJ, Sabers DL. Patient instructors as teachers and evaluators. Acad Med. 1980;55(3):186–93.

6. Stillman PL, Burpeau-Di Gregorio MY, Nicholson GI, Sabers DL, Stillman AE. Six years of experience using patient instructors to teach interviewing skills. J Med Educ. 1983;58(12):941–6.
7. Norman GR, Neufeld VR, Walsh A, Woodward CA, McConvey GL. Measuring physicians' performances by using simulated patients. Acad Med. 1985;60(12):925–34.
8. Barrows HS. An overview of the uses of standardized patients for teaching and evaluating clinical skills. AAMC. Acad Med. 1993;68(6):443–51.
9. Barrows HS. Simulated (standardized) patients and other human simulations. Chapel Hill: Health Sciences Consortium; 1987.
10. Collins JP, Harden RM. AMEE medical education guide no. 13: real patients, simulated patients and simulators in clinical examinations. Med Teach. 1998;20(6):508–21.
11. Churchouse C, McCafferty C. Standardized patients versus simulated patients: is there a difference? Clin Simul Nurs. 2012;8(8):e363–5.
12. Beigzadeh A, Bahmanbijri B, Sharifpoor E, Rahimi M. Standardized patients versus simulated patients in medical education: are they the same or different. J Emerg Pract Trauma. 2016;2(1):25–8.
13. Furman GE. The role of standardized patient and trainer training in quality assurance for high-stakes clinical skills examination. Kaohsiung J Med Sci. 2008;24:651–5.
14. Cleland JA, Abe K, Rethans J. The use of simulated patients in medical education: AMEE guide no 42. Med Teach. 2009;31(6):477–86.
15. May W, Park JH, Lee JP. A ten-year review of the literature on the use of standardized patients in teaching and learning: 1996–2005. Med Teach. 2009;31(6):487–92.
16. Harden RM, Stevenson M, Downie WW, Wilson GM. Assessment of clinical competence using objective structured examination. Br Med J. 1975;1(5955):447–51.
17. Harden RM, Gleeson FA. Assessment of clinical competence using an objective structured clinical examination (OSCE). Med Educ. 1979;13(1):41–54.
18. Stillman PL, Swanson DB. Ensuring the clinical competence of medical school graduates through standardized patients. Arch Intern Med. 1987;147(6):1049–52.
19. Stillman PL, Regan MB, Swanson DB, Case S, McCahan J, Feinblatt J, Smith SR, Willms J, Nelson DV. An assessment of the clinical skills of fourth-year students at four New England medical schools. Acad Med. 1990;65(5):320–6.
20. Stillman P, Swanson D, Regan MB, Philbin MM, Nelson V, Ebert T, Ley B, Parrino T, Shorey J, Stillman A, et al. Assessment of clinical skills of residents utilizing standardized patients. A follow-up study and recommendations for application. Ann Intern Med. 1991;114(5):393–401.
21. Anderson MB, Stillman PL, Wang Y. Growing use of standardized patients in teaching and evaluation in medical education. Teach Learn Med Int J. 1994;6(1):15–22.
22. Lane C, Rollnick S. The use of simulated patients and role-play in communication skills training: a review of the literature to august 2005. Patient Educ Couns. 2007;67(1):13–20.
23. Williams B, Song JJ. Are simulated patients effective in facilitating development of clinical competence for healthcare students? A scoping review. Adv Simul. 2016;1(1):1–9.
24. Anderson MB, Kassebaum DG. Preface. Proceedings of AAMC's Consensus Conference on the use of standardized patients in the teaching and evaluation of clinical skills. Acad Med. 1993;68(6):438.
25. Reznick RK, Blackmore D, Cohen R, Baumber J, Rothman A, Smee S, Chalmers A, Poldre P, Birtwhistte R, Walsh P, et al. An objective structured clinical examination for the licentiate of the Medical Council of Canada: from research to reality. Acad Med. 1993;68(10 Suppl):S4–6.
26. Reznick RK, Blackmore D, Dauphinée WD, Rothman AI, Smee S. Large-scale high-stakes testing with an OSCE: report from the Medical Council of Canada. Acad Med. 1996;71(1 Suppl):S19–21.
27. Tombleson P, Fox RA, Dacre JA. Defining the content for the objective structured clinical examination component of the professional and linguistic assessment board examination: development of a blueprint. Med Educ. 2000;34:566–72.
28. Dillon GF, Boulet JR, Hawkins RE, Swanson D. Simulations in the United States medical licensing examination™(USMLE™). Qual Saf Health Care. 2004;13(Suppl 1):i41–5.
29. Sutnick AI, Stillman PL, Norcini JJ, Friedman M, Regan MB, Williams RG, Kachur EK, Haggerty MA, Wilson MP. ECFMG assessment of clinical competence of graduates of foreign medical schools. Educational Commission for Foreign Medical Graduates. JAMA. 1993;270(9):1041–5.
30. Ziv A, Ben-David MF, Sutnick AI, Gary NE. Lessons learned from six years of international administrations of the ECFMG's SP-based clinical skills assessment. Acad Med. 1998;73(1):84–91.
31. Boulet JR, Smee SM, Dillon GF, Gimpel JR. The use of standardized patient assessments for certification and licensure decisions. Simul Healthc. 2009;4(1):35–42.
32. Khan KZ, Ramachandran S, Gaunt K, Pushkar P. The objective structured clinical examination (OSCE): AMEE guide no. 81. Part I: an historical and theoretical perspective. Med Teach. 2013;35(9):e1437–46.
33. Khan KZ, Gaunt K, Ramachandran S, Pushkar P. The objective structured clinical examination (OSCE): AMEE guide no. 81. Part II: organisation & administration. Med Teach. 2013;35(9):e1447–63.
34. Pell G, Fuller R, Homer M, Roberts T. How to measure the quality of the OSCE: a review of metrics–AMEE guide no. 49. Med Teach. 2010;32(10):802–11.
35. Motola I, Devine LA, Chung HS, Sullivan JE, Issenberg SB. Simulation in healthcare education: a best evidence practical guide. AMEE guide no. 82. Med Teach. 2013;35(10):e1511–30.
36. Nestel D, Burn CL, Pritchard SA, Glastonbury R, Tabak D. The use of simulated patients in medical education: guide supplement 42.1–viewpoint. Med Teach. 2011;33(12):1027–9.
37. Laidlaw A, Hart J. Communication skills: an essential component of medical curricula. Part I: assessment of clinical communication: AMEE guide no. 51. Med Teach. 2011;33(1):6–8.
38. Rosen KR. The history of medical simulation. J Crit Care. 2008;23(2):157–66.
39. About ASPE. The Association of Standardized Patient Educators. Available at: http://www.aspeducators.org/about-aspe. Accessed 2 Jan 2017.
40. Cantillon P, Stewart B, Haeck K, Bills J, Ker J, Rethans JJ. Simulated patient programmes in Europe: collegiality or separate development? Med Teach. 2010;32(3):e106–10.
41. Bromley LM. The objective structured clinical exam-practical aspects. Curr Opin Anesthesiol. 2000;13(6):675–8.
42. Siker ES. Assessment of clinical competence. Curr Opin Anesthesiol. 1999;12(6):677–84.
43. McIndoe A. High stakes simulation in anaesthesia. Contin Educ Anaesth Crit Care Pain. 2012;12(5):268–73.
44. Weller J, et al. Effective management of anaesthetic crises: development and evaluation of a college-accredited simulation-based course for anaesthesia education in Australia and New Zealand. Simul Healthc. 2006;1(4):209–14.
45. Weller JM, Henning M, Civil N, Lavery L, Boyd MJ, Jolly B. Approaches to learning for the ANZCA final examination and validation of the revised study process questionnaire in specialist medical training. Anaesth Intensive Care. 2013;41(5):631–40.
46. Yudkowsky R, Alseidi A, Cintron J. Beyond fulfilling the core competencies: an objective structured clinical examination to assess

communication and interpersonal skills in a surgical residency. Curr Surg. 2004;61(5):499–503.
47. Swing SR. The ACGME outcome project: retrospective and prospective. Med Teach. 2007;29(7):648–54.
48. Levine AI, Swartz MH. Standardized patients: the "other" simulation. J Crit Care. 2008;23:179–84.
49. Webb AR, Young RA, Baumer JG. Emotional intelligence and the ACGME competencies. J Grad Med Educ. 2010;2(4):508–12.
50. Tetzlaff JE. Assessment of competency in anesthesiology. Anesthesiology. 2007;106(4):812–25.
51. Nasca TJ, Philibert I, Brigham T, Flynn TC. The next GME accreditation system—rationale and benefits. N Engl J Med. 2012;366(11):1051–6.
52. Isaak R, Chen F, Hobbs G, Martinelli SM, Stiegler M, Arora H. Standardized mixed-fidelity simulation for ACGME milestones competency assessment and objective structured clinical exam preparation. Med Sci Educ. 2016;26(3):437–41.
53. Van der Vleuten CPM, Swanson DB. Assessment of clinical skills with standardized patients: state of the art. Teach Learn Med. 1990;2:58–76.
54. Colliver JA, Williams RG. Technical issues: test application. AAMC Acad Med. 1993;68(6):454–60.
55. Whelan GP. Educational Commission for Foreign Medical Graduates: clinical skills assessment prototype. Med Teach. 1999;21:156–60.
56. Gorter S, Rethans JJ, van der Heijden D, Scherpbier A, Houben H, Van der Vleuten C, Van der Linden S. Reproducibility of clinical performance assessment in practice using incognito standardized patients. Med Educ. 2002;36:827–32.
57. Sanci LA, Day NA, Coffey CM, Patton GC, Bowes G. Simulations in evaluation of training: a medical example using standardised patients. Eval Program Plann. 2002;25(1):35–46.
58. Adamo G. Simulated and standardized patients in OSCEs: achievements and challenges 1992–2003. Med Teach. 2003;25(3):262–70.
59. Boulet JR, McKinley DW, Whelan GP, Hambleton RK. Quality assurance methods for performance-based assessments. Adv Health Sci Educ. 2003;8(1):27–47.
60. Duffy FD, Gordon GH, Whelan G, Cole-Kelly K, Frankel R. Assessing competence in communication and interpersonal skills: the Kalamazoo II report. Acad Med. 2004;79(6):495–507.
61. Wind LA, Van Dalen J, Muijtjens AM, Rethans JJ. Assessing simulated patients in an educational setting: the MaSP (Maastricht Assessment of Simulated Patients). Med Educ. 2004;38(1):39–44.
62. Williams RG. Have standardized patient examinations stood the test of time and experience? Teach Learn Med. 2004;16(2):215–22.
63. Newble D. Techniques for measuring clinical competence: objective structured clinical examinations. Med Educ. 2004;38(2):199–203.
64. Whelan GP, Boulet JR, McKinley DW, Norcini JJ, van Zanten M, Hambleton RK, Burdick WP, Peitzman SJ. Scoring standardized patient examinations: lessons learned from the development and administration of the ECFMG Clinical Skills Assessment (CSA®). Med Teach. 2005;27(3):200–6.
65. Worth-Dickstein H, Pangaro LN, MacMillan MK, Klass DJ, Shatzer JH. Use of "standardized examinees" to screen for standardized-patient scoring bias in a clinical skills examination. Teach Learn Med. 2005;17(1):9–13.
66. Baig LA, Beran TN, Vallevand A, Baig ZA, Monroy-Cuadros M. Accuracy of portrayal by standardized patients: results from four OSCE stations conducted for high stakes examinations. BMC Med Educ. 2014;14(1):1.
67. Keifenheim KE, Teufel M, Ip J, Speiser N, Leehr EJ, Zipfel S, Herrmann-Werner A. Teaching history taking to medical students: a systematic review. BMC Med Educ. 2015;15(1):1.
68. Brennan RL. Generalizability theory and classical test theory. Appl Meas Educ. 2010;24(1):1–21.
69. Freeth D, Hammick M, Koppel I, Reeves S, Barr H. A critical review of evaluations of interprofessional education. London: Higher Education Academy Learning and Teaching Support Network for Health Sciences and Practice; 2002.
70. Reed DA, Cook DA, Beckman TJ, Levine RB, Kern DE, Wright SM. Association between funding and quality of published medical education research. JAMA. 2007;298(9):1002–9.
71. Sinz E. Simulation-based education for cardiac, thoracic, and vascular anesthesiology. Semin Cardiothorac Vasc Anesth. 2005;9(4):291–307.
72. Lake CL. Simulation in cardiothoracic and vascular anesthesia education: tool or toy? Semin Cardiothorac Vasc Anesth. 2005;9(4):265–73.
73. Kneebone R, Nestel D, Wetzel C, Black S, Jacklin R, Aggarwal R, Yadollahi F, Wolfe J, Vincent C, Darzi A. The human face of simulation: patient-focused simulation training. Acad Med. 2006;81(10):919–24.
74. Nestel DF, Black SA, Kneebone RL, Wetzel CM, Thomas P, Wolfe JH, Darzi AW. Simulated anaesthetists in high fidelity simulations for surgical training: feasibility of a training programme for actors. Med Teach. 2008;30(4):407–13.
75. Hoelzer BC, Moeschler SM, Seamans DP. Using simulation and standardized patients to teach vital skills to pain medicine fellows. Pain Med. 2015;16(4):680–91.
76. Cantrell MJ, Deloney LA. Integration of standardized patients into simulation. Anesthesiol Clin. 2007;25(2):377–83.
77. Nestel D, Bearman M. Simulated patient methodology: theory, evidence and practice. New York: Wiley; 2014.
78. Harless WG, Drennon GG, Marxer JJ, Root JA, Miller GE. CASE: a computer-aided simulation of the clinical encounter. Acad Med. 1971;46(5):443–8.
79. Huang G, Reynolds R, Candler C. Virtual patient simulation at US and Canadian medical schools. Acad Med. 2007;82(5):446–51.
80. Ellaway R, Poulton T, Fors U, McGee JB, Albright S. Building a virtual patient commons. Med Teach. 2008;30(2):170–4.
81. Cook DA, Triola MM. Virtual patients: a critical literature review and proposed next steps. Med Educ. 2009;43(4):303–11.
82. Critchley LA, Wong J, Leung JY. Virtual patients and undergraduate anaesthesia teaching. Med Educ. 2008;42:1120–1.
83. Critchley LA, Kumta SM, Ware J, Wong JW. Web-based formative assessment case studies: role in a final year medicine two-week anaesthesia course. Anaesth Intensive Care. 2009;37(4):637.
84. Leung JY, Critchley LA, Yung AL, Kumta SM. Introduction of virtual patients onto a final year anesthesia course: Hong Kong experience. Adv Med Educ Pract. 2011;2:71.
85. Leung JY, Critchley LA, Yung AL, Kumta SM. Evidence of virtual patients as a facilitative learning tool on an anesthesia course. Adv Health Sci Educ. 2015;20(4):885–901.
86. Schwid HA, Souter KJ. Resident perceptions and cost analysis of a virtual patient application for anesthesia-related critical incidents. J Educ Perioper Med. 2014;16(11):1–14.

Mannequin-Based Simulators and Part-Task Trainers

11

Jacob Schaff and Cortessa Russell

Introduction

History of Mannequin-Based Simulators and Task Trainers

Simulation has been used in military engagements since as early as the sixth century when commanders used the "game" of chess to model battle positions between armies. As centuries passed, more modern simulators and task trainers were adopted by the aviation industry, when in 1929, Edwin Link, a self-taught aviator and inventor, purchased his first plane. He wanted to develop a more realistic way to learn to fly. The Link Trainer was created and could simulate airplane movements and instrument training based in a cockpit. The device soon began to attract commercial airline and military attention, and many Link Trainers were used during World War II [1, 2]. In the 1950s, the Federal Aviation Administration (FAA) made simulation training for pilots mandatory, owing to its success in prior years [1, 3].

Resusci®Anne

The first widely available mannequin-based task trainer was Resusci®Anne, created by Asmund Laerdal in 1960. In the early 1900s, an unknown French girl was found in the river Seine, an apparent suicide victim. As was customary to do at the time, a face cast was made to aid in solving her identity. The cast made showed a peaceful, delicate smile that many around the world associated with innocence and beauty. Laerdal rediscovered this story in the late 1950s and used this face impression on his model, as he was convinced that a life-sized and life-like mannequin would increase user motivation to learn resuscitation [4]. At the suggestion of a colleague, Laerdal would eventually incorporate a spring behind the chest as a trainer for doing high-quality chest compressions, becoming one of the first cardiopulmonary resuscitation trainers.

SIM1

True computer-based, operator-controlled mannequins also had their beginnings in the mid-1960s, with the development of SIM1. Dr. Stephen Abrahamson, an engineer, teamed up with a physician, Dr. Judson Denson, and Aerojet General Corporation and Sierra Engineering to develop the first prototype. For the era, it was remarkably advanced, containing many features that are present on modern-day simulation mannequins including chest rise, eye blinking, pupillary constriction, and the ability to intubate the trachea. The purpose was to train anesthesia residents in endotracheal intubation, and they published a small study demonstrating that simulation training shortened the time to proficiency compared with controls [5]. However, its price point of $100,000 made mass production financially unfeasible [1, 3, 6]. Additionally, its narrow task training focus limited its applicability.

Harvey

Harvey is a cardiology patient simulator created by Dr. Michael Gordon at the University of Miami in 1968. It is a full-sized mannequin capable of replicating the physical exam, auscultatory, and hemodynamic findings of a myriad of cardiovascular diseases. First used to introduce bedside physical exam skills to novice students, Harvey is still in production. Several studies have demonstrated improved

J. Schaff · C. Russell (✉)
Department of Anesthesiology, New York Presbyterian – Columbia University Medical Center, New York, NY, USA
e-mail: cr2235@cumc.columbia.edu

B. Mahoney et al. (eds.), *Comprehensive Healthcare Simulation: Anesthesiology*, Comprehensive Healthcare Simulation,
https://doi.org/10.1007/978-3-030-26849-7_11

medical knowledge and physical exam skills using Harvey as an educational tool. The first pilot studies were done in 1980 to assess its effectiveness in educating medical students and its acceptance among a variety of learners and to demonstrate its technical reliability [7]. In 1987, Ewy et al. performed a study on 208 fourth-year medical students – one group was exposed to interactive training with Harvey, while the other received only conventional teaching. The students that utilized Harvey performed better on post-rotation knowledge quizzes [8]. Harvey was acquired by Laerdal and has been updated for modern and complex cardiovascular training. Currently, the "next-generation Harvey ®" has six breath sound areas and nine cardiac auscultation areas and can simulate 50 different cardiac diseases [9].

Transitioning to the Modern Era

The development of modern-day, technologically advanced simulation mannequins was made possible by advances in computer-based manipulation of physiologic parameters. Several leaders emerged in simulation education by developing advanced platforms. In 1987, Dr. David Gaba of Stanford University created the Comprehensive Anesthesia Simulation Environment (CASE 1.2) [10]. The CASE 1.2 system was designed to completely recreate the anesthesiologist's mental task environment by using a real operating room with all of the standard monitoring equipment. The computer associated with the system allowed for manipulation of noninvasive blood pressure, while various other modules controlled parameters such as invasive pressures, temperature, heart rate, and cardiac rhythm. Contemporaneously, Dr. Michael Good developed the Gainesville Anesthesia Simulator (GAS). This mannequin allowed for complex monitoring of lung function, hemodynamics, and gas analysis aimed at teaching anesthesia residents basic skills before taking care of actual patients [11]. These systems laid the groundwork for the complex and advanced systems that are available today for use in simulation.

Evidence Supporting the Use of Mannequin-Based Simulators and Task Trainers

Introduction

There are many factors which contribute to the success of simulation as a learning tool, including physical, emotional, and conceptual fidelity [12]. Most anecdotal experiences and published studies show that users enjoy simulation. Most report "high satisfaction" after participating in a well-designed simulation with clear objectives, a good level of fidelity, and a well-constructed debriefing [13]. Although most participants "really enjoy" doing simulation, there is an important need to assess objective outcomes beyond the lowest level of the Kirkpatrick Model for evaluating the effectiveness of training [14]. Education research can be very difficult to accomplish when the benchmark is traditional prospective randomized control trials. By utilizing mannequin-based simulations and task trainers, simulation provides a more controlled environment with objective measurements by which to assess educational interventions. This section will summarize the evidence behind the use of mannequin-based simulations and task trainers for education and assessment in the practice of anesthesiology.

Conducting Evidence-Based Simulation Research Using Mannequins and Task Trainers

Generating high-quality, evidence-based education research has long challenged clinicians and researchers. Issenberg et al. published a meta-analysis of studies showing that only approximately 30% of simulation-based studies were randomized control trials, considered the gold standard of research studies. Additionally, the majority of studies reviewed had less than 30 participants, making the power of these studies low and their generalizability questionable. Greater than 70% of these studies described assessment of an educational intervention for teaching a practical procedure. Indeed, mannequin-based simulation and task trainers are particularly well-suited for this purpose. Management skills and clinical skills have also been evaluated – two areas where mannequin-based simulation can also be quite useful [15].

High-Fidelity Versus Low-Fidelity Simulators

Mannequins are used to increase the physical fidelity of simulation. The design of the mannequin should be used to serve a specific purpose and achieve predefined goals and objectives. If the learner-mannequin interaction for a specific aim is too complex, the psychomotor burden on the learner can be too high and the true objective of the simulation may not be achieved due to excessive information.

The advantages of high- vs. low-fidelity mannequin simulators are a topic that frequently arises with respect to balancing educational value with costs. High-fidelity mannequins, such as Laerdal's SimMan 3G or CAE Healthcare's HPS mannequin, offer a vast array of features to add physical validity and, by proxy, emotional validity to the simulation.

Cheng et al. published a meta-analysis evaluating high- vs. low-fidelity mannequin use for advanced life support training. Thirteen of the fourteen studies were randomized controlled trials. The analysis showed that high-fidelity mannequins conferred a moderate benefit in skills performance

[CI 0.13–1.05] initially, at the conclusion of the course; however, no benefit has been compared to low-fidelity simulation at 6 months or 1 year after training. Additionally, there was no difference in knowledge as assessed by pre- and posttest examination [16]. Norman et al. performed a review of the literature and found 24 studies comparing high- and low-fidelity simulation for learning objectives ranging from critical care to weaning from cardiopulmonary bypass. He found that both high- and low-fidelity mannequin-based simulation provided a learning benefit over no intervention; however, most studies showed only a 1–2% difference in skills competency between the two groups [17]. Chandra et al. evaluated the effects of high- vs. low-fidelity fiber-optic intubation in teaching respiratory therapists (novice learners). They found no statistically significant difference between high- and low-fidelity simulation as graded by blinded, independent reviewers [18]. Other procedural tasks such epidural placement have been evaluated as well. Friedman et al. randomized second-year anesthesia residents to one of two arms: a commercially available high-fidelity epidural task trainer or a low-fidelity model that was created at their institution. The investigators then filmed the residents performing epidurals on actual patients over the next 6 months and found no difference in scores based on a Global Rating Scale and Manual Skill Checklist [19].

While many studies show no difference between high- and low-fidelity mannequins for simulation, certain learning goals lend themselves to high-fidelity technology. Transesophageal echocardiography, for instance, is difficult to accomplish with low-fidelity simulation.

High-fidelity mannequins can provide additional realism, potentially helping to engage learners and increase physical and emotional validity. It is reassuring, however, that many learning objectives can be accomplished with relatively low-fidelity mannequins and task trainers, especially when cost and budget are of concern.

Simulation for Airway Management

Successful management of the airway is of paramount importance in the practice of anesthesiology. The difficult airway algorithm published by the American Society of Anesthesiologists (ASA) provides helpful guidance in managing difficult airways. Given that this is a relatively rare occurrence, many practitioners, especially novices and trainees, have limited exposure to these events. This has made mannequin-based simulation for difficult airway management an important option for training.

In 1969, Abrahamson showed that, with a simulation-based training program, anesthesiology residents were able to achieve proficiency in intubating skills in fewer days compared to the cohort that was learning via the apprentice-style method in the operating room [5]. Since then, simulation centers have become excellent research grounds for evaluating new airway equipment. While traditional direct laryngoscopy blades offer a high degree of success for intubation, video laryngoscopes serve as a valuable backup tool for potential difficult intubations. Pieters et al. evaluated seven different video laryngoscopes in a simulation center on mannequins in the hands of both novice and experienced users. They found that most users preferred and had more successful intubations with Macintosh-type blades (C-MAC video laryngoscope included) [20]. Altun et al. also investigated performance with different blades in two separate mannequin-based difficult airway scenarios. They also found that Macintosh-styled blades were associated with the shortest time to intubation, although it was unclear if participants had a bias based on former training [21]. Additionally, Kennedy et al. performed a meta-analysis of 76 studies which employed technology-enhanced simulation. In comparison with non-simulation-based interventions, the mannequin/task trainer airway simulation groups showed increased learner satisfaction, improved skills, and improved patient outcomes; no difference in knowledge was detected [22].

Mannequin-based simulation and trainers have been used for training and assessment of other advanced airway techniques. Cricothyrotomy is extremely rarely performed and can be a life-saving procedure when other options in the difficult airway algorithm have been exhausted. Hubert et al. studied 27 anesthesiology residents before and after a 2-day difficult airway session, including ultimately performing a cricothyrotomy. The participants were assessed pretraining on the mannequin-based simulator and then randomly at one of three time points, 3 months, 6 months, or 12 months post-training, for adherence to the difficult airway algorithm and using a checklist score for cricothyrotomy skills. The investigators found that trainees adhered to the difficult airway algorithm better than they did pretest and were able to perform a cricothyrotomy more quickly and with more skill, using a global rating scale when compared with pretest scores. There were no significant differences at the various time points indicating sustained retention of skills up to 1 year post-training [23]. High-fidelity mannequin-based simulation for unanticipated difficult intubation training has been shown to be effective for attending anesthesiologists as well as trainees. Boet et al. held a training session for 38 anesthesiologists for the management of a "cannot intubate, cannot ventilate" scenario, utilizing a high-fidelity simulation along with a structured debriefing. At a 12-month reassessment, the group was able to demonstrate retention of cricothyrotomy skills as evaluated by independent expert reviewers [24].

Flexible fiber-optic intubation is another indispensable tool for the anesthesiologist for both known and unanticipated difficult intubations. Having an adequate level of expertise and comfort with utilizing this tool is quite important for these situations. Nilsson et al. conducted a randomized trial of 23 anesthesiology residents who were naïve to flexible fiber-optic intubation. Half of the participants were instructed using part-task trainers and the other group whole-task trainers. After training, the learners' performance was evaluated on mannequins in a simulation center. There were no significant differences between the part- and whole-task trainer groups; and the ratings of both groups were similar to experienced, attending anesthesiologists in performing flexible fiber-optic intubation [25].

Simulation for Anesthesia Subspecialties

Cardiothoracic Anesthesia

Cardiothoracic anesthesia is challenging and exciting, particularly for first rotation anesthesiology residents, because the cardiac operating rooms introduce new medications, workflows, and members of the OR team. There is a smooth team dynamic that exists between an experienced anesthesiologist, perfusionist, and surgeon, which can sometimes leave the trainee lost and excluded.

As such, simulation can play an important role to demystify this new environment. One focus for educators and researchers is initiation and discontinuation of cardiopulmonary bypass (CPB). Morais et al. created a training program for anesthesiology trainees, using a HPS mannequin, along with a surgeon, perfusionist, and circulating nurse participating in their real roles during the session. Training included management of arterial blood gas abnormalities while on cardiopulmonary bypass, increased bispectral index (BIS) while rewarming to normothermia, and repeated ventricular fibrillation after aortic cross-clamp release. The trainees were also taught how to distinguish between different types of protamine reactions, assess right heart failure, and ultimately escalate care to provide some type of mechanical support in the setting of cardiogenic shock. Participants felt the simulation improved their knowledge of physiology and pharmacology, ability to manage patients while on cardiopulmonary bypass, confidence in the cardiothoracic operating room, and communication abilities. They also felt stimulated to learn [26].

Simulation is also useful for transesophageal echocardiography (TEE) training. TEE is an invasive procedure that is technically difficult to learn, and there are limited opportunities for trainees to perform and interpret TEE images during a busy operating room case. Several groups have studied the use of simulation and task trainers to teach novices to perform TEE exams as well as assess proficiency. Matyal et al. created a TEE training curriculum for echo-naïve residents, consisting of web-based echo didactics along with weekly hands-on TEE simulator experience. They utilized motion tracking kinetics software to analyze the performance of both novice and expert echocardiographers. Using this analysis, they were able to both distinguish between novice and expert and track performance as the novice group became more proficient in TEE skills [27]. Ferrero et al. randomized 42 anesthesiology residents to either standard, traditional didactics or simulation using a TEE-mannequin simulator. They were able to show that the simulation group had an overall higher quality of image acquisition (83% vs. 67%) as well as a higher percent of images that were acceptable for clinical use (71% vs. 48%). It appeared that clinical anesthesia-1 (CA-1) level residents and echo-naïve participants had the largest performance impact between the two training groups [28]. Others have evaluated TEE simulation as a measure of expertise. Bick et al. performed a multicenter study using the Basic Transesophageal Echocardiography Evaluation Tool (BTEET) using a Heartworks TEE simulator to attempt to distinguish between novice and expert echocardiographers. The investigators were able to consistently and reliably differentiate skill level, making this an exciting prospect for future performance assessment in TEE [29].

Obstetric Anesthesia

Like other anesthesia subspecialties, obstetric anesthesia provides unique challenges to the anesthesiologist, especially those with minimal prior exposure. It is a high-acuity setting where an uncomplicated labor can quickly devolve into an obstetric emergency. It requires constant communication between many players on the team, including the anesthesiologist, obstetrician, nursing staff, and other support staff.

Providing general anesthesia for cesarean section is associated with higher maternal morbidity and mortality [30]. Scavone et al. utilized a high-fidelity patient simulator to validate a checklist for objective performance during a simulated cesarean delivery under general anesthesia. The study demonstrated a high inter-rater reliability coefficient (0.97) [31]. Several years later, Ortner et al. evaluated a training course using lectures and high-fidelity simulation for cesarean section under general anesthesia for anesthesiology residents on their obstetric anesthesia rotation. Utilizing the checklist created by Scavone et al., the group assessed residents and attending anesthesiologists (as the control standard) at 1 week, 5 weeks, and 8 months. At 1 week, the residents expectedly scored significantly lower than the attending anesthesiologists. After the training sessions and mannequin simulations, however, the residents' scores were similar to the attendings' and remained at this level when reassessed at 8 months [32].

Neuraxial anesthesia is commonly employed in the obstetrics suite both for labor analgesia and surgical anesthesia. Epidural placement is typically performed with a loss of resistance technique, where tactile feedback is paramount. Several investigators have evaluated using epidural task trainers to train novices in a safe, convenient environment. Raj et al. demonstrated that items as simple as fruit can be an effective, "low-fidelity" task trainer. They enrolled 50 participants with four concealed fruits as epidural simulators. After accounting for years of experience and needle preference, 63% of participants indicated that a simple banana offered realistic feedback for loss of resistance during epidural placement [33]. Other groups have used more complex task trainers for teaching epidural and spinal anesthesia techniques. Capogna et al. developed an enclosed unit consisting of different layers to approximate the skin, subcutaneous tissue, supraspinous ligament, interspinous ligament, ligamentum flavum, epidural space, and intrathecal space. They were able to use the instrument as a stand-alone task trainer or incorporate it into the back of the SimMom® obstetric patient simulator. Additionally, for more advanced training, bloodlike substance can be added to the epidural space, and simulated CSF (water) can be added to the intrathecal space to simulate complications of epidural placement. Ninety percent of anesthesiologists evaluating the device (with a median of approximately 17 years of experience) thought it accurately simulated the tactile experience encountered in real patients [34]. Magill et al. designed a cable-based actuator device to simulate the experience of placing an epidural needle. By applying varying levels of tension on the cables, the group was able to simulate the different tissue textures encountered by advancing a needle from the subcutaneous layer into the ligamentum flavum and ultimately achieving loss of resistance [35].

Regional Anesthesia

Regional anesthesia is a highly technical and hands-on subspecialty of anesthesiology, lending itself particularly well to simulation-based interventions for education. Over the last decade, the use of ultrasound for performing peripheral nerve blocks has become ubiquitous. Several investigators have published studies regarding the efficacy of mannequin and task trainer-based educational programs. Liu et al. evaluated the use of different phantom models for ultrasound-guided peripheral nerve blockade. Utilizing an opaque model, they found that training on the peripheral nerve block simulator resulted in a decreased number of errors and decreased time to completion versus the group that did not receive task trainer education ($P < 0.05$) [36]. Woodworth et al. performed a multi-institutional study investigating the efficacy of a simulation-based curriculum for teaching anesthesiology residents how to perform a sciatic nerve block. They found that, while test scores significantly improved after the simulation-based educational intervention, hands-on live scanning for nerve identification was not significantly improved [37]. Baranauskas et al. investigated progressively longer training sessions using mannequin-based simulators for teaching peripheral nerve blockade. Those residents who had longer simulation training times were able to perform the nerve block more quickly and with fewer technical flaws than those with abbreviated or no simulator training [38]. Ouanes et al. developed a comprehensive regional anesthesia training program. After multimodal training, including on a phantom simulator, they were able to demonstrate improved written test scores as well as improved objective structured clinical examination (OSCE) scores [39]. While further studies of the use of mannequin- and task trainer-based simulation for regional anesthesia are needed, the majority of the evidence currently suggests a benefit versus traditional didactic or apprentice-type methods of instruction.

Current Mannequin-Based Simulators and Task Trainers

Over the last 15 years, significant advances have been made in improving the quality and fidelity of mannequin-based simulators. Numerous features and control options have been integrated into many of these mannequins. While many companies do have products that are used across various specialties in healthcare, three companies have mannequins that are frequently used in anesthesiology training: Laerdal, CAE Healthcare, and Gaumard.

Programming/Scenario Development

Most high-fidelity mannequin simulators offer several modes of control for manipulating physiologic variables and mannequin responses during a simulation. Essentially, all offer a manual mode or "on-the-fly" programming mode. This is typically very helpful when the scenario is relatively simple and the vital signs need only minor manipulation. For example, a patient is brought to the intensive care unit after open coronary artery bypass surgery and develops atrial fibrillation with rapid ventricular response. While many parameters could be manipulated, only heart rate and rhythm (and possibly blood pressure depending on the goal of the scenario) need to be manipulated. This can be easily achieved with manipulation of vital signs contemporaneously with the scenario.

Most current high-fidelity mannequins also offer options for automated (also known as if…then…) programming. This allows for more complex manipulation of physiologic parameters that might not be possible to accomplish by manual adjustment. For instance, in a patient with worsening acute decompensated heart failure, scenario physiology goals might include decreasing systolic and diastolic arterial blood pressure, increasing central venous pressure, increasing pulmonary capillary wedge pressure, increasing heart rate, decreasing the peripheral oxygen saturation, increasing pulmonary edema (crackles heard during chest auscultation), and adding an S3 or S4 gallop on heart auscultation.

Adjusting all of these parameters contemporaneously is difficult to do manually; however, programming software makes it easy to input characteristics and parameters that will occur at baseline and progress as time elapses during the scenario and in response to interventions, lack of interventions, and medications administered.

Examples of programmable sequences include:

- *After administration of bronchodilator (albuterol), respiratory rate decreases from 45 to 25 and the pulse oximeter reading increases from 88% to 96% over 30 seconds.*
- *Administration of 5–10 mg of ephedrine intravenously increases mean arterial pressure by 20 mmHg and heart rate by 15 beats per minute over one minute.*
- *In a patient with anaphylaxis, administration of dilute epinephrine (10–50 mcg) results in a decrease in mean airway pressures from 45 cm H_2O to 18 cm H_2O, an increase in heart rate from 72 beats per minute to 110 beats per minute, and an increase in blood pressure from 72/32 mmHg to 118/64 mmHg.*
- *In a trauma scenario, administration of a fluid bolus decreases heart rate by 10–20 beats per minute and increases systolic and diastolic blood pressure by 15–25 mmHg. This effect is sustained for 3–5 minutes and then will revert to pre-intervention numbers if further care is not performed.*
- *After mask ventilation of a 6-month-old with sevoflurane, airway pressures increase and the pulse oximeter readings fall from 99% to 84%. Administration of positive pressure ventilation with increased volatile agent increases pulse oximeter reading from 84% to 91% and tidal volumes increase from 10 cc to 100 cc. Administration of succinylcholine intramuscularly resolves abnormal vital signs and respiratory parameters.*

Laerdal

Laerdal was founded by Asmund Laerdal after the creation of the Resusci®Anne CPR training device, as discussed previously. Since then, there have been significant advances in this product line.

The SimMan® 3G has been commercially available for over 5 years and offers a wide range of features for training. It is a high-fidelity, "full-size" mannequin that is both wireless and portable. Battery life typically lasts approximately 4 hours with continuous use and includes a charging station with replaceable batteries. The SimMan® 3G is controlled wirelessly by the Laerdal Learning Application (LLEAP) and allows for both simulation programming and downloading scenario data generated during simulation for use during debriefing. The LLEAP software allows for both automated and manual or "on-the-fly" control of physiologic parameters. The automated feature control system can be programmed based on time, action, or medication administered. It utilizes a radiofrequency identification tag system to automatically identify the medications administered and generate pre-programmed physiologic responses.

The SimMan® 3G has developed technology to mimic many physiologic and pathologic conditions, including responsive pupils, lacrimation, diaphoresis, seizure-like activity, deranged heart and lung sounds, and abdominal sounds. With minimal additions, it can also function as a task trainer for the management of a difficult airway, intravascular central line placement, intraosseous access, needle decompression for tension pneumothorax, and chest tube thoracostomy.

Laerdal also offers a broad range of other simulator devices for subspecialty use. Some of these include:

- SimMan® ALS – Prehospital first-responder training
- SimMom® – Obstetrical emergency training
- SimJunior® – Pediatric medical care training
- SimBaby™/SimNewB® – Infant and neonatal training simulator for airway management and resuscitation
- SimMan® 3G Trauma – Trauma resuscitation training

Additionally, Laerdal acquired the Harvey simulator and has transitioned it to an electronic-based system, complete with over 50 cardiopulmonary pathologic states for diagnostic training. The SonoSim corporation recently partnered with Laerdal to incorporate ultrasound education and assessment into the SimMan® 3G. SonoSim offers an ultrasound training simulator that combines didactics, hands-on training, and knowledge assessment. The SimMan® 3G Skin now has RFID tags embedded in it such that, when the SonoSim ultrasound probe approaches one of RFID tags, it triggers video from ultrasound images obtained from real patients to be displayed. The gyrometer in the ultrasound probe requires that the participant hold the probe in the correct position and angle in order for the image to be displayed correctly. The system offers both a normal anatomy/training mode and a "LiveScan" mode in which pre-programmed cases can be used with various pathologies for the appropriate simulation scenario.

CAE Healthcare

Canadian Aviation Electronics Ltd. (CAE) was founded by Ken Patrick in 1947. The company focused on flight simulation and training after receiving several prominent military contracts. In 2011, CAE broadened their scope of practice into medical simulation and acquired Medical Education Technologies, Inc. (METI). METI corporation had developed METIman, a high-fidelity simulator designed for many uses including prehospital care, nursing, and critical care/"code" situations. In 2016, CAE Healthcare revamped the METIman simulator and renamed it "Apollo," building upon the METIman tradition. The Apollo simulator features a full-sized, wirelessly tethered mannequin with programmable physiologic and physical parameters. While the focus of the device is on the cardiopulmonary systems, the Apollo simulator also offers many other features to increase fidelity during simulation. These include pupillary responsiveness and blinking, a difficult airway with tongue swelling and the ability to manage airway obstruction with jaw thrust, head tilt and chin lift, diverse cardiac and pulmonary pathologies, and even characteristics consistent with trauma. The trauma features include two bleeding sites with a 1.5 liter reservoir, exsanguination linked to changing physiologic parameters, and removable limbs to simulate traumatic amputations. Effective chest compressions are displayed as changes in physiologic parameters (end-tidal CO_2, arterial blood pressure).

Another important mannequin in the CAE Healthcare line is the Human Patient Simulator (HPS). HPS development began in the 1980s under the METI corporation. Since being acquired by CAE Healthcare, HPS remains one of the most advanced high-fidelity units available for use. Its main distinguishing factor is display of gas exchange where the lung interface takes up oxygen and emits carbon dioxide based on pre-programmed patient variables. HPS also includes a gas analyzer, which simulates end-tidal CO_2 monitoring, oxygen delivery analysis, as well as anesthetic gas analysis, making it particularly useful in the field of anesthesiology and critical care. Apart from the gas delivery system, the HPS also has an advanced pharmacologic recognition system using bar codes that automatically record and influence physiologic parameters based on the medications and doses administered. It also provides numerous other neurologic, cardiopulmonary, and genitourinary features. The ability to monitor train-of-four for neuromuscular blockade recovery is also available.

CAE Healthcare also provides a number of other simulators in their product line:

Athena Female patient simulator with many of the same features as the Apollo simulator

Lucina Maternal-fetal simulator, which includes delivery maneuvers for difficult deliveries, simulated fetal monitoring, and obstetrical emergencies

iStan Largely designed for "on-the-field" training and simulation. Offers a wide range of features but focuses on prehospital care and assessment

Caesar A wireless simulator mannequin for use in trauma situations that can provide automated physiologic and bleeding responses when a tourniquet is applied to different sites

PediaSIM A high-fidelity pediatric simulator based on a 6-year-old patient, with integrated physiology management and multiple procedure-enabled features

BabySIM A high-fidelity infant simulator, designed for neonatal trauma and resuscitation as well as critical care management

Gaumard

A World War II trauma physician and chemical engineer formed Gaumard in 1946. He recognized how polymers used in battlefield surgery could create simulators for healthcare education. The company's first product was a synthetic human skeleton followed by a childbirth simulator. Over the next 50 years, Gaumard has made numerous task trainers, but its most notable product is Noelle®, a wireless, advanced maternal and neonatal birthing simulator released in 2000. Noelle® can simulate antenatal care situations, routine and high-risk deliveries, and complex postpartum issues. In addition to the numerous physiologic parameter adjustments, it features an Automated Precision Delivery System that moves the fetus throughout the labor stages for lifelike births. In addition to managing peripartum emergencies, there is also an epidural trainer insert available – it has simulated skin, subcutaneous, ligament, and ligamentum flavum spaces. The system can recognize when the ligamentum flavum is engaged, when the epidural space is entered, and if the needle is advanced too far into the intrathecal space, which can be used during the debriefing session.

The HAL simulator is the most advanced wireless mannequin from Gaumard. Its distinguishing feature is the ability to operate continuously during transport and training from multiple working environments, for example, from the ER to the ICU while trainees continuously diagnose and treat his condition. Via a wireless tag system, the HAL simulator is able to log and automatically respond to over 20 administered medications. The HAL simulator, along with most of the high-fidelity mannequins offered by the Gaumard company, is controlled by the UNI®, Unified Simulator Control Software. It offers many pre-programmed scenario modules, automatic physiologic responses, as well as operator on-the-fly control for changing parameters on an as-needed, second-by-second basis.

Task Trainers

Task trainers provide a focused, limited scope to teach a particular procedure or technique. Given that anesthesiology is a very procedural specialty, these can be of considerable value.

Vascular Access

Several companies offer central venous access trainers including internal jugular, subclavian, and femoral venous cannulation. Most typically have an "arterial" and a "venous" tube to simulate the vessels as well as a removable skin over the area of interest. While some rely on using landmark techniques, most now can be imaged with a high-frequency ultrasound probe to mimic real-time, ultrasound-guided line placement. Several companies, including Laerdal, Simulaids, and Blue Phantom, offer peripheral intravenous trainers for the dorsum of the hand as well as the antecubital fossa. Pressurized, pulsating arterial line placement simulators are also helpful for procedural teaching.

Neuraxial Trainers

Several trainers exist for helping to teach neuraxial anesthetic techniques, that is, spinal, epidural, and combined spinal-epidural procedures. These trainers can either be stand-alone models, dedicated to the task, or an add-on feature for many of the high-fidelity mannequins. Most use layered materials of differing densities to mimic passing the needle through skin, subcutaneous tissue, supraspinous and interspinous ligament, and ligamentum flavum. Most include a small fluid reservoir that aids in identification of the intrathecal space, whether by design (spinal anesthetic procedure) or inadvertently during placement of an epidural catheter. Some trainers also include identification software that can digitally track location of the needle, which can be particularly useful for learner feedback after the exercise.

Airway Trainers

While many high-fidelity mannequins include components of airway management, high cost and bulkiness can limit their usability. Most medical simulation companies offer at least one airway trainer. These range from very basic (teaching direct laryngoscopy skills) to more advanced (emergency/difficult airway management, double-lumen endotracheal tube placement, and confirmation). Double-lumen endotracheal tube placement simulators offer a high-fidelity bronchial tree so that, after placement, the right upper lobe bronchial anatomy can be visualized by fiber-optic bronchoscopy to confirm positioning. Nasal fiber-optic intubation and emergency cricothyrotomy are additional features available on several trainers.

Conclusion and Future Directions

Significant advances have occurred over the past 10 years in high-fidelity mannequins and task trainers. Most of the current focus toward advancing mannequin-based simulation education centers around two ideas: improving and advancing technology to increase the amount of fidelity the mannequin provides and integrating different components of mannequins and task trainers into single units.

Technology

The fidelity of mannequin-based simulators is constantly being increased. Advanced cardiovascular physiology features are being incorporated into devices. Many simulator mannequins can now generate real-time 12-lead electrocardiograms based on the scenario and using an actual electrocardiogram machine. Pulse strength is adjustable for changes in blood pressure as well as other physiologic conditions. Heart sounds are being added to simulate pathologic cardiovascular disease processes. Systems are incorporating real-time simulated gas analyzers, for monitoring end-tidal carbon dioxide, oxygen delivery, and anesthetic gasses. Some modules use a carbon dioxide emission system in order to simulate ventilation of the mannequin as well as assess the quality of chest compressions.

Integration

High-fidelity mannequin simulators often have airway training technology incorporated – this is becoming even more advanced as the field progresses. Some mannequins include an interchangeable skin over the cricothyroid membrane for simulation of emergency cricothyrotomy procedures and retrograde intubation technique. Many institutions have created "home modifications" to existing simulators, adding to the armamentarium for training students. Hirsch et al. incorporated a realistic bronchial tree simulator into a Laerdal ALS simulator mannequin – it allows for placement of up to an 8.0 single-lumen endotracheal tube as well as a left or right 35 French double-lumen endotracheal tube. Fiber-optic bronchoscopy can then be utilized to confirm correct position utilizing the carina and right upper lobe airway anatomy as landmarks [40]. The SonoSim company and Laerdal recently teamed up to advance mannequin-based simulation combining two technologies into one. SonoSim is a corporation that offers ultrasound training and education modules using a computer-based gyroscopic probe. The images displayed are from real patients and are shown relative to the location and orientation of the probe – both normal anatomy and various pathologies are available. Laerdal has incorporated these radiofrequency identification tags into the SimMan 3G tags so that "real-time" point-of-care ultrasound can be used during simulations with greater ease and integration.

As innovators in the field continue to improve technology, one can expect the physical and experiential fidelity of mannequins to continue to increase. Integration of new and existing technologies and task trainers into mannequins also provides an exciting future to mannequin-based simulation.

References

1. Rosen KR. The history of medical simulation. J Crit Care. 2008;23(2):157–66.
2. Training LS. History of Edward Link [Internet]. [cited 2016 Sep 1]. Available from: https://www.link.com/about/pages/history.aspx.
3. Cooper JB, Taqueti VR. A brief history of the development of mannequin simulators for clinical education and training. Postgrad Med J. 2008;84(997):563–70.
4. Laerdal, Inc. The Girl from the River Seine [Internet]. http://www.laerdal.com/us/docid/1117082/The-Girl-from-the-River-Seine. [cited 2016 Aug 30]. Available from: http://www.laerdal.com/us/docid/1117082/The-Girl-from-the-River-Seine.
5. Abrahamson S, Denson JS, Wolf RM. Effectiveness of a simulator in training anesthesiology residents. Acad Med. 1969;44:515.
6. Abrahamson S. Sim one--a patient simulator ahead of its time. Caduceus. Caduceus (Springfield). 1997;13(2):29–41.
7. Gordon MS, Ewy GA, DeLeon AC, Waugh RA. "Harvey," the cardiology patient simulator: pilot studies on teaching effectiveness. Am J Cardiol. 1980;45(4):791–6.
8. Ewy GA, Felner JM, Juul D, Mayer JW, Sajid AW, Waugh RA. Test of a cardiology patient simulator with students in fourth-year electives. J Med Educ. 1987;62(9):738–43.
9. Laerdal, Inc. Next Generation Harvey – The Cardiopulmonary Patient Simulator [Internet]. [cited 2016 Feb 11]. Available from: http://www.laerdal.com/us/harvey#/Specifications.
10. Gaba DM, DeAnda A. A comprehensive anesthesia simulation environment: re-creating the operating room for research and training. Anesthesiology. 1988;69:387.
11. Good M, Lampotang S. Critical events simulation for training in anesthesiology. J Clin Monit Comput. 1988;4(140)
12. Paige JB, Morin KH. Simulation fidelity and cueing: a systematic review of the literature. Clin Simul Nurs. 2013;9(11):e481–9.
13. Agha S, Alhamrani A, Khan M. Satisfaction of medical students with simulation based learning. SMJ. 2015;36(6):731–6.
14. AgencyforHealthcareResearch.InConversationwith...DavidGaba, MD [Internet]. 2013 [cited 2016 Dec 16]. Available from: https://psnet.ahrq.gov/perspectives/perspective/137/in-conversation-with%2D%2Ddavid-m-gaba-md.
15. Issenberg SB, Mcgaghie WC, Petrusa ER. Features and uses of high-fidelity medical simulations that lead to effective learning: a BEME systematic review. Med Teach. 2005;27(1):10–28.
16. Cheng A, Lockey A, Bhanji F, Lin Y, Hunt EA, Lang E. The use of high-fidelity manikins for advanced life support training—a systematic review and meta-analysis. Resuscitation. 2015;93:142–9.
17. Norman G, Dore K, Grierson L. The minimal relationship between simulation fidelity and transfer of learning. Med Educ. 2012;46(7):636–47.
18. Chandra DB, Savoldelli GL, Joo HS, Weiss ID, Naik VN. Fiberoptic oral intubation the effect of model fidelity on training for transfer to patient care. Anesthesiology. 2008;109(6):1007–13.
19. Friedman Z, Siddiqui N, Katznelson R, Devito I, Bould MD, Naik V. Clinical impact of epidural anesthesia simulation on short- and long-term learning curve. Reg Anesth Pain Med. 2009;34(3):229–32.
20. Pieters BMA, Wilbers NER, Huijzer M, Winkens B, van Zundert AAJ. Comparison of seven videolaryngoscopes with the Macintosh laryngoscope in manikins by experienced and novice personnel. Anaesthesia. 2016;71(5):556–64.
21. Altun D, Ozkan-Seyhan T, Orhan-Sungur M, Sivrikoz N, Camci E. Comparison of 4 laryngoscopes in 2 difficult airway scenarios. Simul Healthc. 2016:1–5.
22. Kennedy CC, Cannon EK, Warner DO, Cook DA. Advanced airway management simulation training in medical education. Crit Care Med. 2014;42(1):169–78.
23. Hubert V, Duwat A, Deransy R, Mahjoub Y, Dupont H. Effect of simulation training on compliance with difficult airway management algorithms, technical ability, and skills retention for emergency cricothyrotomy. Anesthesiology. 2014;120(4):999–1008.
24. Boet S, Borges BCR, Naik VN, Siu LW, Riem N, Chandra D, et al. Complex procedural skills are retained for a minimum of 1 yr after a single high-fidelity simulation training session. Br J Anaesth. 2011;107(4):533–9.
25. Nilsson PM, Russell L, Ringsted C, Hertz P, Konge L. Simulation-based training in flexible fibreoptic intubation. Eur J Anaesthesiol. 2015;32(9):609–14.
26. Morais RJ, Ashokka B, Siau C, Ti LK. Simulation of cardiopulmonary bypass management: an approach to resident training. J Cardiothorac Vasc Anesth. 2014;28(5):1387–92.
27. Matyal R, Mitchell JD, Hess PE, Chaudary B, Bose R, Jainandunsing JS, et al. Simulator-based transesophageal echocardiographic training with motion analysis. Anesthesiology. 2014;121(2):389–99.
28. Ferrero NA, Bortsov AV, Arora H, Martinelli SM, Kolarczyk LM, Teeter EC, et al. Simulator training enhances resident performance in transesophageal echocardiography. Anesthesiology. 2014;120(1):149–59.
29. Bick JS, DeMaria S Jr, Kennedy JD, Schwartz AD, Weiner MM, Levine AI, et al. Comparison of expert and novice performance of a simulated transesophageal echocardiography examination. Simul Healthcare. 2013;8(5):329–34.
30. Green M, Tariq R, Green P. Improving patient safety through simulation training in anesthesiology: where are we? Anesthesiol Res Pract. 2016;2016(5):1–12.
31. Scavone BM, Sproviero MT. Development of an objective scoring system for measurement of resident performance on the human patient simulator. Anesthesiology. 2006;105(2):260.
32. Ortner CM, Richebé P, Bollag LA, Ross BK, Landau R. Repeated simulation-based training for performing general anesthesia for emergency cesarean delivery: long-term retention and recurring mistakes. Int J Obstet Anesth. 2014;23(4):341–7.
33. Raj D, Williamson RM, Young D, Russell D. A simple epidural simulator. Eur J Anaesthesiol. 2013;30(7):405–8.
34. Capogna G, Stirparo S, Caniggia S. Evaluation of a new training device to simulate the epidural and subarachnoid spaces for neuraxial anesthesia techniques. Minerva Anestesiol. 2013;79(4):385–90.
35. Magill JC, Byl MF, Hinds MF, Agassounon W, Pratt SD, Hess PE. A novel actuator for simulation of epidural anesthesia and other needle insertion procedures. Simul Healthcare. 2010;5(3):179–84.
36. Liu Y, Glass NL, Glover CD, Power RW, Watcha MF. Comparison of the development of performance skills in ultrasound-guided regional anesthesia simulations with different phantom models. Simul Healthcare. 2013;8(6):368–75.
37. Woodworth GE, Chen EM, Horn J-LE, Aziz MF. Efficacy of computer-based video and simulation in ultrasound-guided regional anesthesia training. J Clin Anesth. 2014;26(3):212–21.
38. Baranauskas MB, Margarido CB, Panossian C. Simulação de bloqueios periféricos guiados por ultra-som: curva de aprendizado dos residentes de anestesiologia do CET-SMA/HSL. Rev Bras. 2008;
39. Ouanes J-PP, Schwengel D, Mathur V, Ahmed OI, Hanna MN. Curriculum development for an advanced regional anesthesia education program: one institution's experience from apprenticeship to comprehensive teaching. Middle East J Anaesthesiol. 2014;22(4):413–8.
40. Hirsch J, Generoso JR, Latoures R, Acar Y. Simulation manikin modifications for high-Fidelity training of advanced airway procedures. A A Case Rep. 2016;6(9):268–71.

Computer- and Web-Based Simulators and Virtual Environments

12

David A. Edwards and Samsun Lampotang

History

Computer technology has revolutionized medical education as it has all other aspects of modern life. Medical students still attend lectures and learn from slide sets and wet labs, but this is now supplemented with video-based demonstrations, virtual and augmented reality, and computer-based simulation. The aim of simulation in medicine is to recreate a medical case which is by nature artificial but with enough realism and efficacy to enhance the acquisition or maintenance of a learning objective or skill, all without the downsides of practicing on real patients. As technology has advanced, computer-based simulators, including mobile devices, are capable of recreating actual clinical experiences in many ways, making it easier for learners to acquire skills and translate what was learned to the real world.

The ability to practice medical cases in a simulated environment has many advantages (Table 12.1). Computer systems have replaced human workers in many industries; likewise, computer-based simulation can nearly replicate cases that otherwise require multiple actors and complicated environments. Learners can acquire knowledge through self-directed practice, on their own time, using computer-based simulation in a lab, at home, or really anywhere when the simulation is based on a smartphone app. The growth in medical knowledge and ever-increasing specialization requires deliberate practice outside of the clinical realm in order for a trainee to acquire sufficient knowledge and skills. Computer-based simulation can also allow for objective measurement of learning if such measurement systems are built into the simulation programming.

Table 12.1 Advantages of computer-based simulation

Advantages
Flexible
Allows for self-directed learning
Is convenient
Promotes deliberate practice
Cost-effective
Can be less resource and personnel intensive
May be free or have a minimal cost of dissemination
Is scalable
Software-based skill assessment
Can measure decision-making process
Can track skill acquisition
Could calibrate objective performance to competency

Early Simulation Examples

Prior to the existence of the personal computer (PC), medical simulation consisted of recreated enactments of medical situations using mannequins and standardized patients. Among the earliest mannequin simulators was Resusci Anne®, developed in the 1960s by the Norwegian toymaker Asmund Laerdal, along with Peter Safar, MD, an anesthesiologist in Baltimore, to teach cardiopulmonary resuscitation (CPR). It was a model of the head and upper torso with a spring-loaded chest that recoiled with chest compressions and included the ability to obstruct the model's naso- and oropharynx as well as the trachea, allowing for practicing mouth-to-mouth ventilation with varying degrees of difficulty. Interestingly, the face of Resusci Anne® was designed after the death mask of a French girl who likely committed suicide in the river Seine. Additionally, the Michael Jackson song "Smooth Criminal" and the phrase "Annie, are you OK?" were inspired by Michael Jackson's experience with CPR training using Resusci Anne® [1, 2].

Early in the advent of computer technology, computer-controlled simulators were developed. In 1966, Stephen

D. A. Edwards (✉)
Department of Anesthesiology, Vanderbilt University Medical Center, The Vanderbilt Clinic, Nashville, TN, USA
e-mail: david.a.edwards@vanderbilt.edu

S. Lampotang
Center for Safety, Simulation & Advanced Learning Technologies, Simulation Innovation, Office of Educational Affairs/Office of Medical Education, Simulation Core, Clinical & Translational Science Insitute, University of Florida, Gainesville, FL, USA
e-mail: slampotang@anest.ufl.edu

B. Mahoney et al. (eds.), *Comprehensive Healthcare Simulation: Anesthesiology*, Comprehensive Healthcare Simulation,
https://doi.org/10.1007/978-3-030-26849-7_12

Abrahamson, PhD, created the first computer-controlled mannequin that simulated vital signs and responded to drug administration [1, 3]. At the time, Dr. Abrahamson was the new Director of Research in Medical Education at the University of Southern California. He was approached by Tullio Ronzoni from Aerojet General Corporation about the possibility of using computers for teaching in medical schools [4]. In the postwar period, military contracts were being cut, and Aerojet General Corp was interested in generalizing its technologies to nonmilitary applications. Dr. Abrahamson posed the possibility of creating a simulator to recreate operating room scenarios an anesthesiologist would face. Judson Samuel Denson, MD, then Chief of Anesthesiology at Los Angeles County General Hospital, joined the team as the content expert. In collaboration with Sierra Engineering and Aerojet General Corp, Dr. Abrahamson's proposal for funding was awarded by the US Office of Education for $272,000, after being turned down by the National Institutes of Health (NIH) and other military sources. On March 17, 1967, the Sim One mannequin patient simulator (MPS) was unveiled.

The purpose of Sim One was to teach anesthesiology residents how to safely intubate patients. The Sim One setup included a computer with an interface unit, an instructor's console, and an anesthesia machine all attached to a mannequin. Sim One could simulate breathing, eye movements, and pupil responses. The pulse could be palpated and blood pressure measured, and the mouth could be opened and manipulated for endotracheal intubation [5]. Dr. Abrahamson reported that anesthesia trainees performed better in the operating room after having practiced on Sim One [6]. Ultimately due to cost, Sim One was not commercialized, and only the original unit was ever constructed [1]. Sim One was also ahead of its time; the computer that ran Sim One occupied an entire wall of the lab (personal communication of JS Gravenstein, MD, to S Lampotang) so that it was not easily transportable as the new crop of MPS that arose in the late 1980s.

A year later, in 1968, the first computer-controlled part-task trainer was developed. It was called "Harvey," after W. Proctor Harvey, MD, of Georgetown University and mentor to Harvey's inventor, Michael Gordon, MD, PhD, who was based at the University of Miami's Center for Research in Medical Education (CRME) [1, 7]. Harvey was able to simulate breath sounds, pulses, jugular venous and arterial blood pressures, and cardiac sounds varying for 27 cardiac conditions. Medical students who trained on Harvey were better able to identify heart conditions by auscultation in patients than peers who did not [7].

In the 1980s, two groups simultaneously developed full-body computer-controlled mannequin simulators. J.S. "Nik" Gravenstein, MD, founder of the Department of Anesthesiology at the University of Florida (UF) and cofounder of the Anesthesia Patient Safety Foundation (APSF), together with Michael Good, MD, an anesthesiologist with a computer science degree who worked at UF, and Samsun "Sem" Lampotang, PhD, were the founding inventors of the Gainesville Anesthesia Simulator (GAS), more recently called the Human Patient Simulator (HPS). This system is currently marketed by Montreal-based CAE Healthcare, formerly Medical Education Technologies Incorporated (METI), in Sarasota, Florida, the latter licensing the HPS technology from UF [1]. The HPS system was initially created to train residents on clinical anesthesia-related skills. Simulation cases range from detecting anesthesia machine faults to complex reenactments of intraoperative emergencies.

On the other side of the country, David Gaba, MD, and colleagues at the Veterans Hospital affiliated with Stanford University in Palo Alto developed the Comprehensive Anesthesia Simulation Environment (CASE) to investigate individual and team performance in anesthesia scenarios. CASE 1.2 (commercially known as "Virtual Anesthesiology Training Simulator System" or VATSS) combined a mannequin simulator with a Macintosh Plus computer that could alter the vital signs such as the blood pressure measured by a noninvasive blood pressure cuff. The models running VATSS were licensed from Howard Schwid, MD, an anesthesiologist and engineer. Simulation scenarios were created to observe and evaluate individual and group performance in critical events. CASE 2.0's components included a mannequin, an interface cart, and simulation computers with parallel processing to run multiple physiological capabilities simultaneously and an instructor's control station. CASE 2.0 was brought to Boston, and collaborative efforts laid the foundation for the establishment of the Boston Anesthesia Simulation Center, now known as the Center for Medical Simulation (www.harvardmedsim.org). The CASE system and software underwent several iterations, the last one being the MedSim-Eagle Patient Simulator, before it was discontinued.

Screen-Based Computer Simulators

Modern full-body mannequin simulators and part-task trainers that incorporate computer-driven features have continued to receive favorable attention; however, they are notably expensive to build and purchase. As a result, their use is limited to a few anesthesiology departments or hospitals with resources to purchase and house them or in cost-sharing simulation centers. This also restricts frequent use by trainees or groups with limited time to attend simulation sessions. Both time and cost have been significant drivers for the development of cheaper, more accessible products (Table 12.1).

In the early 1960s, a prototype screen-based simulator was developed by Entwisle on an LGP-30 digital computer (also known as Librascope General Precision, made by Royal

Precision Corporation, Port Chester, NY) that presented patient scenarios to students and allowed them to determine the diagnosis based upon an array of physical findings [8]. Students would enter a symptom, and the computer would respond "yes" or "no" depending on the case [9]. Ventre and Schwid identify this prototype as the origin of screen-based trainers [9].

The personal computer (PC) was introduced in the early 1980s and the World Wide Web in 1989. These enabled learning to occur at home or anywhere the personal device was located. Software was developed to run as an installable package or within web browsers. Screen-based trainers, a.k.a. computer-based trainers (CBT), were developed to represent a range of simple concepts or complex scenarios. Screen-based trainers display a graphical output onto a computer screen, and many allow for user interaction through input devices such as a mouse, keyboard, controller, or finger through a touch display. Cloud-based computing has allowed for many programs to be run through web browsers such as Chrome, Safari, Firefox, and Internet Explorer.

Advantages of screen-based anesthesia simulators (Table 12.1) and recommended basic technical standards and key attributes put forth by Ventre and Schwid (Table 12.2) remain valid [9]. Screen-based simulators are flexible, in that they allow learners to practice on their own time and in any location. They are scalable and cost-effective, many being delivered for free or at minimal cost. Lastly, because they are software based and employ interactivity, the learner's decision-making process and performance can be tracked to provide feedback to the learner and teacher [9].

Modern CBTs in anesthesiology range from the complex virtual reality (VR) and mixed-reality simulators that replicate multiple tasks and run on sophisticated software engines to the simpler task-specific or model-specific simulators that use basic animation and interactive inputs to teach only a few concepts [10–12]. Many of the most impressive anesthesia CBTs are those that have been developed and updated over the years as technology has advanced. Unfortunately, many of the older CBTs in anesthesia have not been updated or upgraded to keep up with modern operating systems or browsers and their plugins, so they are no longer available or simply won't run and, as a result, are not being used by the modern anesthesiology learner. A highlight of some influential CBTs for anesthesiology follows here (Table 12.3).

Table 12.2 Key attributes of screen-based simulators

1. A graphical user interface
2. An engine of models to predict simulated responses
3. An embedded feedback/help system
4. An automated debriefing and log system
5. A case library
6. Compatibility with learning management systems (LMS)

Data from (Ventre and Schwid, 2013) [9]

Table 12.3 Classic computer-based trainers in anesthesiology

BODY Simulation (1978) – N. Ty Smith
Anesthesia Simulator Recorder (1989) – Schwid and O'Donnell
Anesoft Anesthesia Simulator (1995) – Schwid
Gas Man (1990s) – James Philip
Virtual Anesthesia Machine (1999) – Samsun Lampotang

Examples of Computer-Based Trainers

BODY Simulation (1978)

N. Ty Smith, MD, PhD, (1932–2015), professor of anesthesiology at the University of California San Diego (UCSD), was a visionary who foresaw the use of simulation for anesthesiology training and the advantage that "small simulators" have over the "large" or high-fidelity simulators [13]. He was the founding president of the Society for Technology in Anesthesia and pioneered the use of computers in the operating room. In 1978, he described the invention of an analog precursor of BODY Simulation (BodySim), *Sleeper*. BodySim was a PC-based interactive simulator based on mathematical models of patient physiology and pharmacology and included representations of an anesthesia workstation and the operating room environment. Due to his expertise in anesthesia monitoring, the models built into BODY Simulation presented a sophistication not previously seen in simulation [14].

The current BodySim software can be found online as a 32-bit program that is unable to run on modern 64-bit computers. Its features include two levels of interaction: clinical training and scientific background. The learner can observe and interact with the patient and operating room personnel and manage the anesthetic care of the patient by controlling the anesthesia machine, the drug delivery, the ventilator and monitors, and the anesthesia record to carry out tasks and deal with critical operating room incidents. Further, the user can generate kinetic plots of agent concentrations in body compartments, observe dynamic tables of respiratory variables, follow pressure and flow-volume curves, and more.

Anesthesia Simulator Recorder (1989)

The Anesthesia Simulator Recorder, later named the Anesthesia Simulator Consultant (1990), was developed in 1989 by Howard Schwid, MD, a former fellow in the UCSD labs with N. Ty Smith and then an Assistant Professor of Anesthesiology at the University of Washington, and Daniel O'Donnell, PhD, a systems analyst and programmer [9]. Their work was supported by a grant from the Anesthesia Patient Safety Foundation. The Anesthesia Simulator Recorder was an expansion of an earlier version described in 1987,

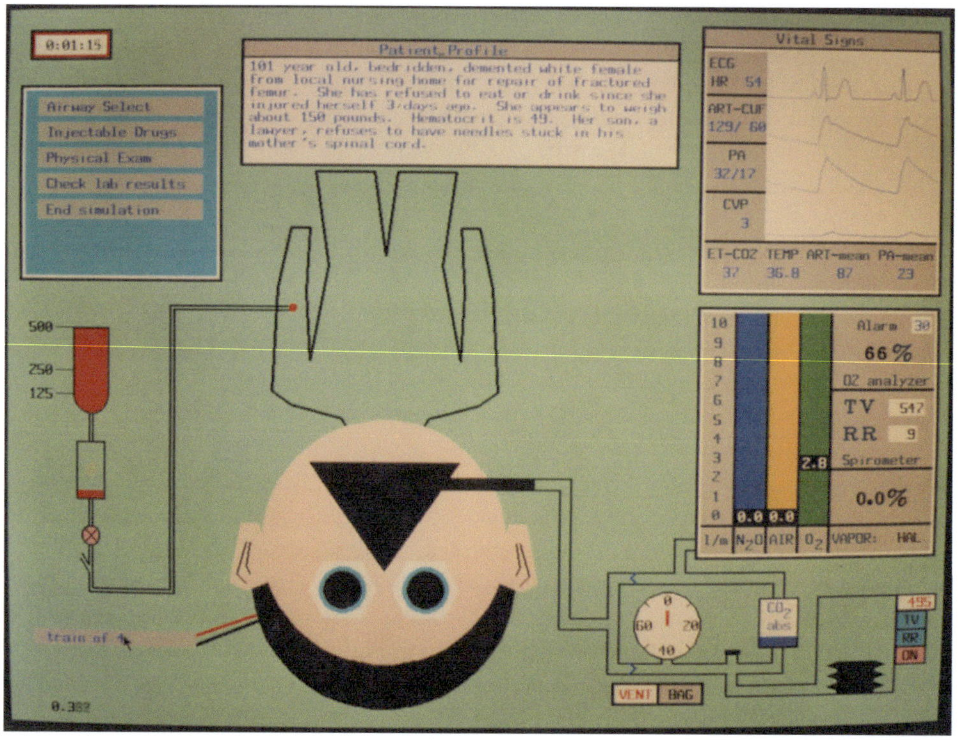

Fig. 12.1 A screen-based simulator for general anesthesia training (1987) designed after contemporary flight simulators. (Reproduced with permission of Schwid [31])

designed after contemporary flight simulators (Fig. 12.1), and a simplification of models developed for BodySim at UCSD [15]. It was designed to run on an IBM PC utilizing a graphical user interface, keyboard, and mouse. The software simulated a patient, the anesthesia machine, and monitors, and integrated mathematical models simulated patient vital signs, physiology, and response to drugs. Simulated critical event scenarios allowed the learner to work through treatment scenarios while recording a summary of the process that could later on be printed for review.

Anesoft Anesthesia Simulator (1995)

The Anesoft Anesthesia Simulator development began over 25 years ago as the Anesthesia Simulator Recorder [16]. Anesoft Corporation was founded in 1995 and has since marketed several screen-based simulators including Anesoft Anesthesia Simulator (Fig. 12.2), Anesoft Sedation Simulator, Advanced Cardiac Life Support (ACLS) Simulator, Pediatric Advanced Life Support (PALS) Simulator, Bioterrorism Simulator, and Critical Care Simulator [9].

The Anesoft Anesthesia Simulator is a case-based simulator that contains over 80 anesthesiology-related patients or case scenarios that include general anesthesia and the specialties of regional, cardiac, pediatric, obstetric, and neurosurgical anesthesia. The interface has a menu that toggles through management options for the user to control the anesthetic care of the patient, the airway, drug delivery, order labs, and more. There is an image of the patient and a dynamic display of vitals and waveforms. The simulation also contains an automated debriefing system and a context-sensitive help system to guide the learner to ensure learning objectives have been met.

Gas Man®

Gas Man® (MED MAN Simulations, Chestnut Hill, MA, USA) is an example of a 2D animation, screen-based simulator (Fig. 12.3) [17]. Dr. James Philip is Director of Bioengineering at Brigham and Women's Hospital and a founding member of the Society for Technology in Anesthesia (STA). He is the creator of Gas Man®, a screen-based simulator, textbook, and learning environment, which teaches the pharmacokinetics of anesthesia administration by demonstrating the uptake into body compartments (the heart, lung, brain) as well as the anesthesia breathing circuit and vaporizers (Fig. 12.3).

The Virtual Anesthesia Machine (1999)

The Virtual Anesthesia Machine (VAM) (University of Florida, Gainesville, FL, USA) was developed in 1999 by Samsun Lampotang, PhD; David Lizdas, BSME; and others as a way for anesthesiologists to conceptualize the working of an anesthesia machine. It was the first widely adopted web-enabled simulator in anesthesiology [18]. The simulation was developed on a Macromedia Director platform, now

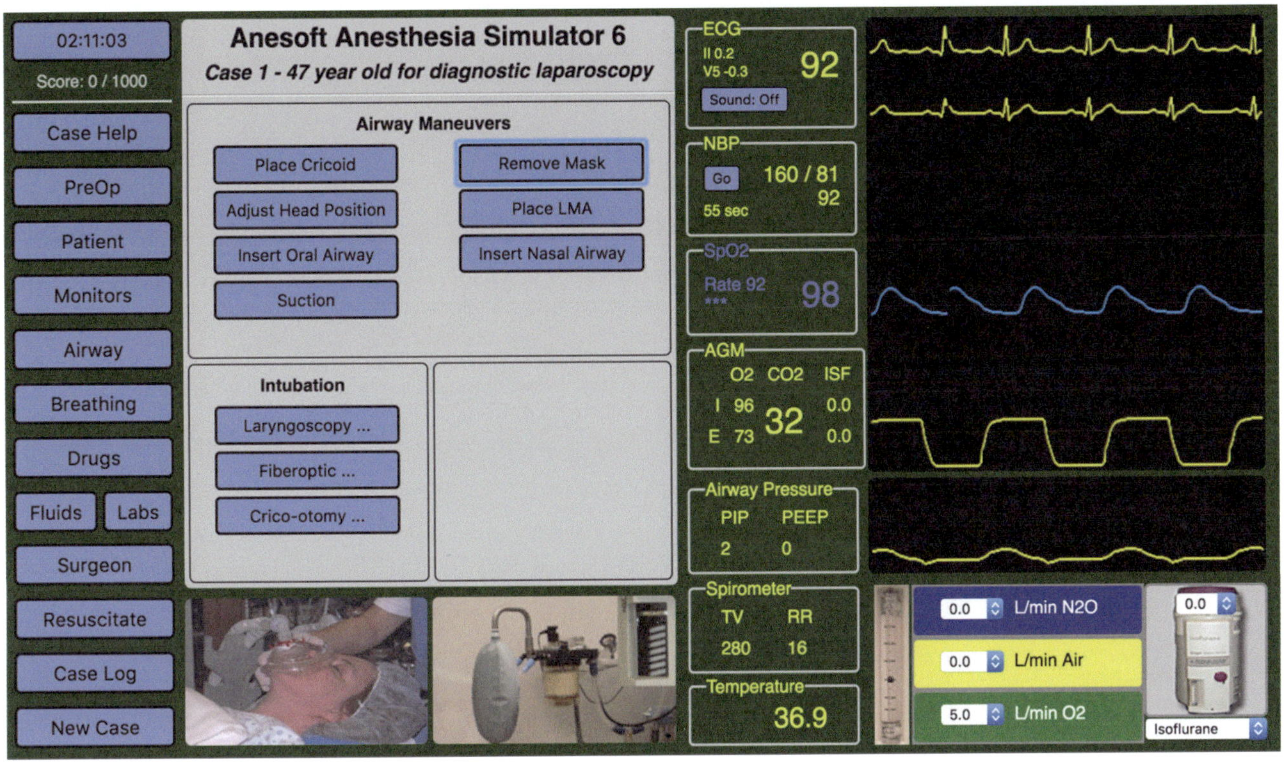

Fig. 12.2 The Anesoft Anesthesia Simulator 6 – a screen-based anesthesia simulator that allows users to practice in a safe environment the complete management of a patient under anesthesia

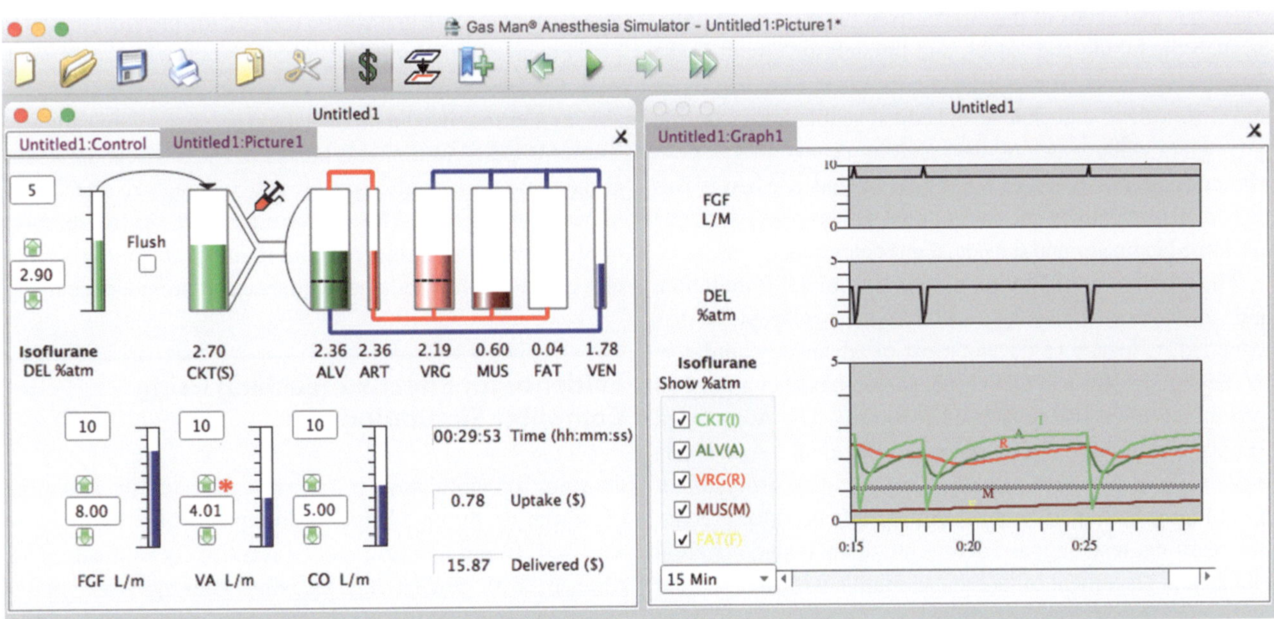

Fig. 12.3 Gas Man® – a screen-based simulation of anesthetic tension in the respective compartments. The user can adjust the vaporizer settings, the fresh gas flow rate, alveolar ventilation, and cardiac output. The software is available at http://www.gasmanweb.com (Philip 2015) [17]

Adobe, because of its powerful animation capabilities and (at that time) royalty-free web distribution as a way to disseminate patient safety information broadly around the world [18]. With funding support from the Anesthesia Patient Safety Foundation, an accompanying workbook was created to explain the fundamental anesthesia machine design considerations and how the VAM can be used and to develop a series of exercises to impart understanding of the anesthesia machine subsystems (high pressure, low pressure, breathing circuit, manual ventilation, mechanical ventilation, and scavenging)

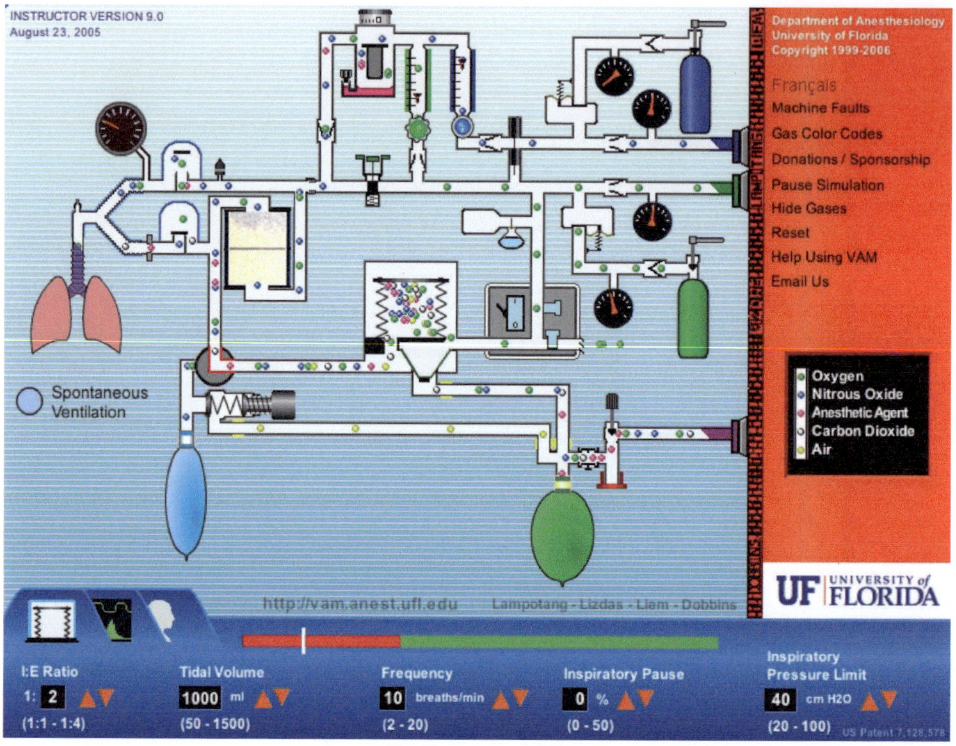

Fig. 12.4 The University of Florida Virtual Anesthesia Machine (VAM) is a 2D interactive, web-enabled simulation that teaches gas flow and machine fault concepts

and common machine faults [18]. Through the animation, the inside of the anesthesia machine is visible as are the color-coded gas molecules as they travel from the wall or gas tank, through the tubing and valves, and through the circuit to the patient (Fig. 12.4). The user is able to squeeze the bag, open and close valves, and change and adjust ventilation mode and parameters while watching the resulting change in gas flow. The considerable reach of VAM was extended when it was translated pro bono by anesthesiologist native speakers into 23 available languages and 6 medical gas color codes.

The University of Florida Center for Safety, Simulation, and Advanced Learning Technologies (CSSALT) has extended its legacy of development of advanced simulators by combining physical and virtual screen-based components into mixed-reality simulators [12, 19, 20]. The Augmented Reality Simulator of Thoracic Regional Anesthesia (Fig. 12.5) is a robust, turnkey, mixed-reality simulator of part of an anatomically correct thorax. It is used for practicing, learning, teaching, and debriefing thoracic paravertebral blocks and placement of thoracic epidurals with and without ultrasound guidance or assistance.

This simulator includes a physical model of a 3D-printed thoracic spine embedded in gel attached to a laptop computer that displays a virtual representation of the physical 3D spine with the addition of subcutaneous structures. Attached to the laptop are several peripherals that allow for interaction with the physical model: an ultrasound probe pressed against the physical model creates a simulated ultrasound image on the laptop screen, a directional pointer allows the learner to adjust the point of view of the 3D visualization on the laptop screen to analyze the virtual anatomy and needle approach, and a Tuohy needle that can be used on the physical model to perform an epidural or paravertebral block with tactile feedback for loss of resistance is tracked in 3D space and viewable as a virtual needle on the laptop screen. All this allows a learner to perform regional blocks of the thoracic spine and at the same time or afterward watch and analyze one's technique on the screen. The software includes several learning modules to allow for independent training, and a scoring system grades the learner's performance and provides feedback.

Evidence for Effective Teaching Using Computer Simulation

One aim of simulation is the recreation of life situations or scenarios through which participants may learn or be assessed. Being able to practice repetitively in a safe environment with few, if any, negative consequences, before applying one's skills or knowledge in the real world, intuitively seems like it would be effective and preferred. However, studies of the efficacy of computer-based simulation are mixed. This is true for several reasons: first, it can be difficult to determine whether enhanced learning is due simply to the increased time spent in education regardless of whether it involves simulation or whether learning is actually enhanced by the process of simulation specifically. Further, learning can be environment or task specific, so attempts to

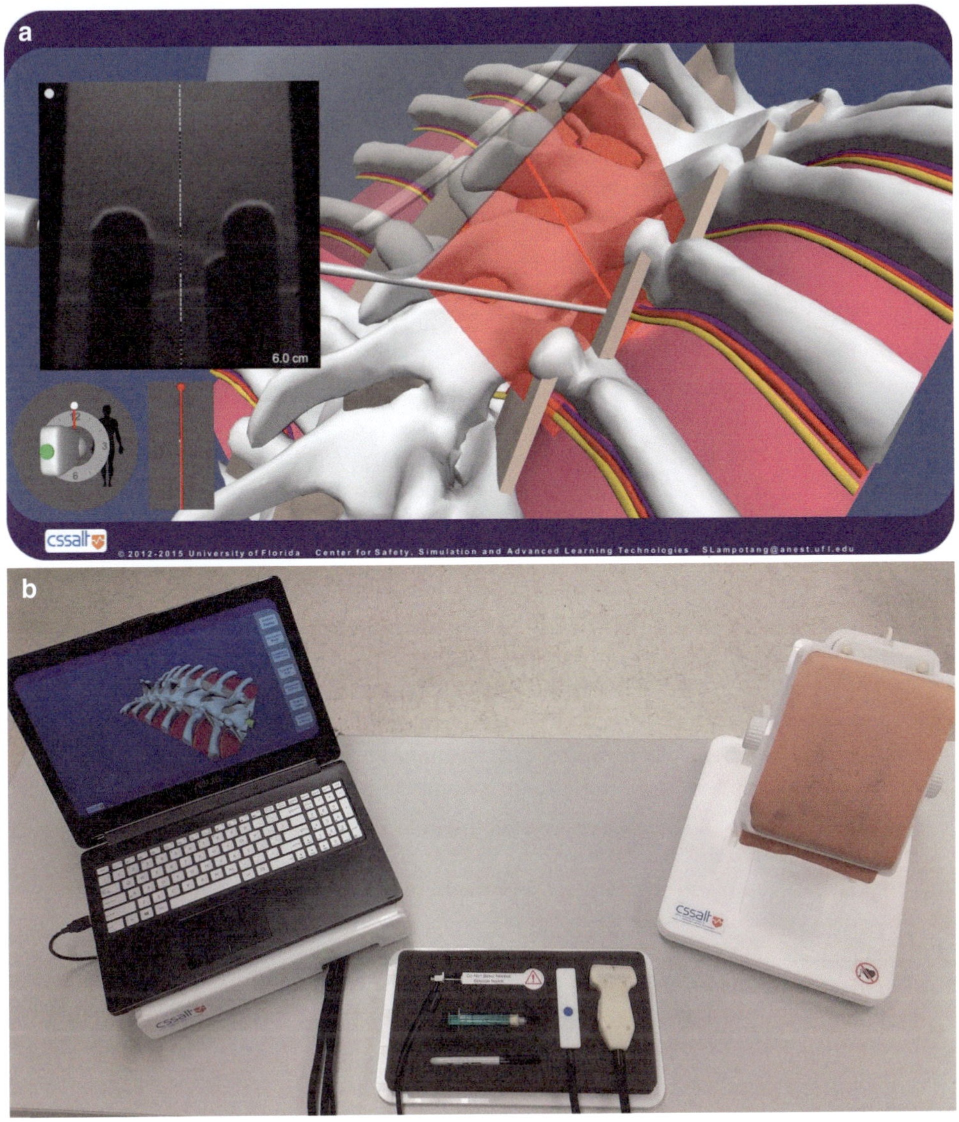

Fig. 12.5 The University of Florida Thoracic Spine Simulator combines physical and virtual screen-based components into a mixed-reality simulator. a) Computer monitor screen showing a simulated ultrasound (inset), and 3-dimensional representation of the thoracic region of the spine. b) Table top setup showing the portable simulator components: the laptop, input devices (needle, ultrasound probe, directionality pointer), and the physical mounted 3-D printed thoracic spine

measure the efficacy of simulation training on improvement in the clinical realm may not translate easily. It has even been shown that in some instances, perception of enhanced learning does not necessarily match actual learning, and a participant's overconfidence can actually result in worsened performance. In addition, methodological issues such as flawed study protocols and uncontrolled confounding influences when assessing the efficacy of simulators can result in erroneous results and conclusions.

Topic-specific simulations and models that teach specific concepts are rarely studied to see if they have that effect. Many screen-based simulations exist, but their impact on the learner has not been measured in anesthesiology [10, 21]. Yavas et al. developed a screen-based topic-specific model of the pharmacokinetics of fospropofol in comparison to propofol [21]. The authors declare that, "such interactive models may provide a realistic and real-time method for practitioners to familiarize themselves with dispensing a new drug." [21]

Schwid and O'Donnell used screen-based simulation to recreate critical events during anesthesia to prospectively observe and potentially quantify the frequency of anesthesiologist error [22]. This approach to assessment shows the versatility of simulation and the benefit of being able to reproduce critical event scenarios in a safe environment. The validity may depend highly on the fidelity of the simulation in these types of experiments. In other words, the errors observed while an anesthesiologist performs in simulation may not be what are actually seen in the operating room environment. There is great value, however, in being able to identify lapses in judgment, knowledge gaps, and failures that are consistent across subjects, especially when debriefing confirms an incorrect or incomplete understanding.

In one study, Schwid and O'Donnell used the Anesthesia Simulator Consultant to evaluate the performance of 30 participants (10 anesthesiology residents, 10 faculty anesthesiologists, 10 private practice anesthesiologists) during

6 critical care cases [22]. Participants managed the care of simulated patients on-screen and were observed to manage either correctly or incorrectly critical events such as myocardial ischemia, anaphylaxis, and cardiac arrest. Many errors were observed even among experienced anesthesiologists. While only 2/30 (both were residents) did not detect esophageal intubation, 60% failed to identify the signs and symptoms of anaphylaxis, and only 30% correctly managed the ACLS protocol for cardiac arrest. No participant who had trained in ACLS greater than 2 years prior successfully managed the protocol.

An example of modern, single-task screen-based simulation is a virtual airway simulation, called iLarynx, developed by De Oliveira et al., at Northwestern University in Chicago [23]. The application was built using the iPhone software development kit (Apple Inc., Cupertino, CA, USA) and Unity 3D gaming engine (Unity Technologies SF, San Francisco, CA, USA) and takes advantage of the accelerometer abilities of the iPhone as a control to maneuver a simulated fiber-optic scope down a virtual airway. Twenty medical students were randomly assigned to instruction plus iLarynx practice versus instruction only and then evaluated on time to fiber-optic placement to the carina on a mannequin. There were 24 failed attempts in the control group and only 4 failed attempts in the trained group. Screen-based virtual part-task trainers may improve task performance of novices. Whether the performance observed represents a legitimate indicator of capability that can translate to the clinic is the obvious next test and has yet to be shown with any screen-based simulation in anesthesiology.

Learning is said to have been enhanced by simulation when knowledge tests show improvement. In the few studies of screen-based simulators in anesthesiology, subjects had a favorable experience and felt that the use of the simulator enhanced their understanding [11, 16, 24, 25]. In pretest and posttest evaluation, scores were higher in subjects who practiced on Gas Man [24]. Retention of ACLS algorithms was better in subjects who practiced with screen-based simulation compared to those who only used a textbook [26]. Those who were trained on the Transparent Virtual Anesthesia Machine scored higher on the posttest, and their knowledge of cause and effect related to anesthesia machine errors was greater [11]. Debriefing after screen-based simulation can improve performance on mannequin-based simulator [27].

Conclusion

The pioneers in medical simulation were progressive academic anesthesiologists who worked at the vanguard of technology to advance the safety of anesthesia. All living anesthesiologists have benefited from the foundation of education these innovators have established. With the hyper-growth of digital technology, exponential increase in processing power, and learning ability of machine algorithms, the task of the modern clinical anesthesiologist is to continue to bring these tools into medical education and practice. Mixed-reality and virtual reality technology promises to further increase simulation fidelity through near-complete immersion [28–30]. The American Society of Anesthesiology and CAE Healthcare have partnered to develop online virtual environments for screen-based simulation training (https://www.asahq.org/education-and-career/educational-and-cme-offerings/simulation-education/anesthesia-simstat). The challenge for academia remains to validate simulation in whatever form, not only for learning but in creating competent anesthesiologists and safer patient outcomes.

References

1. Cooper JB, Taqueti VR. A brief history of the development of mannequin simulators for clinical education and training. Postgrad Med J. 2008;84:563–70. https://doi.org/10.1136/qshc.2004.009886.
2. "Annie, are you OK?". http://www.laerdal.com/us/News/49080368/Annie-are-you-OK. Accessed 29 Dec 2016.
3. Denson JS, Abrahamson S. A computer-controlled patient simulator. JAMA. 1969;208:504–8. https://doi.org/10.1001/jama.1969.03160030078009.
4. Abrahamson S. Essays on medical education: (S.A.'s on Medical Education). New York: University Press of America, Inc.; 1996.
5. Barnes A, Scott RP. Sim one - the first computer-controlled patient simulator - VHA SimLEARN. http://www.simlearn.va.gov/SIMLEARN/FA_2010_4-Sim_One_The_First_Computer_Controlled_Patient_Simulator.asp. Accessed 29 Dec 2016.
6. Denson JS, Abrahamson S, Wolf RM. Effectiveness of a simulator in training anesthesiology residents. 2004;13:395–7. https://doi.org/10.1136/qhc.13.5.395.
7. Woolliscroft JO, Calhoun JG, Tenhaken JD, Judge RD. Harvey: the impact of a cardiovascular teaching simulator on student skill acquisition. Med Teach. 1987a;9:53–7.
8. Entwisle G, Entwisle DR. The use of a digital computer as a teaching machine. J Med Educ. 1963;38:803–12.
9. Ventre KM, Schwid HA. Computer and web based simulators. In: Anonymous the comprehensive textbook of healthcare simulation. 2013th ed. DE: Springer Verlag; 2013. p. 191–208.
10. Edwards DA, Rice M. (2011) 15 minute power lecture: vaporizers and the Copper Kettle. Accessed 30 Dec 2016.
11. Fischler IS, Kaschub CE, Lizdas DE, Lampotang S. Understanding of anesthesia machine function is enhanced with a transparent reality simulation. Simul Healthc. 2008a;3:26–32. https://doi.org/10.1097/SIH.0b013e31816366d3.
12. Robinson AR, Gravenstein N, Cooper LA, Lizdas D, Luria I, Lampotang S. A mixed-reality part-task trainer for subclavian venous access. Simul Healthc. 2014;9:56–64. https://doi.org/10.1097/SIH.0b013e31829b3fb3.
13. Smith NT. Simulation in anesthesia: the merits of large simulators versus small simulators. Curr Opin Anaesthesiol. 2000;13:659–65.
14. Smith NT, Starko KR. The physiology and pharmacology of growing old, as shown in body simulation. Stud Health Technol Inform. 2005;111:488–91.
15. Rosen KR. The history of medical simulation. J Crit Care. 2008;23:157–66. https://doi.org/10.1016/j.jcrc.2007.12.004.

16. Schwid HA, O'Donnell D. The anesthesia simulator-recorder: a device to train and evaluate anesthesiologists' responses to critical incidents. Anesthesiology. 1990;72:191–7. https://doi.org/10.1097/00000542-199001000-00028.
17. Philip JH. Using screen-based simulation of inhaled anaesthetic delivery to improve patient care. Brit J Anesth. 2015;115(Suppl 2):ii94. https://doi.org/10.1093/bja/aev370.
18. Lampotang S. Computer and web-enabled simulations for anesthesiology training and credentialing. J Crit Care. 2008;23:173–8. https://doi.org/10.1016/j.jcrc.2008.01.002.
19. Lampotang S, Lizdas D, Rajon D, Luria I, Gravenstein N, Bisht Y, Schwab W, Friedman W, Bova F, Robinson A. Mixed simulators: augmented physical simulators with virtual underlays. Proceedings of the IEEE Virtual Reality 2013 meeting 978-1-4673-4796-9/13: 7-10, 2013.
20. Sappenfield JW, Smith WB, Cooper LA, Lizdas DE, Gonsalves D, Gravenstein N, Lampotang S, Robinson AR. Visualization improves supraclavicular access to the subclavian vein in a mixed reality simulator. Anesth Analg. 2018 *ecopy ahead of print* https://doi.org/10.1213/ANE.0000000000002572.
21. Yavas S, Lizdas D, Gravenstein N, Lampotang S. Interactive web simulation for propofol and fospropofol, a new propofol prodrug. Anesth Analg. 2008;106:880–3. https://doi.org/10.1213/ane.0b013e3181614fae.
22. Schwid HA, O'Donnell D. Anesthesiologists' management of simulated critical incidents. Anesthesiology. 1992;76:495–501.
23. Oliveira GS, Glassenberg R, Chang R, Fitzgerald P, McCarthy RJ. Virtual airway simulation to improve dexterity among novices performing fibreoptic intubation. Anaesthesia. 2013;68:1053–8. https://doi.org/10.1111/anae.12379.
24. Garfield JM, Paskin S, Philip JH. An evaluation of the effectiveness of a computer simulation of anaesthetic uptake and distribution as a teaching tool. Med Educ. 1989;23:457–62.
25. Schwid HA. Computer simulations and management of critical incidents. Acad Med. 1994;69:213.
26. Schwid HA, Rooke GA, Ross BK, Sivarajan M. Use of a computerized advanced cardiac life support simulator improves retention of advanced cardiac life support guidelines better than a textbook review. Crit Care Med. 1999;27:821–4.
27. Schwid HA, Rooke GA, Michalowski P, Ross BK. Screen-based anesthesia simulation with debriefing improves performance in a mannequin-based anesthesia simulator. Teach Learn Med. 2001;13:92–6. https://doi.org/10.1207/S15328015TLM1302_4.
28. Aïm F, Lonjon G, Hannouche D, Nizard R. Effectiveness of Virtual Reality Training in Orthopaedic Surgery. Arthroscopy. 2016;32:224–32. https://doi.org/10.1016/j.arthro.2015.07.023.
29. Vaughan N, Dubey VN, Wainwright TW, Middleton RG. A review of virtual reality based training simulators for orthopaedic surgery. Med Eng Phys. 2016;38:59–71. https://doi.org/10.1016/j.medengphy.2015.11.021.
30. Yiannakopoulou E, Nikiteas N, Perrea D, Tsigris C. Virtual reality simulators and training in laparoscopic. Surgery. 2015;13:60–4. https://doi.org/10.1016/j.ijsu.2014.11.014.
31. Schwid HA. A flight simulator for general anesthesia training. Comput Biomed Res. 20(1):64–75.

Part III

General Practice of Anesthesiology

Undergraduate Medical Education

13

Jonathan Lipps and Lori Meyers

Introduction

Simulation-based education as a tool for instruction and evaluation has been used successfully across many domains, both within and external to medicine. The military and aviation industry have been innovators in the use of simulation technology to provide personnel with experience in highly stressful, rare, or critical situations which prove difficult to encounter in a real-life training situation. Simulation-based technology has also shown itself to be an invaluable tool in team-based training paradigms such as crew resource management (CRM) through the feature of repetitive practice and refinement of skills in a high-fidelity simulated environment. Ideally, this repetitive practice of high-intensity situations in a safe and controlled environment allows trainees to gain increased competency in protocols and communication skills conferring increased safety to their respective industries. The healthcare industry has worked to leverage these features of simulation technology in order to increase trainee aptitude in domains such as procedural skills, communication, and competency in the management of rare and critical events that may be encountered in clinical practice.

In 1960, Resusci Anne was developed to provide simulation-based training in a newly protocolized life support method, allowing trainees the ability to practice prior to encountering life-threatening emergencies [1]. From this modest beginning, the role of simulation-based training has expanded beyond the practice of life support and into multiple subspecialties of medical practice at the undergraduate, graduate, and postgraduate level. From the earliest stages of general medical education, competency in basic professional interaction with patients, families, and other healthcare professionals can be facilitated through simulation. For the medical student, simulation may first be encountered through its use in the acquisition of skills such as history taking, physical examination, and basic procedural skills through the use of standardized patients, mannequin-based simulators, or partial task trainers. High-fidelity simulation (HFS) has been less frequently encountered in undergraduate medical education given its traditional use in team training and for providing exposure to rare and critical events. While HFS can provide medical students with an immersive environment in which they can participate in scenarios that mimic general critical events such as cardiac arrest, creative use of this tool can also provide innovative and effective methods for teaching basic science principles. Coupled with post-scenario debriefing or even hybrid didactic simulation-based models of instruction, HFS can provide a powerful tool for students during the preclinical and clinical portions of undergraduate medical education.

As a goal of undergraduate medical education and as the Association of American Medical Colleges (AAMC) and similar bodies seek to better ensure medical student preparedness for internship and residency, simulation-based assessment can provide a tool for evaluating preparedness or competency attainment. The 13 Core Entrustable Professional Activities (EPAs) developed by the AAMC provide a discrete set of measurable skills for which some medical schools are currently utilizing simulation as a means of assessment [2].

Such simulation-based assessment would preview for medical students future encounters with simulation as an assessment tool, given its use in medical degree qualification and subspecialty board certification [3].

While anesthesiologists have proven to be early adopters and innovators of simulation-based technology for clinical anesthesia training, we have also begun to show a track record of introducing this art into general medical education. By coupling a large degree of simulation expertise with universal proficiency in pharmacology, physiology, advanced cardiac life support, and critical event management,

J. Lipps (✉) · L. Meyers
Department of Anesthesiology, The Ohio State University Wexner Medical Center, Columbus, OH, USA
e-mail: Jonathan.lipps@osumc.edu; Lori.meyers@osumc.edu

B. Mahoney et al. (eds.), *Comprehensive Healthcare Simulation: Anesthesiology*, Comprehensive Healthcare Simulation,
https://doi.org/10.1007/978-3-030-26849-7_13

anesthesiologists have a great opportunity to contribute to every level of undergraduate medical education as curricula designers, preclinical or clinical instructors, or medical student evaluators.

Rationale for an Anesthesiologist-Driven Undergraduate Education

The general practice of anesthesia has evolved a great deal over the last century through improvements in technology and pharmacology, changes in the nature and setting of surgical interventions, and expansion of the patient population exposed to anesthesia care. Through this development, the practice of anesthesiology has found itself further removed from medical generalists compared to other medical specialties in both knowledge base and practice. This feature of the profession offers both opportunities and challenges for anesthesiologists looking to become involved in undergraduate medical education. While medical student exposure to the practice of anesthesiology during the clinical years can be sporadic, exposure to anesthesiologists in the nonclinical years is virtually nonexistent. Increasing the role of anesthesiologists in undergraduate medical education allows experts in physiology, pharmacology, and technology to provide useful contributions to relevant subjects taught to medical students during both the nonclinical and clinical years of undergraduate medical training.

While most preclinical medical school curricula do not provide any specific focus on topics relevant to the clinical practice of anesthesiology, anesthesiology training requires a strong foundation in basic medical sciences such as pharmacology and cardiopulmonary physiology. Given the merely partial overlap of anesthetic pharmacology with general medical pharmacology or the more limited cardiopulmonary principles relevant to anesthesia practice compared to general cardiac and pulmonary physiology presented to medical students in their preclinical years of training, anesthesiologists rarely instruct such courses. Typically, anesthesiologists' contribution to medical student education has focused on instruction in basic airway management. While this is certainly an appropriate domain for anesthesiologist-driven instruction, the scope of anesthesiologist expertise and practice allows for many other opportunities for anesthesiologists to contribute to the medical school curriculum, and simulation technology can provide an educational context for this instruction. Topics such as physiology and dynamic pharmacology can be effectively reinforced through simulation, and the high-fidelity simulation lab is an ideal arena for the teaching anesthesiologist. Anesthesiologists, specialists for whom real-time changes in physiology and the effects of pharmacology are routine practice, can utilize HFS to imitate the operating room or intensive care unit setting to recreate dynamic physiology and pharmacology for the medical student accustomed to standard didactic instruction.

The benefits of anesthesiologist-driven undergraduate medical education can also be reciprocal. Unsurprisingly, while medical students do not typically decide upon their specialty training until their clinical years, their interactions with physician instructors throughout medical school can have a profound effect on their specialty choice [4–6]. Paiva et al. showed that instructors with whom medical students have had contact, especially full-time faculty members and community physicians who teach part-time, are the most influential factor in specialty preference. While especially true for the clinical years, this effect is also significant for the basic science (preclinical) years [5]. Kassebaum et al. also determined that seeing examples of a physician in a particular specialty had a moderate influence on students' choice of medical specialty [6]. In many medical schools, exposure to anesthesiology is not a core component of the clinical years of training, and in those in which it is, by the time some students have been exposed to the field, he or she may have already chosen a different career path. Integration of anesthesiologist educators through every stage of medical school can provide role models otherwise not encountered by potential future anesthesiologists. DeMaria et al. assessed medical students' attitudes toward anesthesiology before and after participating in simulation-based physiology labs taught by anesthesiology faculty and residents during the first year of medical school. After taking part in the lab, students' perceptions about the specialty improved. Furthermore, they found the field to be more stimulating, hands-on, and rewarding than they had initially believed, and the students also were more likely to consider anesthesiology as a career choice [7].

Anesthesiologist-Driven Education in the Nonclinical Years

Current trends in medical school curricula to provide better clinical fidelity through vertical curricular integration—the blending of basic science principles with practical clinical applications—present a unique opportunity for anesthesiologists to assume a larger role as in preclinical or early undergraduate medical education [8]. Vertical curricular integration serves the purpose of both providing learners with a clinical context for the basic science concepts presented and providing students with early exposure to the clinical specialties involved in the lesson. While learning in situ—the hands-on learning of basic science concepts in the clinical setting—would be the most direct path to achieving vertical curricular integration, practical considerations such as patient safety may prevent extensive application of this strategy [9]. High-fidelity simulation of clinical settings, however, can provide a reproducible experience tailored to the concepts targeted within a controlled and safe environment.

Simulation-based education has long been a part of preclinical undergraduate medical education and is now nearly ubiquitous across medical schools. A survey sponsored by the AAMC in 2011 showed that simulation is being used as an educational modality in 84% and 91% of medical schools in the first and second years, respectively [10]. This shift toward an increased use of simulation-based medical education (SBME) may rest in part on a growing recognition of the opportunity for an immersive experience provided by simulation technology not previously available through more traditional didactic modalities. Simulation technology can engage medical students across three of the most common learning types: visual, auditory, and kinesthetic. SBME allows the students to be actively involved, or hands-on, a critical quality for kinesthetic learners but also effective for visual and auditory learners. By incorporating diverse teaching modalities, learning and retention is enhanced [11]. In recognition of medical students as adult learners, the physician simulation instructor must be familiar with the five key principles of Adult Learning Theory during curriculum design:

1. Adults need to know why they are learning.
2. Adults are motivated to learn by a need to solve problems.
3. Adults' previous experience must be respected and built upon.
4. Adults need learning approaches that match their background and diversity.
5. Adults need to be actively involved in the learning process.

By integrating adult learning principles into a simulation curriculum design, SBME can help to build upon the didactic instruction and reading that has taken place while providing an opportunity to engage with the content in a clinically relevant context within a safe high-fidelity simulated environment. Finally, and critically, simulation can inject an emotional component to learning which is otherwise absent from traditional basic science preclinical course material. Gordon argues that immersive exercises can provide an "affective anchor," promoting memory and enhancing the application of basic sciences in the clinical environment [12].

The content domains most commonly taught through the use of simulation are clinical skills, introduction to clinical medicine, and physical diagnosis (Fig. 13.1). Simulated patient encounters and role modeling using standardized patient actors constitute a large portion of a medical student's earliest clinical experience and are used by over 90% of medical schools [10]. Interpersonal communication, professionalism, and basic physical exam skills are commonly practiced with a standardized patient in a simulated environment. After careful observation and evaluation by medical school faculty in performing such tasks, the students may be better prepared to interact with patients in the clinical years.

While clinical and interpersonal communication skills appear to be obvious targets for incorporating simulation into the preclinical curriculum given the extensive use of standardized patients that exist nationally in medical schools, the basic (hard) sciences, traditionally approached through didactic or problem-based learning focused models, can also be effectively taught through simulation. At first glance, simulation, let alone high-fidelity simulation, may not be the best fit for demonstrating topics such as pharmacology and physiology. However, several educators have successfully utilized HFS to great effect. Physiology has traditionally been proven to be a challenging topic for medical students and educators alike [13]. HFS demonstrations and lab experiences for medical students provide an opportunity for educators to integrate basic physiology principles into simulated clinical scenarios. Several educators have shown simulation-enhanced physiology instruction to be preferred by students and in some cases superior with respect to knowledge acquisition. Euliano et al. replaced the vacancy left by animal-based physiology instruction at her institution in 2000 with simulation-based physiology demonstrations. Their group used an early version of the METI HPS to teach pulmonary physiology concepts including V/Q mismatch, pulmonary compliance, and the oxyhemoglobin dissociation curve [14, 15]. This curricular innovation originating within the anesthesiology department at the University of Florida is an early example of anesthesiologist-led simulation instruction in undergraduate medical education. Gordon et al. in 2006 demonstrated improved understanding of cardiac physiology in a small sample of first-year medical students immediately after a simulated encounter of a patient with a myocardial infarction [16]. Compared to controls receiving a traditional case discussion model of instruction, retention of knowledge remained superior at 1 year following the session. Other groups have shown similar success in the instruction of shock physiology and dynamic pharmacology [17–20].

The authors of this chapter use small group interactive simulation lab experiences as a component of the core cardiac and pulmonary physiology curriculum for first-year medical students. During each anesthesiologist-facilitated session, a group of approximately 10 students interact directly with

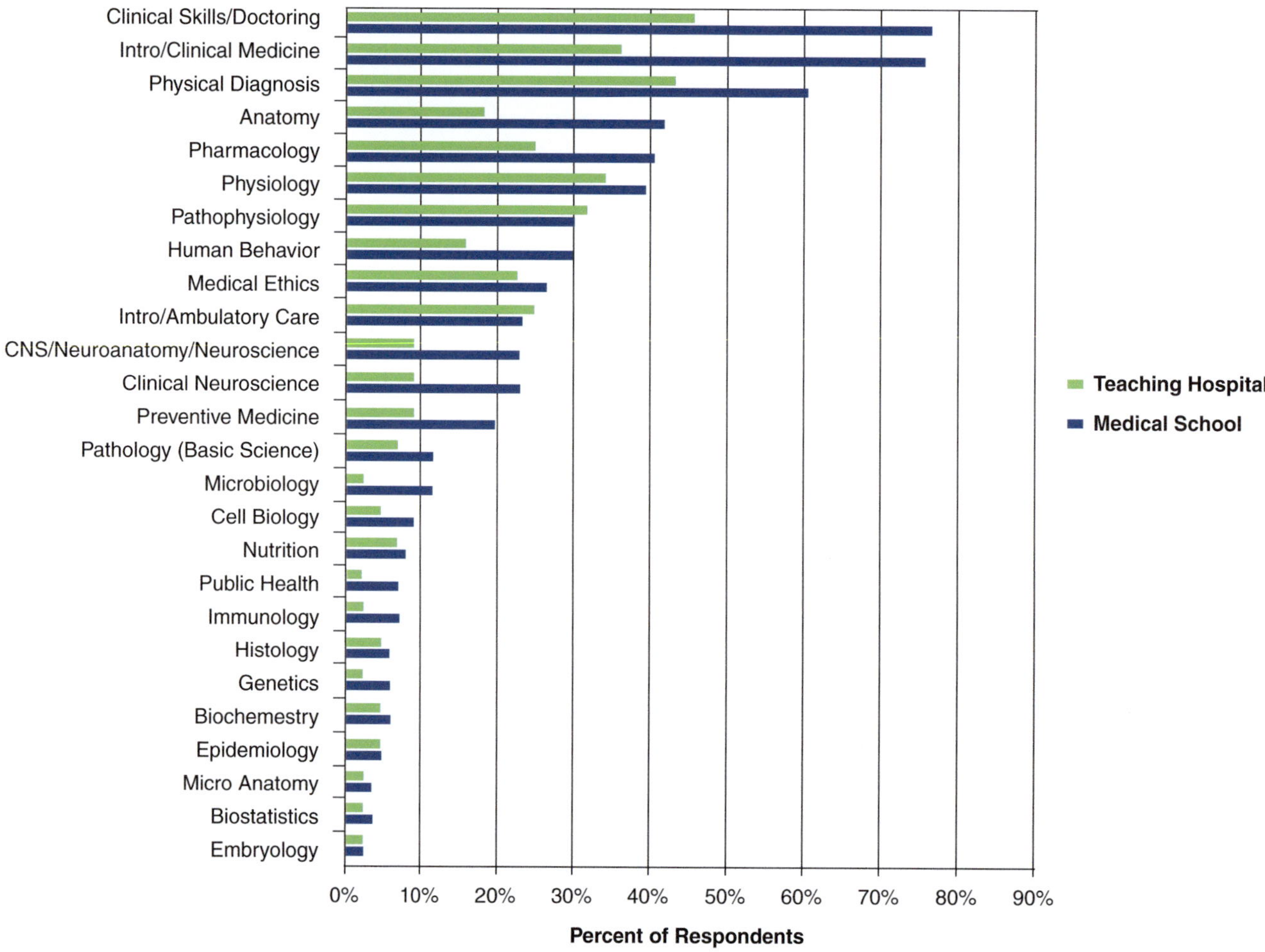

Fig. 13.1 Preclinical content, AAMC survey

a high-fidelity mannequin progressively through different phases of the clinical care of a simulated patient [20]. In our pulmonary physiology sessions, they initially encounter the simulated patient at the scene of a recent trauma and are encouraged to perform lung auscultation and discuss specific pulmonary correlates of the physical examination. The students then follow the patient into the emergency room trauma bay where the patient develops acute respiratory failure. The students discuss principles of pulmonary physiology while being guided toward the management of a life-threatening tension pneumothorax. During this portion of the session, students will place external and invasive monitors, perform arterial blood gas analysis, initiate endotracheal intubation, interpret a chest film, and perform needle decompression. Through these steps, physiologic principles such as ventilation/perfusion mismatch, alveolar to arterial oxygen gradients, and lung mechanics and dynamics are introduced and serially revisited following each intervention. At the conclusion, students follow the simulated patient to the ICU where they adjust ventilator settings and evaluate a capnograph during a discussion of ventilation and the West zones of the lungs (Table 13.1).

In creating these sessions, the incorporation of hands-on procedures and student-mannequin interaction was prioritized as essential for multisensory engagement through a kinesthetic learning experience to maximally exploit the benefits of simulation-based education. While students are not expected in their preclinical years to attain proficiency in the incorporated procedures, the kinesthetic experience allows for active learning and better understanding of abstract concepts through clinical engagement. In addition to the unique nature of content delivery in this manner, the fact that their instruction comes exclusively from faculty anesthesiologists, experts in the clinical applications of these concepts, provides a novel insight for students into the clinical relevance of the topics presented. Of benefit to the field of anesthesiology, students who have had mostly limited or no exposure to the field at this point in their education receive a demonstration of both the scope of anesthesiology practice and role models in academic anesthesiology.

Table 13.1 An example of using high-fidelity simulation to teach basic science to medical students

Title: Pulmonary physiology lab – medical school year 1 or 2			
Audience: First- and second-year medical students			
Objectives – Medical knowledge: Relating basic science pulmonary physiology concepts with pulmonary clinical findings and diagnoses			
Case stem: Brad Luck is a 24-year-old male who has been in a bicycle vs. car accident. He is otherwise a healthy male with no other medical problems			
Scenario setup: There will be three (3) stations for this simulation lab			
Station 1: Scene of accident/trauma			
Station 2: Emergency room setting, projected slides and/or white boards are used in this room to recall and reinforce basic pulmonary physiology concepts			
Station 3: Intensive care unit setting, projected slides and/or white boards are used in this room to recall and reinforce basic pulmonary physiology concepts			
Station 1			
State	**Patient status**	**Teacher instructions/learner actions**	
Immediately post-trauma	Tachypneic breathing, awake but unable to talk. Stridulous breathing sounds heard from patient. Decreased/absent breath sounds on the right side. Patient also appears to have a right femur fracture	Instructor speaks with students about the importance of physical exam and what they can learn about the patient's respiratory status without the use of monitors After physical exam is complete, instructor will state that patient is going to the emergency room where further evaluation can be done with monitoring	Students should discuss visual respiratory findings (patient color, level of consciousness, respiratory rate, equality and depth of chest rise, and use of accessory muscles with breathing), auditory respiratory findings (normal and abnormal breath sounds), and tactile respiratory findings (feeling for actual movement of air and chest rise)
Station 2			
State	**Patient status**	**Teacher instructions/learner actions**	
		Upon entering emergency room simulation setting, the instructor acknowledges to students that extra time will be taken to discuss findings on the simulated patient and pulmonary physiology that goes along with these findings. These discussions will cause a delay in treatment to the mannequin that would not occur on a living patient	
Dyspnea	Patient continues to be tachypneic and unable to talk, but eyes are open	Instructor asks for arterial blood gas (ABG) and chest x-ray upon entering emergency room (which will not be available for several minutes) Instructor facilitates discussion on monitors that will assist in assessment of pulmonary status (we focus on pulse oximetry for this lab, although other vital signs are shown on the monitor to the students)	Students answer questions about pulse oximetry, how it works, and issues that can lead to incorrect readings
Hypoxia	HR (seen on pulse oximetry) 120, BP 82/46, RR 30–35, Sat 82% After O_2 mask is placed: HR 120, RR 30–35, Sats 85%, ABG: 7.5/34/55	Instructor notes that the O_2 saturation is low and asks students what they want to do about it, places O_2 mask on patient, and receives ABG results. Instructor then facilitates discussion on oxygenation: Alveolar gas equation, A:a gradient, oxyhemoglobin dissociation curve, and shunt This is where it is helpful to have slides for diagrams or a white board for the instructor to work through equations with the students	Students actively participate in decision making (placing O_2 mask, interpreting ABG results). They also provide answers to the instructor's questions on oxygenation topics

(continued)

Table 13.1 (continued)

Continuing hypoxia	Patient is still tachypneic and uncommunicative. HR 120, BP 70/40, RR 35, Sat 82% CXR returns with a tension pneumothorax	Instructor asks students to diagnose what is occurring on the chest x-ray. Once diagnosis of tension pneumothorax is made, the instructor also points out that tension pneumothoraces are a clinical diagnosis and a clinician should never wait for a chest x-ray to treat a tension pneumothorax. He also informs the students that they had all the information they needed for diagnosis from the physical exam (absent breath sounds on the right side and the hypoxia, tachycardia, and hypotension seen on the monitor). There is also a discussion on how a tension pneumothorax causes shunt and hypoxemia Instructor leads a student in performing a needle decompression on the mannequin	Students participate in the diagnosis of tension pneumothorax and performance of a needle decompression
Recovery	HR 95, RR 20, Sats 97%	Instructor discusses that a chest tube needs to be placed as a permanent treatment for the tension pneumothorax (which can be painful) and the patient will be going to surgery for his femur fracture and therefore suggests sedating and intubating the patient After the student places the endotracheal tube (ETT), a confederate pushes the endotracheal tube in deep to cause a mainstem intubation while securing the ETT with tape Another confederate "places" a chest tube	Students participate in giving sedating medications and intubating the patient
Hypoxia	HR 95, RR controlled, Sats 87% Breath sounds now absent on the left side	Instructor facilitates evaluation of current hypoxemia. When students realize breath sounds are absent on the left side, instructor guides them to a mainstem intubation diagnosis and discusses how this is also an example of shunt Confederate pulls the endotracheal tube back into the trachea	Students provide differential for hypoxemia. Students should suggest/be led to doing a physical exam and listening to breath sounds
Recovery	HR 95, RR controlled, Sats 100%	Instructor announces that the confederate will continue getting the patient ready for the operating room by placing an a-line and a central line. While this is being done, the instructor facilitates a discussion on lung volumes, especially functional residual capacity, and the effect of different vectors on the lung volumes (topic slides are used here) Confederate places mannequin in Trendelenburg, "places" central line, and leaves the mannequin in the head-down position	Students participate in discussion on lung volumes and FRC

Table 13.1 (continued)

Hypoxia	HR 95, RR controlled, Sats 87%	Instructor notes that the patient has dropped his oxygen saturations again and facilitates the diagnosis of shunt occurring due to atelectasis. Explains how shunt can occur from alveoli collapsing from a long period in the Trendelenburg position, without adequate tidal volumes or positive end-expiratory pressure Confederate takes mannequin out of Trendelenburg position and facilitates student participation to give recruitment breaths to improve oxygenation	Students participate in discussion on lung volumes and shunt caused by atelectasis A student gives recruitment breaths through the bag setting on the ventilator
Recovery	HR 95, RR controlled, Sats 100%	Instructor announces that patient is ready for transport to the operating room, and the students will meet him again after surgery in the intensive care unit	
Station 3			
State	**Patient status**	**Teacher instructions/learner actions**	
Baseline – in ICU immediately after surgery	Patient is still asleep from anesthesia. Patient is intubated and being ventilated by ambu bag on arrival to the ICU. A unit of PRBCs is almost done being transfused with a pressure bag through his central line	Instructor states that the patient was fairly stable through surgery but at one point lost a liter of blood and became hypotensive, and that is why he is being transfused	
	HR 85, BP 125/70, RR controlled, Sats 100% (on FIO_2 100%)	Informs students that at this station we are going to focus on ventilation since we focused on oxygenation in the emergency room	Students participate in discussion on ventilation and the selection of ventilator settings: TV 500 ml, RR 12, FiO_2 60%, PEEP 5
		Instructor asks students about ventilator settings, production of CO_2, and how to determine if minute ventilation is adequate to eliminate the CO_2 that is produced	Students should suggest/be led to getting an arterial blood gas to check pCO_2 for adequate ventilation
Hypercarbia	Patient asleep and on ventilator HR 85, BP 125/70, RR controlled, Sats 100% (on FIO_2 100%) ABG: 7.3/50/300	Instructor has students interpret blood gas and makes suggestions on how to correct the respiratory acidosis After students make changes to minute ventilation, instructor suggests getting another ABG to check pCO_2 again	Students should suggest increasing the TV and/or RR
Awake	Patient's ventilation is still controlled, but blinking eyes and appears awake Vital signs: as above ABG: 7.35/45/250 After attaching mannequin to end-tidal CO_2 monitor TV 500, RR 15, FiO_2 60%, PEEP 5, $EtCO_2$ 35	Instructor talks about noninvasive ways to estimate CO_2 elimination (even though this patient has an a-line, taking multiple blood gases is invasive and painful for patients; lab tests cost money and take time to return results). Instructs students on end-tidal CO_2 monitoring. Explains what end-tidal CO_2 monitoring measures and how it differs from pCO_2. This leads to a discussion about dead space and how increasing dead space decreases $EtCO_2$ (Slides on West zones of the lung and pictures of anatomical dead space, show Bohr equation to calculate amount of dead space)	Students participate in discussion about dead space including where it occurs, the normal gradient between pCO_2 and end-tidal CO_2, and normal percentages of dead space in a tidal volume breath

(continued)

Table 13.1 (continued)

Air embolism	HR 110, BP 75/54, RR 15, Sats 97%, $EtCO_2$ 20, new RBBB on EKG	Instructor turns students' attention to the monitor where the $EtCO_2$ has decreased significantly during the discussion. Suggests getting one last ABG to determine if they are overventilating or something else is happening	Students should provide a differential for the decrease in $EtCO_2$ including overventilation and possible causes for increased dead space
	ABG: 7.3/50/250	Confederate points out that the bag of PRBCs is empty and, because it was being infused under pressure, air has been injected through the IV tubing into the patient	Allow a student to aspirate air out of the central line
Recovery	HR 95, BP 100/64, RR 15, Sats 97%, $EtCO_2$ 37	Instructor allows time for students to ask further questions and concludes the lab	
Discussion points: Pulmonary physiology can be a confusing topic for medical students learning the information for the first time. Relating the didactic information they have learned in lectures with simulated clinical scenarios has potential to reinforce these concepts and help with information retention			
It should be noted that the instructors in this lab acknowledge some of the artificiality of the simulation:			
Instructors admit that, although shunt and dead space are discussed and shown separately in this lab, they can be seen together in a real-life situation			
Instructors point out differences in the simulation setting vs. actual clinical practice (e.g., not waiting for a CXR to treat a tension pneumothorax; not allowing air into bags of fluid/blood; and, if this does occur, not administering the contents under pressure in order to prevent occurrences of air embolism)			
Instructors acknowledge that, although this lab focuses on the respiratory system and therefore mainly focuses on the pulse oximetry and $EtCO_2$ monitors, other vital signs are affected by the pathology seen in the lab (e.g., hypotension and tachycardia with tension pneumothorax and air embolism)			

High-fidelity simulation experiences such as the physiology session described by these authors are valued for providing an opportunity to manage rare and critical scenarios without exposing patients to potential harm; however, the cost and time required to facilitate numerous small group session can limit utility. The pulmonary physiology small group sessions outlined above do require several sessions per day over multiple days in order to provide exposure for every student, a substantial time investment for a topic traditionally taught to all students simultaneously in a large lecture hall. Some simulation educators have described success utilizing a hybrid model with on-site or teleconferenced simulated demonstrations to provide a large group of students with a dynamic and clinical context for these basic science concepts [21, 22]. Fitch, after introducing large group simulated neuroscience demonstrations in 2007, showed posttest performance improvement [21]. A model of this nature can achieve a degree of vertical curricular integration while making some concessions due to simulations' resource-intensive nature.

Clinical Years

While simulation technology can serve to facilitate vertical curricular integration of basic science concepts with simulated clinical exposure early in medical school, it is during the later clinical years of medical training (traditionally starting in the third year), in which simulation technology can most easily be integrated in a manner familiar to most simulationists. As students rotate through core clinical clerkships (internal medicine, surgery, obstetrics-gynecology, pediatrics, psychiatry) as well as subspecialty electives or standard rotations including anesthesiology, clinical faculty utilize simulation technology ranging from part-task trainers to HFS. The use of simulation in medical education in the clinical years is widespread with approximately 90% of US medical schools reporting some degree of simulation-based education for clinical instruction [10] (Fig. 13.2).

The majority of medical schools report the greatest use of simulation technology during internal medicine, pediatrics, and emergency medicine rotations, which would appear at odds with the leadership role played by anesthesiology in the adoption of simulation technology. This can partly be attributed to the fact that, while most medical schools require some degree of exposure to anesthesiology in the third year, many do not provide exposure until the fourth year of undergraduate medical education and often in the form of an elective rotation. Furthermore, despite the widespread use of simulation in the clinical years, the AAMC reported in a 2011 survey that just over half of medical schools reported the use of simulation-based education during anesthesiology rotations [10]. While the resource-intensive nature of high-fidelity simulation can provide a barrier to universal implementation, low-cost simulation technology can also be of great utility to the novice learner.

Much of the focus for the students during their clinical exposure to anesthesiology is on the attainment of procedural skills such as basic airway management—bag-mask ventilation, the use of airway adjuncts such as oral and nasal airway devices, and direct laryngoscopy. Airway management, a high-stakes procedure even when performed by the most

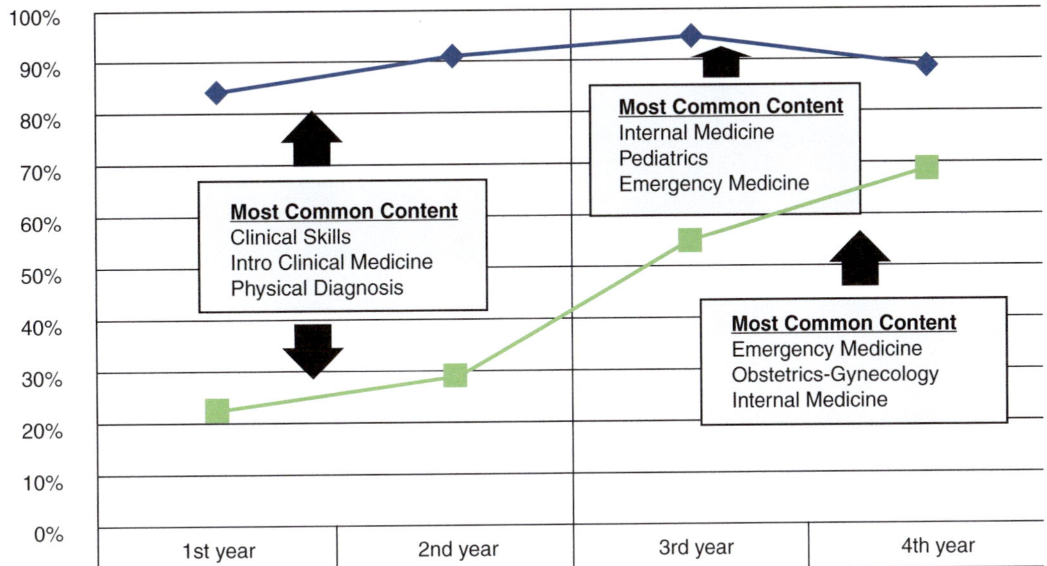

	1st year	2nd year	3rd year	4th year
Medical School	84%	91%	94%	89%
Teaching Hospital	22%	28%	55%	69%

Fig. 13.2 Simulation use with medical students, AAMC survey

senior practitioner, can be introduced to the student through the use of partial task trainers. Task trainers allow the student to become more comfortable with basic techniques before progressing to patient airway management in the perioperative setting. The specific model of task trainer used for medical students will depend on the goals and objectives for their anesthesiology rotation. Airway trainers, consisting of a mobile head with a variable combination of rudimentary upper and lower airway anatomy (oropharynx, larynx, trachea, esophagus, mainstem bronchi, and inflatable lungs), are commonly used to facilitate instruction in bag-mask ventilation, direct laryngoscopy, endotracheal tube placement, and airway adjuvant placement. Some models can also be used to effectively allow for advanced airway techniques such as supraglottic airway placement, video laryngoscopy, or even fiber-optic laryngoscopy and bronchoscopy. While relatively affordable compared to their mannequin-based HFS counterparts, these airway trainers do not typically allow for adjustment in the difficulty of airway anatomy and may provide relatively lower fidelity. For students contemplating a career in anesthesia enrolled in an advanced elective rotation or sub-internship, course objectives may include more advanced procedural skills such as neuraxial anesthetic techniques or vascular access. For initial instruction in spinal and epidural placement, neuraxial trainers are available which consist of a mannequin torso containing a vertebral column containing a fluid-filled space. While the degree of realism and the fidelity of the haptic feedback with most commercially available neuraxial trainers can vary, these trainers all provide students the opportunity to physically rehearse critical steps including sterility procedures, epidural and spinal kit preparation, palpation of anatomy, and loss of resistance techniques, prior to performing in the clinical setting. Task trainers are also available for instruction for peripheral and central venous or arterial vascular cannulation, many of which can provide for ultrasound-guided techniques. Depending on the goals and objectives of the rotation, the incorporation of partial task trainers for regional anesthetic techniques, surgical airway management, and flexible bronchoscopy may be considered as well.

HFS or even intermediate-fidelity simulation can play an effective role in introducing common anesthetic scenarios and complications (see sample scenario). Such individual or small group sessions can ensure exposure to clinical experiences contained within the goals and objectives of the medical student rotation and also provide an opportunity for students to inhabit the role of the primary provider. McIvor describes his experience in instituting a "bag-valve-mask course" for rising third-year medical students in which scenarios were scripted to include changing vital signs in response to student interventions along with built-in breaks and prompts to prevent undue stress [23].

Not surprisingly, some of the earliest descriptions of the use of high-fidelity mannequin-based simulation involved the training of anesthesia residents, a practice which continues to this day [24]. This technology can also be utilized to better prepare medical students for residency (Table 13.2). Hallikainen et al. found that fourth-year medical students trained using full-scale simulation had superior performance measured by a 40-item checklist of clinical actions for induction of a patient for general anesthesia compared to those

Table 13.2 Sample scenario

<table>
<tr><td colspan="4">Title: Induction and intubation of patient with cervical spine injury</td></tr>
<tr><td colspan="4">Audience: Anesthesia medical student</td></tr>
<tr><td colspan="4">Objectives:</td></tr>
<tr><td colspan="4">Medical knowledge: Identify special concerns in securing the airway in a trauma patient with suspected cervical spine injury</td></tr>
<tr><td colspan="4">Patient care: Perform rapid sequence intubation, and secure airway while maintaining manual in-line stabilization</td></tr>
<tr><td colspan="4">Communication: Utilize closed-loop communication to instruct other providers to maintain manual in-line stabilization and apply cricoid pressure</td></tr>
<tr><td colspan="4">Case stem: Trauma alpha is a previously healthy 34-year-old male who presented to the ED as a level 1 trauma following a MVA. He is now in the OR for an ORIF of his left femur. He has no other injuries. He does admit to eating 2 hours prior and also is complaining of neck pain. A CT scan of his neck was unremarkable</td></tr>
<tr><td colspan="4">Scenario setup:
Mannequin on OR table with C-collar in place
IVF connected to 18 g PIV in right AC
Left-sided periorbital ecchymosis
Typical OR environment with anesthesia machine/monitors (NIBP, pulse oximetry, ECG, $EtCO_2$)
Basic induction drugs (propofol, etomidate, succinylcholine, rocuronium), rescue medication (atropine, phenylephrine, epinephrine), and standard airway equipment
Backup airway equipment (glidescope, bougie, LMA) available upon request
Suction</td></tr>
<tr><td>State</td><td>Patient status</td><td>Learner actions</td><td></td></tr>
<tr><td>Baseline
HR 110, BP 110/65, RR 26
SpO_2 94% on RA</td><td>Supine on OR table. Patient anxious and complaining of left leg pain</td><td>Placement of monitors reveals vital signs. Preoxygenation of patient</td><td>SpO_2 will increase to 100% with preoxygenation</td></tr>
<tr><td>Induction
HR 100, BP 90/60, RR 0, SpO_2 100%</td><td>Patient paralyzed, eyes closed. Unresponsive</td><td>Administer induction drugs while directing additional participants to hold manual in-line stabilization and cricoid pressure</td><td>Spontaneous respirations cease with induction medications.
Mask ventilation or failure to apply cricoid pressure will result in aspiration and hypoxia
Transition vitals over 30 seconds or faster if patient is not preoxygenated</td></tr>
<tr><td>Hypoxia
HR 130, BP 140/90, RR 0, SpO_2 85%</td><td>Patient hypoxic from aspiration or inability to secure airway</td><td>Suction patient
Call for help
Employ alternative approach to the airway (mask ventilation, second attempt at intubation, LMA placement)</td><td>Airway can be set to easy or difficult depending on learner ability</td></tr>
<tr><td>Resolution
HR 90, BP 110/65, RR0, SpO_2 95%</td><td>Hypoxia resolved with secure airway</td><td>Administer 100% FiO_2 and ventilator the patient. Secure the endotracheal tube</td><td>SpO_2 will increase to 100% with preoxygenation</td></tr>
<tr><td colspan="4">Discussion points:</td></tr>
<tr><td colspan="4">Are there special concerns for securing the airway in a trauma patient? What are they?</td></tr>
<tr><td colspan="4">What is the preferred technique for holding manual in-line stabilization of cervical spine? Discuss your airway concerns.</td></tr>
<tr><td colspan="4">What are the indications for rapid sequence intubation in this patient? How did you accomplish that? Discuss your choice of induction medications.</td></tr>
<tr><td colspan="4">What did you do when the patient became hypoxic? Did you have the help that you needed? What could you have done differently?</td></tr>
</table>

who underwent more traditional training [25]. Others have reported the use of HFS for teaching third- and fourth-year medical students concepts of both basic and subspecialty anesthesia practice [23, 26, 27].

Simulation for Medical Student Assessment

Increasingly, simulation technology is being utilized in assessment of healthcare professionals at multiple levels of training. The AAMC revealed through a recent survey that simulation is being utilized nationally as a tool for assessment of the core competencies as defined by the Accreditation Council for Graduate Medical Education (ACGME). Those reported as being most often assessed through simulation at the medical student level include patient care, interpersonal communication, and professionalism. Assessment has traditionally been performed in medical education both formatively and summatively. In conducting formative assessment, the goal is to observe and rate performance to provide feedback which can be applied toward improvements in future performance. The majority of simulation-based education involving post-scenario debriefing would meet this definition. Summative assessment, on the other hand, consists of producing a sum-

Table 13.3 List of the AAMC Core Entrustable Professional Activities for Entering Residency

EPA 1: Gather a history and perform a physical examination
EPA 2: Prioritize a differential diagnosis following a clinical encounter
EPA 3: Recommend and interpret common diagnostic and screening tests
EPA 4: Enter and discuss orders and prescriptions
EPA 5: Document a clinical encounter in the patient record
EPA 6: Provide an oral presentation of a clinical encounter
EPA 7: Form clinical questions and retrieve evidence to advance patient care
EPA 8: Give or receive a patient handover to transition care responsibility
EPA 9: Collaborate as a member of an interprofessional team
EPA 10: Recognize a patient requiring urgent or emergent care and initiate evaluation and management
EPA 11: Obtain informed consent for tests and/or procedures

mary of the practitioner's performance for determining whether a predefined standard has been met. An example of this form of assessment through the use of simulation would be the USMLE Step 2 CS exam, which includes standardized patient encounters, which are observed and rated by trained examiners [28]. In the field of anesthesiology, the OSCE-based component of the ABA licensing examination similarly consists of simulation-based tasks designed for summative assessment of diplomates [29]. Simulation provides a useful tool for summative assessment due to its ability to provide specifically designed, controlled, and repeatable clinical scenarios or tasks. Simulation can also be utilized to better ensure attainment of competencies identified by the ACGME and licensing bodies as essential for a practitioner following the completion of training not well assessed through traditional written examinations.

In 2014, the AAMC produced a list of 13 Core Entrustable Professional Activities (EPAs) that a graduating medical school should be able to perform unsupervised prior to entering residency [2] (Table 13.3). These EPAs span multiple clinical competency domains that are not well suited for assessment through the use of traditional multiple choice examination [30]. Simulation can provide a component of an effort to assess whether students have met the standards set forth in the EPAs [2] (Table 13.4). For example, standardized patient encounters are ideal for assessing EPA 1 (Gather a History and Perform a Physical Exam). EPA 12 (Perform General Procedures of a Physician) would be ideally served through the use of partial task trainers to avoid exposing patients to potential harm. Case-based scenarios presented through HFS would meet more complex clinical EPAs. For example, EPA 8 (Give or Receive a Patient Handover to Transition Care Responsibility), EPA 10 (Recognize a Patient Requiring Urgent or Emergent Care and Initiate Evaluation and Management), and EPA 11 (Obtain Informed Consent for Tests and/or Procedures) could all be assessed

Table 13.4 Example of simulation for assessment of EPA 10: recognize a patient requiring urgent or emergent care and initiate evaluation and management

Title: Treatment of tension pneumothorax

Audience: Third or fourth year medical student

Objectives-medical knowledge: Identify need for emergent needle decompression in patient presenting with tension pneumothorax

Patient care: Perform primary survey in trauma patient, identify tension pneumothorax, and perform needle decompression

Communication: *Instruct* other providers to help assess the patient during primary survey of a trauma patient.

Case stem: Trauma Beta is a 24 y/o male who presented to the ED as a level 1 trauma following a MVA. He can speak, but appears dyspneic and states he is having trouble breathing. No other past medical history is known.

Scenario setup:
Mannequin in ER trauma bay
IVF connected to 18 g PIV in right AC
Left-sided contusion to chest wall
Typical ER environment with crash cart, defibrillator, and code medications
Large angiocath for needle thoracostomy
Basic intubation kit

State	Patient status	Learner actions	
Baseline HR 120, BP 95/45, RR 35 SpO_2 84% on NRB	Supine on gurney. Non-rebreather O_2 applied Patient anxious, coughing, states unable to breath	Placement of monitors reveals vital signs Perform primary survey	Breath sounds and chest rise absent on the left Halt patient noises when participant auscultates Progress to decompensation if participant does not perform needle thoracostomy in first minute
Decompensation HR 140, BP 65/34, RR 40, SpO_2 80% on NRB	Patient less responsive, eyes closed	Immediately needle decompress patient	Transition vitals over 30 seconds
Recovery HR 100, BP 105/74, RR 20, SpO_2 95%	Patient awake, less dyspneic	Proceed with primary survey Order CXR Place chest tube	Bilateral breath sounds and chest rise resume with decompression

Discussion points:

What are signs and symptoms of a tension pneumothorax, and how is the diagnosis made?

What is the definitive treatment for this condition?

Discuss next steps for this patient once the tension pneumothorax is resolved.

through the use of a single well-designed scenario. Similar simulation-based assessment is currently underway at some centers in response to competency-based milestones recently produced by the ACGME for anesthesiology residency training [31]. While the 13 EPAs are not specialty specific, anesthesiologists as simulationists could be well positioned to develop and implement a simulation-based assessment program. Similar simulation-based assessment is currently underway at some centers in response to competency-based milestones recently produced by the ACGME for anesthesiology residency training. Morgan et al. developed a series of scenarios for fourth-year medical students for the purpose of assessing both technical and nontechnical skills [26].

Conclusion

The use of simulation through a variety of modalities at the undergraduate level has grown to become almost universal at US medical schools. SBME can be used effectively for the instruction of subjects typically covered in both the preclinical and clinical curricula. Specifically, SBME can help achieve vertical curricular integration during the preclinical years by providing a method for clinical contextualization of basic science content in a dynamic, simulated environment. High-fidelity mannequin-based physiology labs are just one example of how simulation can bridge the gap between the preclinical content and clinical context, by creating a kinesthetic learning experience effective for multiple adult learning styles. In the clinical years, simulation-based techniques allow students to gain early exposure to clinical scenarios and provide an opportunity to practice procedural skills. The safe and controlled setting of the simulation lab with opportunity for repetition allows students to gain confidence and improve skills prior to entering the clinical environment. A great deal of both preclinical and clinical undergraduate content falls within the realm of expertise of the anesthesiologist-educator, thus presenting an opportunity for leadership by anesthesiologist faculty through the use of SBME. The anesthesiologist educator's involvement in early undergraduate medical education can provide the additional benefit of early student exposure to role models in the field of anesthesiology.

Interest in simulation-based technology as a tool for assessment has grown and will continue to do so. Although challenges exist in the creation of any assessment tool, advantages of standardization, repeatability, and customizability argue in favor of the development of simulation-based assessments for the newly proposed Entrustable Professional Activities for medical students entering residency.

References

1. Tjomsland N, Baskett P. Resuscitation greats: Asmund S Lærdal. Resuscitation. 2002;53:115–9.
2. Core Entrustable Professional Activities for Entering Residency: Faculty and Learners' Guide. [Internet] Washington. D.C. 2014. Association of American Medical Colleges. [cited Sept 29]. Available from: https://members.aamc.org/eweb/upload/Core%20EPA%20Faculty%20and%20Learner%20Guide.pdf.
3. theaba.org [internet]. Raleigh. Applied examination, objective structured clinical examination: content outline. Available from: http://www.theaba.org/PDFs/APPLIED-Exam/APPLIED-OSCE-ContentOutline.
4. Burack J, Irby D, Carline J, Ambrozy D, Ellsbury K, Stritter F. A study of medical students' specialty choice pathways: trying on possible selves. Acad Med. 1997;72:534–41.
5. Paiva R, Vu N, Verhulst S. The effect of clinical experiences in medical school on specialty choice decisions. J Med Educ. 1982;57:666–74.
6. Kassebaum D, Szenas P. Factors influencing the specialty choices of 1993 medical school graduates. Acad Med. 1994;69(2):164–70.
7. DeMaria S Jr, Bryson E, Bodian C, Khelemsky Y, Sim A, Schwartz A, et al. The influence of simulation-based physiology labs taught by anesthesiologists on the attitudes of first-year medical students towards anesthesiology. Middle East J Anesthesiol. 2011;21(3):347–53.
8. Wijnen-Meijer MM. Vertical integration in medical school: effect on the transition to postgraduate training. Med Educ. 2010;44(3):272.
9. Koens FF. Analysing the concept of context in medical education. Med Educ. 2005;39(12):1243.
10. Medical simulation in medical education: results of a AAMC survey. [Internet] Association of American Medical Colleges. Washington, D.C. 2011. [cited Sept 29]. Available from: https://www.aamc.org/download/259760/data.
11. Kharb PP. The learning styles and the preferred teaching-learning strategies of first year medical students. J Clin Diagn Res. 2013;7(6):1089.
12. Gordon JAJ. Early bedside care during preclinical medical education: can technology-enhanced patient simulation advance the Flexnerian ideal? Acad Med. 2010;85(2):370.
13. Hasan ZZ. Challenges of teaching physiology in an integrated system-based curriculum. Can Med Educ J. 2012;3(1):e73.
14. Euliano TYT. Teaching respiratory physiology: clinical correlation with a human patient simulator. J Clin Monit Comput. 2000;16(5–6):465.
15. Euliano TYT. Small group teaching: clinical correlation with a human patient simulator. Adv Physiol Educ. 2001;25(1–4):36.
16. Gordon JAJ. Can a simulated critical care encounter accelerate basic science learning among preclinical medical students? A pilot study. Simul Healthc. 2006;1 Spec no:13.
17. Koniaris LGL. Two third-year medical student-level laboratory shock exercises without large animals. Surg Infect (Larchmt). 2004;5(4):343.
18. Helyer RR. Progress in the utilization of high-fidelity simulation in basic science education. Adv Physiol Educ. 2016;40(2):143.
19. Waite GN. Human patient simulation to teach medical physiology concepts: a model evolved during eight years. J Teach Learn Tech. 2013;2(2):79–89.
20. Meyers LL. Integration of simulation into medical school basic sciences. Med Educ. 2016;50(5):577.
21. Fitch MTM. Using high-fidelity emergency simulation with large groups of preclinical medical students in a basic science course. Med Teach. 2007;29(2–3):261.
22. Heitz CC. Large group high-fidelity simulation enhances medical student learning. Med Teach. 2009;31(5):e206.
23. McIvor WRW. Experience with medical student simulation education. Crit Care Med. 2004;32(2 Suppl):S66.
24. Abrahamson SS. Effectiveness of a simulator in training anesthesiology residents. J Med Educ. 1969;44(6):515.
25. Hallikainen JJ. Teaching anaesthesia induction to medical students: comparison between full-scale simulation and supervised teaching in the operating theatre. Eur J Anaesthesiol. 2009;26(2):101.
26. Morgan PJP. Validity and reliability of undergraduate performance assessments in an anesthesia simulator. Can J Anaesth. 2001;48(3):225.

27. Morgan PJP. Applying theory to practice in undergraduate education using high fidelity simulation. Med Teach. 2006;28(1):e10.
28. Step 2 Clinical Skills (CS) Content Description and General Information. [Internet] National Board of Medical Examiners and Federation of State Medical Boards of the United States, Inc [updated 2006 March; cited 2016 Sept 29]. Available from: http://www.usmle.org/pdfs/step-2-cs/cs-info-manual.pdf.
29. Staged Exam Policy Book. [Internet] Raleigh: American Board of Anesthesiology [updated 2016 Feb; cited 2016 Sept 29]. Available from: http://www.theaba.org/PDFs/BOI/StagedExaminations-BOI.
30. ten Cate OO. Entrustability of professional activities and competency-based training. Med Educ. 2005;39(12):1176.
31. Jonker GG. A case for competency-based anaesthesiology training with entrustable professional activities: an agenda for development and research. Eur J Anaesthesiol. 2015;32(2):71.

Graduate Medical Education

14

Bryan Mahoney and Migdalia H. Saloum

Abbreviations

ABA	American Board of Anesthesiology
ACGME	Accreditation Council for Graduate Medical Education
ACLS	Advanced cardiac life support
ACRM	Anesthesia crisis resource management
AHA	American Heart Association
ANTS	Anaesthetists' Non-Technical Skills
ASA	American Society of Anesthesiologists
CASE	Comprehensive Anesthesia Simulation Environment
CRM	Crew Resource Management
EMD	Electromechanical dissociation
FRC	Functional residual capacity
GAS	Gainesville Anesthesia Simulator
HPS	Human Patient Simulator
MOC	Maintenance of Certification
MOCA	Maintenance of Certification in Anesthesiology
OSCE	Objective Structured Clinical Examination
PEA	Pulseless electrical activity
RRC	Residency Review Committee
SBME	Simulation-based medical education
VARK	Visual, auditory, read/write and kinesthetic

B. Mahoney (✉) · M. H. Saloum
Department of Anesthesiology, Perioperative and Pain Medicine, Mount Sinai St. Luke's and West Hospitals, Mount Sinai St. Luke's & Roosevelt Hospital, Icahn School of Medicine at Mount Sinai, New York, NY, USA
e-mail: bryan.mahoney@mountsinai.org; migdalia.saloum@mountsinai.org

Introduction

In 2011 the Anesthesiology Residency Review Committee (RRC) for the Accreditation Council for Graduate Medical Education (ACGME) announced a revision to the program requirements for anesthesiology residency training that represented a milestone in the history of role simulation based for anesthesiology education:

> IV.A.6 Residents must participate in at least one simulated clinical experience each year [1].

The RRC further described requirements for incorporation of the six core competencies as defined by the ACGME along with a description by programs of the formal debriefing mechanisms utilized and the extent to which ancillary personnel are incorporated into the experience. However, the import of this announcement lies, to a large extent, in the factors leading to this announcement not enunciated by the Anesthesiology RRC or ACGME. The year preceding this announcement, the American Board of Anesthesiology (ABA) instituted a required simulation educational activity to satisfy one component of Maintenance of Certification in Anesthesiology (MOCA®) Part IV (Improvement in Medical Practice Component) [2]. These mandates represent a recognition by the accrediting and certifying bodies of the value simulation-based education and assessment can bring to the profession of anesthesiology.

The utilization of simulation-based technology in the profession of anesthesiology, and in anesthesiology residency training in particular, can be traced back to the utilization of "Sim One" at the University of Southern California in the 1960s [3]. Investigators, through the incorporation of the Sim One mannequin, sought to demonstrate an acceleration and enhancement of residents' clinical performance through repetitive and deliberate practice in the simulated environment. In the 1980s, Gaba and colleagues utilized the CASE (Comprehensive Anesthesia Simulation Environment) to

B. Mahoney et al. (eds.), *Comprehensive Healthcare Simulation: Anesthesiology*, Comprehensive Healthcare Simulation,
https://doi.org/10.1007/978-3-030-26849-7_14

investigate anesthesiology resident trainee performance in the simulated environment, elucidating the utility of simulation technology for formative assessment in addition to education [4, 5, 6]. Soon thereafter, in the early 1990s, a team at the University of Florida developed the GAS (Gainesville Anesthesia Simulator) out of a goal to teach resident trainees basic skills in anesthesia practice [7, 8]. This work led to the development of a mannequin-based simulation technology incorporating physiologic modeling driven and drug recognition software which led to an advance in operator-driven manual control of physiologic output data in response to trainee actions.

Looking back on the development of high-fidelity mannequin-based simulation, it would be difficult to argue that the goal of training residents in the clinical practice of anesthesiology was not a critical impetus. In fact, for the last half century, one would not be far-off in characterizing simulation-based medical education (SBME) as the handmaiden of anesthesiology resident training. In recent years, educators have found an array of challenges effectively addressed through simulation-based education, assessment, and training. Simulation has provided a mechanism for the transfer of valuable skills from other high-stakes industries such as the airline industry such as Crew Resource Management (CRM) to anesthesia trainees. In fact, since the 1990s, there has been a great deal of literature in the instruction of anesthesiology residents in anesthesia crisis resource management (ACRM) skills [9] or other non-technical skill sets such as the Anaesthetists' Non-Technical Skills (ANTS) system (task management, teamworking, situation awareness, and decision-making) [10]. Educators have utilized the simulated clinical environment in order to provide exposure to rare critical events for which clinical exposure during the standard period of training is unlikely [11], a technique which has become a mainstay of simulation education for resident trainees. Simulation training has even been used as a mechanism for the reintroduction of the impaired anesthesia trainee to clinical training and eventual practice [12].

This chapter is intended to provide a practical guide to the development of simulation curricula for a general graduate anesthesiology training program. While a curriculum for basic anesthesia skills and rare and critical scenarios aimed at the introduction of subspecialty techniques and clinical management and can be found in the chapters on undergraduate medical education (Chap. 13) and the subspecialties of anesthesiology (Chaps. 16, 17, 18, 19, 20, 21, 22, 23, 24, 25, 26, and 27), respectively, here focus will be placed on the development of simulation curricula designed to provide a mechanism for the progressive acquisition of skills in clinical anesthesiology practice that reflects the competency-based milestones approach to anesthesiology training as mandated by the ACGME. Toward that end, this chapter will provide a review of simulation-based curriculum development for anesthesiology training followed by a description of practical considerations for the department seeking to integrate simulation as a component of their graduate anesthesiology training program. Three general categories of curricula will be covered to reflect the progressive nature of graduate anesthesiology education: simulation-based education for an introduction to anesthesiology curriculum, simulation-based formative assessment for training-level specific competency-based milestone attainment, and simulation-based summative assessment for advancement based on competency-based milestone attainment.

General Considerations for Simulation-Based Curriculum Development

Simulation can serve as a valuable component of the broader residency curriculum, and the specific role it will serve is best elucidated a posteriori in the process of global residency curriculum design. This reflects the historical development of SBME in tandem with an attempt to meet the needs of educating anesthesiology resident trainees. The educator developing a simulation curriculum must maintain a focus on the unique benefits of SBME compared to more traditional methods of education or assessment to identify the content best served by this tool and to most effectively apply SBME to the content identified. This focus will ensure the creation of the most appropriate goals and objectives for the simulation-based curriculum as the first step in an effective curriculum design, construction, and execution. Many leaders in residency education and educators in general have looked upon the promise of this tool with a sense of great opportunity only to be humbled when encountering the resource-intensive nature of SBME. A recognition of these limitations and departmental resources must also be accounted for when contemplating the integration of a simulation-based curriculum, and multiple strategies have been described to aid in those creating curricula de novo. However, the first step in the process of curriculum development is the incorporation of the benefits of SBME to the adult learner in anesthesia.

Learning Theory and Curricular Content Selection

The Adult Learner

While an extensive review of the role adult learning theory plays in SBME is beyond the scope of this chapter, a brief recapitulation is necessary to highlight the relevant concepts to the topic of graduate anesthesiology education for the educator developing a simulation-based curriculum for education or assessment. The development of the CASE and

GAS simulation technologies developed for anesthesiology residency education coincided with the description by Knowles of a necessary shift from pedagogy to andragogy or the art and science of adult learning [13]. This is fortuitous given Knowles' recognition of the need for educators to address four principles he had identified to effective adult learning: an understanding of the rationale behind the learning, experiential learning allowing for mistakes, relevance of the material to their professional or personal life, and problem-centeredness, as opposed to content-centeredness. These authors propose inscribing these four principles into residency simulation curriculum development through the following four principles for simulation curriculum development:

1. Provide learners with the goals and objectives for the simulation-based learning exercise or module in relation to anesthesiology residency competency-based milestones.
2. Maximize the experiential and active components of SBME and minimize the potential for each exercise to devolve into didactics. Debriefing should also learner reflection and minimize educator instruction.
3. Ensure that learners are confronted with simulation-based exercises or modules relevant to their training level and/or subspecialty rotation.
4. Focus on competencies over "keywords" in developing curricular content, or preferentially utilize SBME to develop competencies as opposed to medical knowledge.

Learning Styles

Additional concepts have been studied in an effort to focus on learner styles and optimize curricular development, VARK typology being one of the more relevant to SBME [14, 15]. This system categorizes learning styles into four discrete categories: visual, auditory, reading, and kinesthetic or learning through carrying out physical categories [16]. Work has been done to identify the predominant learning style identified by adult students in medical education, and while a mixed style predominates, the kinesthetic style represents the most common unimodal preference, and teaching strategies employing a kinesthetic approach were the most preferred [17]. The obvious application of this insight to the development of a simulation curriculum for graduate anesthesiology training would be the maximization of "hot seat" exposure for each trainee when utilizing high-fidelity mannequin-based scenarios (serving the role of primary anesthesia care provider in the scenario). This principle is reflected in the requirement for MOCA Part 4 course ensuring that each participant is placed in "hot seat" at least once during each course [18]. Utilization of partial task trainers as part of high-fidelity scenarios or at discrete "stations" would be an additional strategy for maximizing kinesthetic learning.

Competency Attainment

In determining the content for a learning objective met through a simulation-based curriculum, the educator must identify the function this component will serve within a broader curricular context. In matching design to goals, be they educational, formative assessment, or summative assessment, Miller's taxonomy of clinical competence can provide guidance in matching content and structure to goals [19]. This concept envisions a pyramid of clinical competence describing progression from "novice" to "expert," the base of which is described as "knows," or knowledge, underlying "knows how" or competence, followed by "shows how" or performance, and capped by "does" or action. Simulation can serve as an ideal format for facilitating progression in competency attainment, and the design of any curricular component would ideally reflect the trainee's dynamic position in this progression. This chapter will reflect this principle in its presentation of differing modes of simulation-based curricula for graduate residency education as presented in Table 14.1.

Kneebone described the inherent benefits of SBME in four parts: (1) the ability to tailor the training to the needs of the learner, (2) the provision of a safe environment in which the learner is permitted to fail, (3) the ability to

Table 14.1 Application of Miller's taxonomy to specific components of a simulation-based graduate anesthesiology curriculum

Curricular component	Miller's level(s) of clinical competence	Application of goals to design
Introduction to anesthesiology	Knows → knows how	Fluid and open-ended scenarios and structure provide a forum for applying principles in the clinical setting. Debriefing provides an opportunity for linking basic concepts to practice
Formative assessment for progression	Knows how → shows	Format and scenarios scripted with specific learning objectives designed to facilitate trainee self-assessment. Opportunities for repetition and reflection during debriefing accelerate milestone attainment in a safe environment
Summative assessment for advancement	Shows → does	Emphasis on standardization of scenarios or Objective Structured Clinical Examinations (OSCEs) and validation of scoring tools to allow examiner assessment of competency attainment

provide objective evidence of performance, and (4) the capacity to provide immediate feedback [20]. The educator will emphasize certain of these SBME benefits over others in recognition of the learners' expected progression through Miller's taxonomy, and this emphasis should manifest in a very specific manner through curriculum design. For example, during an introduction to anesthesia curriculum for junior residents at the start of the academic year, scenarios may be less structured to allow learners to experience the consequence of certain actions, or inaction, as a scenario progresses. Debriefing may be interposed at intervals throughout a single scenario to highlight relevant concepts. Partial task trainers may be utilized in isolation to introduce learners to new technical skills. A curriculum designed to complement progressive milestone attainment for the non-novice may utilize more tightly scripted scenarios to allow for more objective measure of trainee performance with an emphasis on reflection during the debriefing process. Partial task trainers may be incorporated into large-scale mannequin-based scenarios to incorporate technical skills into the simulated clinical experience. Finally, when employing simulation for summative assessment, great emphasis must be placed on standardization of content as well as scoring tools to ensure a valid tool for potentially high-stakes assessment.

Clinical Competency in Anesthesiology Training

Miller's taxonomy is reflected in the recent development of competency-based milestones which represent the result of an ongoing effort on the part of the ACGME to ensure the ability of graduating residents to provide patient care and work effectively in the healthcare system. A brief background on the genesis of this framework can help to identify the role SBME can play in competency attainment and assessment to help anesthesiology residency programs fulfill the mandate set for them by the ACGME.

In 1998, the ACGME initiated the Outcome Project to provide graduate medical training programs with guidance in the competencies expected of trainees by the conclusion of their graduate medical training [21]. This initiative also made accreditation contingent on programs' trainees' ability to demonstrate the educational outcomes identified through this project: the six core competencies are patient care, medical knowledge, practice-based learning and improvement, interpersonal and communication skills, professionalism, and systems-based practice. While the ACGME provided residency training programs with more specific components within each competency domain, however, these sub-competencies were general or not specific to any specialty training.

In 2009, the ACGME reached the culmination of the Outcomes Project through the introduction of a mandate for specialty-specific competency-based milestones [22]. Milestones are ultimately described within the broader context of the previously defined six core competencies. Within each competency domain, specialty-specific sub-competencies are described, and five progressive levels of competency demonstration utilized as the framework in which specific milestones provide specific performance descriptions for progressive sub-competency attainment within each core competency domain (Fig. 14.1). An example of this framework is presented in Fig. 14.1. Milestones for anesthesiology were introduced in 2014 and like milestones for other subspecialties are intended to provide benefits on three levels [23, 24]:

- *Accreditation*: Milestones serve as an objective metric for program evaluation, provide accountability to the public of training standards, and provide a context for further research and improvement of training standards.

Patient Care 1: Preanesthetic Patient Evaluation, Assessment, and Preparation

Has Not Achieved Level 1	Level 1	Level 2	Level 3	Level 4	Level 5
	Performs general histories and physical examinations Identifies clinical issues relevant to anesthetic care with direct supervision Identifies the elements and process of informed consent	Identifies disease processes and medical issues relevant to anesthetic care Optimizes preparation of noncomplex patients receiving anesthetic care Obtains informed consent for routine anesthetic care; discusses likely risks, benefits, and alternatives in a straightforward manner; responds appropriately to patient's or surrogate's questions; recognizes when assistance is needed	Identifies disease processes and medical or surgical issues relevant to subspecialty anesthetic care; may need guidance in identifying unusual clinical problems and their implications for anesthesia care Optimizes preparation of patients with complex problems or requiring subspecialty anesthesia care with indirect supervision Obtains appropriate informed consent tailored to subspecialty care or complicated clinical situations with indirect supervision	Performs assessment of complex or critically ill patients without missing major issues that impact anesthesia care with conditional independence Optimizes preparation of complex or critically ill patients with conditional independence Obtains appropriate informed consent tailored to subspecialty care or complicated clinical situations with conditional independence	Independently performs comprehensive assessment for all patients Independently serves as a consultant to other members of the health care team regarding optimal preanesthetic preparation Consistently ensures that informed consent is comprehensive and addresses patient and family needs

Fig. 14.1 Example of milestones stratified within levels in a single sub-competency. (From the Anesthesia Milestone Project, December 2013. Copyright (c) 2013 The Accreditation Council for Graduate Medical Education and The American Board of Anesthesiology; reproduced with permission)

- *Graduate Medical Training Programs*: Milestones provide a framework for clinical competency committees, guide curriculum development and assessment, and provide a mechanism for early identification of trainee struggle.
- *Graduate Medical Trainees*: Milestones provide explicit expectations, assist in self-directed learning, and provide a context for effective feedback.

The benefits intended by the ACGME overlap to a large extent with those provided by SBME. An effective simulation curriculum for graduate anesthesiology education would ideally identify those sub-competencies and milestones best addressed through the experiential and kinesthetic aspects of simulation-based training while tailoring each session to training level and associated expectations for relevant milestone attainment. Furthermore, an SBME curriculum can be effectively guided by the milestones framework while also providing a tool for assessment, both formative and summative, through milestones performance within the simulated environment.

Challenges in SBME Curriculum Implementation

The clinical educator seeking to integrate SBME into the overall graduate anesthesiology training program quickly encounters the challenges inherent in this mode of instruction. In recent surveys of medical schools and anesthesiology training programs, just over half of medical student anesthesiology rotations incorporated SBME, while 55% of anesthesiology residencies incorporated SBME into intern training, 83% as part of clinical anesthesia year 1 (CA-1) training, and 96% as part of one or more rotations during residency [25, 26]. The main barriers to universal implementation cited in these surveys were time, financial, and human resources. To ensure the success of a curriculum for graduate anesthesiology education, these limitations must be taken into account and institutional resources must be realistically assessed and incorporated into the specific design of SBME implementation. While some strategies to overcome these obstacles will be presented here and in other section of this text, there are specific issues which must be addressed by each department seeking to integrate an SBME curriculum into their residency.

Simulation Facilities and Staffing

Those simulation centers endorsed by the ASA for ABA MOCA Part 4 simulation courses represent the spectrum of strategies through which anesthesiologist/educators have developed and implemented high-quality SBME curricula. On one end of this spectrum lie simulation centers housed within anesthesia departments fully staffed by faculty who provide the manpower for curriculum design, scenario development and scripting, hardware and software operation, confederate actors in immersive scenarios, debriefing, and even administrative tasks such as scheduling. This arrangement, while providing priority to the SBME initiatives of the anesthesiology department, depends a great deal on anesthesia faculty with heavy clinical workloads who demand relatively more financial resources for their time than non-physicians. Alternatively, many anesthesiology simulation programs interface with an institutional simulation center operated independently by their associated medical school or hospital. These centers often provide simulation technicians, administrative staffing, and a variety of other resources not available to anesthesia department-based simulation centers. This can drastically reduce the demands placed on the anesthesiologist/educator, but the SBME priorities of an anesthesiology residency program will be balanced against those of other departments and potentially an associated medical school. Many of the curricula presented in this chapter have been successfully implemented in both settings by making necessary modifications to staffing, scheduling, and format. A curriculum will be presented that was developed as a solution for those programs for whom no intra-institutional simulation center was available as well.

Simulation Hardware and Software

A variety of mannequin-based simulators, operating software, and partial task trainers exist representing a good deal of variability in cost and capability. The two most widely used models for mannequin-based simulation are the SimMan® manufactured by Laerdal Medical and the Human Patient Simulator (HPS®) manufactured by CAE Healthcare. SimMan® provides operator-dependent vital signs output coupled with a number of physiologically accurate cardiopulmonary findings on physical examination and allows basic airway management and effective fidelity for advanced cardiac life support coupled with a lower cost (around $60,000 for the popular SimMan® 3G model) and a low barrier or entry for educators intending to operate the software. The HPS® provides similar opportunities to the trainee for airway management and ACLS while incorporating physiologic modeling and direct interface between the mannequin and the anesthesiology workstation providing greater fidelity for the anesthesiology trainee. The HPS® couples these large advantages in fidelity and physiology with a much higher barrier to entry for the instructor intending to operate the software and a higher cost (over $200,000). Both Laerdal Medical and CAE Healthcare provide a variety of other models to represent the pediatric, neonatal, parturient, and other patients.

Educators looking to utilize scenarios and scripts created at one institution must consider that major revisions in design or implementation may be necessary if transferring from one model to another. Furthermore, certain goals of a simulation-based exercise for anesthesiology residents may be constrained based on the model utilized, as the practice of anesthesiology arguably places greater demands on a high degree of fidelity in SBME than the majority of medical practice.

Partial task trainers can greatly enhance a simulation curriculum through freestanding use for acquisition, practice, and assessment of technical skills or through incorporation into a mannequin-based immersive scenario. These can range greatly in cost and fidelity and would also be necessary for the educator looking to incorporate many essential skills in anesthesia training into an SBME such as neuraxial techniques, advanced airway techniques such as realistic lung isolation or bronchoscopy, central venous or arterial access, regional anesthetic techniques, ultrasound-guided needle manipulation, and echocardiography. More details on these products can be found in the chapters describing subspecialties of anesthesia in this text (Chaps. 16, 17, 18, 19, 20, 21, 22, 23, 24, 25, 26, and 27) as well as in the chapters on mannequin-based simulators and part-task trainers (Chap. 11).

A variety of other tools exist for SBME that can provide solutions for departments with more limited resources and include options such as standardized patient encounters and screen-based simulation products such as the Virtual Anesthesia Machine, a web-based interactive application run on the Adobe Shockwave Player [27]. Serious gaming may provide a future tool for educators, but this technology is currently in its infancy [28].

Simulation Faculty Expertise

More critical than human resource considerations such as simulator operation, administration of a simulation center, and confederate roles in scenarios, all of which were mentioned previously in consideration of simulation facilities and staffing, effective simulation educators require a great deal of training and experience. A successful SBME program for graduate anesthesiology training is not possible without trained simulation educators on faculty within the department providing the instruction. A number of simulation fellowship training programs exist to train simulation faculty in a variety of subspecialties [29]. Furthermore, a large number of programs for the training of current anesthesiology faculty are offered. The existence of these training programs reflects the complexity and skill involved in SBME curricular development and effective debriefing and the necessity of these skills for the success of a simulation program.

Time

The most widely reported challenge educators face in realizing their aspirations for a simulation curriculum is time. For an anesthesia residency training program in which the simulation educators also serve as clinical anesthesiologists and the simulation students also serve as trainee anesthesiologists capable of providing patient care under supervision, time spent in the simulation lab is time spent away from the provision of anesthetic care the department is tasked with. Given the revenue producing function of healthcare provision in modern medicine, this time can also be quantified monetarily, or in other words, time spent in the simulation lab costs the department an equal measure of time which those faculty or residents could be performing clinical duties and producing income for the department. To account for this additional demand on faculty and trainee time, a department must be sufficiently staffed to meet the educational mission in addition to the clinical functions of running an academic department. The challenge in provisioning time for simulation education not as commonly met with a traditional didactic session stems as the result of a feature of simulation commonly perceived as a pedagogical benefit. The small group format standardly utilized to facilitate kinesthetic learning, "hands-on" experience, and "hot seat" or primary management of the simulated clinical event is extremely inefficient from the point of view of one attempting to provide some targeted content to the largest possible audience over the shortest possible duration. The potential efficiency of didactic instruction is flexible and undeniable. Morning or afternoon sessions prior to or following scheduled anesthetic care provision are an extremely common strategy across graduate anesthesiology training programs for this reason.

While no formal systematic review has been conducted to assess strategies for scheduling simulation activities in graduate anesthesiology training, it is important to recognize that as one increases the efficiency of exposure (increasing the number of learners within a single session) one necessarily loses some of the benefits of this tool. A short, non-exhaustive list of some commonly observed strategies are listed in Table 14.2.

Introduction to Anesthesiology

Simulation is utilized across many specialties as a tool for the transition from medical school to residency training with many curricula described [30–32]. Despite the prevalence of simulation training in anesthesiology, a relative deficit of literature exists describing specific curricula designed for this purpose. A recent survey of anesthesia residency training programs revealed that 83% utilized SBME as part of orientation for junior anesthesiology residents [26], revealing

Table 14.2 Commonly utilized strategies for SBME scheduling in a graduate anesthesiology training program with relevant considerations and disadvantages

Simulation scheduling strategy	Strategy shortcomings
Morning small group sessions	Duration limited due to the scheduled start of anesthetic care. May conflict with existing morning didactic curriculum
Afternoon small group sessions	Requires a reliable method of faculty and trainee relief from clinical duties. May conflict with existing afternoon didactic curriculum
Education days (days on which faculty and trainees are relieved of clinical duties)	Requires sufficient global staffing for the removal of faculty and trainees from the labor pool
Telecasting of a high-fidelity simulation scenario to a larger audience during a morning session or departmental grand rounds	A minority of participants receive hands-on exposure or engage in effective debriefing
Workshops with "stations" through which participants rotate during time set aside for a departmental "grand rounds"	Limited primarily to interaction with part-task trainers or modified OSCEs. Takes the place of other departmental educational priorities served during "grand rounds" sessions
Day-long weekend simulation workshops	Less popular with trainees. Faculty participation requires additional compensation

high degree of penetrance. Therefore, this section will focus on considerations for providing the most effective introduction to anesthesiology curriculum and provide a sample curriculum.

Goals for the Junior Learner

The integration of SBME into a graduate anesthesiology training program's introductory curriculum must reflect a recognition of learners' novice level of clinical competency attainment, potential unfamiliarity with the anesthetic and perioperative environment, and a relative deficit of the medical knowledge relevant to anesthesia practice. In Miller's model, these learners find themselves at the starting point of the transition from "knows" to "knows how." Goals of an introductory simulation-based curriculum would focus on those novice competency domains or introductory principles best addressed through SBME's experiential, kinesthetic approach compared to other methods of pedagogy. General goals and learning objectives effectively addressed as part of an SBME introduction to anesthesiology curriculum include:

- Gain familiarity with the operating room environment and anesthesia equipment.
- Display an understanding of the workflow of a general anesthetic.
- Apply relevant medical knowledge to basic anesthesia care.
- Perform basic airway management of the anesthetized patient.
- Participate in institutional safety initiatives such as screening relevant patients for pregnancy, universal time-out, and postoperative debriefing.

Multiple level 1 milestones of patient care can be introduced and practiced effectively in the simulated environment as a component of the curriculum, some examples of which are presented in Table 14.3 [23]. In some instance, level 2 milestones may be relevant to the novice learner as well.

General Strategies for an Introduction to Anesthesiology Curriculum

The characteristics of the novice learner and goals consisting of an introduction to multiple aspects of clinical anesthesia care, institutional practices, and applied medical knowledge impose a structure and form on SBME for an introductory curriculum that will differ from a standard SBME curriculum for anesthesiology residency. While no ideal format has been identified, these authors suggest integrating the following strategies for bringing learner characteristics in line with educational goals as part of the overall introductory curriculum:

- *Open-ended scenarios:* Allowing for a multitude of interval or final outcomes serves multiple purposes for the novice learner. Given lack of familiarity and experience, learner actions will be extremely unpredictable and difficult to script. This provides the educator with an opportunity to allow learners to experience the potential consequences of certain actions or omissions as they occur in a safe environment. Examples include patient desaturation in response to omission of manual or controlled ventilation following intubation, evidence of awareness with omission of anesthesia administration following intubation, or even evidence of anaphylaxis following antibiotic administration if patient allergies were not assessed during the preoperative assessment. These techniques may be more appropriate for scenarios involving an introduction to basic induction or emergence.
- *Deliberate practice through scenario rewind:* In the event of learner error, following manifestation of clinical consequences (e.g., unrecognized esophageal intubation leading to patient hypoxia and instability), return to the point in the scenario directly preceding the error allowing appropriate management and the ability to proceed through additional learning objectives.

Table 14.3 Level 1 milestones appropriate for integration into an introduction to anesthesiology simulation curriculum

Sub-competency	Milestone(s)
Patient care 1: Pre-anesthetic patient evaluation, assessment, and preparation	Performs general histories and physical examinations Identifies clinical issues relevant to anesthetic care with direct supervision Identifies the elements and process of informed consent
Patient care 2: Anesthetic plan and conduct	Formulates patient care plans that include consideration of underlying clinical conditions, past medical history, and patient, medical, or surgical risk factors
Patient care 4: Management of peri-anesthetic complications	Performs patient assessments and identifies complications associated with patient care; begins initial management of complications with direct supervision
Patient care 5: Crisis management	Recognizes acutely ill or medically deteriorating patients; initiates basic medical care for common acute events; calls for help appropriately
Patient care 8: Technical skills: airway management	Recognizes airway patency and adequacy of ventilation based on clinical assessment Positions patient for airway management; places oral and nasal airways; performs bag-valve-mask ventilation
Patient care 9: Technical skills: use and interpretation of monitoring and equipment	Demonstrates the correct use of standard monitoring devices, including blood pressure (BP) cuff, electrocardiogram (ECG), pulse oximeter, and temperature monitors Interprets data from standard monitoring devices, including recognition of artifacts
Practiced-based learning and improvement 1: Incorporation of quality improvement and patient safety initiatives into personal practice	Has knowledge that patient safety issues exist in medicine and that they should be prevented (e.g., drug errors, wrong site surgery)
Practiced-based learning and improvement 2: Analysis of practice to identify areas in need of improvement	Identifies critical incidents or potentially harmful events pertaining to one's patients and brings them to the attention of the supervisor

- *Integrated debriefing or scenario pauses:* The novice anesthesiology resident is tasked with acquiring the requisite knowledge in parallel with its application, and the simulated clinical environment can provide an ideal forum for this process. Some examples of this practice include pausing the scenario: while patient monitors are placed to assess trainee knowledge of their utility and function, during preoxygenation to assess trainee knowledge of the principles of de-nitrogenation and patient positioning for ventilation and intubation, or after intubation to assess trainee knowledge of evidence successful intubation and adequate ventilation. During sessions on management of common complications such as hypoxia or hypotension, an in-depth discussion of cardiopulmonary concepts can be introduced at clinically relevant portions of the scenario, integrating traditional didactic instruction with experiential simulation-based learning.
- *Focus less on specific pathology and more on general principles:* While the educator may envision a specific pathophysiology to achieve the desired clinical presentation, the purpose of the clinical scenario highlights a general diagnostic and management approach as opposed to identification and management of a rare and critical event. For example, a perioperative myocardial infarction *should* be utilized as a strategy to provide an example of hypotension due to decreased cardiac output as part of a discussion basic cardiovascular physiology and *should not* be used for formative assessment of clinical management.

As with any group, an introduction to learning in the simulated environment at the outset of simulation-based instruction will ensure maximal utility of SBME for the novice learner. Given the role simulation will play throughout their training, an effective introduction is essential and should include an introduction to the simulation hardware and environment, a discussion of the safe learning space, and a general discussion of the general goals of SBME in residency training.

An explanation of the importance of "hot seat" learning, a delineation of the boundaries of the simulated and real world, and instructions for calling for help should also be provided.

A Sample "Introduction to Anesthesiology" Simulation-Based Curriculum

The following curriculum is adapted from the "Introduction to Clinical Anesthesia" simulation-based course first developed at the Human Emulation, Education, and Evaluation Lab for Patient Safety and Professional Study at the Icahn School of Medicine at Mount Sinai Hospital [33]. An adapted form of this course is currently being utilized by multiple anesthesiology training programs including the Department of Anesthesiology at the Wexner Medical Center at the Ohio State University as well as the Department of Anesthesiology, Perioperative, and Pain Medicine at Mount Sinai St. Luke's and West Hospitals. This curriculum incorporates many of the principles and strategies described above based on decades of experience in instruction and multiple revisions to format and content. The complete course consists of five sessions over the first month of training. Each session is 2 hours in duration, consists of three scenarios, and is intended to involve 3–4 CA-1 resident learners with 2–3 faculty or senior resident educators. All scenarios will have roles including the patient, circulating nurse, and surgeon. This curriculum is intended to provide a progression from basic to more advanced topics relevant to the junior anesthesia resident.

Sessions 14.1 and 14.2 are an introduction to the basic practice of clinical anesthesia. *Scenario pauses* allow the learner to review knowledge to apply to recent or upcoming actions, *simulation rewinds* following learner errors allow a demonstration of consequences, and *open-ended scenarios* allow for wider variation in learner performance to take advantage of unanticipated learning opportunities. Each scenario will vary subtly in order that each participant can meet the learning objectives, and the instructor should draw upon the list of relevant content for assessment of relevant knowledge during pauses in the scenario.

Session 14.1. Preoperative Evaluation and Induction of General Anesthesia

Learning objectives	Perform a preoperative evaluation and physical examination. Obtain informed consent. Obtain appropriate preoperative testing. Perform a preoperative anesthesia machine check and room preparation. Properly apply external patient monitors. Participate in universal protocol or "time-out" Provide appropriate premedication. Perform airway management including preoxygenation, manual ventilation, intubation, and controlled ventilation. Administer appropriate medications for induction and paralysis. Initiate a balanced anesthetic.
Relevant knowledge	Components of a basic patient history Mallampati classification Indications for preoperative testing Interpretation of data from external patient monitors and how each monitor functions Reasoning behind preoxygenation and proper performance Doses, concentration, indication, and mechanism of action for medications administered Appropriate position for ventilation/intubation Types of laryngoscopes and relation to airway anatomy Laryngoscopy: Anatomy, views, and grading Modes of ventilation and ventilator settings Characteristics of volatile anesthetics
Scenario 1	**Healthy young male requires general anesthesia for scheduled laparoscopic cholecystectomy.**
Case stem:	Our patient is a 30-year-old male undergoing scheduled laparoscopic cholecystectomy. His past medical history is significant for biliary colic. He reports no other past medical history. He takes no medications. He has experienced throat swelling from cephalexin. He has had no prior surgeries or anesthetic care.
Physical examination:	Healthy, non-obese male, normal physical examination, Mallampati 1 airway. 20-gauge antecubital intravenous line in place.
Scenario details:	Learners are expected to perform learning objectives described above. Learner actions will determine scenario progression (learner errors will lead to appropriate consequence), and a scenario rewind can take place following an error to allow learners a chance to make appropriate interventions and proceed to scenario completion when appropriate (*scenario is terminated following mechanical ventilation of the patient and initiation of a balanced anesthetic*).
Scenario 2	**Healthy young woman requires general anesthesia for scheduled breast augmentation.**
Case stem:	Our patient is a 25-year-old female undergoing a breast augmentation. Her past medical history is negative. She takes no medications. She has no allergies to medications. She reports an appendectomy as a child with no complications from anesthesia.
Physical examination:	Healthy, non-obese female, normal physical examination, Mallampati 3 airway. 20-gauge antecubital intravenous line in place.
Scenario details:	Learners are expected to perform learning objectives described above. Manual ventilation will require insertion of an oral airway. Highlight the requirement of a preoperative pregnancy screen (if omitted, have circulating nurse discover omission following intubation). Learner actions will determine scenario progression (learner errors will lead to appropriate consequence), and a scenario rewind can take place following an error to allow learners a chance to make appropriate interventions and proceed to scenario completion when appropriate (*scenario is terminated following mechanical ventilation of the patient and initiation of a balanced anesthetic*).
Scenario 3	**Healthy young male requires general anesthesia for emergent exploratory laparotomy.**
Case stem:	Our patient is a 31-year-old male undergoing an exploratory laparotomy. His past medical history is negative. He takes no medications. He has no allergies to medications. He reports no prior surgeries. He was stabbed in the abdomen during an argument while enjoying a pizza dinner. He is currently hemodynamically stable, but CT shows evidence of bowel perforation.
Physical examination:	Healthy, non-obese male, clear abdominal wound, rebound tenderness, and guarding. Normal cardiopulmonary physical examination findings. Mallampati 1 airway. 16-gauge antecubital intravenous line in place.
Scenario details:	Learners are expected to perform learning objectives described above. Rapid sequence intubation is required; omission will lead to regurgitation and aspiration. Learner actions will determine scenario progression (learner errors will lead to appropriate consequence), and a scenario rewind can take place following an error to allow learners a chance to make appropriate interventions and proceed to scenario completion when appropriate (*scenario is terminated following mechanical ventilation of the patient and initiation of a balanced anesthetic*).

Session 14.2. Emergence from General Anesthesia

Learning objectives	Determine extent of neuromuscular blockade. Perform reversal of neuromuscular blockade. Provide for adequate postoperative analgesia. Initiate and accelerate elimination of volatile anesthetic. Provide nausea and emesis prophylaxis. Identify and review extubation criteria. Identify stage 2 anesthetic plane during emergence. Perform oropharyngeal suction prior to extubation. Identify an appropriate patient postoperative disposition.
Relevant knowledge	Dosing and duration action of opioid agents Opioid alternatives for postoperative analgesia Analysis of train-of-four neuromuscular stimulation Relative effects of neuromuscular blockade on different muscle groups Characteristics of phase 1 vs. phase 2 blockade Sites for peripheral nerve stimulation Dosage, concentration, and mechanism of action of neuromuscular blockade reversal agents Factors that accelerate clearance and elimination of volatile anesthetic Risks of hypercarbia and hypoventilation Stages of anesthesia Antiemetic agent dosing and mechanisms of action Strategies for aspiration prevention Strategies for prevention of negative pressure pulmonary edema Causes of delayed emergence
Scenario 1	**Healthy young female requires general anesthesia for scheduled laparoscopic cholecystectomy.**
Case stem:	Our patient is a 40-year-old female undergoing scheduled laparoscopic cholecystectomy. Her past medical history is significant for cholelithiasis. She reports no other past medical history. She takes no medications. She has experienced throat swelling from cephalexin. She has had no prior surgeries or anesthetic care. The surgeon reports 10 minutes are remaining for skin closure.
Physical examination:	Healthy, non-obese female, normal physical examination, intubated under general anesthesia. Airway. 20-gauge antecubital intravenous line in place.
Scenario details:	Learner actions will determine scenario progression (learner errors will lead to appropriate consequence), and a scenario rewind can take place following an error to allow learners a chance to make appropriate interventions and proceed to scenario completion when appropriate (*scenario is terminated following patient extubation and stabilization*).
Scenario 2	**Obese woman undergoing gastric bypass for treatment of obesity**
Case stem:	Our patient is a 38-year-old female undergoing gastric bypass surgery. Her past medical history is positive for morbid obesity, OSA, DM type II. She takes metformin, glargine insulin, and tramadol. She is supposed to wear a CPAP at night, but is noncompliant. She has no allergies to medications. She had an uncomplicated cholecystectomy 5 years ago and a C-sect. 2 years ago. The surgeon reports 10 minutes are remaining for skin closure.
Physical examination:	Morbidly obese female, intubated, under general anesthesia with clear bilateral breath sounds. The patient has an 18-gauge antecubital intravenous line in place.
Scenario details:	Learners are expected to perform learning objectives described above. Emphasis will be placed on issues of hypoventilation and obesity, the impact of obesity on volatile anesthetic elimination. The patient will undergo a significant period of stage 2 emergence, and extubation criteria should be emphasized. Learner actions will determine scenario progression (learner errors will lead to appropriate consequence), and a scenario rewind can take place following an error to allow learners a chance to make appropriate interventions and proceed to scenario completion when appropriate (*scenario is terminated following successful patient extubation and stabilization*).
Scenario 3	**Delayed emergence in the setting of multiple risk factors**
Case stem:	Our patient is a 73-year-old female undergoing cholecystectomy. Her past medical history is positive for type I diabetes, fibromyalgia, generalized anxiety disorder, and CRPS of the right lower extremity related to previous trauma. She takes gabapentin as well as valium and percocet on an as-needed basis in addition to insulin and atorvastatin. She states she's allergic to morphine. She had an ORIF for a broken ankle 5 years ago complicated by severe postoperative nausea requiring an overnight stay. The patient has received a larger than normal dose of opioids in anticipation of higher requirements due to chronic pain therapy and a larger dose of benzodiazepine premedication due to anxiety. The surgeon reports 10 minutes are remaining for skin closure.
Physical examination:	Thin female, intubated, and under general anesthesia. Normal cardiopulmonary physical examination findings. 18-gauge antecubital intravenous line in place.
Scenario details:	Learners are expected to perform learning objectives described above. Delayed emergence will occur and following elimination of volatile anesthetic and reversal of neuromuscular blockade, learners are expected to contemplate reversal of opioids and benzodiazepines. Instructor may choose to allow for hypoglycemia discovered on laboratory analysis or an intracranial event to be the culprit. A full review of a delayed emergence management algorithm will be explored (*scenario is terminated following either successful extubation or once the decision is made to obtain intracranial imaging*).

Sessions 14.3 and 14.4 serve to provide an early conceptual framework for understanding pulmonary and cardiac physiology through the management of hypoxia and hypotension, respectively. These sessions utilize a "hybrid" format of immersive simulation in which planned "pauses" are utilized to reflect upon the clinical condition of the simulated patient and the learner's interpretation and management to clinical findings. These interval pauses are exploited to incrementally introduce a conceptual framework through application of the relevant principles of physiology to the clinical scenario. This curriculum integrates accessory materials such as displays of equations and diagrams during these interval scenario pauses. The session descriptions that follow will make note of these pauses and the content applicable to each one.

Session 14.3. Hypoxia

Learning objectives	Perform a differential diagnosis for intraoperative hypoxemia. Identify and correct a mainstem endotracheal intubation. Identify and treat intraoperative hypoxemia due to pulmonary alveolar atelectasis. Appropriately communicate the presence of patient hypoxemia with operating room staff. Identify an oxygen supply failure and utilize an alternative method of patient oxygenation. Provide a differential diagnosis for hypoxemia with a concomitant reduction in expired carbon dioxide concentration. Manage intraoperative pulmonary air embolism.
Medical knowledge objectives	Define oxygenation, ventilation, and respiration. Identify all lung volumes and capacities. Understand the determinants of functional residual capacity (FRC). Calculate the rate of oxygen consumption for a 70 kg patient. Describe the alveolar gas equation. Develop and apply an algorithm for management of intraoperative hypoxemia. Describe shunt and dead space physiology at the alveolar level. Understand pulmonary perfusion and ventilation. Describe the pulmonary west zones according to arterial, venous, and alveolar pressure relationships. Describe the relationship between FRC and closing capacity. Recognize the utility of continuous or bi-level positive airway pressure. Calculate and estimate an alveolar to arterial oxygen tension gradient.
Scenario 1	**Hypoxia during robotic laparoscopic hysterectomy**
Case stem:	Our patient is a 45-year-old female undergoing a robotic hysterectomy. Her past medical history is significant for obesity, hypertension, uterine fibroids, and OSA (home CPAP). She reports no other past medical history. She takes hydrochlorothiazide. She has no known drug allergies. She has had no prior surgery or anesthetic.
Physical examination:	Obese female, intubated, under general anesthesia currently supine prior to incision. The patient has an 18-gauge antecubital intravenous line in place.
Scenario details:	Learner encounters the patient under general anesthesia and receives a report from the prior anesthesia care provider. An uncomplicated induction and intubation is reported, antibiotics have been administered, and neuromuscular blocking agents and loading dose of opioid analgesics have been administered. Pre-surgical "time-out" completed just prior to learner arrival. Prior care anesthesia provider leaves the operating room. Endotracheal tube depth should be surreptitiously deeper than appropriate.
Event 1:	Surgical port placement, insufflation, and placement of patient into steep Trendelenberg positioning lead to rapid desaturation (SpO_2 mid-80s).

Pause	Define oxygenation, ventilation, respiration. Review lung volumes with an emphasis on FRC and its determinants. Calculate alveolar oxygen tension. Introduce an algorithm for hypoxia management
	1. 100 FiO_2
	2. √ other vitals ($ETCO_2$)
	3. $ETCO_2$ (+):
	  1. √ breath sounds/tube depth
	  2. √ inspired volume vs. expired volume
	  3. Diagnose cause of shunting
	$ETCO_2$ (−):
	  1. Switch off vent and attempt to hand bag
	    1. **Can** bag: Problem is in the ventilator
	    2. **Cannot** bag: Problem is proximal to the ventilator
	    Inspect ETT, elbow, circuit, etc.
	  2. If problem cannot be identified, utilize a self-inflating manual resuscitating bag with external oxygen or room air.

Event resolution	Learner should identify unilateral right-sided breath sounds, and resolution of hypoxia occurs with withdrawal of endotracheal tube to an appropriate depth.

Event 2:	The operator informs the learner that a fair deal of time has passed and lowers the oxygen saturation incrementally over the passage of time such that SpO_2 settles to the mid-80s following a simulated passage of 1 hour of time.
Pause	Define shunt and dead space at the alveolar level. Identify the west zones and the relationship of arterial and venous pressures to alveolar pressure. Define anatomic and physiologic dead space. Discuss the relationship of closing capacity and FRC and the impact on arterial oxygenation.
Event resolution	Learner should identify the role of alveolar atelectasis and shunt in clinical hypoxemia, initiate an alveolar recruitment maneuver, and utilize positive end-expiratory pressure (PEEP) to increase patient FRC.
Pause	Discuss the role of CPAP and BIPAP in oxygenation and ventilation and their use in the perioperative setting. *This will serve as the conclusion of the scenario.*
Scenario 2	**Loss of central oxygen supply intraoperatively**
Case stem:	We continue with our patient, a 45-year-old female undergoing a robotic hysterectomy. Her past medical history is significant for obesity, hypertension, uterine fibroids, and OSA (home CPAP). She reports no other past medical history. She takes hydrochlorothiazide. She has no known drug allergies. She has had no prior surgery or anesthetic.
Physical examination:	Obese female, intubated, under general anesthesia currently supine prior to incision. The patient has an 18-gauge antecubital intravenous line in place. Trendelenberg position.
Scenario details:	Between scenarios, advise learners to take a brief "break" during which time the central oxygen supply will be disconnected and the rear oxygen tank will be removed from the operating room/simulation theater. Upon return from their break, have the scenario paused and the anesthesia machine shut down, and have the first participant provide "sign-out" to the incoming learner. Following sign-out, the anesthesia machine can be powered on and the scenario un-paused.
Event 1	Progressive hypoxemia will occur in the setting of an inability to ventilate or oxygenate due to loss of central oxygen supply.
Pause	Reintroduce the previously discussed hypoxia algorithm.
Event resolution	Using the hypoxia algorithm, the participant should utilize a self-inflating manual resuscitating bag and potentially an external (tank) source of oxygen.
Pause	Review the volume and pressure relationship of an "E" cylinder of oxygen. Review the role of pressure from central gas supply to drive positive pressure ventilation with many models of anesthesia workstations. Discuss the impact of an anesthesia machine mounted oxygen "E" cylinder. *Scenario terminates following this discussion*
Scenario 3	**Intraoperative pulmonary embolism**
Case stem:	We continue with our patient, a 45-year-old female undergoing a robotic hysterectomy. Her past medical history is significant for obesity, hypertension, uterine fibroids, and OSA (home CPAP). She reports no other past medical history. She takes hydrochlorothiazide. She has no known drug allergies. She has had no prior surgery or anesthetic.
Physical examination:	Obese female, intubated, under general anesthesia currently supine prior to incision. The patient has an 18-gauge antecubital intravenous line in place. Trendelenberg position.
Scenario details:	This scenario will be a continuation of the prior two, now with operating oxygen supply restored. Learner 2 will provide a patient sign-out to learner 3. The surgeon informs the team of an hour or more remaining.
Event 1	Following a few minutes, the circulating nurse announces that the sequential compression devices had not been running and turns them on. Over the next few minutes, the patient will become progressively hypoxic, hypotensive, and the expired carbon dioxide tension will decrease.
Pause	Utilize the hypoxia algorithm. Calculate an alveolar to arterial oxygen gradient. Estimate arterial oxygen tension based on SpO_2 and a normal oxyhemoglobin dissociation curve. Discuss dead space physiology and its impact on ventilation. Briefly discuss the management options for pulmonary embolism. *Scenario is concluded after this discussion.*

Session 14.4. Hypotension

Learning objectives	Perform a differential diagnosis for intraoperative hypotension. Identify the pathophysiology of hypotension due to myocardial ischemia. Treat demand ischemia in the perioperative setting. Identify and treat intraoperative hypotension due to hemorrhage. Identify and treat intraoperative hypotension due to distributive shock from sepsis.
Medical knowledge objectives	Relate Ohm's law to the systemic and pulmonary circulation. Identify the components of stroke volume (preload, afterload, contractility). Describe the determinants of myocardial oxygen supply and demand. Review the role of the frank-Starling curve on stroke volume. Understand the role of decreased cardiac output on dead space ventilation and expired carbon dioxide tension.
Scenario 1	**Postoperative demand ischemia**

Case stem:	Our patient is a 65-year-old male status post open partial colectomy due to adenocarcinoma of the colon. His past medical history is significant for obesity, hypertension, and coronary artery disease with stents 2 years prior, obstructive sleep apnea on home CPAP, hyperlipidemia, and non-insulin-dependent diabetes mellitus. He has been off of clopidogrel for 8 days and takes aspirin, metoprolol, atorvastatin, metformin, and hydrochlorothiazide. He has no known drug allergies.
Physical examination:	Obese male, in obvious distress, tachycardic, hypertensive, diaphoretic, and dyspneic. He has an 18-gauge antecubital intravenous line in place. All other access has been removed.
Scenario details:	The learner is called to the postoperative care unit to evaluate a patient. The nurse informs our participant that the patient had received a colectomy and was ready for discharge to the floor. Monitors and all intravenous and arterial access lines have been removed but for a single peripheral venous line. The nurse informs the learner that the patient is complaining of unbearable pain at the surgical incision site. Patient information available from bundled chart if requested by participant (intraoperative management includes conservative use of analgesics out of concern for postoperative respiratory complications)
Event 1:	ECG (if connected) reveals sinus tachycardia with ST depressions in the anterolateral distribution. Patient initially hypertensive and complaining of severe pain at the surgical site and difficulty breathing. If a 12-lead ECG is available, have available an example of anterolateral ischemia and sinus tachycardia.
Pause	Discuss management of ischemia encouraging the participant to independently describe MONA-B management. Discuss the likely etiologies of perioperative ischemia and infarctions in the context of the intraoperative, immediate postoperative, and general postoperative time periods. Discuss the concept of myocardial supply and demand mismatch and the components of both myocardial oxygen supply and demand.
Event 2:	As the learner requests administration of medical and other interventions for cardiac ischemia, begin to lower the patient blood pressure to a low normal level (systolic pressure in the low 90's) while the nurse confederate attempts to retrieve beta-blocker treatment (if requested) with the goal of forcing the participant to evaluate the etiology of decreased cardiac output in the setting of worsening demand ischemia.
Pause	Introduce Ohm's law (V = IR) and relate the variables to those in the systemic cardiovascular circuit generally (MAP-CVP = CO x SVR). Have participants describe how to calculate cardiac output (SV x HR) and define the components of stroke volume (preload, afterload, and contractility). Identify the etiology of hypotension in the context of demand ischemia, and interrogate the rationale for the specific interventions represented in MONA-B treatment as they serve to optimize myocardial supply and demand and how this improves cardiac output utilizing the framework of Ohm's law and the relevant components in the systemic cardiovascular circuit.
Event resolution	The learner should recognize the utility of medical rate control with vasopressor support while also considering the need for coronary intervention.
Scenario 2	**Hypotension due to acute urosepsis**
Case stem:	Our patient is a 37-year-old woman with a medical history relevant for multiple episodes of nephrolithiasis and ureteral obstruction requiring cystoscopy and stone removal. She has no other past medical or surgical history. She takes no medications and has no allergies.
Physical examination:	Thin female, tachypneic, tachycardic, febrile, with low normal blood pressure. Favorable airway examination.
Scenario details:	The learner is called to the emergency room to conduct a pre-anesthetic evaluation for an urgent cystoscopy and ureteral stone removal. Emergency room staff confederate will inform the learner that the patient has received two liters of crystalloid via an 18 G peripheral venous catheter, as well as large doses of parenteral hydromorphone for pain. Antibiotics ordered by the urology service have been administered as well. Upon request, laboratory findings revealing leukocytosis and a negative pregnancy test will be provided.
Event 1	Learner is provided time to meet and evaluate patient in the emergency room. Attending anesthesiologist confederate will "call" the learner to receive a report on the patient and request the learner's anesthetic plan.
Pause	Utilize the conceptual framework of Ohm's law and the systemic cardiac circuit, and evaluate the etiology of hypotension in the context of this patient's history. Reserve an in-depth discussion of the role of tachycardia in compensating for intravascular depletion for later in this scenario.
Event 2	Arrival to operating room and induction of general anesthesia. Patient hemodynamic assessment reveals tachycardia and systolic pressure in the low 90s. The learner should be provided with the intravenous access, invasive or external blood pressuring monitoring they request. Learner should be allowed to perform the induction technique of their choosing. The goal of this portion of the scenario is to illustrate the effect of iatrogenic insult to the patient's compensatory response to evolving sepsis. If a non-judicious induction plan is utilized, severe hypotension will result. If a judicious induction plan is utilized, the attending anesthesiologist confederate may choose to (inappropriately) administer an agent such as esmolol in response to increased tachycardia to induce severe hypotension to facilitate the forthcoming event pause discussion.
Pause	Revisit the patient condition in the setting of the framework of Ohm's law, the role of preload, afterload, and contractility on stroke volume, and place emphasis on the role of heart rate in compensating for preload reduction and drop in systemic vascular resistance. This should serve to reinforce a systematic approach to perioperative hypotension performed by identifying within the concepts and formulas previously introduced. Learners should be encouraged to identify the "source" of derangement within the equations being utilized, i.e., SVR and/or cardiac output, if cardiac output, HR and/or stroke volume, and if stroke volume, preload, afterload, and/or contractility. Further discussion should involve the appropriate interventions to address the derangements.

Event 3 (optional)	Allow participant to employ interventions discussed during the previous event pause to stabilize hemodynamics to pre-induction conditions and continue to cystoscopy. Immediately following renal stone extraction, severe hypotension resistant to vasopressor support will ensue. This can allow for a post-scenario discussion of the dangers of urosepsis and the importance of preoperative and intraoperative resuscitation.
Scenario 3	**Hypotension secondary to hemorrhage**
Case stem:	Our patient is a 28-year-old female with no past medical or surgical history presenting for emergency laparoscopy for ruptured ectopic pregnancy. She takes no medications and has no allergies.
Physical examination:	Thin female, tachypneic, tachycardic, hypotensive, and afebrile with a favorable airway.
Scenario details:	Learner will encounter this patient just as they are brought to the operating room by the obstetrics and gynecology team. Two large-bore peripheral venous catheters are in place. Blood products are available if requested. Laboratory data obtained in the emergency room reveals a hematocrit of 36.
Event 1	Induction of anesthesia. Learner is allowed to develop a plan for induction and Maintenance of anesthesia.
Pause	Returning to the framework of Ohm's law presented earlier, discuss the cause of hypotension, existing compensatory changes, the impact of induction and maintenance of general anesthesia, and relevant considerations to preserve tissue perfusion.
Event resolution	Stabilization of vital signs following utilization of vasopressors, fluid administration, and potentially blood products after induction of general anesthesia.
Event 2	After the start of the procedure, large hemoperitoneum is discovered via laparoscopy. Deterioration of hemodynamics occurs upon initiation of pneumoperitoneum. This will manifest as severe hypotension, tachycardia, and a pronounced drop in expired carbon dioxide.
Pause	Revisit the cause of hypotension within the conceptual framework utilized in this exercise. Bring attention to the reduction of expired carbon dioxide tension. Introduce the application of Ohm's law as a model for the pulmonary circulatory circuit and correlate the relevant variables to those in the systemic circuit. Reintroduce the lung zones discussed during the preceding "hypoxia" session (ideally show diagrams previously utilized). Show the role played by cardiac output in the increase or decrease of zone 1 physiology and the impact on dead space ventilation that occurs as a result. Encourage the learner to connect this to the change in expired carbon dioxide tension in order to bring attention to the utility of capnography in detecting changes in cardiac output.
Event resolution	Administration of blood products (massive transfusion protocol) and aggressive vasopressor administration.

Sessions 14.5, "Arrhythmias," serves to reinforce the principles from the "Hypotension" sessions while incorporating advanced cardiac life support algorithms for managing unstable tachycardias, bradycardia, and pulseless rhythms. This session will continue to utilize a hybrid model of immersive simulation with intermittent "pauses" for the introduction of concepts and algorithms. This allows learners to gain an introduction to management principles and algorithms within the context of the relevant pathology while also allowing for deliberate practice through a "pause, discuss, reset, re-attempt" approach to experiential learning.

Session 14.5. Arrhythmias

Learning objectives	Evaluate hemodynamic instability in the context of a cardiac dysrhythmia. Identify and manage dysrhythmias including unstable tachycardias, bradycardias, and pulseless rhythms. Apply knowledge of treatable causes of pulseless electrical activity. Appropriately communicate the presence of an unstable arrhythmia with operating room staff. Understand the interaction between arrhythmias and cardiac output as it impairs coronary and other tissue perfusion.
Medical knowledge objectives	Describe the American Heart Association (AHA) algorithm for management of unstable tachycardias. Describe the AHA algorithm for management of unstable bradycardia. Describe the AHA algorithm for management of pulseless rhythms.
Scenario 1	**Management of symptomatic bradycardia**
Case stem:	Our patient is a 35-year-old male presenting for surgical treatment of a ruptured globe. He has no past medical or surgical history, takes no medications, and has no allergies. He reports that his injury was the result of a mishap in his workshop occurring just after lunch.

Physical examination:	Healthy male with an obvious foreign body and injured left eye. Mildly tachypneic, tachycardic, hypertensive with an 18 G peripheral venous catheter in his right hand.
Scenario details:	Learner encounters the patient in the operating room in preparation for urgent repair of a ruptured globe. Additional assessment can be made at this time. The learner will develop and conduct an anesthetic plan independently. While there are many salient issues raised by this case including the utilization of a rapid sequence induction and the choice of paralytic agent, these issues are secondary to the main learning objectives.
Event 1:	Following sterile preparation, draping, and surgical "time-out," surgical manipulation leads to mild bradycardia (high 40s) without resultant hypotension.
Event resolution	Prior to learner treatment (if intended), with cessation of surgical stimulation bradycardia resolves.
Event 2:	The surgeon confederate announces that further traction will be necessary to proceed with the procedure. This will result in severe bradycardia to 28 beats per minute with resultant hypotension. If the learner requests cessation of surgical traction, our confederate will comply (with resolution of bradycardia), however stating that further similar traction will be necessary to achieve their surgical goals.
Pause	Reintroduce the concept of Ohm's law and the systemic cardiac circuit to explain the role of bradycardia in this instance hemodynamic instability. A diagram displaying the frank-Starling curve and the effects of increasing preload on stroke volume should be discussed as well.
Event 3:	With ongoing surgical manipulation, heart rate decreases to 21 beats per minute with severe hypotension. Requests by the learner to cease surgical manipulation are met with a response by the surgical confederate to "treat it or something, I have to retrieve this foreign body!"
Pause	Display the AHA bradycardia algorithm. Discuss the current scenario insofar as it is addressed by the bradycardia algorithm. Discuss alternative scenarios in which symptomatic bradycardia may occur and the rationale behind the guidelines.
Event resolution	Learner administers 0.5 milligrams of atropine.
Scenario 2	**Management of unstable tachycardia**
Case stem:	Our patient is a 34-year-old female presenting for scheduled liposuction and breast augmentation. Her past medical history is significant for anxiety. She takes alprazolam daily and reports no drug allergies.
Physical examination:	Mildly overweight, anxious female with a favorable airway and a 20 G peripheral venous catheter in the left arm.
Scenario details:	The learner will meet the patient in the preoperative area and conduct a preoperative evaluation and develop an anesthetic plan. Anesthetic induction should proceed without incident as will the initiation of the surgical procedure.
Event 1	"Fast forward" the scenario into the midst of liposuction (45 minutes into the procedure). The patient's cardiac rhythm will progress from mild tachycardia to a rapid supraventricular rhythm with concomitant hypotension not responsive to phenylephrine.
Pause	Revisit the concept of systemic cardiac circuit and the role of heart rate and stroke volume on maintenance of cardiac output and mean arterial blood pressure.
Event 2	Allow the learner to attempt multiple interventions. The surgical team should initially discourage suggestions of cardioversion given then current surgical field preparations (however this would be the sole intervention leading to resolution).
Pause	Provide the AHA tachycardia (with pulse) algorithm and discuss the current patient condition in the context of the algorithm. Discuss alternative scenarios in which an unstable tachycardia may occur and the rationale behind the guidelines.
Event resolution	Learner utilizes synchronized cardioversion to treat the unstable tachycardia.
Scenario 3	**Management of pulseless rhythms**
Case stem:	Our patient is a 65-year-old male undergoing a laparoscopic right partial nephrectomy. His past medical history is significant for coronary artery disease with stent placement 5 years ago, hypertension, non-insulin-dependent diabetes, obesity, nephrolithiasis, and a right renal mass. He takes metoprolol, clopidogrel, aspirin, furosemide, metformin, and glyburide and has no known drug allergies. He had a left knee replacement 10 years ago without complications.
Physical examination:	Obese male, intubated, under general anesthesia currently in left lateral decubitus position. He has a left radial arterial line in place, and two 18 G peripheral venous lines (one in each hand).
Scenario details:	This scenario will begin intraoperatively with a hand-off from an anesthesia care provider confederate requiring relief for the end of their shift. The learner will receive a full report for transition of care including information that antiplatelet therapy has been discontinued for more than 1 week, but metoprolol was taken the morning of surgery. Preoperative hematocrit and glucose were 43 and 143, respectively, and a recent arterial sample revealed new values of 39 and 123. The procedure has been underway for an hour and has been without incident thus far.
Event 1	Following a few minutes, the patient monitor will reveal frequent premature ventricular contractions. If the learner inquires about the status of surgery, the surgical confederates will state that the procedure has progressed well and without complication.
Pause	Discuss the clinical significance, meaning, causes, and treatment of premature ventricular contractions. This is a good opportunity to define terms such as couplet, triplet, bigeminy, and trigeminy.

Event 2	Patient deteriorates over a few minutes into pulseless electrical activity (PEA). This will be unresponsive to vasopressors as it progresses.
Pause	Briefly discusses the definition of PEA drawing a comparison between electromechanical dissociation (EMD) PEA and non-EMD PEA and the clinical presentation.
Event 3	Rhythm progresses to ventricular tachycardia.
Pause	Present the AHA algorithm for pulseless cardiac arrest. Allow learner to review management in the context of patient status.
Event 4	Progress to ventricular fibrillation despite management.
Event resolution	Application of defibrillation. This will convert the rhythm to PEA.
Pause	Discuss the causes of PEA and potential management. Discuss the likely causes of arrest in this patient (cardiogenic shock secondary to myocardial infarction, embolism, etc.)

Simulation Training for Formative Assessment

SBME has already achieved a high degree of penetrance in graduate anesthesia education with a majority of ACGME-accredited programs utilizing this technology [26]. While debate exists regarding the wisdom and feasibility of utilizing SBME as a tool for assessing resident competency [34], survey data reveals that 79% of training programs have developed or plan to develop this tool as a means of assessing milestone attainment. While concerns about performance data from simulation-based training being utilized by clinical competency committees in resident assessment are well-founded and deserve further consideration in the training community, this does not preclude the use of milestones as means for development of an SBME curriculum for *formative* assessment. The simulated environment provides an ideal setting for allowing residents to "show" (using Miller's taxonomy) attainment of specific milestones which have been incorporated into SBME exercises in a manner that provides clear performance metrics. These authors prefer to utilize the phrase "facilitated self-assessment" to best describe the goals of such a curriculum.

General Strategies for a Simulation-Based Curriculum for Graduate Anesthesia Training

The simulated learning environment offers educators a tool for attaining goals in resident training less easily met through didactic or clinical means:

- *Tightly scripted scenarios with clear performance metrics:* If relevant information of performance is to be provided to the learner, simulated clinical scenarios must be standardized and structured in a way that clear outcomes metrics can be assessed. SBME is an ideal vehicle for providing opportunities for residents to receive feedback for practice improvement based on real-time performance assessment.
- *Deliberate practice through scenario repeat:* Toward the goal of learner improvement, following a simulated clinical exercise and debriefing, learners can revisit each scenario. This allows learners to apply lessons learned from feedback in debriefing and "better" manage each scenario. This will encourage active self-reflection and deliberate practice to reinforce the content and competencies assessed.
- *Exposure and practice with rare and critical events:* This is both a benefit and potential pitfall for the educator developing a simulation-based curriculum. The advice of these authors is to *not* develop a series of scenarios representing a wide swath of rare and critical events, but *do* start with general learning goals and objectives (ideally based on training-level specific milestones) and utilize a simulated clinical scenario that incorporates those goals and objectives. A wide variety of rare scenarios can easily serve a dual purpose of clinical exposure and provide residents the opportunity to practice general skills such as advanced resuscitation and crisis resource management.
- *Integration of competency-based milestones:* While an exhaustive list of the milestones well-suited to simulation-based assessment would be too large to reprint in this space, within multiple competency domains (patient care,

Table 14.4 Non-exhaustive list of sub-competencies appropriate for formative assessment of milestone attainment through simulation for graduate anesthesiology trainees

Anesthesiology sub-competency	Sub-competency description
Patient care 1	Pre-anesthetic evaluation, assessment, and preparation
Patient care 2	Anesthetic plan and conduct
Patient care 3	Peri-procedural pain management
Patient care 4	Management of peri-anesthetic complications
Patient care 5	Crisis management
Patient care 6	Triage and management of the critically ill patient in a non-operative setting
Patient care 8	Technical skills: airway management
Patient care 9	Use and interpretation of monitoring and equipment
Patient care 10	Technical skills: regional anesthesia
Systems-based practice 1	Coordination of patient care within the healthcare system
Practice-based learning and improvement 4	Education of patient, families, students, residents, and other health professionals
Professionalism 1	Responsibility to patients, families, and society
Professionalism 2	Honesty, integrity, and ethical behavior
Professionalism 4	Receiving and giving feedback
Interpersonal and communication skills 1	Communication with patients and families
Interpersonal and communication skills 2	Communication with other professionals
Interpersonal and communication skills 3	Team and leadership skills

communication, professionalism, practice-based learning), educators can use the milestones as a guiding superstructure in the development of a simulation-based curriculum for graduate anesthesia training. The structure of the competency-based milestones as developed by the ACGME also provides the advantage of developing a milestones-driven curriculum tailored to resident training level. The description of milestones progression provided within many sub-competencies (Table 14.4) can easily be reflected in a deliberately constructed curriculum consisting of training-level relevant scenarios.

A Sample Training-Level Specific Simulation-Based Curriculum for Formative Assessment

A simulation-based curriculum for formative assessment in graduate anesthesiology education is dependent to a large extent on the institutional and departmental simulation resources available and the level of departmental faculty expertise. The curriculum described here was developed in order to meet the needs of multiple training programs clustered within a single region, most of which had no access to a simulation center when the inclusion of a simulated clinical experience was included in the revised program requirements by the Anesthesiology Residency Review Committee in 2011. This curriculum consists of a 1-day workshop for each level of clinical anesthesia training. Each workshop is divided into "modules" consisting of three separate scenarios/stations through which small groups of trainees rotate to maximize the opportunity for exposure within a limited time period alternating in the role of the "hot seat." Between modules, brief didactic or discussion sessions were utilized to reinforce relevant topics such as the ASA difficult airway algorithm, the AHA algorithm for pulseless cardiac rhythms, or team training and communication. The details for the scenarios utilized (scripts, supporting documents) are less important than the extent to which fidelity to milestones and competency-based objectives is served by the scenarios utilized or developed.

Workshop for Formative Assessment of Clinical Anesthesia Year 1 (CA-1) Trainees

Our group has developed a series of modules (Modules 17.1) designed to address level 1 and 2 milestones within sub-competencies in the domains of patient care, interpersonal and communication skills, professionalism, and systems-based practice. Specific anesthetic issues will focus on core topics such as airway management, ACLS, and common intraoperative issues such as hypotension and hypoxia.

Module 17.1. A Simulation-Based Workshop for Formative Assessment of Clinical Anesthesia Year 1 (CA-1) Trainees

Learning objectives	Perform a standard preoperative anesthetic assessment. Perform a standard anesthetic induction and emergence. Evaluate and treat common causes of intraoperative hypoxia. Evaluate and treat common causes of intraoperative hypotension. Evaluate and treat intraoperative arrhythmias. Display the ability to apply supraglottic airway techniques. Display the ability to apply videolaryngoscopic techniques.
Medical knowledge objectives	Describe the American Heart Association (AHA) algorithm for pulseless rhythms. Describe the ASA difficult airway algorithm.
Module 1	**Partial task trainer stations** *Placement and management of supraglottic airways* Using a variety of head or airway mannequins, trainees can display appropriate placement, securement, and use of a supraglottic airway device. *Flexible and rigid video-assisted laryngoscopy* Using a variety of head or airway mannequins, trainees can display endotracheal tube placement with the assistance of videolaryngoscopy and flexible fiberoptic bronchoscopy. *Neuraxial anesthetics and sterile technique* With the use of low or high-fidelity mannequin-based partial task trainer, trainees can demonstrate spinal and epidural anesthetic technique as well as sterile technique.
Module 2	**High-fidelity simulated airway management** *Non-urgent difficult airway management* This scenario should allow trainees an opportunity to perform a standard induction of anesthesia, work through multiple steps of the difficult airway algorithm (at the discretion of the instructors) and conduct a safe emergence from anesthesia. Elements of communication and professionalism can also easily be integrated into this scenario, and many of the following scenarios. *Emergent critical airway management* This scenario should allow provide trainees with an opportunity to manage a difficult airway working through all steps of the difficult airway algorithm concluding with cricothyrotomy. Our group utilized a scenario involving a patient in the surgical intensive care unit following a complex cervical spine procedure requiring transfusion of multiple blood products. The trainee encounters the patient in response to a "STAT" anesthesia page. The patient's cervical spine is immobilized in a cervical collar and has self-extubated. *Emergent intubation in a non-clinical location* This scenario should provide the trainee an opportunity to encounter a patient requiring intubation away from the standard operating room or critical care unit environment in order that the trainee can display the ability to obtain the appropriate tools necessary and coordinate assistance from those present. This can be achieved involving a scenario in which a colleague is found unconscious in a call room with vomitus present in the airway.
Module 3	**Management of hypoxia, hypotension, and pulseless cardiac arrest** *Hypoxia* In this scenario, trainees will diagnose and treat multiple causes of hypoxia within a single scenario. Our group utilizes a scenario involving a laparoscopic hysterectomy in an obese patient. Following initiation of pneumoperitoneum and Trendelenberg positioning, a right mainstem bronchus intubation occurs. After diagnosis and treatment of mainstem intubation, the patient experiences insidious and slow developing hypoxia due to progressive atelectasis from habitus, pneumoperitoneum, and positioning effects of functional residual capacity. *Hypotension* This scenario should provide trainees with an opportunity to distinguish between causes of hypotension. Ideally, the scenario will provide an example of hypotension due to a decrease in vascular tone as well as hypotension due to a decrease in cardiac output. Our group utilizes a scenario involving an elderly hypertensive woman undergoing a partial colectomy. Following induction, an anesthesia-mediated decrease in systemic vascular resistance leads to hypotension (perhaps from overzealous dosing by a senior). Later, unrecognized bleeding leads to a decrease in cardiac output. *Pulseless rhythms* This scenario provides trainees with an opportunity to manage pulseless rhythms in the operating room. The specific scenario details are of less importance than simulating rhythms that can be effectively defibrillated as well as those that cannot. Our group utilizes a scenario involving a patient with severe coronary artery disease with recent drug-eluting stent placement undergoing emergent surgery for gastric bleeding. The electrocardiogram devolves from evidence of ischemia with ectopy to pulseless electrical activity, ventricular tachycardia, and ventricular fibrillation. The instructor can cycle through rhythms as is deemed appropriate.

Workshop for Formative Assessment of Clinical Anesthesia Year 2 (CA-2) Trainees

For trainees in the second year of training, simulation-based formative assessment should reflect the progression of clinical training house staff have experienced. Therefore, subspecialty simulations can play a role to expand the breadth of competencies assessed. While core concepts such as airway management and ACLS are readdressed, milestones assessed should be those between levels 2 and 3 of the relevant sub-competencies (patient care, interpersonal and communication skills, professionalism, and systems-based practice). Some technical skills are readdressed through the use of part-task trainers to allow for a demonstration of progression of technical skills (see Module 17.2).

Module 17.2. A Simulation-Based Workshop for Formative Assessment of Clinical Anesthesia Year 2 (CA-2) Trainees

Learning objectives	Perform a complex preoperative anesthetic assessment relevant to subspecialty anesthetic care. Perform a subspecialty anesthetic induction and emergence Evaluate and treat uncommon complications that arise within subspecialty anesthetic care. Evaluate and treat common causes of intraoperative hypotension Lead a team in the management of pulseless cardiac arrest. Display the ability to apply advanced airway techniques. Display the ability to perform cricothyrotomy and transtracheal jet ventilation.
Medical knowledge objectives	Describe the American Heart Association (AHA) algorithm for pulseless rhythms. Describe the ASA difficult airway algorithm.
Module 1	**Partial task trainer stations** *Placement and management of supraglottic airways* Using a variety of head or airway mannequins, trainees can display appropriate placement, securement, and use of a supraglottic airway device. *Flexible and rigid video-assisted laryngoscopy* Using a variety of head or airway mannequins, trainees can display endotracheal tube placement with the assistance of videolaryngoscopy and flexible fiberoptic bronchoscopy. *Cricothyrotomy and transtracheal jet ventilation* Through the use of a head or airway mannequin, trainees can perform cricothyrotomy with an angiocatheter or surgical cricothyrotomy kit in order to provide oxygenation through transtracheal jet ventilation or a more secure tracheostomy.
Module 2	**High-fidelity simulated complications in anesthesia subspecialties** *High spinal anesthesia in an obstetric patient with a difficult airway* This scenario should allow trainees an opportunity to recognize the development of a high spinal anesthetic through characteristic changes in hemodynamics and patient symptoms. This will require communication with the obstetric team regarding prioritization of fetal delivery or maternal support as a difficult airway is encountered requiring application of the difficult airway algorithm. *Venous air embolism during a craniotomy* This scenario will provide trainees with an opportunity to recognize the development of a high spinal anesthetic through characteristic changes in hemodynamics and patient symptoms. This scenario can easily integrate issues such as surgical complaints regarding the interventions required for treatment and the impact on the surgical field and surgical progress. *Postoperative respiratory arrest due to narcotic overdose* In this scenario, trainees encounter an obtunded patient in the post-anesthesia care unit. This patient has a complex history of chronic pain, and perioperative analgesic management has been conducted under the guidance of the pain management service and includes long-acting opioids and a battery of non-opioid analgesics.
Module 3	**Management of advanced life-threatening anesthetic complications** *Malignant hyperthermia in a pediatric patient* In this scenario, trainees will conduct a standard induction of anesthesia for a pediatric patient, be expected to diagnose and treat malignant hyperthermia, and direct the postoperative management and disposition. Particular attention should be paid to directing the acquisition and administration of therapeutic agents. *Local anesthetic systemic toxicity (LAST) following a regional anesthetic block* This scenario should focus on the identification and management of LAST resulting in cardiovascular collapse. In order to integrate milestone representative of the competency of systems-based practice, debriefing should focus on locating and obtaining lipid therapy within the perioperative environment. *ACLS leadership* Our group utilizes a scenario in which the trainee is expected to lead ACLS in the postoperative care unit. This scenario should focus on resource allocation, leadership, and communication in addition to command of the AHA algorithms.

Workshop for Formative Assessment of Clinical Anesthesia Year 3 (CA-3) Trainees

For trainees in the final year of training, simulation-based formative assessment should reflect a transition to supervision of anesthetic care management of multiple patients as may occur in the postoperative care unit. Simulated scenarios will be designed to allow for practice and end performance of these skills. Given the critical role of airway management and ACLS, these topics are revisited through partial task trainers and scenarios with an emphasis on supervision and team leadership. Transthoracic and transesophageal echocardiography are introduced through partial task training as well. Milestones assessed should be those between levels 3 and 4 of the relevant sub-competencies (patient care, interpersonal and communication skills, professionalism, and systems-based practice) (see Module 17.3).

Module 17.3. A Simulation-Based Workshop for Formative Assessment of Clinical Anesthesia Year 3 (CA-3) Trainees

Learning objectives	Perform oversight if the administration of an anesthetic with a junior practitioner. Display the ability to prioritize and delegate care of multiple critical patients. Recognize and effectively manage an operating room fire. Evaluate and treat postoperative complications that may occur in the post-anesthesia care unit. Lead a team in the management of pulseless cardiac arrest or other unstable cardiac arrhythmias. Display the ability to supervise or perform advanced airway techniques.
Medical knowledge objectives	Understand and acquire key transesophageal and transthoracic echocardiographic views of cardiac anatomy and function. Describe advanced airway techniques as part of the ASA difficult airway algorithm.
Module 1	**Partial task trainer stations** *Transesophageal and transthoracic echocardiography* Through the use of a partial task trainer, trainees will obtain and evaluate key views and describe function of cardiac anatomy. *Flexible fiberoptic bronchoscopy* Using a variety of head or airway mannequins, trainees can perform endotracheal tube placement with the assistance of flexible fiberoptic bronchoscopy. Participants will also utilize a virtual bronchoscopy partial task trainer to obtain views of glottic and tracheobronchial anatomy. *Cricothyrotomy and transtracheal jet ventilation* Through the use of a head or airway mannequin, trainees can supervise and instruct another in the performance of cricothyrotomy with an angiocatheter or surgical cricothyrotomy kit in order to provide oxygenation through transtracheal jet ventilation or a more secure tracheostomy.
Module 2	**High-fidelity simulated situations in anesthetic supervision and administration** *Supervision of a difficult junior resident* This scenario should allow trainees an opportunity to supervise a junior resident lacking proficiency in diagnosis, management, and procedural competence during a difficult ventilation and intubation upon induction of anesthesia. This will require the trainee to strike a balance between education and patient safety. *Postoperative bleeding in the postoperative care unit* In this scenario, trainees encounter a hemodynamically unstable patient status post renal transplantation in the postoperative care unit. The trainee will have to diagnose hemorrhage and direct the surgical team to return to the operating room. This scenario will transition to the hemorrhage scenario in the operating room. This scenario will focus on communication in addition to management of an unstable patient. *Hemorrhage* In this scenario, the trainee will transition the patient from the prior PACU scenario into the operating room where they will be required to oversee the anesthetic with a junior resident while receiving requests from the PACU nursing regarding other postoperative patients. This scenario emphasizes team leadership, OR management, teamwork, communication, task delegation, and resource allocation.
Module 3	**Management of rare or complex life-threatening perioperative complications** *Intraoperative airway fire during tracheostomy placement in the operating room* In this scenario, poor communication will occur between the surgical team and the trainee regarding the use of electrocautery during in the setting of a high fraction of inspired oxygen. The trainee can be led to provide high FiO_2 through the simulation of a patient with tenuous arterial oxygenation due to ARDS. This scenario will focus on both the management of an airway fire and communication. *Hematoma and respiratory distress following tracheostomy in the PACU* In this scenario, the trainee will be called to evaluate a patient experiencing respiratory distress following thyroidectomy. They will discover an expanding hematoma compromising oxygenation and ventilation. Focus should be placed on communication with the surgical team, marshalling airway supplies and support, and difficult airway management. *ACLS leadership* In this scenario, the trainee(s) will be asked to assume alternating roles during ACLS. Trainees should practice leadership, closed-loop communication, speaking up, mutual support, and other crisis resource management skills.

Simulation for Summative Assessment

Beyond its role in instruction for graduate medical education, simulation technology offers an opportunity for summative assessment of clinical competency. Unlike formative assessment, in which trainees are given feedback to prompt self-reflection and promote further learning, summative assessment is utilized to evaluate trainees prior to attainment of a certain status or matriculation. This can vary from attainment of specific milestones or competencies to the more critical question of whether the trainee is ready to graduate and to independently practice.

The high-fidelity simulated environment allows the opportunity to evaluate residents in ACGME defined competency-based milestone domains difficult to assess using typical written exams. These milestones represent the highest layer of Miller's pyramid, in which the student "does." [19] Communication, teamwork, technical skills, complex diagnostic and therapeutic abilities, and performance in crisis situations are areas that are challenging to objectively measure [35]. Typically, training programs rely on clinical performance evaluations or input from faculty and the Clinical Competency Committee to measure performance in these competencies. However, these methods can be subjective among other shortcomings.

Although simulation has been seen as a tool in anesthesiology education since the 1950s, interest in using simulation as an evaluative tool has arisen more recently. This has resulted partly from the response of academic institutions and professional organizations (i.e., ASA, Anesthesia Patient Safety Foundation) to the public demand for assurance practitioner competency. The shift in the graduate medical education from a time-based to an outcomes-based model has included a shift toward recognition that specific milestones must be met and competencies demonstrated before advancement and certification [36, 37]. Medical licensing and professional accrediting bodies have accepted the role of performance assessments as a component in professional licensure and accreditation. In addition to the introduction of a mandatory, simulation-based component to Maintenance of Certification (MOC) by the American Board of Anesthesiology (ABA), summative assessments using simulation or OSCE have been adopted by the National Board of Medical Examiners (NBME), The Medical Council of Canada, The Fellow Royal College of Anesthesiologists, and The Israeli National Board Examination in Anesthesiology [38]. Furthermore, an Objective Structured Clinical Examination (OSCE) component has been added to the ABA APPLIED Board Examination as an adjunct to the oral exam. Through the development of these standardized, patient-based simulations, a wealth of experience and expertise has been gained regarding examination design, test administration, logistics, quality assurance, and psychometrics [39]. This has provided a foundation for the development of summative assessment through the use of simulation. For these high-stakes assessments in which decisions are made regarding the competency and/or the advancement status of a trainee, quality assurance measures and precision in scoring are essential.

Since the ACGME finalized the transition to a competency-based education model with the "milestone project," residency programs have each been charged with developing their own approach to assessment competency-based milestone attainment. In response to this charge, many anesthesiology residency training programs have found simulation to be a valuable tool in assessment of competency attainment [40]. A survey of 132 US academic anesthesiology residency programs revealed that of those institutions that responded (66%), 40% utilize simulation for resident assessment and remediation. A far greater share of those responding (89%) utilize standard simulation for resident education. Many of the programs that have begun to use simulation for summative assessment are explicitly assessing milestone attainment to trigger transition between training levels and remediation. Some of these programs have focused on the competency domains of communication and professionalism, while others have incorporated checklists of complex clinical tasks into their evaluations. The biggest challenges reported by training programs in instituting and maintaining simulation into summative evaluations are insufficient time, simulation-trained personnel, and money. Others have expressed concern that using simulation for any reason than training or formative assessment is in conflict with the principle that the simulation environment should provide a "safe space for learning." [26]

Key Steps in Developing a Simulation-Based Program for Summative Assessment

There are several important issues to consider when developing a curriculum for simulation-based assessment. One must define the purpose of the assessment (advancement in training level, data collection for the clinical competency committee), choose the appropriate clinical competencies to measure, create scenarios that elicit performances reflecting the targeted competencies, and develop measurement tools that can provide reliable and valid assessment scores.

Identifying the Purpose of the Assessment

The first step in developing a simulation-based assessment program is identifying the specific purpose of the assessment. For example, in resident education, a critical question is whether trainees have acquired the necessary competencies to independently provide safe anesthesia care following completion of their training. Once the aim of the assessment is clearly defined, one can develop the components of the test that will provide date to meet this goal (i.e., which specific clinical competencies will be assessed). A conventional way to choose competency-based milestones or competency domains for summative assessment is to utilize those already detailed in a training program's curriculum (i.e., goals and objectives) based on those enumerated by the ACGME Anesthesiology Milestone Project. In addition, The Joint Council on In-Training Examinations, a committee of the American Board of Anesthesiology, publishes a content outline comprised of a detailed description of the basic and clinical topics in which an anesthesiology consultant should be competent. When creating objectives for a simulation-based assessment program, it is imperative to select only those milestones or skill domains that can be reasonably assessed in the simulated environment to collect accurate information regarding trainee competence. Several methods for development of simulation-based assessment programs and the relevant skill domains have been described in the literature. One method is the creation of a list of perioperative events that a resident should be able to effectively manage following the completion of their training and cross-referencing this list with topics in the American Board of Anesthesiologists content outline to assure that they conform to the attributes of a consultant as determined by the ABA. Using this method, Murray et al. [41] developed a set of six clinical cases for assessment: (1) postoperative anaphylaxis, (2) intraoperative myocardial ischemia, (3) intraoperative atelectasis, (4) intraoperative ventricular tachycardia, (5) postoperative stroke with intracranial hypertension, and (6) postoperative respiratory failure (Table 14.5). Another method described by Blum et al. involves the creation of a list of behavioral domains [42]. In this method, a panel of experts from one's institution composed of clinically experienced board-certified anesthesiologists involved in residency education are asked, "What traits characterize residents who, upon graduation, have not achieved a minimum level of competency?". Then, using a modified Delphi process,[1] these responses can be reduced to a list of key behaviors that are lacking in an underperforming senior resident. Blum et al. identified five key behaviors through this method: (1) synthesizes information to formulate a clear anesthetic plan, (2) implements a plan based on changing conditions, (3) demonstrates effective interpersonal and communication skills with patients and staff, (4) identifies ways to improve performance, and (5) recognizes own limits. Seven scenarios were then designed based on these five behavioral domains with clinical material incorporated using the ABA examination content outline and the ACGME core competencies. The resulting scenarios were (1) preoperative assessment of a patient scheduled for urgent exploratory laparotomy, (2) operative management of a patient with perforated ulcer and hemorrhage, (3) monitored anesthesia care for a patient with discomfort during basal cell carcinoma surgery, (4) post-anesthesia care for a patient with aspiration after basal cell carcinoma surgery, (5) management of anaphylaxis in a patient with transurethral resection of the prostate and bladder biopsy, (6) care for a patient with delayed awakening in the operating room after transurethral resection of the bladder, and (7) identification and management of mainstem intubation secondary to coughing in a patient undergoing total thyroidectomy [43].

Scenario Development

Once competency domains and scenario topics have been identified, it is important to develop simulation scenarios that best target the specific skills or behaviors one intends to observe or measure. To minimize simulation artifact and optimize the precision of the assessment, scenarios should maintain fidelity to the clinical environment by providing those usual supplies, equipment, and patient characteristics with which the trainee is familiar. Scenarios that work well within the technical limitations of the simulation equipment while targeting the expected training level of the examinees are most successful. Summative assessment curricula are often composed of scenarios that focus on critical clinical situations for many valid reasons. First, the field of anesthesiology, by its nature, deals with rare yet catastrophic events that can lead to severely adverse patient outcomes if the practitioner is ineffective in their management. Secondly, rare and critical scenarios may provide an opportunity to identify residents that are struggling earlier in training given the inability to reveal some deficits through the performance of routine anesthetic care. Additionally, acute care simulation scenarios typically test difficult to evaluate skill sets that are frequently lacking in "borderline residents" such as prioritization, generating of a differential diagnosis, processing knowledge, assigning probabilities, isolating essential from non-essential information, integrating competing issues, acknowledging limits, and knowing when to call for help [44].

[1] *The modified Delphi technique is a well-described method in education of obtaining consensus among several experts on a subject* [43]. *In this case, it involves distributing a list of tasks/behaviors that are believed to be lacking in an underperforming resident to a panel of experts. Each behavior is rated in importance by each panel member, and any additional comments or additions/deletions of behaviors are accepted. The data is gathered and median scores and ranges for each behavior are calculated. This data is then redistributed to the panel of experts, and each expert can change any scores that deviate from the median or explain why they do not wish to change their scores. The medians and ranges are the recalculated and the data is redistributed. This process is repeated until an acceptably small range of variation is present.*

Table 14.5 Scoring items

Scenario	Checklist scoring items	Time-based scoring items
Anaphylaxis – PACU	Establish neuromuscular recovery (1 point), examine/inquire airway/ blood loss/secretions (1 point), FIO_2 of 100% rebreathing mask or Ambu bag and mask (1 point), auscultate chest (1 point), diagnose bilateral wheeze/coarse breath sounds (1 point), increase intravenous fluids (1 point), anaphylaxis diagnosed within 3 min (2 points), anaphylaxis diagnosis (2 points), epinephrine within 3 min (3 points), epinephrine any dose (1 point), epinephrine correct dose (>50 μg, <300 μg) (1 point)[a], pharmacologic treatment of hypotension (1 point), inhaled β agonists (1 point), intravenous diphenhydramine (1 point), intravenous steroids (1 point)	(a) Time to diagnosis of anaphylaxis (b) Time to treatment regimen for suspected anaphylaxis (c) Time to dose of epinephrine
MI – intraoperative	Diagnose ischemia (2 points), confirm ischemia (rhythm strip, ST analysis, check other leads) (2 points), increase FIO_2 to 100% (1 point), increase anesthetic depth (1 point), maximum heart rate during scenario less that 110 beats/min (1 point)[b], maximum heart rate during scenario less than 120 beats/min (1 point), nitroglycerin therapy (1 point), titrate nitroglycerin (1 point), β-blocker therapy (2 points), titrate β-blocker therapy (1 point), inform surgery team of ischemia (1 point), heart rate less than 100 beats/min at end of scenario (1 point), heart rate less than 95 beats/min at end of scenario (1 point)[b], systolic blood pressure less than 150 beats/min, diastolic blood pressure less than 100 beats/min at end of scenario (1 point)	(a) Time to diagnose ischemia by ST analysis or electrocardiographic rhythm strip (b) any treatment directed at improving ischemia (c) Time to reduce heart rate less than 100 beats/ min
Atelectasis – intraoperative	FIO_2 to 100% (2 points), review ventilator settings (1 point), diagnose hypoventilation/atelectasis (2 points), increase tidal volume/PEEP (2 points), mechanical to hand ventilation (1 point), auscultate chest (1 point), diagnose diminished breath sounds bilaterally (1 point), effective ventilation by hand (increase oxygen saturation to 90%, increase chest excursion) (1 point), lowest oxygen saturation greater than 80% (2 points), pass suction catheter via endotracheal tube (2 points), oxygen saturation to 90% at any time during scenario (1 point), oxygen saturation to 95% before 120 s (1 point), oxygen saturation to 95% at any time during scenario (2 points)	(a) Time to 100% FIO_2, hand ventilation, and auscultation (b) Time to reverse decline in oxygen saturation and improve oxygen saturation to 90% or greater (c) Time to oxygen saturation greater than 95%
Ventricular tachycardia – intraoperative	Diagnose ventricular tachycardia (1 point), palpate pulse or auscultate heart sounds (1 point), indicate patient is unstable or need for immediate shock (1 point), FIO_2 to 100% (1 point), defibrillator to bedside (1 point), correct joule (200+) (1 point), correct procedure for shock (1 point), administer shock within 60 s (1 point)[c], administer shock within 3 min (1 point), administer shock (2 points), abort operative procedure (1 point), lidocaine bolus/infusion (2 points), laboratory tests and 12-lead electrocardiogram (1 point)	(a) Time to diagnosis of ventricular tachycardia (b) Time to initiate any correct therapy (lidocaine/shock) (c) Time to shock
Cerebral hemorrhage – PACU	Establish patient is unresponsive (1 point) or unresponsive to pain (2 points), auscultate (1 point), conduct neurologic evaluation (1 point), indicate neurologic event (1 point), indicate potential increased ICP (1 point), neurology consult/CT scan (1 point), diagnosis within 2 min (1 point), prepare for intubation (1 point), FIO_2 to 100% (1 point), intubate (2 points), ventilate and auscultate (1 point), does not attempt to lower blood pressure (1 point)	(a) Time to establish patient unresponsive to verbal/pain or neurologic examination (b) Time to diagnose cerebral event/CT scan (c) Time to intubation
Aspiration – PACU	Establish patient is unresponsive to verbal (1 point), auscultate chest (1 point), request arterial blood gas (1 point), diagnose respiratory failure (2 points), prepare to intubate (1 point), Ambu bag and mask oxygen before intubation (1 point), sedation/anesthesia before or after intubation (1 point), laryngoscopy and intubation technique (1 point), intubated in less than 2 min (2 points), effective ventilation after intubation (2 points), indicate ventilator/PEEP required (1 point)	(a) Time to diagnose respiratory failure (b) Time to intubation (c) Time to effective ventilation after intubation

From Ref. 41

CT computed tomography, *FIO_2* fraction of inspired oxygen, *ICP* intracranial pressure, *MI* myocardial ischemia, *PACU* post-anesthesia care unit, *PEEP* positive end-expiratory pressure

[a]Anaphylaxis

[b]MI: If the resident received a point for maximum heart rate less than 110 beats/min, he/she also received a point for maximum heart rate less than 120 beats/min. If the resident received a point for heart rate less than 95 beats/min at the end of the scenario, he/she also received a point for heart rate less than 100 beats/min

[c]Ventricular tachycardia: If the resident received a point for administering a shock within 60 s, he/she also received a point(s) for administering a shock with 3 min and administering a shock during scenario

Given existing evidence of the effectiveness of the OSCE format [45] coupled with the recent integration an OSCE component into part II of the ABA APPLIED Examination, it is reasonable to utilize this format as a component in the design of a curriculum for summative assessment. OSCEs may be brief simulation scenarios in which a trainee would be required to quickly diagnose and perform key therapeutic actions, brief interactions with standardized patients or care team members, or partial task trainers integrated into a clinical scenario. Compared to high-fidelity simulated clinical scenarios with multiple learning objectives, there is evidence that a series of short OSCE-based scenarios with clearly defined objectives more accurately reflect a trainee's abilities [2]. Moreover, many of the psychometric concerns associated with high-fidelity, mannequin-based assessments can be overcome with this style of testing [46].

Metrics

One of the most critical steps in constructing a high-stakes simulation-based curriculum for summative assessment is the creation of appropriate metrics. One must be certain that the scoring tools that are used accurately reflect the trainee's abilities.

Two scoring methods have been most widely described anesthesia simulation literature – checklists and global assessments. Generally, checklists composed of key actions are considered a more objective measure of performance such as clinical diagnosis and management, while global assessments tend toward greater subjectivity while allowing more utility in assessing complex behavioral traits such as judgment, teamwork, and communication [47]. To create a valid scoring tool, it is important to understand the advantages and limitations of each system. Generally, a valid and comprehensive summative evaluation may use various scoring methods in combination.

Checklist Scoring In this scoring method, a comprehensive list of actions is created comprising the essential steps for successful management of a scenario. For example, in a case of anaphylactic shock, steps in the diagnosis of anaphylaxis (i.e., examine the airway, auscultate the chest, elicit wheezing, etc.) and critical steps in the treatment (i.e., administer IV fluids, administer epinephrine, treat hypotension, administer diphenhydramine, administer steroids, etc.) would constitute the anaphylaxis checklist. While checklists are considered an objective scoring system, they suffer from subjectivity in their construction [48]. Typically, faculty convene and determine which actions are essential to successful trainee performance based in the scenario. To work toward a valid checklist, experts frequently integrate patient care guidelines and practice standards, but considerable debate may remain regarding those actions which are essential or inessential in a scenario. One may utilize a Delphi technique to achieve a consensus among experts to produce an objective and valid scoring tool [49].

Though checklist scoring can provide objective data in summative assessments, it is imperative to recognize the shortcomings of this scoring method. With checklist scoring, it is difficult to account for timing and sequence. In many scenarios, as in clinical practice, it is not only important what actions are performed but also the order and the timing of the actions. In the example of anaphylactic shock, for example, a resident may perform all the items in the checklist correctly, but if the time to give treatment is delayed or if epinephrine is given prior to diagnosis of anaphylaxis, clinical performance would be considered a substandard. To address the issue of timing, one may incorporate a time limit or a "time to action" component into the scoring rubric [50]. Checklist items that use a time limit for various actions are particularly useful in discriminating between more and less experienced trainees. An additional drawback to checklist scoring is a tendency to promote rote behaviors and reward "completeness" as opposed to the prioritization and performance of more critical steps over less critical steps. In clinical situations, a competent physician identifies the most critical steps to be performed in order to effectively manage the critical situation. Using a simple checklist would penalize residents who rapidly assess a patient and effectively manage the condition with the most critical steps but do not perform certain ancillary actions placed on the scoring sheet. On the other hand, a resident could perform the majority of actions on a checklist but fail to perform those most critical to effectively diagnosing and treating the patient. Creating a weighted checklist, in which more value is added to the most important checklist items, helps to address this concern. In addition, shortening of checklists to essential "key actions" ensures the examinees are primarily evaluated on the ability to perform the most critical steps in diagnosis and management. For example, in a case of anaphylactic shock, the checklist may be reduced to three essential steps: (a) diagnosis of anaphylaxis, (b) any treatment regime for suspected anaphylaxis, and (c) any dose of epinephrine given. In addition, a "time to key action" can be beneficial in long scenarios where accounting for time plays an important role.

Global Rating Scoring A global assessment is an evaluation of the entire performance, as a whole. For example, the rater will decide on a Likert scale of 0 to10 the level at which a resident has performed. Typically, there are descriptors assigned to the values (i.e., level 0 = unsatisfactory, level 7 = performance of a competent consultant, level 10 = outstanding). Global assessments are a more subjective scoring tool than the checklist method, appropriate for measuring non-technical skills such as communication and teamwork that are, by their nature, less objective in nature. Given this subjective character, the main concern practitioners have in using global rating scales is the potential for inter-rater variability. This potential shortcoming can be minimized through proper scenario construction and effective rater training. Despite the criticism that global ratings are generally more subjective than analytical checklists, there is literature suggesting that holistic ratings have similar reliability and reproducibility [2]. Global ratings can be an effective and reliable tool for assessing complex and multidimensional skills such as teamwork and communication [51]. In some instances, such as when a competency is assessed across multiple scenario assessments, it may be acceptable to sacrifice a degree of score precision for a greater score validity in assessing non-technical skills such as judgment, communication, planning, situational awareness, and teamwork. Holistic ratings are particularly advantageous over analytical checklists in allowing evaluators to assess the sequence of actions taken by the trainee while accounting for inappropriate actions and unnecessary patient management. This approach can also liberate the rater from a long list of checklist items that can be taxing to complete and provide for uninterrupted observation.

The most challenging aspect of integrating global ratings into a summative evaluation is ensuring that raters are qualified, proficient, and reliable evaluators. Although faculty physicians involved in clinical education typically serve as raters, they are not necessarily qualified. Establishing an effective rater training program is crucial, especially when the appropriateness of behaviors that are scored is open to interpretation. Videotaping the performance of the examinee and later allowing raters to evaluate the session is beneficial as it permits time for a careful review and documentation of debatable performance.

While here is significant disagreement regarding the most effective scoring rubric, various studies have looked at the relationship between scoring modalities with some concluding a similarity in ranking of examinee performances regardless of the holistic or analytical method [52]. The importance of utilizing a scoring modality appropriate to the competencies being assessed is without debate. A combination of checklists, key actions, and global ratings can be used for a comprehensive assessment of resident performance of technical skills, acute care scenarios, communication, and teamwork skills, all of which are important elements of anesthesia practice.

Reliability and Validity

As opposed to formative assessments which aim to assist a trainee in his or her development, summative assessments serve a role in assuring the public that the trainee has met competency standards and is fit to practice independently. It is, therefore, imperative that summative assessments are valid and reproducible. In developing a simulation-based summative assessment, one need be certain of reliability or precision, repeatability, and reproducibility of the results. Reliability imparts confidence that the scores obtained fairly serve as a true reflection of the examinees' abilities. However, examiner variability, candidate performance variability, or errors in measurement associated with the content of the assessment can negatively affect reliability through the introduction of error. Although inter-rater variability can be a significant source of error, there are several tactics that can help to mitigate this effect: selecting the appropriate skills or competencies for assessment, the method of assessment (i.e., live vs. video review), the scoring methods (i.e., checklists vs. global), use of rater training protocols, and utilizing multiple raters for any given examinee [49]. As one increases the quantity of assessment for each examinee, one better ensures that the performance measured reflects the examinees' true clinical abilities. This can be achieved by incorporating multiple scenarios or tasks. In general, for multi-scenario performance-based assessments, issues regarding inadequate score reliability can be best addressed by increasing the number of simulated tasks rather than increasing the number of raters per simulated scenario [51]. Furthermore, with proper rater training and well-specified scoring rubrics, the impact of inter-rater variability on reliability can be minimized.

An assessment is valid if it measures what it sets out to measure. The ideal benchmark for validity of a simulation-based assessment is the ability to correlate performance with patient outcomes. Establishing a causal link between simulation performance and patient outcomes is challenging, and although strong evidence in the literature is lacking, numerous studies have concluded that the skills acquired in simulation can transfer to actual clinical practice. Based on this growing evidence, simulation-based training courses for faculty have been used to reduce malpractice insurance premiums [53, 54, 55]. If we want to make inferences (ability to practice independently) based on assessments of performance, validity is critical. Scientific literature regarding simulation-based performance assessments has argued that these assessments have validity and therefore inferences about clinician competency can be reliably based on the resultant scoring [56, 57]. To ensure the validity of a simulation-based assessment, scenarios should be designed to resemble clinical practice as closely as possible. This involves scripting cases and modeling simulated patients to mimic the clinical setting to which the examinee is accustomed. In addition, the specific tasks to be measured should be carefully chosen to reflect practice-based guidelines or expert opinion. One would expect a valid test to corroborate with other assessment tools such as in clinical evaluations and that examinees who perform better in a simulation-based assessment would outperform lower-performing examinees in the clinical setting as assessed through clinical evaluations. In fact, most studies investigating simulation-based summative assessments show that if the scoring systems are appropriate and the scenarios incorporate the appropriate content, individuals with more clinical training and advanced experience perform better in these simulation-based assessments. If the scores obtained from a simulation assessment do not reflect this clinical reality, the validity of the assessment results should be questioned. An additional factor that could lead to such a disparity includes examinee unfamiliarity with the simulated clinical environment. Most programs will introduce simulation-based summative evaluations only after trainees have had requisite exposure to the simulation environment through prior training or formative assessments.

By ensuring fidelity to the clinical environment and trainee familiarity with the simulated setting, a simulation-based summative assessment incorporating the appropriate targeted competencies and assessment strategies can play a role in aiding anesthesiology residency training programs in making critical decisions regarding trainee advancement.

References

1. RRC/ACGME A. Simulation: new revision to program requirements. Chicago; 2011. p. 1–2.
2. Levine AI, Flynn BC, Bryson EO, Demaria S. Simulation-based Maintenance of Certification in Anesthesiology (MOCA) course optimization: use of multi-modality educational activities. J Clin Anesth. 2012;24(1):68–74. https://doi.org/10.1016/j.jclinane.2011.06.011.
3. Abrahamson S, Denson JS, Wolf RM. Effectiveness of a simulator in training anesthesiology residents. Acad Med. 1969;44(6):515–9.
4. Gaba, David M., DeAnda BS A comprehensive anesthesia simulator environment: re-creating the operating room for research and training. Anesthesiology 1988;69:387–394.
5. Gaba DM, DeAnda A. The response of anesthesia trainees to simulated critical incidents. Anesth Analg. 1989;68:444–51.
6. Gaba DM, Lee T. Measuring the workload of the anesthesiologist. Anesth Analg. 1990;71:354–61.
7. Good M, Gravenstein JS. Anesthesia simulators and training devices. Int Anesthesiol Clin. 1989;27(3):161–6. http://www.ncbi.nlm.nih.gov/pubmed/15128631.
8. Good M, Gravenstein J, Mahla M, et al. Can simulation accelerate the learning of basic anesthesia skills by beginning residents? (abstract). Anesthesiology. 1992;77(3A):A1133.
9. Howard SK, Gaba DM, Fish KJ, Yang G, Sarnquist F. Anesthesia crisis resource management training: teaching anesthesiologists to handle critical incidents. Aviat Space Environ Med. 1992;63(9):763–70.
10. Yee B, Naik VN, Joo HS, et al. Nontechnical skills in anesthesia crisis management with repeated exposure to simulation-based education. Anesthesiology. 2005;103(2):241–8. https://doi.org/10.1097/00000542-200508000-00006.
11. Smith HM, Jacob AK, Segura LG, Dilger JA, Torsher LC. Simulation education in anesthesia training: a case report of successful resuscitation of bupivacaine-induced cardiac arrest linked to recent simulation training. Anesth Analg. 2008;106(5):1581–4. https://doi.org/10.1213/ane.0b013e31816b9478.
12. Bryson EO, Levine A. One approach to the return to residency for anesthesia residents recovering from opioid addiction. J Clin Anesth. 2008;20(5):397–400. https://doi.org/10.1016/j.jclinane.2007.10.011.
13. Knowles M. The modern practice of adult education: From pedagogy to andragogy (2nd ed.). New York, NY: Cambridge Books; 1980.
14. Curry RH, Hershman WY, Saizow RB. Learner-centered strategies in clerkship education. Am J Med. 1996;100(6):589–94. https://doi.org/10.1016/S0002-9343(97)89424-7.
15. Fleming ND. Teaching and learning stlyes: VARK strategies. Hershey, PA: IGI Global; 2001.
16. Fleming ND. The V.A.R.K. questionnaire. Retrieved from URL: http://vark-learn.com/the-vark-questionnaire/.
17. Kharb P, Samanta PP, Jindal M, Singh V. The learning styles and the preferred teaching-learning strategies of first year medical students. J Clin Diagn Res. 2013;7(6):1089–92. https://doi.org/10.7860/JCDR/2013/5809.3090.
18. MOCA 2.0® Part 4: quality improvement. The American Board of Anesthesiology. http://www.theaba.org/MOCA/MOCA-2-0-Part-4. Accessed 9 Feb 2017.
19. Miller GE. The assessment of clinical skills/competence/performance. Acad Med. 1990;65(9):S63–7. https://doi.org/10.1097/00001888-199009000-00045.
20. Kneebone R. Simulation in surgical training: educational issues and practical implications. Med Educ. 2003;37(3):267–77. https://doi.org/10.1046/j.1365-2923.2003.01440.x.
21. Swing SR. The ACGME outcome project: retrospective and prospective. Med Teach. 2007;29(7):648–54. https://doi.org/10.1080/01421590701392903.
22. Swing SR, Beeson MS, Carraccio C, et al. Educational milestone development in the first 7 specialties to enter the next accreditation system. J Grad Med Educ. 2013;5(1):98–106. https://doi.org/10.4300/JGME-05-01-33.
23. Culley DEA. The anesthesiology milestone project. J Grad Med Educ. 2014;6(1 Suppl 1):15–28. https://doi.org/10.4300/JGME-06-01s1-30.
24. Milestones. ACGME. http://www.acgme.org/What-We-Do/Accreditation/Milestones/Overview. Accessed 3 Sept 2017.
25. Passiment M, Sacks H, Huang G. Medical simulation in medical education: results of an AAMC Survey. Assoc Am Med Coll. 2011;(September):1–48. https://www.aamc.org/download/259760/data.
26. Rochlen LR, Housey M, Gannon I, Tait AR, Naughton N, Kheterpal S. A survey of simulation utilization in anesthesiology residency programs in the United States. A A Case Rep. 2016;6(11):335–42. https://doi.org/10.1213/XAA.0000000000000304.
27. Virtual Anesthesia Machine. University of Florida. https://vam.anest.ufl.edu/.
28. Wang R, DeMaria S, Goldberg A, Katz D. A systematic review of serious games in training health care professionals. Simul Healthc. 2016;11(1):41–51. https://doi.org/10.1097/SIH.0000000000000118.
29. Kotal ER, Sivertson RM, Wolfe SP, Lammers RL, Overton DT. A survey of simulation fellowship programs. J Emerg Med. 2015;48(3):351–5. https://doi.org/10.1016/j.jemermed.2014.10.004.
30. Parent RJ, Plerhoples TA, Long EE, et al. Early, intermediate, and late effects of a surgical skills "boot camp" on an objective structured assessment of technical skills: a randomized controlled study. J Am Coll Surg. 2010;210(6):984–9. https://doi.org/10.1016/j.jamcollsurg.2010.03.006.
31. Cohen ER, Barsuk JH, Moazed F, et al. Making July safer. Acad Med. 2013;88(2):233–9. https://doi.org/10.1097/ACM.0b013e31827bfc0a.

32. Malekzadeh S, Malloy KM, Chu EE, Tompkins J, Battista A, Deutsch ES. ORL emergencies boot camp: using simulation to onboard residents. Laryngoscope. 2011;121(10):2114–21. https://doi.org/10.1002/lary.22146.
33. Human emulation, education, and evaluation lab for patient safety and professional study: courses for anesthesia house staff. Icahn School of Medicine at Mount Sinai. https://anesweb02.mountsinai.org/simulator/main.html. Accessed 3 Sept 2017.
34. Wen LY, Gaba DM, Udani AD. Summative assessments using simulation requires safeguards. Anesth Analg. 2017;124(1):369. https://doi.org/10.1213/ANE.0000000000001705.
35. Murray DJ, Boulet JR, Kras JF, McAllister JD, Cox TE. A simulation-based acute skills performance assessment for anesthesia training. Anesth Analg. 2005;101(4):1127–34. https://doi.org/10.1213/01.ane.0000169335.88763.9a.
36. Steadman RH, Huang YM. Simulation for quality assurance in training, credentialing and maintenance of certification. Best Pract Res Clin Anaesthesiol. 2012;26(1):3–15. https://doi.org/10.1016/j.bpa.2012.01.002.
37. Scalese RJ, Obeso VT, Issenberg SB. Simulation technology for skills training and competency assessment in medical education. J Gen Intern Med. 2008;23(1 SUPPL):46–9. https://doi.org/10.1007/s11606-007-0283-4.
38. Ziv A, Rubin O, Sidi A, Berkenstadt H. Credentialing and certifying with Simulation. Anesthesiol Clin. 2007;25(2):261–9. https://doi.org/10.1016/j.anclin.2007.03.002.
39. Boulet JR, Mckinley DW, Whelan GP, Hambleton RK. Quality assurance methods for performance-based assessments. Adv Heal Sci Educ. 2003;8(1):27–47. https://doi.org/10.1023/A:1022639521218.
40. Ebert TJ, Fox CA. Competency-based education in anesthesiology. Anesthesiology. 2014;120(1):24–31. https://doi.org/10.1097/ALN.0000000000000039.
41. Murray DJ, Boulet JR, Kras JF, Woodhouse JA, Cox T, McAllister JD. Acute care skills in anesthesia practice: a simulation-based resident performance assessment. Anesthesiology. 2004;101(5):1084–95. https://doi.org/10.1097/00000542-200411000-00007.
42. Blum RH, Boulet JR, Cooper JB, Muret-Wagstaff SL. Simulation-based assessment to identify critical gaps in safe anesthesia resident performance. Anesthesiology. 2014;120(1):129–41. https://doi.org/10.1097/ALN.0000000000000055.
43. Clayton MJ. Delphi: a technique to harness expert opinion for critical decision-making tasks in education. Educ Psychol. 1997;17(4):373–86. https://doi.org/10.1080/0144341970170401.
44. Wilkinson TJ, Harris P. The transition out of medical school – a qualitative study of descriptions of borderline trainee interns. Med Educ. 2002;36(5):466–71. https://doi.org/10.1046/j.1365-2923.2002.01209.x.
45. Rathmell JP, Lien C, Harman A. Objective structured clinical examination and board certification in anesthesiology. Anesthesiology. 2014;120(1528–1175 (Electronic)):4–6.
46. Norcini J, Boulet J. Status of standardized patient assessment: methodological issues in the use of standardized patients for assessment. Teach Learn Med. 2009;15(4):293–7.
47. Morgan P, Cleave-Hogg DA. Comparison of global ratings and checklist. Acad Med. 2001;76(10):1053–5.
48. Boulet JR, Van Zanten M, De Champlain A, Hawkins RE, Peitzman SJ. Checklist content on a standardized patient assessment: an ex post facto review. Adv Heal Sci Educ. 2008;13(1):59–69. https://doi.org/10.1007/s10459-006-9024-4.
49. Scavone BM, Sproviero MT, McCarthy RJ, et al. Development of an objective scoring system for measurement of resident performance on the human patient simulator. Anesthesiology. 2006;105(2):260–6. https://doi.org/10.1097/00000542-200608000-00008.
50. Hunt EA, Walker AR, Shaffner DH, Miller MR, Pronovost PJ. Simulation of in-hospital pediatric medical emergencies and cardiopulmonary arrests: highlighting the importance of the first 5 minutes. Pediatrics. 2008;121(1):e34–43. https://doi.org/10.1542/peds.2007-0029.
51. Boulet JR, Murray DJ. Requirements for practical implementation. Med Care. 2010;287:1041–52. https://doi.org/10.1097/ALN.0b013e3181cea265.
52. Gordon JA, Tancredi DN, Binder WD, Wilkerson WM, Shaffer DW. Assessment of a clinical performance evaluation tool for use in a simulator-based testing environment: a pilot study. Acad Med. 2003;78(10 Suppl):S45–7.
53. Weller JM, Merry AF, Robinson BJ, Warman GR, Janssen A. The impact of trained assistance on error rates in anaesthesia: a simulation-based randomised controlled trial. Anaesthesia. 2009;64(2):126–30. https://doi.org/10.1111/j.1365-2044.2008.05743.x.
54. Blum RH, Raemer DB, Carroll JS, Sunder N, Feinstein DM, Cooper JB. Crisis resource management training for an anaesthesia faculty: a new approach to continuing education. Med Educ. 2004;38(1):45–55. https://doi.org/10.1046/j.1365-2923.2004.01696.x.
55. Okuda Y, Bryson EO, DeMaria S, Jacobson L, Quinones J, Shen B, Levine A. The utility of Simulation in medical education: what is the evidence? Mt Sinai J Med. 2009;76(2):330–43. https://doi.org/10.1002/MSJ.
56. Downing SM. Validity: on the meaningful interpretation of assessment data. Med Educ. 2003;37(9):830–7. https://doi.org/10.1046/j.1365-2923.2003.01594.x.
57. Kane MT. Current concerns in validity theory. J Educ Meas. 2001;38(4):319–42. https://doi.org/10.1111/j.1745-3984.2001.tb01130.x.

15 Faculty and Allied Health Providers

Michael Kushelev and Kenneth R. Moran

Introduction

Today's patient care needs are more complex with ever-expanding advances in technology, knowledge, and innovations in healthcare delivery. Historically, anesthesiologists have been recognized for leading the way in furthering patient safety initiatives. In line with the field's notable reputation, practitioners have embraced simulation technology as a tool for developing a new generation of anesthesiology professionals. The challenges in providing anesthetic care can be particularly well reproduced in the high-fidelity simulated environment. Skill sets that can be enhanced through targeted simulation exercises include crisis resource management, team training, resource optimization, and medical knowledge. Although trainees have been the most commonly targeted group for simulation education, experienced practitioners such as those seeking reentry following a prolonged clinical absence can also experience significant gains through assessment and potential retraining using simulation modalities. Practitioners can participate in structured multispecialty team training shown to minimize "medical errors" and lead to savings in malpractice premiums. Technical skills such as ultrasound-guided regional anesthesia or echocardiography can be modeled and improved upon utilizing a combination of high- and low-fidelity simulation. Furthermore, there are a variety of routes to further faculty development through simulation. Training simulationists, expert in building scenarios and debriefing, allows for development of clinical educators capable of utilizing these skills in the simulation lab and the clinical environment. Anesthesiologists can utilize simulation technology to institute safety initiatives using experiential learning models inherent in this modality. Practitioners entering an unfamiliar healthcare system are able to undergo expeditious integration including electronic medical record training and familiarization with hospital emergency resources. All of these simulation innovations provide fertile ground for future research and quality improvement projects. This chapter focuses primarily on the utilization of simulation technology for experienced anesthesia care providers, highlighting existing and future directions in the pursuit for optimization of patient care and professional development.

M. Kushelev
Department of Anesthesiology, The Ohio State University Wexner Medical Center, OSU East Hospital, Columbus, OH, USA

K. R. Moran (✉)
Department of Anesthesiology, The Ohio State University Wexner Medical Center, Columbus, OH, USA
e-mail: Kenneth.Moran@osumc.edu

Anesthesiologists as Simulationists

The Role of Anesthesiologists in the History of Simulation

As simulation technology began to develop in its various forms, anesthesiologists quickly recognized its application to their field. The earliest mannequin simulators, including Resusci Anne, involved the participation of anesthesiologists [1]. In 1960, a Norwegian toy company led by Asmund Laerdal paired with Norwegian anesthesiologist, Dr. Bjorn Lind, to create a mannequin that could be used to train individuals in mouth-to-mouth resuscitation. The idea for Resusci Anne's creation was inspired by Dr. Peter Safar's work as an anesthesiologist at Baltimore City Hospital [2]. Safar would later encourage Laerdal to put a spring in the mannequin's chest to allow for chest compressions. With the help of these innovative anesthesiologists, Laerdal created what would become the birth of modern-day simulation mannequins. While at the University of Pittsburgh, Dr. Safar worked with other notable anesthesiologists such as Dr. Rene Gonzales and Dr. John Schaefer in developing a simulator mannequin that would later be acquired by Laerdal. Laerdal would eventually create the modern-day SimMan simulation mannequin that is commonly used today [2].

B. Mahoney et al. (eds.), *Comprehensive Healthcare Simulation: Anesthesiology*, Comprehensive Healthcare Simulation,
https://doi.org/10.1007/978-3-030-26849-7_15

As the technology of simulation mannequins progressed, anesthesiologists continued to breathe life and fidelity into their development. In the 1960s, Dr. Judson Denson, Chairman of Anesthesiology at the University of Southern California, began to integrate computer control into a mannequin with the help of engineer Dr. Stephen Abrahamson [1]. Their work was recognized by the Society for Technology in Anesthesia following a demonstration of their work at their annual conference [2]. Multiple anesthesiology societies of the time promoted and encouraged the integration of simulation technology into the field and began to shape the recognition of this teaching modality as a tool in medical education.

Meanwhile, other anesthesiologists such as Drs. Philip, Sikorski, Smith, and Schwid began to work on various projects integrating computer models capable of predicting or reproducing physiological responses greatly improving the fidelity of models used for anesthesiology training [2].

The first high-fidelity mannequin models that would eventually define the standard for simulation modeling today came from the work of anesthesiologists such as Dr. Gaba (Comprehensive Anesthesia Simulation Environment (CASE)) and Drs. Gravenstein and Good (Gainesville Anesthesia Simulator (GAS)). The GAS system would later be renamed the Medical Education Technologies (METI) Human Patient Simulator (HPS), which together with the Laerdal SimMan are the most commonly found models in modern anesthesiology simulation labs [1, 3].

As the fidelity of simulation technology improved, anesthesiologists began to shift their focus from task trainer skills such as Advanced Cardiac Life Support (ACLS) and procedural techniques to more advanced simulation-based training and assessment incorporating rapidly changing clinical scenarios, rare clinical events, and quality improvement exercises such as crew resource management [1, 4–6]. In the early 1990s, research began to demonstrate the potential for simulation as a tool to enhance education and training for anesthesiology residents, and its use as a method to orient new residents to clinical practice became more common [3, 7].

National and regional anesthesiology societies played a large role in the advancement of simulation technology as a tool for training and assessment. In the 1980s and 1990s, simulation was announced as a topic of interest at conferences hosted by the Anesthesia Patient Safety Foundation, the University of Rochester Simulators in Anesthesiology Education meetings, the Society for Technology in Anesthesia, and the Society for Education in Anesthesiology [3, 7]. These meetings brought together anesthesiologists and simulation experts to discuss and collaborate on methods to better integrate new and developing technology in simulation.

Perhaps one of the greatest influences anesthesiologists have had on the growth of simulation in medical education and training is its wide acceptance as a tool for education despite a lack of definitive evidence for its utility as a means in improving clinical performance or patient safety. An often-quoted anesthesiologist on the topic once declared, "no industry in which human lives depend on skilled performance has waited for unequivocal proof of the benefits of simulation before embracing it" [3, 5, 8]. The use of simulation in anesthesiology residency training became so widespread that the American College of Graduate Medical Education (ACGME) has made simulation education a required part of the curriculum for all anesthesiology residency programs. In addition, the American Board of Anesthesiologists briefly made it a requirement that all physicians seeking Maintenance of Certification must take a simulation-based course. Currently, while not a requirement of all anesthesiologists, simulation can be used as one of the options to meet MOCA requirements. (http://www.theaba.org/PDFs/MOCA/MOCA-2-0-Part-4-Requirements).

A Field Particularly Well Suited for Simulation

Integral to the process of becoming an anesthesiologist, residency training demands regular exposure to high-stakes events that can often result in significant patient morbidity or mortality without a prompt and appropriate response by practitioners. Educators often struggle to provide adequate exposure through clinical training given the unexpected nature and rare occurrence of such events. Allied health providers such as Certified Registered Nurse Anesthetists (CRNAs) and Anesthesiology Assistants (AA) are also required to provide anesthesia care in an environment where inadequate preparation and training can result in harm to patients, particularly during the early phases of their education. Even long-practicing physicians face similar challenges as they learn new techniques, apply new technologies, or require evaluation and assessment of their clinical skills. Given that interventions common to anesthesia care frequently have an immediate effect on the cardiopulmonary and other systems of a patient, the introduction of new techniques and technologies can sometimes put patients at risk for adverse events until practitioner competency is achieved. The simulated environment allows for the introduction of new techniques and equipment prior to practitioner application or use on patients [9]. In addition, anesthesiologists serve as members of multidisciplinary patient care teams and leaders in quality improvement and patient safety requiring them to be proficient in collaboration and team-based efforts to accomplish common goals. Required expertise in performing high-stakes procedures, working cohesively as a team, and responding to rapidly changing physiologic and hemodynamic states all while minimizing risk to patients make anesthesiology an ideal field for simulation education allowing recipients to acquire complex skills in a protected environment shielding patients from harm [1].

Crisis Management

Anesthesiologists and anesthetists are frequently required to manage crisis situations. Intubation, invasive intravenous access and monitoring, administration of drugs that cause hemodynamic change, trauma, blood loss, and surgical intervention all result in rapidly changing clinical conditions that require an experienced hand to effectively and decisively maintain the stability of a patient. Prior to simulation, the "see one, do one, teach one" model of medical education required young physicians to deal with critical clinical scenarios after watching another, more experienced physician in a similar situation. Unfortunately, this model forced trainee physicians to practice previously unmastered skills with varying supervision putting patients at potential risk of harm. In addition, anesthesiology often consists of long stretches of monotonous monitoring followed by unexpected and sometimes startling events requiring decisive intervention. Given that these crises are often difficult to predict and do not come with great frequency, anesthesiologists will spend long hours of vigilant waiting before a test of their crisis management skills occurs. Simulation has been used as a useful tool to practice events in crisis management outside of the clinical environment [1]. Simulation provides the advantage of being able to practice in a safe environment with no risk of harm to patients in a repetitive manner that can be evaluated and standardized [5].

Teamwork and Communication

Anesthesiologists, particularly in a time of crisis, are expected to work effectively as a member of an interdisciplinary team. Communication with nurse anesthetists, anesthesiology assistants, anesthesiologists, nurses, scrub techs, surgeons, consultants, and schedulers are all critical to the success of anesthesia administration. Similarly, anesthetists are required to communicate effectively with the OR team when clinical support and rapid decision-making are required. During these events deficits in communication, a critical skill in order to safely care for patients, may become evident. Often referred to as non-technical or soft skills, communication, teamwork, situational awareness, and task management are all best developed through experience. While recreating stress-inducing clinical scenarios, lessons in communication and teamwork can be integrated into a simulation-based exercise in order that providers can identify and practice the skills required for effective team-based care [10].

Pharmacology and Physiology

Vasoactive drugs, controlled ventilation, surgical trauma, and anesthetics all have an immediate impact on human physiology. Most physiological effects of anesthetics are immediate and can be monitored. These interactions and cause/effect relationships, inherent to the field of anesthesiology, make anesthesiologists content experts in many of the principles of pharmacology and physiology that are essential to medical education. With modern-day simulation mannequins and the integration of computer-based technologies, complex interactions of physiology and pharmacology can be recreated and practiced by anesthesia providers without risking patient harm.

Quality Improvement and Patient Safety

The field of anesthesiology is well-regarded for its leadership in advancing patient safety. As anesthesiologists find safer drugs, techniques, equipment, and algorithms for anesthesia administration and monitoring, the rates of morbidity and mortality associated with anesthesia have fallen precipitously. As early as 1969, research has shown that simulation can be used to decrease the amount of clinical time required for learners to gain proficiency during the early phase of their clinical training [11]. Simulation can be used to practice handoff of care and crew resource management protocols, and to target specific safety practices designed to improve the quality of anesthetic care. It also allows for the testing and introduction of new technology and equipment in a safe manner [5].

Effective simulation allows learners to see one, do one, and even teach one without placing patients at risk, particularly when gaining experience in complex, rare, and crisis situations.

Assessment and Retraining

New Age of Assessing Physicians

Whether due to extremities of age, disability, impairment, or time away from training, a physician's ability to safely practice medicine can be adversely affected by a myriad of life events. Few universal standards exist to determine when a physician is no longer able to practice. Similarly the pathway to retraining from a temporary lapse in clinical skills is not universally defined. Nonetheless, hospitals and clinical practices are commonly faced with the dilemma of determining a physician's ability to safely return to practice.

In the process of diagnosing, treating, and curing patients, modern healthcare providers have the potential to cause great harm. An often-cited report by the Institute of Medicine, "To Err is Human," highlighted potential quality failures in healthcare delivery. The headline of the report was a statistic that estimated that 44,000 to 98,000 yearly preventable deaths are caused by medical errors [12]. Additional research has identified medical error as the third leading cause of death in the United States [13]. Despite scrutiny of these data for potential bias and overreach, it remains clear that medical mistakes are associated with significant mortality and morbidity. Attempting to minimize medical errors is an enormous undertaking that demands scrutiny of the entire healthcare delivery process.

Growing public demand for safe, capable, and cost-neutral medical care has placed a greater focus on identifying efficacious assessment tools for examining healthcare providers. Ideally, physician performance and skills would be assessed in the clinical setting. However, a myriad of financial restraints, safety concerns, standardization issues, and difficulties in capturing rare events has made assessment in the clinical environment challenging, if not impossible [14]. Fortunately, there is abundant educational literature directed at building assessment tools for residents and medical students as they proceed through their medical training. One of the methods that has become particularly valuable and has gained greater popularity utilizes a combination of both high- and low-fidelity simulation in assessing trainees. Simulation assessment may present the best surrogate for assessing a practitioner in the clinical setting.

Assessing Anesthesiologists

Since 1938 the American Board of Anesthesiologists (ABA), a member of ABMS, has served as the certifying body for anesthesiologist. The self-stated mission of the ABA is to "advance the highest standards of the practice of anesthesiology" [15]. The ABA oversees the board certification of candidates and administers the maintenance of certification in anesthesiology (MOCA) program to provide a mechanism for practicing anesthesiologists to exhibit continued competence. The ABA has not only utilized simulation as a major part of MOCA, but starting in 2018, board certification of candidates included a simulation-based assessment of communication skills and professionalism.

In order to build effective simulation assessments, one must consider the multifaceted skill sets that are required of anesthesiologists, set a defined goal for the simulation activity, and clearly define the stakes. Anesthesia care providers must excel in a variety of both technical and non-technical skills in a challenging and complex perioperative environment that requires vigilance and preparedness for the unexpected. Simulation exercises may focus on activities as diverse as intraoperative crises management, team training on the labor and delivery floor, optimizing hospital-wide resource utilization in managing simulated level 1 traumas, or simply an evaluation of the difficult airway algorithm. The varying professional demands placed on anesthesiologists can be individually or collectively assessed using simulation.

Retraining Anesthesiologists

Access continues to be a challenge in underserved populations with primary care and general surgery services lacking [16]. Healthcare provider shortages place an increasing strain on the delivery of high-quality medical care. The physician shortage in all medical specialties by the year 2020 has been estimated to be as high as 90,000 individuals [17]. The RAND corporation estimates the anesthesiologist deficit to be 4400 by the next decade [18].

Robust programs aimed at physician retraining have been proposed as a possible remedy in rectifying physician shortages. Since 2005, the American Medical Association (AMA) through its Initiative to Transform Medical Education (ITME) has advocated on behalf of formalized reentry programs for physicians. The AMA defines physician *reentry* as: "A return to clinical practice in the discipline in which one has been trained or certified following an extended period of clinical inactivity not resulting from discipline or impairment" [19]. The term *reentry*, as defined by the AMA, specifically refers to physicians that have left clinical practice in good standing, as opposed to retraining physicians who have been somehow disciplined for a variety of reasons. The AMA has gone on to define a set of guiding principles for reentry programs. The number of physicians seeking to return to clinical practice is difficult to verify, but one study estimated the number to be close to 10,000 individuals per year [20].

In addition to voluntary clinical inactivity, there exists a variety of causes for gaps in clinical practice. Anesthesiologists, more so than other medical specialties, have been particularly susceptible to substance abuse [21]. Additionally, there can be legal or contractual reasons for involuntary gaps in clinical practice. Family crises, pregnancy, childrearing responsibilities, and temporary disability can also require extended absences from clinical practice. The abundance of physicians seeking reentry after a gap in clinical practice combined with growing physician shortage crises has prompted motivation for formal anesthesiologist reentry programs [22].

For anesthesiologists considering a return to clinical practice, the conventional methodology for assessing anesthesiologists through the ABA, MOCA, and continuing medical education (CME) system is inadequate. A 2-year gap in clinical practice has been suggested as the benchmark requiring a formalized retraining program [23]. A first step to designing a retraining program must be to consider the cause of the gap in clinical practice. A voluntary absence should be addressed differently than a physician that has been restricted due to substance abuse or licensure restriction. Traditionally, most retraining programs have consisted mostly of clinical observership. Such programs have many obstacles including patient safety concerns, legal/licensing/accreditation challenges, and the overall staffing costs of a prolonged observership. Nationally, programs such as the Center for Personalized Education for Physicians (Denver, CO), Physician Assessment and Clinical Education Program (San Diego, CA), and the Drexel Medicine Physician Refresher/Re-entry course (Philadelphia, PA) (Fig. 15.1) [16] have been designed to combine a variety of modalities including preceptorships, web-based modules, reading curriculum, and examinations over a varying length of time in an attempt to certify a reentry process [19]. However, most of these programs are not specifically structured for anesthesiologists. One of the unique challenges in retraining anesthesiologist through conventional methods as compared to some other medical specialties is reproducing the clinical actions and rapid decision-making required of anesthesiologists. Assessing a practitioner's skill in crises management, interprofessional communication skills, professionalism, team leadership, technical abilities, etc. can be challenging over the course of 4-year residency, let alone during a limited educational program.

Simulation assessment as a modality has several advantages compared to observership or classroom-based reentry programs. First, the simulated clinical setting can closely replicate the chaotic perioperative environment with multiple sensory inputs barraging a clinician tasked with managing a critical situation. Second, high-fidelity, mannequin-based simulation technology can reproduce most rare events that would be unlikely to occur during a brief preceptorship. Third, the participant's actions can be observed in order to assess real-time decision-making and not simply knowledge assessed through standardized written or oral examinations. Most significantly, scenarios can be constructed specifically to address the nature of the participant's clinical gap in practice.

The Federation of State Medical Boards has noted that retraining through simulation allows curricula to "replicate cognitive and procedural skills and simulate team interaction" [24]. Additionally, a high-fidelity simulation program fulfills most of the AMA guiding principles in structuring a reentry program [25]. DeMaria et al. reported on a unique simulator-based assessment and retraining program at the Mount Sinai Human Education, Emulation, and Evaluation Lab for Patient Safety and Professional Study Center (MSSM HELPS) in New York, NY, specifically designed for anesthesiologists seeking return to clinical practice [25].

The Mount Sinai Anesthesiology Retraining Program

A group of experienced simulationists has created a unique and comprehensive simulation assessment/retraining program at the Icahn School of Medicine at Mount Sinai (New York, NY) specifically designed for anesthesiologists seeking retraining. This program allows participants to undergo an assessment followed by an option to participate in a more prolonged retraining. Each participant's experience is tailored to best address the indication for their referral into the program [26].

The evaluation begins with a *preassessment* designed to identify the nature surrounding the anesthesiologist's gap in clinical practice. At this time all stakeholders involved, such as licensing bodies or employers, are identified, and a specific goal is set for the retraining course. Additionally, the simulation team attempts to identify the participant's baseline clinic skill set and experience. The anesthesiologist is introduced to the simulation environment and allowed to

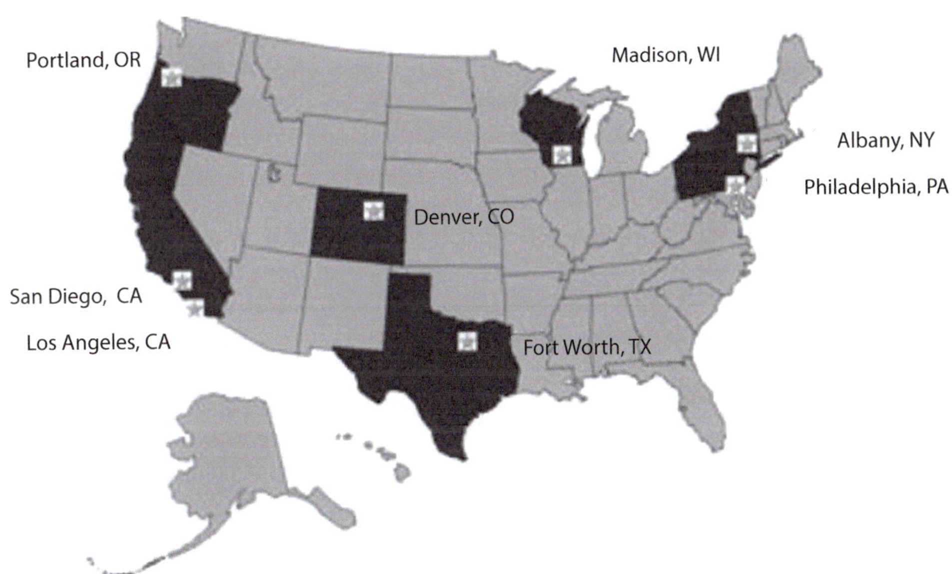

Fig. 15.1 Location of physician reentry programs in the USA. (Reproduced from Kenagy et al. Fig. 1 Page 118 [16])

"walk through" several basic simulated scenarios. Ideally, the *preassessment* succeeds in setting clear expectations for the participant and minimizes "simulation artifact" [26].

Following the *preassessment*, the simulation team begins the *assessment* through a combination of multiple-choice examinations and live simulations. Participants complete the anesthesia knowledge test (AKT) 6 and 24 combined with the American Heart Association (AHA)/Advanced Cardiopulmonary Life Support Protocols (ACLS) examination. The goals of the examinations are to highlight gaps in knowledge that can be further addressed through the tailored course. Two days of summative simulation evaluations are carried out by two board-certified anesthesiologists with the assistance of two anesthesiology confederates with simulation experience. Initial simulation scenarios are well established and standardized to help assess baseline skill level. Following initial simulations, subsequent scenarios are specifically designed to address the identified gaps in clinical practice. Participants are graded on Anesthetists' Nontechnical Skills (ANTS) system, University of Toronto technical rating scale, and global rating Likert scale. Following the completion of the scenarios, a report is generated that details performance for each individual scenario, the assessment tools used by the raters, and a list of clinical deficits. Successful performance during the course corresponds to the clinical skills exhibited by clinical anesthesia year 3 resident (CA-3). Completion of the *assessment* allows the simulation team to provide a statement that the anesthesiologist "practices within the standards of care in the *simulated environment*." Interestingly, no statement judging the participant's clinical competence is made at the conclusion of the course [26].

Following the *assessment*, certain participants move on to participate in voluntary *retraining*. The period of *retraining* varies between 1 and 6 weeks depending on the deficits that have been identified and the goals of the retraining. The goal of the retraining period is to complete 20–40 hours of simulation training covering 10–15 topics per week. The simulation experience is combined with an observership of one of the simulation faculty in the clinical environment. Table 15.1 demonstrates a sample curriculum for *retraining*. After completion of the course, regular follow-up is scheduled with the participant and simulation faculty [26]. One year following course completion, 73% of participants self-reported having been able to return to clinical practice [25].

Considering the presumed abundance of anesthesiologists contemplating a return to practice, it is instructive to consider that only 20 participants completed the course between 2000 and 2011 [25]. Such a small number of participants in the course are notable despite the substantial expertise of the Mount Sinai simulation team, the significant resources devoted to the program, and the unique design specifically targeting anesthesiologists. Additionally, it can be argued that a simple return to clinical practice does not necessarily indicate having achieved adequate clinical competence. The relatively low participation numbers highlight some of the challenges that must be overcome to replicate programs similar to the ISMMS HELPS center program throughout the country. First, the resource utilization of the ISMMS HELPS center is significant. Four trained anesthesiologists participate in the *assessment* over a 2-day period. Additionally, if *retraining* is attempted this program may last anywhere from 1 to 6 weeks with subsequent follow-up. During the *retraining* phase, participants are expected to spend 20–40 hours in the simulation lab combined with clinical observership. Second, an institution must consider the liability associated with offering a simulation *assessment* and *retraining* course. Participants who successfully complete the ISMMS HELPS center program are judged solely on their performance in the simulated environment, and the team of simulationists is careful not to make a determination of clinical competence [27]. Finally, high-stakes summative evaluation requires standardization of assessment metrics, frequent rater train-

Table 15.1 Sample curriculum for retraining

Week	Topic
1. Induction week: lectures focus on issues pertaining to the induction of general anesthesia	Anesthetic induction 1. Non-problematic induction 2. Aspiration event 3. Rapid-sequence induction
2. Emergence week: lectures focus on issues pertaining to emergence from general anesthesia	Anesthetic emergence 1. Non-problematic emergence 2. Delayed emergence 3. Laryngospasm/urgent reintubation
3. Hypoxia week: lectures focus on safeguards and safety features designed to prevent the accidental delivery of a hypoxic mixture	Perioperative hypoxia 1. Hypoxemia during laparoscopy 2. Bronchospasm 3. Mechanical ventilator failure
4. Hypotension week: lectures focus on the differential diagnosis of intraoperative hypotension	Perioperative hypotension 1. Hypovolemia 2. Intraoperative MI 3. Pulmonary embolism
5. Dysrhythmia week: lectures focus on the recognition and treatment of malignant arrhythmias. ACLS course	Dysrhythmias 1. Inadequate anesthesia 2. Supraventricular tachycardias 3. Malignant arrhythmias/ACLS management
6. Difficult airway workshop	Difficult airway 1. Unanticipated difficult ventilation 2. Unanticipated difficult intubation 3. Awake intubation

Reproduced with permission of *Journal of Clinical Anesthesia* (2010) 22, 294–299
ACLS Advanced Cardiac Life Support, *MI* myocardial infarction

ing, demonstration of inter-rater reliability, and correlation of simulation performance with clinical practice. For these reasons, there have been no other institutions, to our knowledge, that have chosen to develop a program similar to that of the ISMMS HELPS center.

Methodology of Simulation-Based Assessment

We would be remiss to examine the topic of simulation-based assessment and potential retraining of anesthesiology professionals, without highlighting some of the inherent difficulties in methodology of such simulation evaluations. The most prominent criticism centers on the relative lack of research supporting the ability of simulation activities to accurately assess anesthesiologist performance [28]. These concerns are heightened when simulation exercises are intended for high-stakes assessment, for licensure, or for public verification of an anesthesiologist's skill level determination. Studies demonstrating a positive association between performance in the simulated environment and clinical sphere have been reported [29]. Clinical improvement following simulation training and assessment of medical students and residents has been demonstrated in improving application of cricoid pressure, weaning from cardiopulmonary bypass, and minimizing central line infections [30–32]. However, other studies such as the one performed by Hatala et al. demonstrate a low correlation of internist's performance in the simulation lab with management of real patients in relation to cardiac physical examination skills [33]. The divergence of some of the available literature on this topic highlights the growing demand to demonstrate the validity and reliability of simulation-based assessment metrics [34]. In fact, a recent review of 417 simulation-based assessment studies concluded that "validity evidence for simulation based assessments is sparse and is concentrated within specific specialties, tools, and sources of validity evidence. The methodological and reporting quality of assessment studies leaves much room for improvement" [35]. Additionally, most studies on this topic recruit nurses, midlevel providers, medical students, residents, and fellows, posing the legitimate question of applicability to experienced practitioners.

There are further anesthesiology-specific challenges in simulation-based assessment. Building simulation scenarios that encompass all aspects of clinical anesthesiology is a nearly impossible task. Assessment of a provider's skill level can be very task specific. For example, an anesthesiologist may demonstrate competence in managing difficult airway scenarios, but perform poorly in managing malignant hyperthermia. Weller et al. have suggested that 12–15 simulated anesthesia emergency scenarios are required to evaluate anesthesiology trainees [36]. Additionally, there are multiple diverse skill sets in communication, professionalism, and technical expertise other than management of emergency situations that are required of a general anesthesiologist.

An editorial by Dr. Gaba examined the difference between studies designed by pharmaceutical companies in pursuit of Food and Drug Administration (FDA) drug approval and simulation studies attempting to demonstrate improvement in healthcare delivery. In this article Dr. Gaba highlights many of the complex obstacles that prevent simulation literature from ever achieving the same level of rigor in study design and methodology as seen in the pharmaceutical industry [37]. In spite of the methodological challenges present in studies of simulation-based training and assessment, there continues to be a need to train and assess physicians and the systems within which they function, and few modalities present the safety, fidelity, and reproducibility of simulation-based tools.

Faculty Training and Malpractice Coverage

Competency of Experienced Physicians

While established systems in judging trainees have been validated, assessments of experienced medical providers have lagged significantly [38]. The need for continuing assessment tools that ensure quality and safety in healthcare delivery is nearly universally agreed upon; however, the methodology and objectives of such evaluation vary greatly [38]. Examples of such assessment systems can be found in the United Kingdom under the National Health Service and in Canada where regulation relies heavily on peer assessments [39]. In the United States, assessment is performed with large retrospective studies attempting to identify error rates or an analysis of closed-claims databases linked to medico-legal actions. A review of closed-claims databases demonstrates technical errors, communication gaps, and system design flaws. In one review, 73% of technical errors occurred in the hands of "experienced" surgeons and 84% occurred while performing "routine" operations [40]. In the surgical closed-claims database, communication errors leading to malpractice claims were most likely to involve the attending surgeon [41]. Within the field of anesthesiology, the closed-claims database demonstrates an abundance of communication and technical errors leading to a significant number of preventable events [42]. It appears that simply having significant clinical experience as a practicing physician does not preclude providers from committing mistakes. In order to address this issue, a variety of educational instruments including surgical safety checklist formation, teamwork training, and simulation-based exercises have been developed [43–45].

Anesthesiologists as Patient Safety Experts

While making up only 5% of the physicians within the United States, anesthesiologists are recognized as a leading medical specialties in addressing patient safety concerns [46]. A variety of reasons have been proposed for this association between anesthesiology and healthcare quality assurance including the characteristics of the physicians that the field attracts, the effect of soaring malpractice costs within the field of anesthesiology in the 1970s and 1980s, and support from organizations such as the Anesthesia Patient Safety Foundation (APSF) [47]. The frequency of "nonroutine" events, occurring in 30% of the anesthetics that are administered, further emphasizes the importance of patient safety matters in the minds of anesthesia care providers [48].

Despite the emphasis on vigilance in anesthesiology and a specialty-wide focus on patient safety concerns, various publications have demonstrated existing gaps in knowledge of both professional guidelines and standards of care within the field. Certain studies have confirmed relatively poor performance of anesthesia providers in the management of a variety of clinical, procedural, and non-technical skills including management of malignant hyperthermia, ability to perform cricothyroidotomy, and perioperative management of patients with Do-Not-Resuscitate orders [49–51]. Fortunately, simulation-based exercises can identify existing deficiencies in clinical skill or practice and subsequently improve physician performance. A recent meta-analysis concluded that "technology-enhanced simulation training in health professions education is consistently associated with large effects for outcomes of knowledge, skills, and behaviors and moderate effects for patient related outcomes" [52].

Malpractice Coverage Within the Harvard Medical Institutions

In 1976, the Harvard Medical Institutions founded the Controlled Risk Insurance Company (CRICO) malpractice insurance company [53]. Currently, CRICO represents the largest medical professional liability carrier in Massachusetts. In 1979, CRICO established the Risk Management Foundation (RMF) of the Harvard Medical Institutions, designed to apply a data-driven methodology to malpractice claim management [53]. CRICO/RMF aims to identify the causative factors that are brought forward from the malpractice cases within the Harvard system and apply these teachings to the everyday practice of the Harvard medical providers [54]. While a full description of the CRICO/RMF program is well beyond the scope of this chapter, the reliance of the program on simulation training deserves particular attention.

Within three different specialties, including anesthesiology, CRICO has developed a plan which reduces malpractice insurance premiums for providers who have participated in and completed a series of simulation-based training scenarios and interdisciplinary team training exercises. Starting in 2000, anesthesiologists in the Harvard system were incentivized to complete a voluntary simulation training program at the Massachusetts-based Center for Medical Simulation. Over a 6-year period, actuarial data demonstrated a 24% reduction in claims for faculty who had completed the simulation training (Fig. 15.2). By 2006, 100 percent of anesthesiologists within the Harvard system had completed the training with a subsequent 25% reduction in anesthesia providers' malpractice premiums. Following the success of the CRICO system to reduce claims and provider malpractice

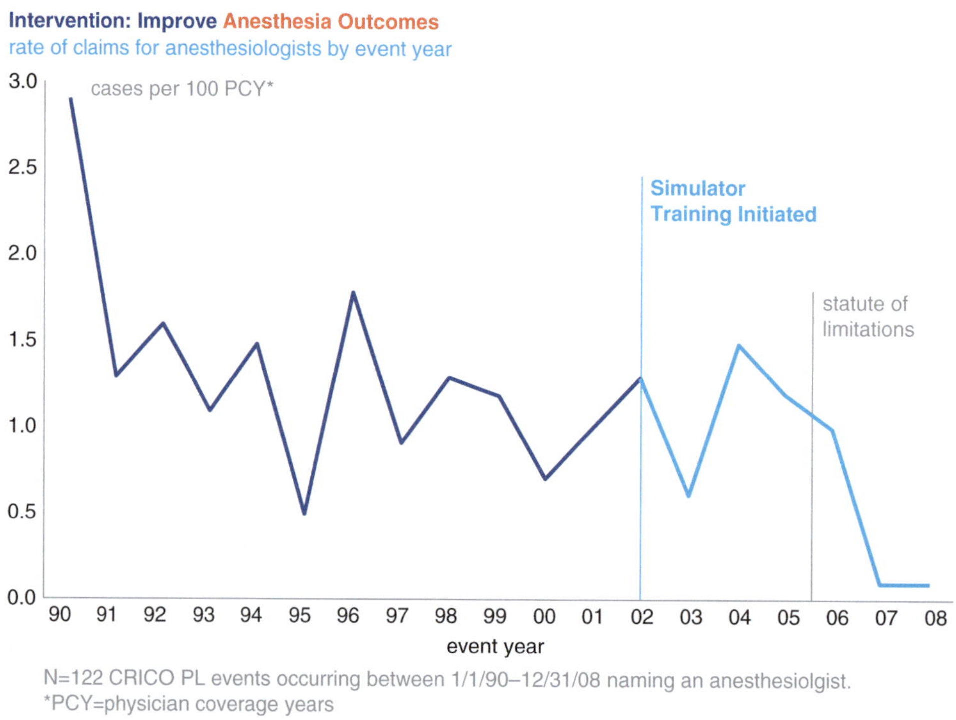

Fig. 15.2 Rate of anesthesia cases before and after initiation of simulation training. (Reproduced with permission from: PSQH: Shannon DW. How a Captive Insurer Uses Data and Incentives to Advance Safety. November 2009)

premiums for anesthesiologists, simulation programs targeting obstetricians and general surgeons have been developed with similar decreases in malpractice premiums [54].

In 2010, CRICO/RMF initiated an ambitious simulation training program focusing on communication and team training. The participation of personnel from various specialties required coordination between leadership of the departments of surgery, anesthesia, and nursing. Each simulation exercise was designed to include an attending surgeon, anesthesiologist, and operating room nurse to work together in resolving perioperative crises management scenarios. Surgeons participating in this program were incentivized with a $4500 malpractice premium discount, while anesthesia providers and nurses were excused from operating room duties. The costs to administer such program were substantial including malpractice premium reductions, a $25,000 grant to each participating anesthesiology department, and a $250,000 grant to each participating institution. The majority of participants (92.6%) felt that completion of the simulation training exercises allowed them to provide safer patient care for their patients. Despite the substantial costs and administrative challenges, CRICO/RMF has plans to expand this training curriculum with a goal of training providers across ten other Harvard institutions [55].

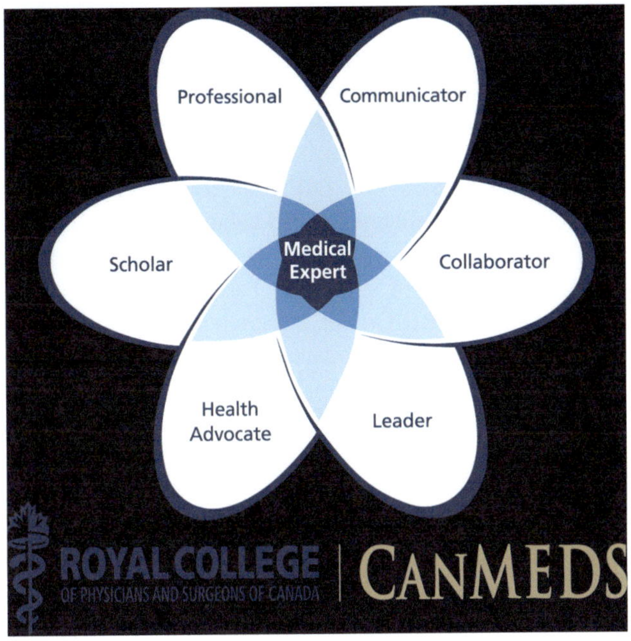

Fig. 15.3 Skills required of physicians in order to provide high-quality care (CanMEDS report) from Royal College of Physicians and Surgeons of Canada. (Copyright © 2015 The Royal College of Physicians and Surgeons of Canada. http://rcpsc.medical.org/canmeds. Reproduced with permission)

Simulation and Faculty Development

Defining Faculty Development

The term "faculty development" can have a variety of meanings depending on the goals of the physician and the employer. In one example, a CanMEDS report produced by the Royal College of Physicians and Surgeons of Canada illustrates the skills required of physicians in order to provide high-quality care (Fig. 15.3). More specifically, an anesthesiologist's responsibilities can vary significantly beyond providing safe and quality patient care and include roles in education, administration, and research [56]. The growing number of roles assigned to anesthesiologists, evolving standards of care, and growth in research and discovery all require providers to continuously broaden their knowledge base and skill set. It has been estimated that medical knowledge will double every 73 days by 2020, as compared to 1950 when the body of information would double every 50 years [57]. Certainly, initial board certification and subsequent MOCA, as administered by the ABA combined with CME activities, are designed to promote continuous faculty development. Despite these activities, scientific literature has demonstrated a decline in practitioners performance as they are further removed from residency and fellowship training [58]. To combat this decline in clinical skills, a variety of educational modalities have been proposed to promote more interactive and engaged learning by physicians. In 2004 an ASA survey showed that 82% of anesthesiologists declared interest in simulation activities to promote faculty development [59].

Continuing Medical Education through Simulation

Simulation can play a significant role in both the development of knowledge, technical competencies, and "soft skills." Training in interprofessional communication, team dynamics, and professionalism allows physicians to provide more effective care in the medical care delivery system. Initiatives such as the World Health Organization surgical safety checklist have been widely accepted to improve patient safety [43]. A well-designed study by Neily et al. demonstrated decreased surgical mortality by healthcare provider participation in the Veterans Health Administration (VHA) Medical Team Training program [60]. The Institute of Medicine (IOM) has designated healthcare provider's ability to function well in interprofessional teams as a core competency [61]. Simulation training has been shown as an effective tool to facilitate interprofessional team training and communication [62].

The experiential nature of the simulated-learning environment is well suited for interprofessional team training for a variety of reasons. Participants often consider the simulated environment to be nonthreatening, encouraging participants to "speak up," while maintaining the fidelity of the operating room environment and allowing for presentation of rare, clinical events in rapid succession. While the majority of literature supporting simulation team training exercises has been drawn from trainees, considerable gains have been shown with experienced cardiac and trauma surgery teams [63, 64] [65]. Additionally, a study by Weller et al. has demonstrated validity of team training within a simulation environment by anesthesiologists [66]. While the benefits of simulation-based team training are significant, the CRICO/RMF experience demonstrates the significant logistical and financial commitments that such programs would require.

In addition to communication and team training gains, professionalism can be assessed and improved upon through time spent in the simulation lab. Professionalism is a core competency recognized by the AMA, ACGME, ABA, and other organizations. One challenge in assessing professionalism lies in the divergent views of individuals regarding "professional behavior" [67]. The main findings by Mazor et al. highlight a need for multiple assessment points by a variety of raters from all walks of life in determining the standards of "professional behavior" [67]. In investigations by Ginsburg et al. utilizing video recordings of professionally challenging simulated patient-physician encounters, the authors hypothesize that the behavior demonstrated in these recordings was more likely to correlate to clinical practice as compared to either text-based or interview examinations [68, 69]. Simulation activities allow modeling and repetition of professionally challenging encounters followed by debriefing sessions that focus on building consensus among observers on the appropriate course of action.

Rapid adoption of technologies such as ultrasound guidance for regional anesthetic procedures and the growing role of intraoperative echocardiography demonstrate the need for continuous skill acquisition for anesthesia providers. Although traditional CME activities offered through conferences, workshops, and web-based tutorials are abundant, their utility in achieving change in clinical practice has been challenged [70, 71]. In comparison, simulation-based CME has been self-reported to achieve greater change in anesthesiologist's practice patterns [72–74]. More consistent and substantial gains with simulation-based CME appear consistent with established adult educational theory which emphasizes the importance of experiential "hands-on" learning [75]. Complex skills such as weaning a patient from cardiopulmonary bypass or establishing intraosseous vascular access have been mastered at a higher level with simulation training as compared to more traditional educational activities [50, 76]. In a high-profile example of utilization of simulation training, the FDA has mandated high-fidelity simulation training as part of their approval process for certain interventional vascular stent procedures [77].

Health System Integration

By 2020, the majority of the healthcare workforce is expected to be from the millennial generation [78]. Millennials expect utilization of experiential learning techniques, peer-to-peer educational modalities, and near-immediate feedback [79]. Additionally, the new generation of medical practitioners has been trained with the ubiquitous presence of electronic health records (EHRs). Three quarters of academic anesthesia departments had adopted anesthesia information management systems (AIMS) by 2014 [80]. Unfortunately, this explosion of EHRs has also corresponded to a large number of software alternatives that have varying capabilities and often require extensive training. The simulation environment can allow training specific to the needs of individual physicians. For example, newly hired anesthesiology faculty can be trained on their health system's AIMS in a simulated OR environment. Simulations can highlight the electronic steps, specific to each institution, required to initiate a massive transfusion protocol, highlight the documentation required to temporarily suspend a patient's DNR status during the perioperative period, or label a patient as "difficult airway" for all subsequent operating room visits. Additionally, simulation modalities can emphasize certain health center-specific initiatives for faculty joining a new medical center. Protocols for "off-site" anesthesia emergencies, airway fire safety, and treatment of malignant hyperthermia are just a few examples of scenarios that may differ significantly among different institutions. Previously, these messages would often be disseminated via email or at a departmental meeting; however, experiential learning modalities in the simulation lab would most likely be more effective in creating a behavioral change which can positively impact patient safety. Additionally, new faculty entering the medical system may not be aware of the recent history of sentinel events leading to internal process changes. Dedicating 1 or 2 days in the simulation lab at the beginning of a new anesthesiologist's employment at a specific center can more effectively accomplish computer training, highlight quality of care programs, and emphasize initiatives for crisis management.

Training Faculty as Simulationists

Historically, as academic medical centers began to form, there existed an assumption that an attending physician's standing within academic medicine would assure adequate skills as an educator [81]. However, progressive development of medical educational literature has highlighted the need for the field of pedagogy (the science of teaching) [82]. The influential 100-year update of the original Flexner report, describing the standards in medical education, further highlighted the existing gaps in physician education and faculty development [83]. One particular topic emphasized in the new Flexner report was the growing pressure of clinical productivity that serves as the main revenue generator in most academic departments [84]. The combination of a growing fund of knowledge and skills that trainees must acquire with shrinking resources to support educational missions of academic anesthesiology departments places growing pressure on the educational system of residency. One proposed solution that has been adopted and supported by the ACGME is a growing reliance on simulation education. Simulation allows time compression of rare clinical events for training in a safe and experiential learning environment.

While the educational benefits of simulation training provided by departmental faculty may appear to be a modality which should be adopted universally, effective simulation training requires extensive development of anesthesia faculty as simulationists. Prebriefing, scenario execution, and the subsequent debriefing session must all be addressed with skill derived from training to ensure the goals of the educational activity are met without alienating the learner [85]. Debriefing, in particular, is a complex skill that invariably requires practice and continuous reevaluation to achieve expertise. Developing expert simulationists requires a combination of formal course work, formative and summative evaluations, self-assessment, and peer reflection [86]. National organizations such as the Society for Simulation in Healthcare and Veterans Administration have offered immersive courses with the express purpose of training physicians as expert simulationists [87, 88]. Additionally, anesthesiologists may pursue a variety of multiday courses, graduate certificate programs, and even degree programs in simulation education. Most importantly, participating in simulationist training ensures that experienced physicians reflect upon and analyze their own style of teaching. Robust development of simulationists allows for more effective educational initiatives in the simulation lab, OR instruction, and more traditional educational activities. Finally, the relative novelty of simulation research provides academic faculty opportunities to engage in research initiatives and pursue career advancement by focusing their energy on simulation-based initiatives.

Conclusion

Commonly associated with trainee education, simulation-based technology offers extensive benefits in post-graduate training and assessment for practicing anesthesiologists and allied health providers. Anesthesiologists' unique combination of challenges and circumstances provides an ideal audience for simulation efforts. Experienced anesthesiologists may be assessed and retrained when attempting to return from a gap in clinical practice. Simulation can be used to rectify gaps in knowledge or communication within healthcare teams preventing disastrous intraoperative events and litigation. Finally, simulation can further faculty development in the ever-changing world of medicine, allowing a laser-like focus in pursuing career development. The field is still in its infancy and, as Dr. Gaba hypothesized, may result in overwhelming success or dismal failure depending on the path the medical community chooses to pursue [89].

References

1. Bradley P. The history of simulation in medical education and possible future directions. MEDU Med Educ. 2006;40(3):254–62.
2. Cooper JB, Taqueti VR. A brief history of the development of mannequin simulators for clinical education and training. Qual Saf Health Care. 2004;13(Suppl 1):i11–8.
3. Rosen KR. The history of medical simulation. J Crit Care. 2008;23(2):157–66.
4. Gaba DM, Howard SK, Fish KJ, SMith BE, Sowb YA. Simulation-based training in crisis resource management (ACRM). Simul Gaming. 2001;32(2):175–93.
5. Wootten RL, Sorensen G, Burwinkle T. The role of simulation in anesthesia. YYAAN Adv Anesth. 2008;26:213–24.
6. Morgan PJ, Cleave-Hogg D. A worldwide survey of the use of simulation in anesthesia. Can J Anaesth. 2002;49(7):659–62.
7. Good ML, Gravenstein GJ, Mahla ME, et al. Can simulation accelerate the learning of basic anesthesia skills by beginning anesthesia residents? Anesthesiology. 1992;77:A1133.
8. Gaba DM. Improving anesthesiologists' performance by simulating reality. Anesthesiology. 1992;76(4):491–4.
9. Singh PM, Kaur M, Trikha A. Virtual reality in anesthesia "simulation". Anesth Essays Res. 2012;6(2)
10. Matveevskii AS, Gravenstein N. Role of simulators, educational programs, and nontechnical skills in anesthesia resident selection, education, and competency assessment. J Crit Care. 2008;23(2):167–72.
11. Abrahamson S, Denson JS, Wolf RM. Effectiveness of a simulator in training anesthesiology residents. J Med Educ. 1969;44(6):515–9.
12. Kohn LT, Corrigan J, Donaldson MS. To err is human: building a safer health system. Washington, D.C.: National Academy Press; 2000.
13. Makary MA, Daniel M. Medical error-the third leading cause of death in the US. BMJ. 2016;353:i2139.
14. Cook DA, West CP. Perspective: reconsidering the focus on "outcomes research" in medical education: a cautionary note. Acad Med. 2013;88(2):162–7.
15. About the ABA. http://www.theaba.org/ABOUT/About-the-ABA.
16. Kenagy GP, Schneidman BS, Barzansky B, Dalton C, Sirio CA, Skochelak SE. Guiding principles for physician reentry programs. J Contin Educ Health Prof. 2011;31(2):117–21.
17. Kirch DG, Henderson MK, Dill MJ. Physician workforce projections in an era of health care reform. Annu Rev Med. 2012;63:435–45.
18. An Analysis of the Labor markets for Anesthesiology. http://www.rand.org/pubs/technical_reports/TR688.html.
19. Physician Re-entry Page. http://www.ama-assn.org/ama/pub/education-careers/finding-position/physician-reentry.page?.
20. Grace ES, Korinek EJ, Weitzel LB, Wentz DK. Physicians reentering clinical practice: characteristics and clinical abilities. J Contin Educ Health Prof. 2010;30(3):180–6.
21. Bryson EO, Silverstein JH. Addiction and substance abuse in anesthesiology. Anesthesiology. 2008;109(5):905–17.
22. Larson CP Jr, Steadman RH. An advanced specialty training program in anesthesiology: a special educational fellowship designed to return community anesthesiologists to clinical practice. Anesth Analg. 2006;103(1):126–30, table of contents

23. Mark S, Gupta J. Reentry into clinical practice: challenges and strategies. JAMA. 2002;288(9):1091–6.
24. Federation of State Medical Boards: Report of the Special Committee on Reentry to Practice. https://www.fsmb.org/siteassets/advocacy/policies/special-committee-reentry-practice.pdf.
25. DeMaria S Jr, Samuelson ST, Schwartz AD, Sim AJ, Levine AI. Simulation-based assessment and retraining for the anesthesiologist seeking reentry to clinical practice: a case series. Anesthesiology. 2013;119(1):206–17.
26. Goldberg A, Samuelson S, Levine A, DeMaria S. High-stakes simulation-based assessment for retraining and returning physicians to practice. Int Anesthesiol Clin. 2015;53(4):70–80.
27. Levine AI, Schwartz AD, Bryson EO, Demaria S Jr. Role of simulation in U.S. physician licensure and certification. Mt Sinai J Med. 2012;79(1):140–53.
28. Farrell SE. Evaluation of student performance: clinical and professional performance. Acad Emerg Med. 2005;12(4):302e306–10.
29. Tamblyn R, Abrahamowicz M, Dauphinee D, Wenghofer E, Jacques A, Klass D, Smee S, Blackmore D, Winslade N, Girard N, et al. Physician scores on a national clinical skills examination as predictors of complaints to medical regulatory authorities. JAMA. 2007;298(9):993–1001.
30. Domuracki KJ, Moule CJ, Owen H, Kostandoff G, Plummer JL. Learning on a simulator does transfer to clinical practice. Resuscitation. 2009;80(3):346–9.
31. Burden AR, Torjman MC, Dy GE, Jaffe JD, Littman JJ, Nawar F, Rajaram SS, Schorr C, Staman GW, Reboli AC. Prevention of central venous catheter-related bloodstream infections: is it time to add simulation training to the prevention bundle? J Clin Anesth. 2012;24(7):555–60.
32. Bruppacher HR, Alam SK, LeBlanc VR, Latter D, Naik VN, Savoldelli GL, Mazer CD, Kurrek MM, Joo HS. Simulation-based training improves physicians' performance in patient care in high-stakes clinical setting of cardiac surgery. Anesthesiology. 2010;112(4):985–92.
33. Hatala R, Issenberg SB, Kassen B, Cole G, Bacchus CM, Scalese RJ. Assessing cardiac physical examination skills using simulation technology and real patients: a comparison study. Med Educ. 2008;42(6):628–36.
34. Boulet JR, Murray D, Kras J, Woodhouse J. Setting performance standards for mannequin-based acute-care scenarios: an examinee-centered approach. Simul Healthc. 2008;3(2):72–81.
35. Cook DA, Brydges R, Zendejas B, Hamstra SJ, Hatala R. Technology-enhanced simulation to assess health professionals: a systematic review of validity evidence, research methods, and reporting quality. Acad Med. 2013;88(6):872–83.
36. Weller JM, Robinson BJ, Jolly B, Watterson LM, Joseph M, Bajenov S, Haughton AJ, Larsen PD. Psychometric characteristics of simulation-based assessment in anaesthesia and accuracy of self-assessed scores. Anaesthesia. 2005;60(3):245–50.
37. Gaba DM. The pharmaceutical analogy for simulation: a policy perspective. Simul Healthc. 2010;5(1):5–7.
38. Klass D. Assessing doctors at work–progress and challenges. N Engl J Med. 2007;356(4):414–5.
39. Norton PG, Faulkner D. A longitudinal study of performance of physicians' office practices: data from the peer assessment program in Ontario, Canada. Jt Comm J Qual Improv. 1999;25(5):252–8.
40. Regenbogen SE, Greenberg CC, Studdert DM, Lipsitz SR, Zinner MJ, Gawande AA. Patterns of technical error among surgical malpractice claims: an analysis of strategies to prevent injury to surgical patients. Ann Surg. 2007;246(5):705–11.
41. Greenberg CC, Regenbogen SE, Studdert DM, Lipsitz SR, Rogers SO, Zinner MJ, Gawande AA. Patterns of communication breakdowns resulting in injury to surgical patients. J Am Coll Surg. 2007;204(4):533–40.
42. Davies JM, Posner KL, Lee LA, Cheney FW, Domino KB. Liability associated with obstetric anesthesia: a closed claims analysis. Anesthesiology. 2009;110(1):131–9.
43. Haynes AB, Weiser TG, Berry WR, Lipsitz SR, Breizat AH, Dellinger EP, Herbosa T, Joseph S, Kibatala PL, Lapitan MC, et al. A surgical safety checklist to reduce morbidity and mortality in a global population. N Engl J Med. 2009;360(5):491–9.
44. Awad SS, Fagan SP, Bellows C, Albo D, Green-Rashad B, De la Garza M, Berger DH. Bridging the communication gap in the operating room with medical team training. Am J Surg. 2005;190(5):770–4.
45. Holzman RS, Cooper JB, Gaba DM, Philip JH, Small SD, Feinstein D. Anesthesia crisis resource management: real-life simulation training in operating room crises. J Clin Anesth. 1995;7(8):675–87.
46. Leape LL. Error in medicine. JAMA. 1994;272(23):1851–7.
47. Gaba DM. Anaesthesiology as a model for patient safety in health care. BMJ. 2000;320(7237):785–8.
48. Oken A, Rasmussen MD, Slagle JM, Jain S, Kuykendall T, Ordonez N, Weinger MB. A facilitated survey instrument captures significantly more anesthesia events than does traditional voluntary event reporting. Anesthesiology. 2007;107(6):909–22.
49. Murray DJ, Boulet JR, Avidan M, Kras JF, Henrichs B, Woodhouse J, Evers AS. Performance of residents and anesthesiologists in a simulation-based skill assessment. Anesthesiology. 2007;107(5):705–13.
50. Siu LW, Boet S, Borges BC, Bruppacher HR, LeBlanc V, Naik VN, Riem N, Chandra DB, Joo HS. High-fidelity simulation demonstrates the influence of anesthesiologists' age and years from residency on emergency cricothyroidotomy skills. Anesth Analg. 2010;111(4):955–60.
51. Burkle CM, Swetz KM, Armstrong MH, Keegan MT. Patient and doctor attitudes and beliefs concerning perioperative do not resuscitate orders: anesthesiologists' growing compliance with patient autonomy and self determination guidelines. BMC Anesthesiol. 2013;13:2.
52. Cook DA, Hatala R, Brydges R, Zendejas B, Szostek JH, Wang AT, Erwin PJ, Hamstra SJ. Technology-enhanced simulation for health professions education: a systematic review and meta-analysis. JAMA. 2011;306(9):978–88.
53. CRICO. https://www.rmf.harvard.edu/About-CRICO.
54. Hanscom R. Medical simulation from an insurer's perspective. Acad Emerg Med. 2008;15(11):984–7.
55. Arriaga AF, Gawande AA, Raemer DB, Jones DB, Smink DS, Weinstock P, Dwyer K, Lipsitz SR, Peyre S, Pawlowski JB, et al. Pilot testing of a model for insurer-driven, large-scale multicenter simulation training for operating room teams. Ann Surg. 2014;259(3):403–10.
56. Souter KJ. What is faculty development? Int Anesthesiol Clin. 2016;54(3):1–17.
57. Densen P. Challenges and opportunities facing medical education. Trans Am Clin Climatol Assoc. 2011;122:48–58.
58. Choudhry NK, Fletcher RH, Soumerai SB. Systematic review: the relationship between clinical experience and quality of health care. Ann Intern Med. 2005;142(4):260–73.
59. ASA Workgroup on Simulation Education White Paper. https://education.asahq.org/drupal/sites/default/files/asasimwhitepaper.pdf.
60. Neily J, Mills PD, Young-Xu Y, Carney BT, West P, Berger DH, Mazzia LM, Paull DE, Bagian JP. Association between implementation of a medical team training program and surgical mortality. JAMA. 2010;304(15):1693–700.
61. Greiner AC, Knebel E. Health professions education: a bridge to quality. Washington D.C.: Institute of Medicine, National Academies Press; 2003.

62. Beaubien JM, Baker DP. The use of simulation for training teamwork skills in health care: how low can you go? Qual Saf Health Care. 2004;13(Suppl 1):i51–6.
63. Paige JT, Garbee DD, Brown KM, Rojas JD. Using simulation in interprofessional education. Surg Clin North Am. 2015;95(4):751–66.
64. Stevens LM, Cooper JB, Raemer DB, Schneider RC, Frankel AS, Berry WR, Agnihotri AK. Educational program in crisis management for cardiac surgery teams including high realism simulation. J Thorac Cardiovasc Surg. 2012;144(1):17–24.
65. Capella J, Smith S, Philp A, Putnam T, Gilbert C, Fry W, Harvey E, Wright A, Henderson K, Baker D, et al. Teamwork training improves the clinical care of trauma patients. J Surg Educ. 2010;67(6):439–43.
66. Weller J, Henderson R, Webster CS, Shulruf B, Torrie J, Davies E, Henderson K, Frampton C, Merry AF. Building the evidence on simulation validity: comparison of anesthesiologists' communication patterns in real and simulated cases. Anesthesiology. 2014;120(1):142–8.
67. Mazor KM, Zanetti ML, Alper EJ, Hatem D, Barrett SV, Meterko V, Gammon W, Pugnaire MP. Assessing professionalism in the context of an objective structured clinical examination: an in-depth study of the rating process. Med Educ. 2007;41(4):331–40.
68. Ginsburg S, Regehr G, Lingard L. The disavowed curriculum: understanding student's reasoning in professionally challenging situations. J Gen Intern Med. 2003;18(12):1015–22.
69. Ginsburg SR, Regehr G, Mylopoulos M. Reasoning when it counts: students' rationales for action on a professionalism exam. Acad Med. 2007;82(10 Suppl):S40–3.
70. Mansouri M, Lockyer J. A meta-analysis of continuing medical education effectiveness. J Contin Educ Health Prof. 2007;27(1):6–15.
71. Davis D, O'Brien MA, Freemantle N, Wolf FM, Mazmanian P, Taylor-Vaisey A. Impact of formal continuing medical education: do conferences, workshops, rounds, and other traditional continuing education activities change physician behavior or health care outcomes? JAMA. 1999;282(9):867–74.
72. McIvor W, Burden A, Weinger MB, Steadman R. Simulation for maintenance of certification in anesthesiology: the first two years. J Contin Educ Health Prof. 2012;32(4):236–42.
73. Wakefield JG. Commitment to change: exploring its role in changing physician behavior through continuing education. J Contin Educ Health Prof. 2004;24(4):197–204.
74. Steadman RH, Burden AR, Huang YM, Gaba DM, Cooper JB. Practice improvements based on participation in simulation for the maintenance of certification in anesthesiology program. Anesthesiology. 2015;122(5):1154–69.
75. Lorello GR, Cook DA, Johnson RL, Brydges R. Simulation-based training in anaesthesiology: a systematic review and meta-analysis. Br J Anaesth. 2014;112(2):231–45.
76. Hallas P, Folkestad L, Brabrand M. How many training modalities are needed to obtain procedural confidence in intraosseous access? A questionnaire study. Eur J Emerg Med. 2011;18(6):360–2.
77. Medical Devices. Acculink Carotid Stent System. http://www.fda.gov/MedicalDevices/ProductsandMedicalProcedures/DeviceApprovalsandClearances/Recently-ApprovedDevices/ucm080874.htm.
78. http://www.bls.gov.
79. Boysen PG 2nd, Daste L, Northern T. Multigenerational challenges and the future of graduate medical education. Ochsner J. 2016;16(1):101–7.
80. Stol IS, Ehrenfeld JM, Epstein RH. Technology diffusion of anesthesia information management systems into academic anesthesia departments in the United States. Anesth Analg. 2014;118(3):644–50.
81. McLean M, Cilliers F, Van Wyk JM. Faculty development: yesterday, today and tomorrow. Med Teach. 2008;30(6):555–84.
82. O'Sullivan PS, Irby DM. Reframing research on faculty development. Acad Med. 2011;86(4):421–8.
83. Ludmerer KM. Abraham Flexner and medical education. Perspect Biol Med. 2011;54(1):8–16.
84. Irby DM, Cooke M, O'Brien BC. Calls for reform of medical education by the Carnegie Foundation for the Advancement of Teaching: 1910 and 2010. Acad Med. 2010;85(2):220–7.
85. Rudolph JW, Simon R, Dufresne RL, Raemer DB. There's no such thing as "nonjudgmental" debriefing: a theory and method for debriefing with good judgment. Simul Healthc. 2006;1(1):49–55.
86. Cheng A, Grant V, Dieckmann P, Arora S, Robinson T, Eppich W. Faculty development for simulation programs: five issues for the future of debriefing training. Simul Healthc. 2015;10(4):217–22.
87. http://www.ssih.org/Certification/CHSE.
88. How to be a Simulation Instructor. http://www.simlearn.va.gov/SIMLEARN/rsrc_9-how_to_be_a_simulation_instructor.asp.
89. Gaba DM. The future vision of simulation in health care. Qual Saf Health Care. 2004;13(Suppl 1):i2–10.

Part IV

Subspecialties of Anesthesiology

Simulation in Pediatrics

16

Kimberly R. Blasius, Agathe Streiff, Devika Singh, Priti G. Dalal, Elizabeth Sinz, Chelsea Willie, and Shivani Patel

Abbreviations

ABA	American Board of Anesthesiology
ACGME	Accreditation Council for Graduate Medical Education
ACRM	Anesthesia crisis resource management
AHA	American Heart Association
CA-1	Clinical anesthesia year 1
CPR	Cardiopulmonary resuscitation
CRM	Crisis resource management
ECG	Electrocardiogram
ED	Emergency department
GERD	Gastroesophageal reflux disease
GRS	Global rating scale
HFS	High-fidelity simulation
ICU	Intensive care unit
IM	Intramuscular
IO	Intraosseous
IOM	Institute of Medicine
IV	Intravenous
LAST	Local anesthetic systemic toxicity
MDT	Multidisciplinary team training
MRI	Magnetic resonance imaging
NBME	National Board of Medical Examiners
NRP	Neonatal resuscitation program
OR	Operating room
OSCE	Objective Structured Clinical Examination
PACU	Post-anesthesia care unit
PALS	Pediatric advanced life support
PICC	Peripherally placed central catheter
POCA	Pediatric perioperative cardiac arrest
TeamSTEPPS	Team strategies and tools to enhance performance and patient safety

Introduction

The pediatric population presents unique challenges in skill acquisition for healthcare providers. The pediatric and neonatal physiologies differ vastly from those of adults. The newborn heart consists of immature myocytes that are less contractile, which may result in a cardiac output that is largely heart rate dependent. In the developing neonatal body, with the higher rate of oxygen consumption coupled with a relatively fixed

K. R. Blasius (✉)
Department of Anesthesiology, University of North Carolina Children's Hospital, Chapel Hill, NC, USA
e-mail: kblasius@aims.unc.edu

A. Streiff
Department of Anesthesiology, Montefiore Medical Center, Bronx, NY, USA
e-mail: astreiff@montefiore.org

D. Singh
Department of Anesthesiology and Critical Care, The Children's Hospital of Philadelphia, Philadelphia, PA, USA
e-mail: Singhd1@email.chop.edu

P. G. Dalal · E. Sinz
Department of Anesthesiology and Perioperative Medicine, Penn State Health Hershey Medical Center, Hershey, PA, USA
e-mail: pdalal@pennstatehealth.psu.edu; esinz@pennstatehealth.psu.edu

C. Willie
Department of Anesthesiology, Medical College of Wisconsin/Children's Hospital of Wisconsin, Milwaukee, WI, USA
e-mail: cwillie@mcw.edu

S. Patel
Department of Pediatric Anesthesiology and Critical Care Medicine, Johns Hopkins University, Baltimore, MD, USA
e-mail: Skadaki1@jhmi.edu

B. Mahoney et al. (eds.), *Comprehensive Healthcare Simulation: Anesthesiology*, Comprehensive Healthcare Simulation,
https://doi.org/10.1007/978-3-030-26849-7_16

stroke volume, maintenance of cardiac output through heart rate becomes critical. Additionally, with the maturation of a parasympathetic nervous system preceding that of the sympathetic, neonates and infants are particularly prone to heightened vagal tone manifesting as bradycardia and hypoxia. The care of this patient population requires a high degree of specialization by the medical, nursing, and allied health practitioners. These teams must function in a well-orchestrated manner during neonatal and pediatric emergencies in which time may be of utmost importance. This multidisciplinary perioperative pediatric team may collaborate in a wide breadth of settings and procedures including pediatric inpatient floors, pediatric units within adult hospitals, outpatient surgical and procedural centers, and emergently in the field. In this chapter, we describe the role of simulation in the instruction, development, and assessment of critical pediatric anesthesia skills across these domains.

Part Task Trainers and Skill Acquisition

There are many characteristics unique to the pediatric population that produce a significant challenge for the healthcare provider in mastering procedures common in clinical care (Table 16.1). Pediatric part task trainers may play a role unique from that of adult patient procedural training in providing procedural exposure and competency development.

For the anesthesia care provider, pediatric and neonatal airway management provides anatomic challenges due to characteristics such as greater subglottic narrowing and superior glottic position relative to the adult airway, physiologic differences such as increased susceptibility to laryngospasm, and a higher rate of pathophysiologic differences including congenital malformations which may alter normal anatomy and respiratory physiology. Following endotracheal intubation or placement of a supraglottic device, pediatric ventilation management also differs from that of adults, and training and familiarity with pediatric ventilation management strategies are crucial.

Pediatric healthcare providers must become facile in potentially challenging vascular access. Required access includes peripheral intravenous, intraosseous, central venous, and peripheral intra-arterial line placement. Due to the smaller anatomy of children and neonates, possible congenital vascular malformations, shorter neck length, and differences in subcutaneous tissue distribution from that of adults, the approach to central and peripheral vascular access in this population may be extremely challenging.

Pediatric and neonatal resuscitation require specific certification due to the major differences in physiology- and algorithm-based management compared to adults. The quality of resuscitation in the first minute of life in neonates has a clear impact on long-term outcomes. Therefore, the neonatal resuscitation program aims to educate healthcare providers for the preparation and successful execution of neona-

Table 16.1 Differences in pediatric procedures and anatomy compared to that of adults

Type of skill	Considerations in pediatric population
Airway	Anatomic: superior location of the larynx, omega-shaped glottis, vocal cords angled over laryngeal inlet, narrowest portion is the subglottic region at the cricoid cartilage Miller blade may be preferable More specific endotracheal tube sizing and type (cuffed versus uncuffed) Higher occurrence of upper respiratory infections and laryngospasm
	Faster desaturation rate from increased oxygen consumption Decreased radius of airway under normal conditions results in higher airway resistance in an edematous airway
Ventilation management	Pressure-controlled ventilation with judicious monitoring of tidal volumes achieved Smaller circuit size
Intravenous access	Smaller veins and arteries Fat pads on the dorsum of the hands creating difficulty with visualization Congenital conditions associated with difficult intravenous access (i.e., Down syndrome)
Intraosseous access	More frequently required compared to adult patients Ideal sites for placement: tibial plateau, distal tibia, and femur
Central line placement	Considerations for length of central venous line catheter and gauge needed Internal jugular access is difficult in infants due to short and thick neck
Lumbar puncture and neuraxial anesthesia	Shallow epidural location More inferior termination of spinal cord Delayed myelination of nerve fibers Cartilaginous bones and vertebrae resulting in higher risk of penetration and direct trauma Different curvatures of the spine and hence orientation of neuraxial needles High risk of inadvertent spinal injection Caudal technique unique to pediatrics
Resuscitation	Dosing of emergency medications by weight Voltage setting for automated external defibrillators by weight
Regional anesthesia techniques and local anesthetic administration	Increased systemic absorption of local anesthetic from: Increased regional blood flow Increased cardiac output and heart rate Lower plasma protein concentrations to decrease unbound free fraction of local anesthetics Enzymatic immaturity Need for general anesthesia for placement of nerve block injections

tal resuscitation by recommending that trainees undergo a simulated resuscitation every 2 years [1]. In such a critical domain where constant proficiency is required, retention of both knowledge and practical skills is key.

Specific to the pediatric anesthesiologist, neuraxial techniques such as caudal nerve blocks and regional techniques differ in the patient's anatomy and dose of local anesthetic and are more frequently performed under general anesthesia. Reducing medication errors is especially crucial in the pediatric population, and these procedural skills may benefit from rehearsal with simulation technology prior to application in the clinical setting.

Part task trainers offer unique advantages in acquisition of the skills mentioned above. They provide specific elements of the procedure or skill being learned. While they cannot fully replicate performing the task on living patients, they do allow learners to acquire these basic skills in isolation from the experience of performing it on a live human being. In fact, part task trainers consist of models that are used primarily for diagnostic skill practice, such as a thoracic model for CPR.

Part task trainers have a key role in simulation-based medical education as an effective method of procedural skill acquisition [2]. While sometimes referred to as low-fidelity simulators, there are inherent challenges in categorizing part task trainers as high or low fidelity. Depending on the key physical features, training task, objectives, learners' education, and emulated scenario, the same part task trainer may be classified in either category [3]. For instance, a pediatric airway mannequin may be considered high fidelity in practicing intubation technique for rising anesthesiology residents but would be considered low fidelity for a cardiopulmonary (CPR) scenario requiring airway and intravenous procedural skills for a multidisciplinary simulation group. Hence, for the scope of this chapter, part task trainers will be defined independently of their fidelity status, which is largely context dependent.

Part task trainers are useful as an alternative to learning in the real-life clinical setting and provide several advantages over direct learning, such as during a clinical encounter. First, they provide an allowance for failure, a key advantage in teaching inexperienced providers pediatric procedures, given that the probability of a successful procedure is negatively correlated with the number of prior attempts. Failure despite multiple attempts creates stress for learners, especially when this procedure is essential for the patient to receive care. Part task trainers allow isolation of the task from the overall situation in part by removing this emotional component. Computer-based training systems for the instruction of neonatal resuscitation have yielded a higher level of satisfaction by medical student learners, who noted that the system allowed for practice without the emotional component of the task affecting their learning [1]. An additional advantage of part task trainers lies in cost, and this compares to higher-fidelity mannequin-based simulation technology, which may cost several thousand dollars and may not be as readily available at a given institution [2]. Part task trainers for the uses preciously mentioned currently range from $300 to $3000, and examples of these are listed in Table 16.2.

Indeed, compared to the full-body mannequin with tactile and verbal responses, part task trainers are easier to maintain and require less expertise to be used in simulation centers. While part task trainers with virtual reality and computer-lead training exist, the vast majority does not require computer software and may be utilized in a wide variety of environments outside of the simulation lab.

Feedback of procedural success is a challenge of part task trainer design. Examples of strategies to meet this challenge include the use of colored reservoirs of fluid that confirm successful venipuncture, chests that rise, bronchi that inflate upon successful endotracheal intubation, and verbal and visual feedback of correct performance with virtual reality software.

Part task trainers have shown some evidence for efficacy in the teaching and maintenance of rarely performed skills. A meta-analysis of pediatric simulation education across a variety of procedural skills and training level demonstrated a higher degree in efficacy in procedural skill acquisition compared to learning over the course of a standard clinical curriculum. While the magnitude of this impact varied between high-fidelity settings compared to, for instance, virtual reality settings, a positive impact was seen across all subgroups [4].

Assessment of the pediatric patient is greatly aided by observation of physical examination findings, such as capillary refill, sunken fontanels, tachycardia, poor turgor of the skin, irritability, and nasal flaring. While providing these findings seems critical in the suspension of disbelief (a common barrier to simulation learning), systematic studies have demonstrated that this is not the case and that, in fact, the quality of learning is often independent of simulator fidelity [3]. Simulator fidelity is defined as the degree to which a simulator feels, appears, and behaves as a human patient [3]. Hamstra et al. explain that the functional correspondence between the simulated scenario and the clinical setting has a greater impact than the physical attributes of the simulator itself. Despite these findings, fidelity is a challenge inherent to part task trainer, as is realism, which is a separate entity. Realism consists of various factors: physical, conceptual, and emotional [4]. This concept encompasses many aspects of the clinical situation being simulated, such as navigating conversations with the patient's guardians, logistics of preparation for the task, and other components of the experience of performing the procedure that are separate from the procedure itself.

Table 16.2 Commercially available part task trainers by clinical setting

Category	Company	Product	Description	Studies
Airway	Laerdal Medical (Stavanger, Norway)	Neonatal Intubation Trainer	–	[6]
		Infant Airway Management Trainer	–	–
	Life/form® (Fort Atkinson, WI)	Child Airway Management Trainer with Stand	–	–
	Syndaver Labs (Tampa, Florida)	Newborn Airway trainer	–	[6]
		Pediatric Airway Trainer	–	–
	Simulaids (Woodstock, NY)	3-Year-Old Airway Management Trainer with Board	–	–
	TruCorp (Belfast, Ireland)	AirSim® Baby, Pierre-Robin, Child (6 years)	–	[6]
Cardiopulmonary resuscitation (CPR)	Life/form®	CPR prompt BLUE child mannequins	Consists of a set of five mannequins and nylon bag	–
		Advanced child CPR/airway management torso with defibrillation features	–	–
Intraosseous access	Life/form®	Intraosseous simulator	–	–
	Laerdal Medical	Infant IO leg	–	[7]
Vascular access	Laerdal Medical	Pediatric IV simulator	Available in pediatric head (temporal, jugular veins), infant IM/IV arm, infant IV leg	–
		Pediatric multi-venous IV training arm kit	–	–
		Infant virtual IV	Computer software and intravenous part task trainer for self-directed learning. Provides clinical scenario, 3D visual images, records performance, and provides feedback	–
	Meadows medicalsupply™ (Quogue, NY)	Pediatric IV hand simulation	One year old, 3 year old, drip infusion	–
	Simulab (Seattle, WA)	Vascular access child task trainer	–	[5]
	VATA Inc. (Canby, OR)	Nita Newborn Model 1800	Venous flashback with intravenous access success including umbilical vein access. Replaceable vein skins. Additionally, nasal suctioning, gavage features included	–
Neuraxial technique	Simulab	Lumbar puncture baby	–	–
	Laerdal medical	Baby stap	–	–
	Life/form®	Pediatric lumbar puncture simulator	–	–
Ultrasound	SonoSim (Santa Monica, CA)	SonoSim® ultrasound training solution laptop-based ultrasound trainer	Integrated didactic instruction, hands-on ultrasound scanning, and performance assessment	–

Part task trainers in the pediatric setting suffer from a paucity of strong evidence. Due to difficulties in comparison of part task trainers and other mannequin-based simulation tools with real-life critical events, most investigations have compared efficacy of this model to no intervention, rendering the true impact of these methods in comparison to the current gold standard, clinical bedside teaching difficult [4]. Future work is needed on the most effective pedagogical and assessment tools in order to clarify the utility of part task trainer use in education. Additionally, methods of assessment of various part task trainers cannot be generalized between studies, and hence it presents difficulty in quantifying the educational value of this tool.

Categories of Part Task Trainers

Airway Part Task Trainers

Airway part task trainers allow learners to gain hands-on practice in airway management techniques, such as bag mask ventilation, oral airway placement, supraglottic airway placement, and oral and nasal endotracheal intubation. They may contain a lung model to confirm correct tube placement by chest inflation, a lifelike feel when performing Sellick's maneuver, as well as negative feedback features, such as stomach inflation (i.e., Laerdal Medical Neonatal Intubation Trainer). These trainers often consist of a model from the oropharynx to the chest mounted on a board with an oropharynx and larynx. Airway part task trainers require some consumable products such as lubricant to allow for passage of airway devices in addition to some maintenance of the model. These models differ in their design, pediatric age represented (neonatal versus infant versus child models), and fidelity of the mannequin skin (Fig. 16.1). These part task trainers also provide a wide range in fidelity in their imitation of the pediatric larynx with some models creating products that very closely resemble human appearance and feeling (Fig. 16.2). For example, TruCorp has produced a pathophysiologic model of a child with Pierre Robin syndrome, a condition that poses unique airway management challenges (Fig. 16.3).

Cardiopulmonary Resuscitation Part Task Trainers

A variety of cardiopulmonary resuscitation part task trainers exist. They frequently include the entire torso and are designed for mastery of chest compressions and oral administration of breaths. These trainers are composed of soft plastic and padded with foam to resemble the same pressure and texture encountered in performing pediatric chest compressions. Disposable components such as single-use inflation bags make the mannequins easy to maintain between uses in the CPR Sim BLUE mannequins. The Life/form® Advanced Child CPR/Airway management torso includes the ability to place advanced airways, such as endotracheal tubes, and provides negative and positive feedback for intubation, defibrillation practice, and electrocardiography (ECG) sites. It also includes the option to add arms and legs to convert to a higher-fidelity mannequin for intravenous (IV) or intraosseous (IO) access in order to run full-code scenarios (Fig. 16.4).

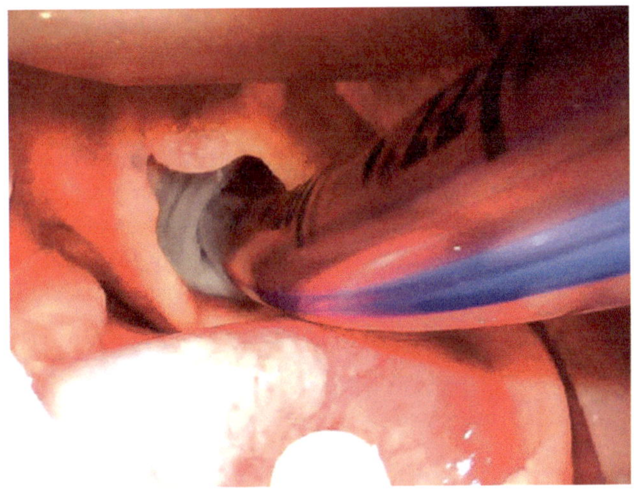

Fig. 16.2 SynDaver Labs Pediatric Airway Trainer with associated view during intubation. (Photo courtesy of SynDaver Labs)

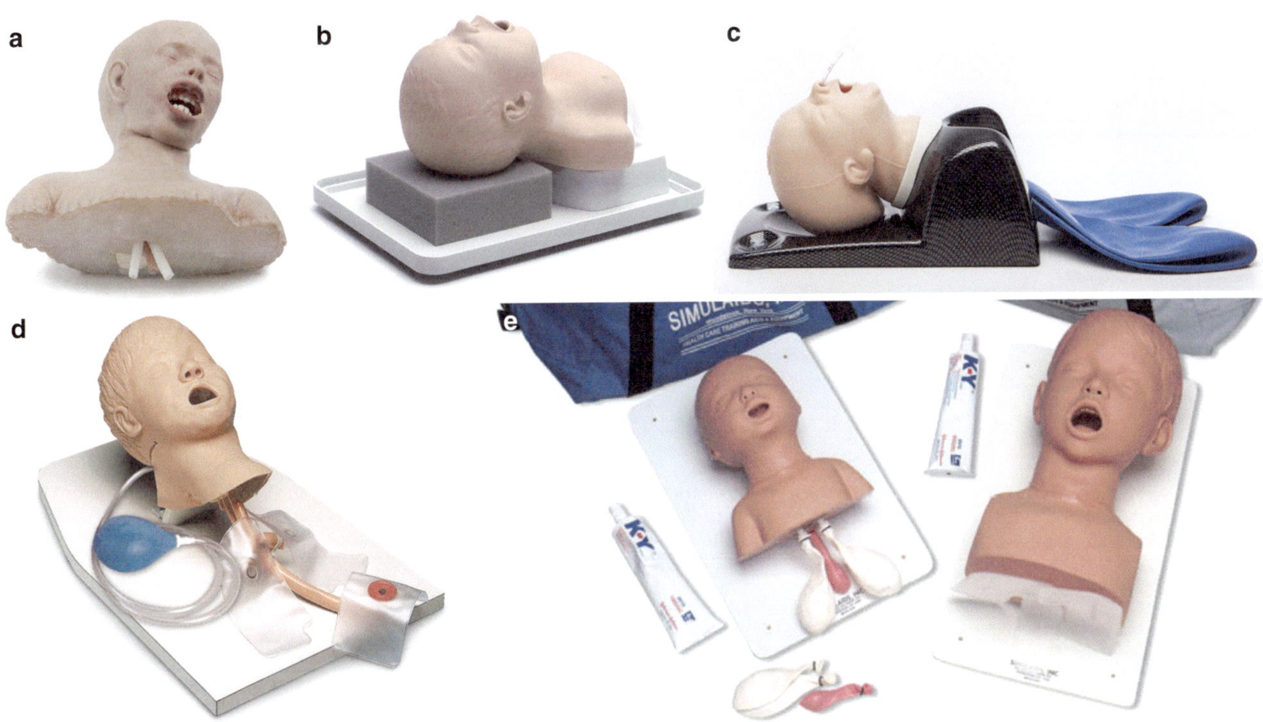

Fig. 16.1 Part task airway trainers. (**a**) SynDaver Labs Newborn Airway Trainer. (Photo courtesy of SynDaver Labs). (**b**) Laerdal Medical Neonatal Airway Intubation Trainer. (Photo courtesy of Laerdal http://www.laerdal.com/us/item/250-00101 accessed September 10, 2016). (**c**) TruCorp AirSim. (Photo courtesy of TruCorp). (**d**) Life/form® Child Airway Management Trainer with Stand. (Photo courtesy of Life/form®). (**e**) Simulaids 3 year-old and Infant Airway Management Trainer With Board. (Photo courtesy of Simulaids)

Vascular Access Part Task Trainers

Vascular access part task trainers include features such as fluid-filled compartments to provide positive feedback to the learner when venous cannulation is successful. Arterial and venous vasculatures are demonstrated using red- and blue-colored fluid, respectively. This feature provides visual feedback for correct or inadvertent puncture of vessels. These models differ in their goal of simulating central or peripheral access and, like airway part task trainers, differ in the degree of fidelity in their simulation of the look and feel of real skin. Some part task trainers are ultrasound compatible, and the venous vessels demonstrate compressibility, while the arterial vessels appear pulsatile, in simulation of in vivo vasculature, such as the Simulab Vascular Access Child task trainer. One single trial demonstrated that in 26 pediatric residents, 60 to 90 minutes of ultrasound-guided central venous catheter simulation training on this simulator resulted in improved central venous catheter placement assessed using a checklist completion score [5].

Neuraxial Part Task Trainers

Neuraxial part task trainers may be used to teach novice anesthesiology residents neuraxial techniques in the pediatric population as well as to teach pediatric residents lumbar puncture (Figs. 16.5 and 16.6). They often feature a mannequin in the lateral decubitus position, palpable landmarks imitating the lumbosacral region, fluid reservoirs to imitate cerebrospinal fluid collection, ability to measure cerebrospinal fluid pressure, and a replaceable lumbar pad. The Simulab mannequin also includes a flexible body form that imitates the interspinous processes opening when positioned correctly and ultrasound compatibility to provide feedback on needle placement.

Virtual Reality Simulators

Virtual reality simulators consist of a subgroup of part task trainers that facilitate the acquisition of psychomotor

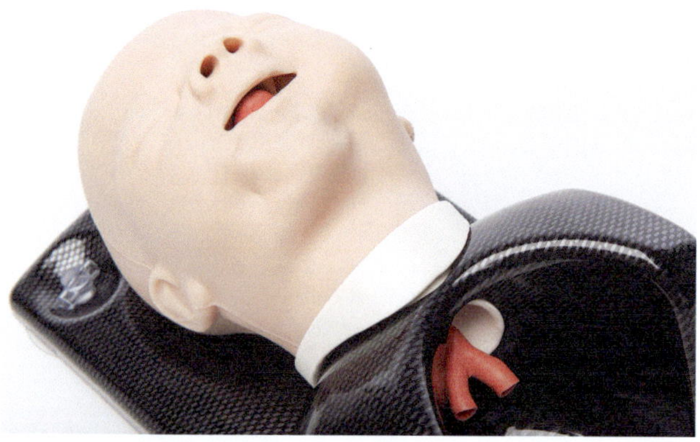

Fig. 16.3 TruCorp AirSim Pierre Robin. (Photo courtesy of TruCorp)

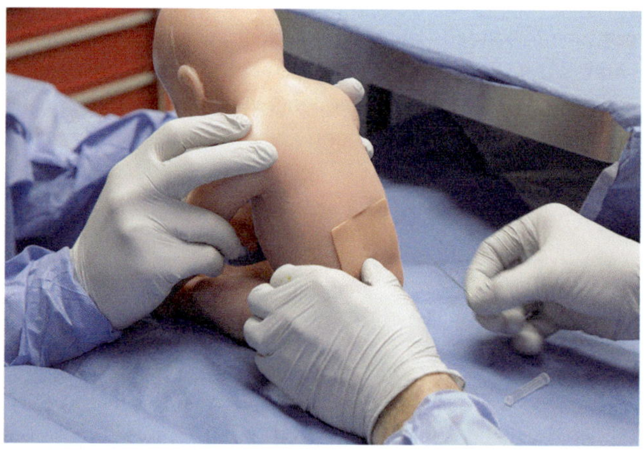

Fig. 16.5 Simulab Lumbar Puncture Baby System. (Photo courtesy of Simulab)

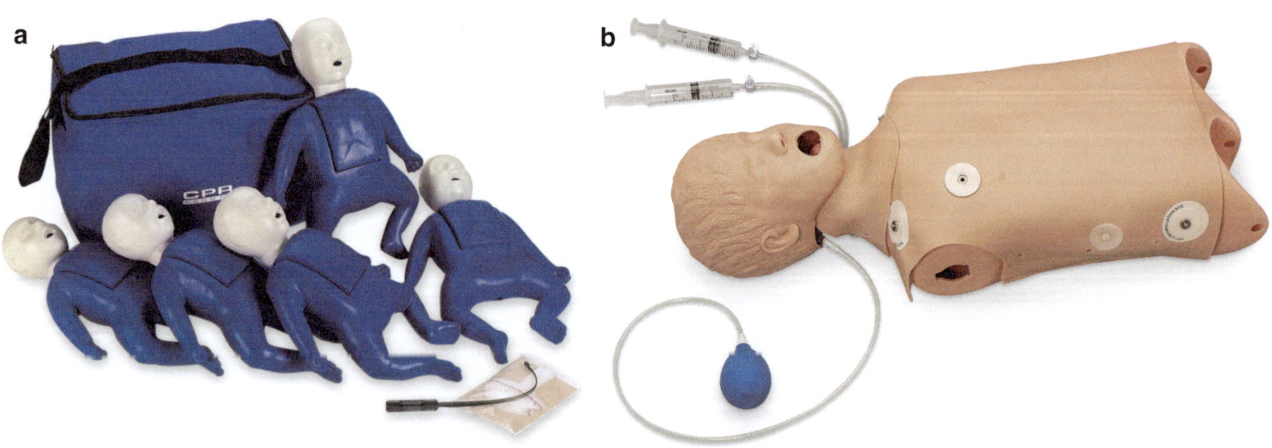

Fig. 16.4 Two different part task trainers for cardiopulmonary resuscitation. (**a**) Life/form® CPR Prompt BLUE Child Manikins, (**b**) Life/form® Advanced Child CPR/Airway Management Torso with Defibrillation Features

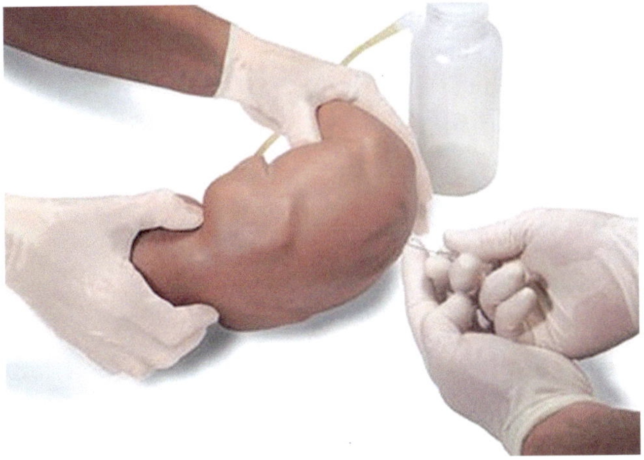

Fig. 16.6 Laerdal Medical Baby Stap lumbar puncture part task trainer. (Photo courtesy of Laerdal http://www.laerdal.com/us/doc/141/Baby-Stap accessed Sep 16, 2016)

skills utilizing, in part, a physical landscape created by a computer program. For instance, the AccuTouch Flexible Bronchoscopy Simulator has been shown to be effective in teaching novice pediatric residents fiber-optic bronchoscope skills, shortening the time to successful intubation and reducing the number of complications [8]. This tool senses the user's touch, but, instead of the controls moving the head of the bronchoscope, the program displays the anatomic image that would be seen from such movements. The software allows feedback, such as the quality of image the learner obtains by maneuvering, a cough elicited from the "patient" for insufficient local anesthetic topicalization, and a count of the bronchial segments viewed by the learner. This simulator training along with a software-driven tutorial demonstrated increased competency in video bronchoscopy technique in emergency medicine residents not only for regular pediatric airway models but also with simulated airway obstruction and Pierre Robin syndrome models [9].

Unlike virtual simulators that include a psychomotor skill component, some virtual simulators consist of an entirely digital world and scenarios that aim to teach skills, protocols, and clinical knowledge. One study examined the effectiveness of a virtual reality environment in Second Life (Linden Lab, San Francisco, CA) to teach pediatric residents pediatric sedation through pre- and post-training test performance [10]. Studies on these programs are limited and have shown mixed results compared to traditional didactic teaching methods [10].

Future of Part Task Simulators in Pediatrics

The pediatric simulation field has been developed out of adult simulation technology, and, as advancements in technology are made, the field may anticipate the ongoing development of part task trainers targeted at a greater variety of age ranges and pathologies specific to pediatrics, including dermatological and vascular conditions. Future developments in technology will also be able to render greater functional fidelity to existing models in a lower-cost format. We anticipate a proliferation of part task trainers with challenging pathology specific to the pediatric population, such as Pierre Robin syndrome (Fig. 16.3). Some institutions have created homemade models of such airways using mold adapted to regular pediatric part task trainers [11].

Cheng et al. demonstrate in their meta-analysis of a variety of simulation settings including procedural training that the degree of realism does not significantly impact learning outcomes [4]. This finding suggests that, even in the absence of available high-fidelity scenarios, part task trainers have an important role in simulation education. Indeed, part task trainers provide a lower-cost, simulation-based curriculum, which has significant implications in resource-limited settings, rural centers, and reality of the contemporary cost of medical education.

High-Fidelity Simulation for Exposure

High-fidelity simulation-based training plays an important role in the education of pediatric anesthesiologists. Currently available simulation technology has allowed educators to develop simulation activities that enable pediatric anesthesiologists to acquire higher proficiency for multiple learning outcomes. Maximizing environmental fidelity and realism may immerse the anesthesiologist into the management of a critically ill child, requiring accurate assessment and timely intervention, but also team leadership and communication skills for successful management. Varying debriefing strategies are implemented in high-fidelity simulation, the importance of which is resonated by learner satisfaction and outcome.

Current goals within the anesthesia community for simulation-based education are to maximize patient care and safety while balancing learner satisfaction and confidence building through the provision of effective experiential learning. Anesthesiologists are often tasked with caring for medically complex pediatric patients during acute clinical events. In these situations, critical thinking, effective decision-making, and proficient psychomotor skills are essential. Although pediatric anesthesiology has become increasingly safe overtime and the frequency of crisis events has decreased, these stakes remain high. In addition to a potential reduction in exposure to rare and critical events during clinical training due to the increasing safety of anesthesia care, a further deficiency in trainees' knowledge, decline in exposure, and skill acquisition may increase with reduced duty and on-call hours [12]. High-fidelity simulation meets a growing need to create situations where the trainee may practice management of critical events in a realistic setting to help remedy these deficiencies. Various modalities ranging from task trainers to living, standardized patients and from screen-based simulation to highly sophisticated mannequin-based technology [13] are available to enable the creation of realistic or "high-fidelity" simulation scenarios (Table 16.3, Figs. 16.7, 16.8, 16.9, 16.10, 16.11, and 16.12). An example of the use of high-fidelity simulation (HFS) in pediatric anesthesiology would be an opportunity to practice a pediatric inhalational induction on sophisticated mannequin in a controlled fashion with the ability to pause, fast-forward, or rewind while at the same time providing an opportunity to hone in on pediatric critical event management skills. Education using HFS provides a way to decrease errors and improve clinical judgment and is also useful for teaching and evaluating specific clinical skills that are essential to improving the care of pediatric patients [14, 15].

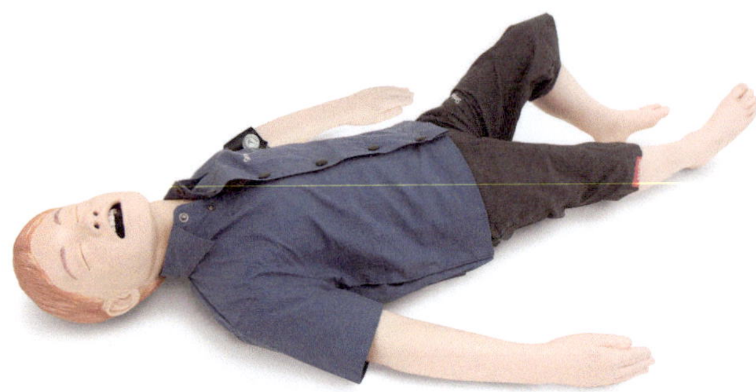

Fig. 16.8 Laerdal Medical SimJunior®. (Photo courtesy of Laerdal http://www.laerdal.com/us/SimJunior accessed September 12, 2016)

Table 16.3 Examples of high-fidelity mannequins

Company	Name	Description
Laerdal medical	SimJunior®	Mannequin that represents a 6-year-old boy. Features vital signs, ability to talk, breath sounds, chest rise, realistic intubation views, ability to create arrhythmias, palpable pulses, ability to create vascular access, change pupil size. See Fig. 16.8
Laerdal medical	SimBaby™	Similar to above except for infant, with vital signs appropriate to infant normal ranges and features, such as grunting. See Fig. 16.9
Laerdal medical	SimNewB®	Similar to above except for neonate, with vital signs appropriate to neonate normal ranges and features, such as possible needle thoracentesis, umbilical venous and arterial access, umbilical pulse. See Fig. 16.10
Laerdal medical	MegaCode kid	Similar to above, specifically designed for code situations. IO lines can be placed with aspiration simulated
Gaumard	HAL® S3005 5 year old pediatric simulator	Mannequin of 5-year-old that includes intubation views, chest rise, gastric insufflation for excess bag masking, chest recoil, ability to perform tracheostomy, skin color corresponding to hypoxia, controllable vital signs and eyelids and pupils, IM, IO and IV access. See Fig. 16.11
Gaumard	HAL® S3001 1 year old pediatric simulator	Similar features as above except for 1-year-old, including appropriate vital signs. See Fig. 16.12

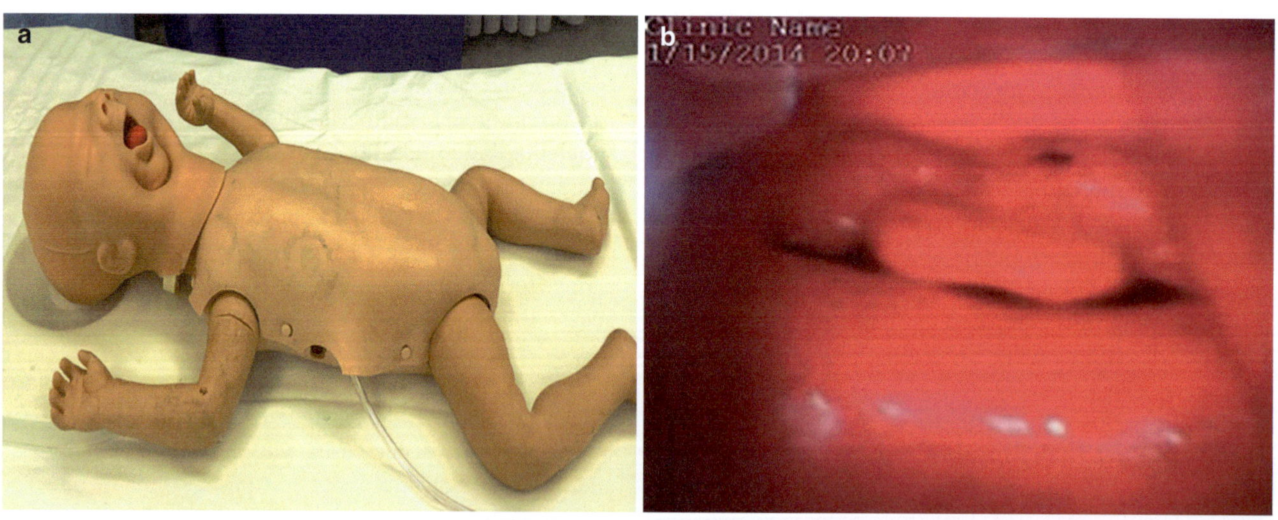

Fig. 16.7 (**a**) Homemade Pierre Robin sequence airway trainer designed for difficult airway simulation [11]. (**b**) Glottic view with the intubation. (Photo courtesy of Poling et al.)

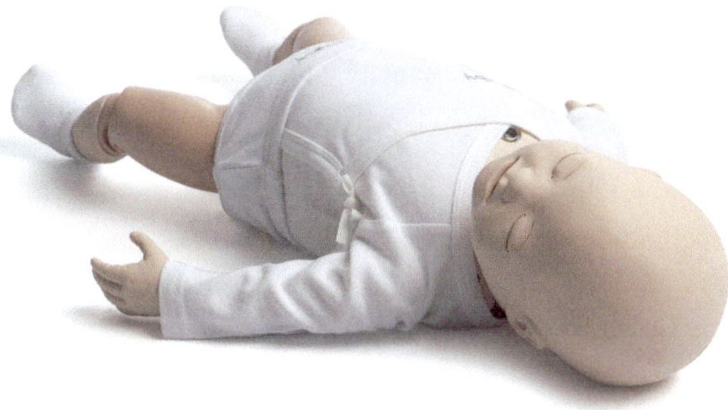

Fig. 16.9 SimBaby®. (Photo courtesy of Laerdal http://www.laerdal.com/us/SimBaby accessed September 11, 2016)

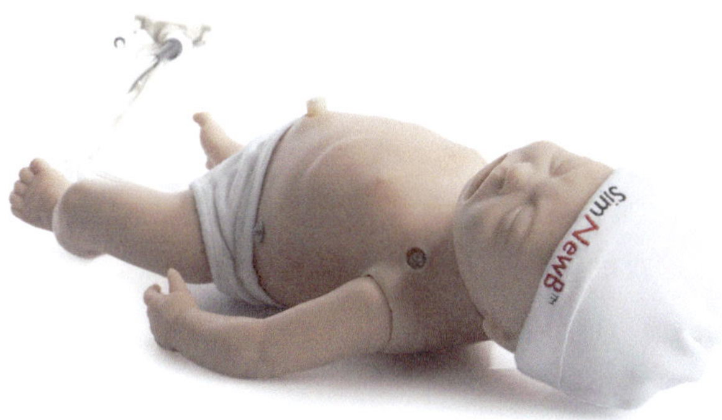

Fig. 16.10 SimNewB®. (Photo courtesy of Laerdal http://www.laerdal.com/us/doc/88/SimNewB accessed September 10, 2016)

HFS has been described as impacting learning outcomes across three domains [16, 17]:

1. Cognitive outcome – knowledge, basic and clinical science such as pediatric anatomy, physiology, pathophysiology, pharmacology including drug dosing.
2. Skill-based (psychomotor) proficiency – this domain includes specific skills, such as pediatric airway management, neuraxial techniques, central venous catheter insertion, and more advanced procedural skills (i.e., difficult airway management, pediatric or neonatal cardiopulmonary resuscitation).
3. Affective outcome – this domain includes learning how to apply the knowledge, skills, and procedures effectively into patient care in a multidisciplinary pediatric perioperative care team (nontechnical skills such as communication, situational awareness, task distribution, and leadership or followership).

HFS facilitates the learning outcomes above for the specific needs of anesthesiologists caring for pediatric patients. HFS offers active participation and real-time formative feedback, which are key aspects in Kolb's experiential learning cycle. Specific and directed feedback promotes real-time review of decision-making and subsequent improvement in performance. This feedback may be followed with repetition or deliberate practice of critical thinking or with focused training of specific skill acquisition, refinement, and maintenance based on facilitated

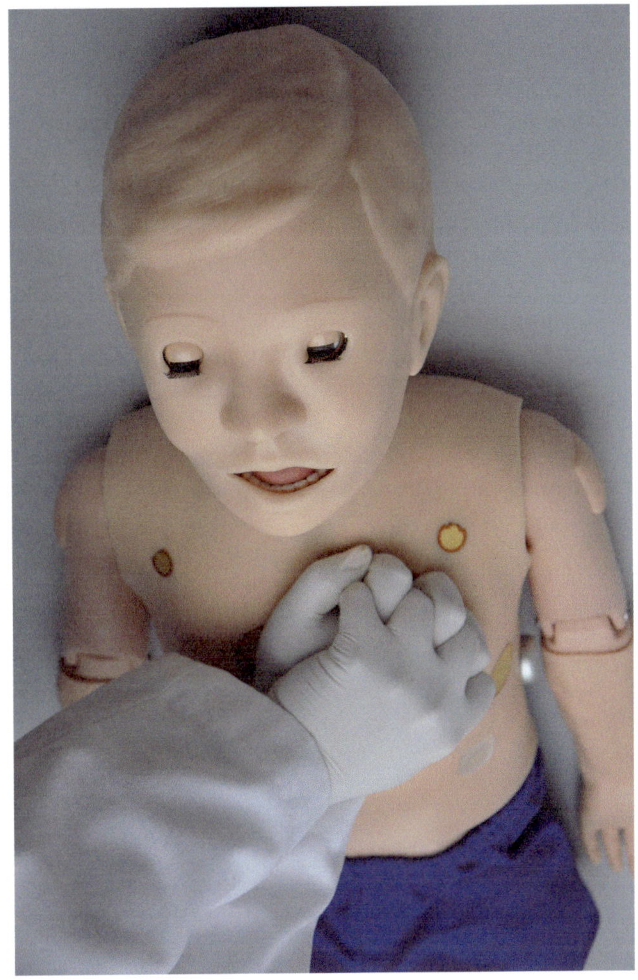

Fig. 16.11 HAL® S3005 5 Year Old Pediatric Simulator. (Photo courtesy of Gaumard)

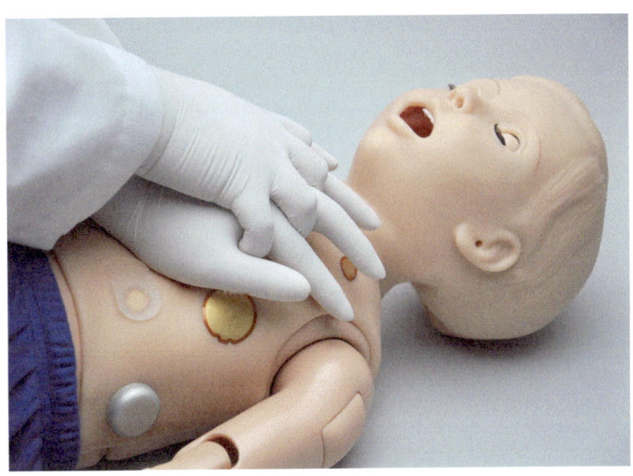

Fig. 16.12 HAL® S3004 1 Year Old Pediatric Simulator. (Photo courtesy of Gaumard)

self-assessment. These elements, readily available in HFS, are the foundational components of Ericsson's educational theory of deliberate practice [18–20].

Despite the impressive nature of technology involved in mannequin-based HFS, critical elements of the learning experience lie in the hands of the trained simulationist [21, 22]. Multiple "nonphysical" elements are vital to effective learning, most notably, feedback methodology. Long considered the "heart and soul" of simulation, facilitated debriefing following an HFS scenario is often thought to be the most crucial aspect of the experience [23]. In addition, the facilitators should create a controlled and suitable learning environment that ensures the psychological safety of the learner during simulation. Psychological safety is essential, especially when caring for the pediatric patient given that caring for this population comes with a unique set of psychological challenges. Ensuring this psychological safety requires facilitators that are experienced with utilizing debriefing as a reflective tool. Furthermore, debriefing should immediately follow the HFS and should clearly delineate the learning objectives. Learning objectives should be specific, should be well defined, and, in some circumstances, should be presented in the pre-brief session. Consideration should also be given to the physical setting for the debriefing. Participants often benefit from a change in location to place distance between them and the stressors present in the scenario that may be distracting during the debriefing session.

An example of HFS use for a frequently encountered pediatric anesthesiology clinical situation is described in Table 16.4. The events that unfold are uncommon yet life-

Table 16.4 A sample pediatric anesthesiology scenario

Room setup	High-technology mannequin that is representative of an 8-month-old Operating table set high at surgeon's request Surgical tray with gauze and instruments set up on the left side of the patient Surgical microscope on the right side of the patient
Actors needed	Circulating nurse, otolaryngology resident, surgical scrub technician, and anesthesiologist who begins the handoff
Case stem	An 8-month-old male infant with trisomy 21 presents for insertion of bilateral ear tubes. The patient is about to be induced when a hurried provider handoff occurs from a scenario actor to the participant
Progression of scenario	The participant assumes patient care and continues with planned inhalational anesthetic induction. One minute into induction, the patient develops bradycardia with pulse slowing from 128 to 95 beats per minute. Blood pressure is stable at 90/48 mmHg. At this point, the participant is expected to decrease the inspired anesthetic concentration to decrease the risk of profound bradycardia. Regardless of this action, laryngospasm ensues with hypoxemia to an oxygen saturation of 75% followed by bradycardia to a pulse of 45 beats per minute and a blood pressure of 50/30 mmHg initially and then becoming subsequently not measurable. The provider should recognize life-threatening bradycardia in this infant and should initiate chest compressions in accordance with published resuscitation guidelines. In the meantime, the bradycardia will not respond to routine treatment, such as atropine
Resolution	Only proper airway management along with cardiopulmonary resuscitation will resolve the cardiopulmonary arrest
Learning objectives for debriefing	Review with facilitators prior to the pre-briefing: 1. Was it safe for the handoff to have occurred at induction? Elicit a discussion around this topic from the group, remembering that there is no definitive right or wrong answer (a) Did the verbal handoff contribute to this patient's problem, and are there better ways to handoff care of patients under anesthesia? (b) Would this scenario have been different if this was an otherwise healthy 8-month-old patient? 2. What are the risks and benefits of decreasing inhalational anesthetic concentration in this patient? 3. Is there a role for prophylactic atropine in this (or any) patient population? 4. Should intravenous access have been established for this patient with trisomy 21? 5. Were resources utilized appropriately in this crisis? (a) Did the participant have enough people in the room or should he or she have called for help? (b) What resources are available in the settings where the participants work? 6. What is the role of succinylcholine in the management of hypoxemia? (a) What dose would be appropriate? (b) Are there contraindications to succinylcholine administration? 7. What special risks should be considered with invasive airway placement for the infant with trisomy 21? (a) Cervical instability (b) Difficult intubation (c) Increased risk of undiagnosed pulmonary hypertension and poor tolerance for hypoxia and hypercarbia 8. Was the management of bradycardia consistent with published guidelines? 9. Were cognitive aids available? (a) If so, were they used? (b) How were they used? 10. What were the barriers to starting chest compressions in this patient? (a) Uncertainty about need (b) Physical obstruction by surgical instruments or microscope (c) Height of operating table

threatening and require expert and proficient management with a limited margin.

A scenario such as the one listed in Table 16.4, when set in a realistic learning environment, promotes problem-centered learning followed by real-time feedback. The participant may safely practice decision-making in a high-acuity clinical setting with no consequences to living patients. With no direct risk to the actual patient, there is less likely to be a negative emotional reaction associated with this teaching technique. Through a structured and guided debriefing, the importance of team-based anesthesia crisis resource management (ACRM) skills may be highlighted in order to create anticipation and early calls for help, leadership and followership skills, prevention of fixation error and other cognitive biases, mobilization of available resources, and appropriate use of cognitive aids [24–26].

Within each institution, HFS should be systematically integrated into the subspecialty of pediatric anesthesiology. Such an approach will help to ensure a curriculum that, while relying on universal traits, maintains utility to the learner in covering topics relevant to the subspecialty of pediatric anesthesiology. Little is known about the cognitive implications of simulated learning, which requires ongoing evaluation. Poling et al. created a difficult airway Pierre Robin neonate model within their institution using components of commercially available equipment to design a part task trainer that accurately recreates a specific airway difficulty while maintaining the realism of a neonate (Fig. 16.7) [11]. This model is truly remarkable in that it allows for practicing of a "cannot intubate, cannot ventilate" pediatric event. Prior to this design, it was challenging to find a pediatric model that could reproduce this scenario.

High-Fidelity Simulation for Assessment

HFS offers a unique opportunity to assess a trainee's performance in situations that closely mimic real life [27]. Unlike written or oral exams, trainees may be evaluated on demonstrated clinical skills and judgment in addition to fund of knowledge. Interactive mannequins and part task trainers may incorporate preprogramed scenarios to facilitate performance assessment across a variety of skill domains. This assessment method may be useful for formative assessment, identification of performance gaps, preparation for low- and high-stake examinations, and summative assessments. Perhaps, the pediatric advanced life support (PALS) mega-code is the most familiar simulation-based test in the field of pediatrics. The American Board of Anesthesiology (ABA) will soon add simulation to their board examination process in the form of Objective Structured Clinical Examinations (OSCEs), which has already occurred for other high-stake examinations, such as the Israeli Anesthesiology Board examinations and the National Board of Medical Examiners (NBME) in the United States. Assessments utilizing simulation technology allow the faculty the chance to provide a consistent evaluation of different trainees over a wide variety of situations and skills without risk of harm to any patient. Simulation may also be helpful in assessing both an anesthesiology resident's and a pediatric anesthesiology fellow's performances in different domains as required by the ACGME. With the recent implementation of the Anesthesiology Milestone project, many institutions have developed simulation programs to assess these milestones. Both clinical and professionalism milestones lend themselves well for assessment with simulation, particularly for those milestones that are challenging to assess in daily practice with limited and inconsistent exposure to individual faculty members.

Technical, procedural, communication, teamwork, and diagnostic skill domains may all be evaluated with high-fidelity simulation. The use of checklists and key actions may be useful in the assessment of technical skills, such as endotracheal intubation or establishing intravenous access. However, for the assessment of nontechnical skills, such as teamwork, behavior, professionalism, and communication, the use of global rating scales may be more useful [28]. Mastery of pediatric anesthesiology practice may be challenging. While there is a minimum training period for pediatric anesthesiology training as determined by the ABA in both residency and potential fellowship training, there is an opportunity for this training to be supplemented with formative simulation education and simulation-based performance assessment [13].

Methods to Assess Performance

There are several methods described in the literature to assess performance of a trainee including [27, 29]:

1. Checklists
2. Key actions performed
3. Time to key action
4. Global scoring systems

There are advantages and disadvantages of each assessment method, and any single method may be inadequate in gauging performance, necessitating a multimodal approach. While global scores are used commonly for simulation performance assessment, there are several disadvantages to this approach: decreased granularity is evaluated by the correct sequence of actions and the rapidity with which the problem is diagnosed and the correct treatment is given. A global scoring system measures overall performance as assessed by an expert observing the encounter, who may utilize a scoring tool incorporating these granular aspects of performance. Some of the disadvantages of this method include inter-rater discrepancy and subjectivity although studies have shown the method to be valid and reliable [28]. Furthermore, these scoring methods do not assess the inner thought process and rationale of the participant.

Overall, the scoring systems described in the literature may be divided into two categories: explicit or implicit. Explicit process scores include the use of checklists or key actions. These checklists are based on expert assessment, who may use standardized guidelines to determine the expected appropriate actions. For example, in scoring performance during a scenario of anaphylaxis during induction of anesthesia, each action taken will be scored; however, the key action of administering fluids and epinephrine in the case of severe anaphylaxis may have more weight in the scoring rubric. A disadvantage of explicit techniques lies in achieving consistent inter-rater reliability in situations in which rater-dependent perception may not take into account order and timing of actions. For example, in a "cannot intubate, cannot ventilate" scenario, the participant who rapidly recognizes the situation and moves correctly through the difficult airway algorithm and ultimately to transtracheal cannulation or cricothyrotomy should be scored higher than a participant who fails to recognize the situation within a predetermined time limit, placing the patient at risk of hypoxia. Thus, while the sequence of interventions is more important when the timing of interventions is not close, if interventions are appropriately occurring simultaneously, the precise sequence may not matter.

Implicit scoring systems evaluate performance as a whole. Although concerns of inter-rater reliability have also been appropriately raised with this system, available literature does suggest that scoring systems using a global rating scale may be very effective and useful in more complex situations in which teamwork is a major learning objective [28, 30]. Global rating scales (GRS) may use three components to assess the performance: knowledge base, behavior, and overall performance score (Table 16.5). Criteria for the knowledge component that may be considered include utilization of appropriate diagnostic and therapeutic algorithms in a timely and correct sequence. Criteria that may be utilized for the behavior component include problem anticipation, planning, calling for help, effective utilization of team and resources, prioritizing, clear closed-loop communication, and management of conflict. For each of these criteria, rating scales may be utilized. Overall performance may be rated using a composite of knowledge and behavior. Although the use of extensive checklists may appear to be an objective method of assessment, subjectivity on the part of the rater may play an important role in the final performance evaluation [29]. Previous studies in pediatric trainee and pediatric anesthesiology trainee scenarios, however, have found a high level of agreement between raters suggesting that GRS is a valid means of assessing performance [30, 31]. Others have shown that multiple scenarios may be needed to reliably assess trainees on their management abilities in a simulation environment [29]. While it is easy to recognize a well-performing trainee compared to one that is poorly performing, the problem arises in the cases of those who do not fall well in either end of the spectrum. Assessment of a multitude of simulated encounters may help to overcome this difficulty. Furthermore, the purpose of the assessment must also be considered, i.e., formative or summative, enhancing performance, raising standards, or achieving a specified level of competence.

Table 16.5 Example of a common pediatric simulation scenario and scoring

Case stem	Laryngospasm in a 5-year-old child undergoing magnetic resonance imaging (MRI) with propofol sedation			
Scoring sheet				
Checklist scoring:	Recognizes that there is a problem		yes	no
	Communicates to MRI team to stop scanning		yes	no
	Calls for help		yes	no
	Time to recognize laryngospasm:			
	<60 sec	>60 sec	fails to recognize	
	Administers 100% inspired oxygen		yes	no
	Deepens level of anesthesia		yes	no
	Attempts bag-valve ventilation		yes	no
	Administers muscle relaxant		yes	no
	Considers transporting child out of scanner if intubation or resuscitation is needed		yes	no
	Verbalizes further options regarding further management		yes	no
	Total score out of 10		**/10**	
Global score	1. Knowledge base (scale 0–5) (a) Gathers relevant information (b) Reaches a diagnosis (c) Initiates correct treatment (d) Initiates timely treatment (e) Sequence of tasks is appropriate 2. Behavior (scale 0–5) (a) Calls for help (b) Reevaluates the situation (c) Utilizes team and resources effectively (d) Prioritizes appropriately (e) Uses clear closed-loop communication 3. Overall performance (scale 0–5)			

Raters and Evaluators

When developing rating scales for global or overall performance, it is important to consider the background of the evaluator in terms of knowledge, experience, and expectations.

Although subjectivity will always play some role, error in judgment may be minimized by specialized training, use of quality measures, and development of meaningful rubrics to ensure the validity of assessment [27].

Any assessment may provide inaccurate information, and high-fidelity simulation as a tool is no exception. Despite the degree of realism that may be achieved, a realism gap remains, and trainees may perform better or worse in the actual clinical setting than in a simulated situation. One particular risk of simulation-based assessment for complex scenarios is that of hindsight bias. This bias is the result of the educator knowing the outcome of a case that he or she is facilitating. In actual patient care, the path to a diagnosis is not often linear. From the perspective of a clinician encountering an unknown case, the response to particular treatments or subtle aspects of the patient's physical examination may be important clues to figuring out the problem. Even high-fidelity simulation is limited in how accurately a real case may be mimicked. The educator may fault a student for reaching the incorrect conclusion even if they propose a plausible diagnosis. Conversely, they may believe a student has reached the correct diagnosis even if their answer was derived from faulty reasoning. The instructor must remember that the goal is not for the student to become an expert at simulation but to become an expert clinician for actual patients. Simulation is but one means to reach this goal.

Multidisciplinary Team Training

Multidisciplinary team (MDT) training has become more than a "buzz" phrase; it has morphed into a potential lifesaving concept. Traditionally, healthcare providers spent multiple hours learning clinical care in a vacuum, either by sitting alone in the library or studying among colleagues in the same field, such as nurses with nurses, physicians with physicians, and so on. Clearly, we do not practice in silos and therefore undergo a paradigm shift to transition to efficient teamwork in the clinical setting. The importance of effective teamwork becomes most evident when facing a patient emergency, as the clinical care team is required to respond rapidly and precisely to prevent further deterioration or successful treatment of the patient condition [32].

This focus on multidisciplinary teams which became the highlight of patient safety in 2000 when the Institute of Medicine (IOM) found that patient harm in healthcare was often a result of poor multidisciplinary teamwork and communication. There was further emphasis that, for critical areas with higher stakes such as the emergency department (ED), intensive care units (ICU), and operating rooms (OR), team training incorporating crisis resource management (CRM) techniques should be established [34]. These recommendations were further emphasized 10 years later with the European Helsinki Patient Safety Declaration which stated that human factors played a large part in the delivery of safe care to patients and OR teams (surgeons, nurses, and other healthcare providers) had to come together to reliably provide safe care [33]. Here, we will discuss the importance of multidisciplinary training specifically focused on the pediatric anesthesia environment. This patient population comes with its own unique challenges, but the dedication to providing safe care still aligns with the fundamental goals of simulation. Simulation training should ideally be multidisciplinary, and decision-making should be practiced in realistic clinical environments [34].

Differences in Pediatric Simulation

Whereas adult simulation may typically be performed using a single mannequin, pediatric simulation is best accomplished with several mannequins to represent the varying ages from the preterm neonate to the adolescent. This diversity leads to a higher degree of complexity and expense. Some of the more intricate details that have been incorporated into adult mannequins may be difficult to duplicate in the smaller pediatric mannequins, leading to less fidelity and unrealistic experience when using pediatric simulators [13]. Due to different patient ages and sizes, there must also be a variety of equipment available during simulations, such as endotracheal tubes, venipuncture equipment, monitors, drug doses, and so forth. This preparation becomes a challenge for both the simulation team and participants.

One of the most valuable opportunities for simulation training lies in team dynamics and improving team communication. Using simulation for team training in pediatrics helps to overcome some of the hurdles of managing both common minor emergencies with ease and rare situations with increased comfort. There may be members of the team that are well-versed in adult emergencies, but these skills may not always be generalizable to pediatric patients; thus, multidisciplinary team training helps members respond to emergencies in a united and consistent manner.

Pediatric Environments

Pediatric patients are challenging not only due to their age and size variation but also because they are cared for in a variety of locations. Out of operating room, anesthesia locations are a significant component of pediatric anesthesia care. Multidisciplinary simulation training may facilitate this need by allowing teams to practice responding to emergencies, mobilizing help, and uncovering systems issues and lead to improvement of resource availability and standardization of processes. As all teams may not work together frequently and team members may be in an unfamiliar environment, simulation may help hone in on crisis resource management (CRM) skills so that the clinical care team may work efficiently and effectively in the face of a pediatric emergency despite the location of care.

The MRI suite, a common location for pediatric anesthesia delivery, carries specific concerns due to the distance of the provider from the patient and limitations with monitoring. Patients are at an increased risk for airway compromise and hemodynamic concerns, which may require interruption of diagnostic studies and rapid intervention. This delayed access may lead to further endangerment of the patient as providers rush to aid without proper removal of items sensitive to the magnet. Another location presenting difficult patient access is the radiation oncology suite. Patients may have airway and hemodynamic compromise in the context of additional obstruction, such as head molds. While caring for patients in the vascular interventional suite or the interventional cardiac suite, although patient access may be more reasonable, there may be a variety of providers who have less experience with pediatric patients, and even those with pediatric expertise may have find it difficult to mobilize resources during a critical situation. Tofil et al. demonstrated MDT collaboration in the radiology suite with radiology residents and radiology technicians in a simulation of severe contrast reaction in pediatric patients [35]. This reaction is a rare entity but may be life-threatening if there fails to be rapid and appropriate responses. Participants improved noticeably after undergoing a simulation scenario and debriefing that included CPR skills and administration of intramuscular (IM) epinephrine (pretest versus posttest scores for residents were 57% versus 82%, respectively and for technologists were 47% versus 72%, respectively). This single example exemplifies in situ simulation as a tool that may enable team members to take the proper precautions, acquire the necessary resources, and work together to help a pediatric patient in case of an emergency.

Pediatric anesthetic care is provided in numerous locations in which sedation is required for a variety of procedures. The hematology oncology clinic typically requires sedation services for lumbar punctures and bone marrow aspirates. Other pediatric hospital sedation teams may be under the supervision of anesthesiology groups, pediatric critical care teams, or hospitalist groups. These teams may vary in their experience and comfort level caring for pediatric patients. MDT may be beneficial in these locations that incorporate a variety of providers with varying backgrounds. Additional settings in which MDT may be extremely beneficial include the post-anesthetic recovery room, pediatric and neonatal intensive care units, emergency department, or pediatric inpatient unit for rapid responses and pediatric codes.

Hospital Settings

Pediatric patients not only receive care in many environments within a free-standing children's hospital but also across a variety of non-children's hospital settings. These locations include pediatric wards within adult hospitals, community and academic centers, urgent care centers, and outpatient office settings. This range creates an inconsistency in provider experience that may be detrimental to patient care. There are more than nine million children seen in the emergency room each year for traumatic injuries, with more than 80% of them cared for in a non-children's hospital setting. In a focus group-based study, 107 providers made up of 32 physicians and 75 nonphysicians felt that barriers to adequate pediatric trauma care included lack of pediatric trauma experience, inadequate pediatric trauma training, and lack of confidence with the assessment of the pediatric trauma patient. Participants desired onsite practice sessions to refine resuscitation skills and team decision-making during scenarios. It was determined that HFS may be one solution to help narrow the gap in comfort levels among providers [36].

Multidisciplinary training in the operating room requires a variety of providers with varying areas of expertise, situational awareness by team members, high-stake communication, and shared decision-making. Training to care for the pediatric trauma patient is no different. Traumatic injury remains the leading cause of pediatric mortality, and the teams entrusted with their care must meet a high standard of team dynamics. These teams may commonly involve members who do not commonly work together (i.e., surgeons, emergency room physicians, emergency room nurses, pediatric critical care physicians, anesthesiologists, respiratory therapists, radiology technicians, paramedics). In a study conducted at Cincinnati Children's Hospital, researchers aimed to improve the functioning of the pediatric trauma team with multidisciplinary education and simulation for training and evaluation. After 1 year, 160 individuals in 6 team groups consisting of pediatric surgery faculty, emergency medicine faculty, surgical and pediatric residents, nurses, critical care fellows, paramedics, and respiratory therapists underwent 23 two-hour pediatric trauma simulations. There was a noticeable improvement in overall performance of tasks and team performance between the early and late groups [37]. Although high-fidelity simulation was only part of a larger program to improve team performance and communication during all aspects of trauma education in a multidisciplinary environment, this work demonstrates the feasibility and utility of performing multidisciplinary simulations to improve care of the pediatric trauma patient.

Pedagogical Tools for Multidisciplinary Simulation Training

There are many types of teaching tools that may be used to reinforce skills and concepts during multidisciplinary simulation exercises. Participants may undergo a teaching workshop before or after to reinforce skills that are essential during an emergency situation. For example, participants may undergo a simulation requiring initiation of chest compressions. It may be noticed that there are a range of speeds and depths at which participants perform compressions; hence, after the simulation, a part task trainer may be used to reinforce proper technique and speed for chest compressions. Similarly, participants may exhibit discomfort with the use of the defibrillator, such that a hands-on workshop may be used to review the defibrillator. The combination of debriefing and recognition of skill gaps with training stations to help with skill reinforcement will greatly enrich the simulation process. With frequent simulation sessions, MDT teams may become accustomed to debriefing and may begin to incorporate debriefing into the daily clinical workflow as well as improve communication and teamwork.

Furthermore, cognitive aids, such as emergency algorithms, PALS, and the neonatal resuscitation program (NRP), help facilitate actions during a pediatric emergency. At the University of North Carolina, an intraoperative simulation session was completed using a local anesthetic systemic toxicity (LAST) cognitive aid adapted from the Society of Pediatric Anesthesiology Pediatric Critical Event Checklists. The MDT included a simulated scenario during which the surgeon injected excess local anesthetic, resulting in LAST. The teams received education about the use of cognitive aids before the simulation and were given checklists to use during the exercise. Simulation may act as a mechanism for the development and integration of tools that may aid providers during the state of cognitive overload common in pediatric emergencies (Fig. 16.13).

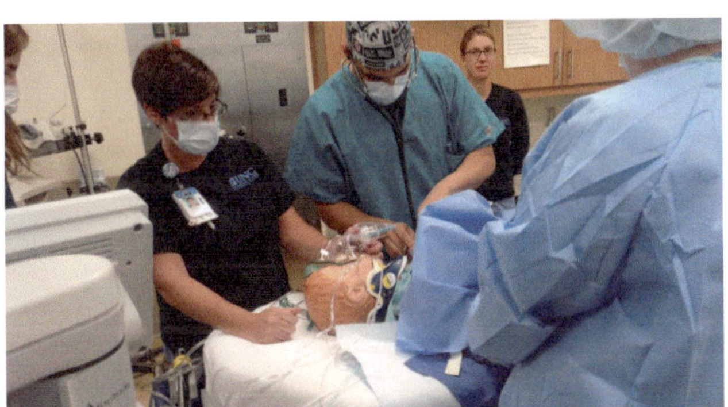

Fig. 16.13 MDT simulation of an 8-year-old with cystic fibrosis developing respiratory distress during a sedation for a peripherally inserted central catheter (PICC) line placement

Sample Scenario

Below is an example of development of a simulation scenario (Tables 16.6, 16.7). Having a structured plan allows the team to hone in on the skills and team dynamics to be accomplished during the scenario. The case content may range from simple to complex, depending on the goals and participants in the scenario.

This simple scenario includes at least five participants (surgeon, circulating nurse, scrub technician, anesthesiology resident, anesthesiology attending) and may be expanded to include more (medical student, surgery resident, additional responders when help is called, etc.). With participants from different backgrounds, communication tools and a team building strategy such as TeamSTEPPS (Team Strategies and Tools to Enhance Performance and Patient Safety) may be demonstrated, practiced, and refined in preparation for real-life events.

Multidisciplinary team training in the simulated environment may help refine team functioning during pediatric emergencies. It provides a mechanism for discovering gaps in skills, knowledge, and system processes that may be practiced, remediated, and streamlined to better care for

Table 16.6 Simulation scenario toolkit

Objectives	1. Establish situational awareness and systematic response during pediatric emergencies 2. Improve perioperative staff performance of initial management steps during a pediatric emergency 3. Promote an increased comfort level of perioperative staff during pediatric emergencies
Critical actions to be performed by participant	1. Recognize rhythm change to asystole and ventricular tachycardia 2. Initiate compressions 3. Attain the code cart. Note the time taken to bring cart in room 4. Attach defibrillator pads. Note the time taken to place pads 5. Dial directed joules on defibrillator 6. Carry out defibrillation. Note the time taken to deliver shock 7. Utilization of closed-loop communication
Patient name	Charlie
Age and gender	2-year-old male
Weight and height	15 kg, 35 inches
Chief complaint	Chronic otitis media
Past medical history	Former 36-week-old premature birth, gastroesophageal reflux disease (GERD)
Past surgical history	Circumcision
Allergies	None
Medications	Ranitidine, multivitamin
Key item in recent history	Cold 2 weeks ago with postnasal drip. Learner should identify that risk of laryngospasm is likely

Table 16.7 Scenario development tool

Scenario background	Patient presents for bilateral myringotomy and ear tube placement. "Dr. B," attending anesthesiologist, is starting the case with a clinical year 1 (CA-1) resident. The patient is overall healthy and appears to be tolerating mask ventilation well for the right ear tube. As the CA-1 is on her last week of the pediatric rotation, Dr. B feels it is safe to leave the resident alone for the left ear tube placement and she exits the operating room. The CA-1 turns the sevoflurane off as directed during the final ear tube. She turns the nitrous oxide to 3 liters per minute. Meanwhile, the patient transitions to a lighter plane of anesthesia and begins to laryngospasm	
Progression	Ventilation becomes ineffective and the oxygen saturation precipitously falls from 98% to 60%. The CA-1 still cannot ventilate and the patient undergoes a hypoxic arrest	
Primary survey	Level of consciousness: Glasgow coma scale 3 Airway: Mask in place Breathing: Initially abdominal muscle movement, no chest rise	
Secondary survey	Head, ear, eye, nose, throat exam: Eyes closed Cardiovascular: No pulses palpable Lungs: No breath sounds auscultated Abdomen: Abdominal muscle contractions initially and then cease Extremities: Cool, pale	
Labs	None	
Radiology	None	
ECG	Bradycardia with progression to asystole and further deterioration to ventricular tachycardia after epinephrine injection	
Case chronology of events		
Scenario status	**Patient status**	**Actions to be performed by participants**
Initial bag mask ventilation for left ear tube	Hemodynamically stable	Nurse charting, scrub, and nurse beginning to count
Finishing right ear tube	Laryngospasm	CA-1 trying to ventilate, nurse calling out for help
Patient progresses to cardiac arrest	Pulseless ventricular tachycardia	Nurse getting code cart, scrub tech initiating compressions
	Pulseless ventricular tachycardia	IV established, pads attached, defibrillator turned on and 2 joules per kilogram dialed in, patient defibrillated

the pediatric patient during a critical event. There continues to be debate about whether improvements documented in simulated exercises may be extrapolated to improved performance in clinical situations. Despite proof of this correlation, MDT is a tool that does provide exposure to rare events in pediatric patients and better equips providers to respond.

Curriculum Development and Resources

With advances in technology, more complex procedures are being performed in younger children, emphasizing the need for robust training in order to reduce perioperative morbidity and mortality. In addition, the scope of practice of pediatric anesthesia has been expanded beyond the operating room into many remote locations, such as MRI, interventional radiology, interventional cardiology, radiation oncology, nuclear medicine, and so forth. Strong clinical skills, sound clinical judgment, and decision-making along with robust leadership, teamwork, and communication skills are necessary to manage pediatric crises in any situation and to ensure patient safety.

Current Education System

As per ACGME requirements, each resident must demonstrate competency in the anesthetic management of children under the age of 12 undergoing surgery or procedure under anesthesia. The minimum pediatric case log for anesthesiology residents is 100 cases, with 20 children under the age of 3 years and 5 children under the age of 3 months [38].

Current Education Modalities

Most of the education and clinical experience that anesthesiology residents achieve during the pediatric subspecialty rotation is via direct exposure to clinical work environment under medical supervision by the faculty. Other educational methods include lectures, simulation, workshops, presentations, or small-group sessions.

Needs Assessment: Why Do We Need Simulation-Based Curriculum?

1. *To bridge the knowledge gap*: The incidence of perioperative cardiac arrests reported by the Pediatric Perioperative Cardiac Arrest (POCA) registry varies from 1.4 cardiac arrests per 10,000 pediatric anesthetics to 3.3–4.6 cardiac arrests per 10,000 by a single institution [39–41]. Because such events are so rare, combined with ACGME compliance with duty hours and subspecialty requirements, the graduating resident

might not have adequate exposure to such a crisis or an opportunity to develop and demonstrate mastery of pediatric crisis management. A study conducted to assess pediatric resuscitation skills of anesthesiology residents demonstrated knowledge gaps in this area [39]. Another conducted by Hunt et al. demonstrated delays and errors in pediatric resuscitation by pediatric residents in a simulated cardiac arrest [42]. In addition, there are a wide variety of cases that one may encounter during their practice involving pediatric patients, to some of which the practitioner may not have sufficient exposure during their training. Case-based simulation may provide a unique opportunity to bridge the curricular gap.

2. *To promote patient safety and satisfaction*: With the publication of *To Err is Human: Building Safer Health System* in 1999, the Institute of Medicine brought to light the frequency of iatrogenic adverse outcomes and errors made in hospitals. Since then, large efforts have been directed toward providing a higher quality of care, improving patient satisfaction and outcomes, and enhancing patient safety. Simulation-based education provides a safe, nonjudgmental, reproducible, and realistic environment where mistakes may be made without consequences to patients and skills may be demonstrated, acquired, and practiced until mastery is achieved.
3. *To complement the current education system*: Some ACGME competencies or milestones such as interpersonal communication and professionalism are difficult to teach and assess. The use of standardized patients or case-based confederates offers a unique platform where those skills may be taught and assessed.

Curriculum Design and Objectives

1. *Anticipatory education through an introductory boot camp.*

Several medical specialties utilize an introductory "boot camp" in both undergraduate and graduate medical education to allow for a smooth transition of the provider in their new clinical role. The purpose of this training is to orient the new learners to clinical workflow and expectations, develop procedural skills, and expose them to common pediatric emergencies that they might encounter. Use of simulation-based education provides an ideal platform to achieve these goals via experiential learning. Hospitals such as Massachusetts General Hospital and the University of North Carolina have developed a simulation-based orientation for anesthesia residents at the start of their pediatric anesthesia rotation [43]. A similar introductory boot camp has been developed for pediatric anesthesiology fellows to teach basic technical skills such as ultrasound-guided pediatric vascular access and difficult pediatric airway management, clinical decision-making using simulation, interactive group discussions, and teamwork during crisis management [44].

2. *Introduction and demonstration of proficiency in technical skills.*

Part task trainers may be used to develop complex psychomotor skills. As described in the previous section, common skills that may be acquired are basic airway skills such as bag mask ventilation, direct laryngoscopy, fiberoptic intubation, cricothyrotomy, placement of vascular access both peripherally and centrally with and without the use of ultrasound, lumbar puncture, placement of intraosseous needle, and regional anesthesia techniques [13, 43].

3. *Demonstrate critical thinking, reasoning, decision-making skills, teamwork, and leadership during crisis management.*

Pediatric emergencies may occur both in and out of the operating room setting, such as MRI, interventional radiology, or the post-anesthesia care unit (PACU). The use of in situ simulation is valuable for training learners to manage crises in such locations, where obtaining skilled help is often challenging. Common examples of simulated pediatric emergencies are laryngospasm, bronchospasm, bradycardia with inhalational induction, hyperkalemic arrest during massive transfusion, management of malignant hyperthermia, anaphylaxis, venous air embolism, or accidental extubation [13, 30].

Each scenario is designed with:

(a) Predetermined objectives.
(b) Predefined tasks, skills, or critical decision-making elements to meet those objectives. These tasks or skills defined should be based on current guidelines or expert opinion.
(c) Simulation scenario where the participants have the opportunity to demonstrate those tasks and skills and explain their decision-making process.

These clinical scenarios help to meet the educational objectives and expose learners to rare high-risk situations that they might encounter in their practice. These scenarios may also be used for simulation-based assessment of technical and nontechnical skills and to provide a platform for formative feedback and to create the opportunity to learn by deliberate practice.

4. *To supplement existing pedagogical tools.*

Per ACGME requirements, anesthesiology residents must demonstrate strong professionalism and interpersonal communication skills (Table 16.8). These competencies are difficult to teach and assess in the clinical work environment. Standardized patients are trained individuals who may assume the role of patient or family member in variety of clinical situations. They are commonly used to teach history taking, physical exam, and communication skills such as informed consent, difficult conversations, or delivery of bad news, such as wrong site surgery or nerve block injection, known complications of procedure such as pneumothorax following line placement, unknown complication, or unexpected adverse event, giving feedback to junior resident or medical students and end-of-life conversations.

5. *For assessment.*

Simulation may be used for assessing both technical and nontechnical skills. Common methods used for assessment include checklists; critical actions; time to critical actions, such as time to initiate chest compressions following an arrest or time to shock following diagnosis of ventricular fibrillation; and, lastly, the use of global scoring system which assesses performance as a whole [24, 30, 45]. Simulation-based assessment has also been in incorporated into the certification process. Objective Structured Clinical Examination (OSCE) has been incorporated into the Israeli National Board Examination for Anesthesiology [46, 47]. As previously discussed, in March of 2018, the American Board of Anesthesiology will launch the OSCE as a part of the applied examinations in the third and final stage of the exam series in addition to traditional oral board examinations for initial certification [48].

6. *To evaluate and remediate areas of deficiency in trainees struggling to progress to the next milestone level.*

Occasionally, a resident may struggle to progress along the milestone grid in one or more areas of clinical competencies as defined by the ACGME. Such deficiencies may manifest into clinical errors thereby compromising patient safety, increasing trainee and faculty frustration and stress, lowering self-esteem, and increasing self-doubt in the trainee. Simulation provides a unique opportunity to identify deficiencies and to develop an individualized educational plan for remediation [49, 50].

Table 16.8 Aligning simulation-based curriculum with ACGME milestones and clinical competencies

Simulation curriculum	ACGME milestones and competencies	Simulation-based educational method
Introductory boot camp	Patient care Medical knowledge System-based practice Practice-based learning and improvement Professionalism Interpersonal communication skills	Standardized patient Human patient simulator Partial task trainer Hybrid simulation
Technical skills	Patient care: technical skills Practice-based learning and improvement	Partial tasks trainers Human patient simulator Hybrid simulation
Clinical scenario (critical thinking, judgment, and crisis resource management)	Patient care Medical knowledge System-based practice Practice-based learning and improvement Interpersonal communication skills Professionalism	Human patient simulator (high-fidelity simulation) Hybrid simulation Screen-based simulation, such as pediatric advanced life support (PALS) certification by American Heart Association (AHA)
Nontechnical skills	Professionalism Interpersonal communication skills Practice-based learning and improvement System-based practice	Standardized patient Hybrid simulation
Assessment: checklist, critical action, global rating	Patient care Medical knowledge System-based practice Professionalism Interpersonal communication skills Practice-based learning	Standardized patient Human patient simulator (high-fidelity simulation) Hybrid simulation Partial task trainer
Remediation	Patient care Medical knowledge System-based practice Practice-based learning and improvement Professionalism and interpersonal communication	Human patient simulator Hybrid simulation Screen-based simulation Part task trainer Standardized patient

Conclusion

Collaboration with multidisciplinary teams is vital in the pediatric setting where teams must draw on each other's expertise and function seamlessly under pressure. Educators face the challenge of training rising anesthesiologists how to care for the pediatric patient in emergent settings as well as how to perform procedures proficiently. Simulation in the pediatric context comes with many challenges but has been shown to be an indispensable tool in imparting competencies, knowledge, and attitudinal skills. Pediatric anesthesiology simulation may be incorporated in fulfilling core competencies demanded by accreditation bodies such as the ACGME. The field of pediatric simulation is relatively young, and its growth is greatly aided by advocacy groups such as the International Pediatric Simulation Society (IPSS), the International Network for Simulation-based Pediatric Innovation, Research, and Education (INSPIRE), and others for furthering ongoing research collaborative efforts such as those in growing within the Society of Pediatric Anesthesiology (SPA).

References

1. Curran VR, Aziz K, O'Young S, Bessell C. Evaluation of the effect of a computerized training simulator (ANAKIN) on the retention of neonatal resuscitation skills. Teach Learn Med. 2004;16(2):157–64.
2. Lopreiato JO, Sawyer T. Simulation-based medical education in pediatrics. Acad Pediatr. 2015;15(2):134–42.
3. Hamstra SJ, Brydges R, Hatala R, Zendejas B, Cook DA. Reconsidering fidelity in simulation-based training. Acad Med. 2014;89(3):387–92.
4. Cheng A, Lang TR, Starr SR, Pusic M, Cook DA. Technology-enhanced simulation and pediatric education: a meta-analysis. Pediatrics. 2014;133(5):e1313–23.
5. Thomas SM, Burch W, Kuehnle SE, Flood RG, Scalzo AJ, Gerard JM. Simulation training for pediatric residents on central venous catheter placement: a pilot study. Pediatr Crit Care Med. 2013;14(9):e416–23.
6. Sawyer T, Strandjord TP, Johnson K, Low D. Neonatal airway simulators, how good are they? A comparative study of physical and functional fidelity. J Perinatol. 2016;36(2):151–6.
7. Oriot D, Darrieux E, Boureau-Voultoury A, Ragot S, Scépi M. Validation of a performance assessment scale for simulated intraosseous access. Simul Healthc. 2012;7(3):171–5.
8. Rowe R, Cohen RA. An evaluation of a virtual reality airway simulator. Anesth Analg. 2002;95(1):62–6, table of contents.
9. Binstadt E, Donner S, Nelson J, Flottemesch T, Hegarty C. Simulator training improves fiber-optic intubation proficiency among emergency medicine residents. Acad Emerg Med. 2008;15(11):1211–4.
10. Zaveri PP, Davis AB, O'Connell KJ, Willner E, Aronson Schinasi DA, Ottolini M. Virtual reality for pediatric sedation: a randomized controlled trial using simulation. Cureus. 2016;8(2):e486.
11. Poling S, Blum R, Dodson A, Patel S, Koka R. A better training mannequin for intubating neonates with Pierre Robin sequence. Poster session presented at: International Meeting on Simulation in Healthcare (IMSH), 2014 Jan 25–29; San Francisc.
12. Grant VJ, Cheng A. Comprehensive healthcare simulation: pediatrics. Cham: Springer; 2016.
13. Fehr JJ, Honkanen A, Murray DJ. Simulation in pediatric anesthesiology. Paediatr Anaesth. 2012;22(10):988–94.
14. Bearnson CS, Wiker KM. Human patient simulators: a new face in baccalaureate nursing education at Brigham Young University. J Nurs Educ. 2005;44(9):421–5.
15. Halamek LP, Kaegi DM, Gaba DM, Sowb YA, Smith BC, Smith BE, Howard SK. Time for a new paradigm in pediatric medical education: teaching neonatal resuscitation in a simulated delivery room environment. Pediatrics. 2000;106(4):E45.
16. Krage R, Erwteman M. State-of-the-art usage of simulation in anesthesia: skills and teamwork. Curr Opin Anaesthesiol. 2015;28(6):727–34.
17. Kraiger K, Ford JK, Salas E. Application of cognitive, skill-based, and affective theories of learning outcomes to new methods of training evaluation. J Appl Psychol. Apr 1993;78(2):311–28.
18. Ericsson KA. Summing up hours of any type of practice versus identifying optimal practice activities: commentary on Macnamara, Moreau, & Hambrick (2016). Perspect Psychol Sci. 2016;11(3):351–4.
19. Udani AD, Harrison TK, Mariano ER, Derby R, Kan J, Ganaway T, Shum C, Gaba DM, Tanaka P, Kou A, Howard SK, ADAPT (Anesthesiology-Directed Advanced Procedural Training) Research Group. Comparative-effectiveness of simulation-based deliberate practice versus self-guided practice on resident anesthesiologists' acquisition of ultrasound-guided regional anesthesia skills. Reg Anesth Pain Med. 2016;41(2):151–7.
20. Wang JM, Zorek JA. Deliberate practice as a theoretical framework for interprofessional experiential education. Front Pharmacol. 2016;7:188.
21. Harder BN, Ross CJ, Paul P. Instructor comfort level in high-fidelity simulation. Nurse Educ Today. 2013;33(10):1242–5.
22. Yelon SL, Ford JK, Anderson WA. Twelve tips for increasing transfer of training from faculty development programs. Med Teach. 2014;36(11):945–50.
23. Rall M, Manser T, Howard S. Key elements of debriefing for simulator training. Eur J Anaesthesiol. 2000;17:516–7.
24. Gaba DM, Howard SK, Fish KJ, Smith BE, Sowb YA. Simulation-based training in anesthesia crisis resource management (ACRM): a decade of experience. Simul Gaming. 2001;32:175–93.
25. Manser T, Harrison TK, Gaba DM, Howard SK. Coordination patterns related to high clinical performance in a simulated anesthetic crisis. Anesth Analg. 2009;108(5):1606–15.
26. Gaba DM. Crisis resource management and teamwork training in anaesthesia. Br J Anaesth. 2010;105(1):3–6.
27. Boulet JR, Murray DJ. Simulation-based assessment in anesthesiology: requirements for practical implementation. Anesthesiology. 2010;112:1041–52.
28. Jepsen RM, Dieckmann P, Spanager L, et al. Evaluating structured assessment of anaesthesiologists' non-technical skills. Acta Anaesthesiol Scand. 2016;60:756–66.
29. Weller JM, Bloch M, Young S, et al. Evaluation of high fidelity patient simulator in assessment of performance of anaesthetists. Br J Anaesth. 2003;90:43–7.
30. Fehr JJ, Boulet JR, Waldrop WB, et al. Simulation-based assessment of pediatric anesthesia skills. Anesthesiology. 2011;115:1308–15.
31. McBride ME, Waldrop WB, Fehr JJ, et al. Simulation in pediatrics: the reliability and validity of a multiscenario assessment. Pediatrics. 2011;128:335–43.
32. Institute of Medicine (US) Committee on Health Care in America. In: Kohn LT, Corrigan JM, Donaldson MS, editors. To err is human: building a safer health system. Washington, D.C.: National Academies Press (US); 2000.

33. WMA Declaration of Helsinki – Ethical Principles for Medical Research Involving Human Subjects. WMA General Assembly. South Africa. June 1964.
34. Gaba DM. Improving anesthesiologists' performance by simulating reality. Anesthesiology. 1992;76:491–4.
35. Tofil NM, White ML, Grant M, et al. Severe contrast reaction emergencies: high-fidelity simulation training for radiology residents and technologists in a children's hospital. Acad Radiol. 2010;17:934–40.
36. Falgiani T, Kennedy C, Jahnke S. Exploration of the barriers and education needs of non-pediatric hospital emergency department providers in pediatric trauma care. Int J Clin Med. 2014;5:56–62.
37. Falcone RA, Daugherty M, Schweer L, et al. Multidisciplinary pediatric trauma team training using high-fidelity trauma simulation. J Pediatr Surg. 2008;43:1065–71.
38. ACGME Program Requirements for Graduate Medical Education in Anesthesiology [Internet]. Accreditation Council for Graduate Medical Education [February 9, 2015]. Available from: https://www.acgme.org/Portals/0/PFAssets/ProgramRequirements/040_anesthesiology_2016.pdf.
39. Howard-Quijano KJ, Steigler MA, Huang YM, et al. Anesthesiology residents' performance of pediatric resuscitation during a simulated hyperkalemic cardiac arrest. Anesthesiology. 2010;112:993–7.
40. Morray JP, Geiduschek JM, Ramamoorthy C, et al. Anesthesia –related cardiac arrest in children. Initial findings of the pediatric perioperative cardiac arrest registry. Anesthesiology. 2000;93:6–14.
41. Morray JP. Cardiac arrest in anesthetized children: recent advances and challenges for the future. Pediatr Anesth. 2011;21:722–9.
42. Hunt EA, Vera K, Diener-West M, et al. Delays and errors in cardiopulmonary resuscitation and defibrillation by pediatric residents during simulated cardiopulmonary arrests. Resuscitation. 2009;80:819–25.
43. Mai CL, Szyld D, Cooper JB. Simulation in pediatric anesthesia. In: Cote CJ, Lerman J, Anderson B, editors. Practice of anesthesia for infants and children: Elsevier; 2013. p. 1089–96.
44. Ambardekar A, Singh D, Lockman J, et al. Pediatric anesthesiology fellow education: is a simulation based boot camp feasible and valuable. Pediatr Anesth. 2016;26:481–7.
45. Everett TC, Ng E, Power D, et al. The managing emergencies in Paediatric Anaesthesia global rating scale is a reliable tool for simulation-based assessment in pediatric anesthesia crisis management. Pediatr Anesth. 2013;23:1117–23.
46. Berkenstadt H, Ziv A, Gafni N, et al. Incorporating simulation-based objective structured clinical examination into Israeli National Board Examination in anesthesiology. Anesth Analg. 2006;102:853–8.
47. Ben-Menachem E, Ezri T, Ziv A, et al. Objective structured clinical examination of regional anesthesia skills: the Israeli National Board Examination in anesthesiology experience. Anesth Analg. 2011;112:242–5.
48. TheABA.org [internet]. The American Board of Anesthesiology: APPLIED (Staged Exams). [cited 2016, Sep 26]. Accessed from: http://www.theaba.org/TRAINING-PROGRAMS/APPLIED-(Staged-Exam)/About-APPLIED-(Staged-Exam).
49. Rosenblatt MA, Abrams KJ. The use of a human patient simulator in the evaluation of and development of a remedial prescription for an anesthesiologist with lapsed medical skills. Anesth Analg. 2002;94:149–53.
50. Haskvitz LM, Koop EC. Students struggling in clinical? A new role for the patient simulator. J Nurs Educ. 2004;43:181–4.

Simulation in Cardiothoracic and Vascular Anesthesia

17

Wendy K. Bernstein and David L. Schreibman

Introduction

For many years, resident physicians learned from actual patients in a graded operative experience, essentially a "see one, do one, teach one" supervised model. Competency was assumed to develop with time spent on clinical rotations designed to help the trainee demonstrate ability and proficiency with complex tasks prior to independent practice. However, in a high-stress operating room environment not necessarily conducive for teaching, this assumption may be ill-founded. In addition, unpredictable clinical occurrences prevent standardization of curriculum resulting in a learning experience difficult to structure and organize. Not every trainee can have a consistent exposure to similar patient encounters and medical conditions during their clinical rotations given that exposure to technical procedures is based on patient availability.

While this traditional apprenticeship model has served medicine moderately well for the past 100 years, societal pressures to enhance patient safety and changes in training regulations have demanded modifications in the way in which we train future physicians. In 2003, the Accreditation Council for Graduate Medical Education (ACGME) restricted house staff duty hours to address concerns that overwork and sleep deprivation were adversely impacting residents' ability to function well and effectively care for patients [1]. As a result, already inconsistent clinical exposure became further limited, reducing experience with certain clinical situations and procedural practice opportunities. It has now become difficult for trainees to "see one" in the case of certain rare events and procedures, let alone "do" the many competencies that are required in more advanced cardiac and vascular skills. Therefore, new educational modalities must be incorporated into training programs with an increased focus on competency-based education [2].

Simulation-based technology can provide a solution to this dilemma. Its widespread use in the field of anesthesiology enables repetitive practice for unlimited training opportunities. While, previously, trainees would learn advanced skills using patients as their practice model, with simulation technology, no patient need be harmed or placed at risk by inexperienced practitioners [3]. Trainees can practice clinical and procedural skills repetitively in order to better prepare for real clinical encounters. Simulation-based learning can also provide engagement in a controlled environment, accommodating a low-stress environment for both the trainee and the educator.

Use of Part Task Trainers and Skill Acquisition

Many skills required in anesthesia practice must be acquired through hands-on experience rather than traditional lectures, problem-based learning, or clinical performance examinations. Cardiothoracic and vascular anesthesiology requires complex skills that can benefit from task trainers which provide a promising alternative to bedside teaching. Part task trainers are simulation technologies that replicate only a portion of a process or system and serve as a precursor to computer-based simulation. Some of these skill sets include central line access, bronchoscopy, invasive monitoring, or other aspects of the management of complex cardiac, thoracic, and vascular cases. There is a variety of simulation-based technologies relevant to cardiothoracic and vascular

W. K. Bernstein (✉)
Division of Cardiac Anesthesiology, Department of Anesthesiology and Perioperative Medicine, University of Rochester Medical Center, Rochester, NY, USA
e-mail: wendy_bernstein@urmc.rochester.edu

D. L. Schreibman
Department of Anesthesiology, University of Maryland School of Medicine, University of Maryland Medical Center, Baltimore, MD, USA

B. Mahoney et al. (eds.), *Comprehensive Healthcare Simulation: Anesthesiology*, Comprehensive Healthcare Simulation,
https://doi.org/10.1007/978-3-030-26849-7_17

anesthesiology training including anesthesia management software, vascular access trainers, bronchoscopy simulators, full-sized mannequins, and cardiopulmonary bypass simulators.

With the training of technical or procedural skills, it is necessary to identify the abilities required, review the process to perform a procedure, develop a consensus on the sequence of the steps, identify major performance milestones, ensure that trainees acquire the skills for each step prior to advancement, define common complications, and design strategies to reduce frequency of errors. Curricula should be designed to support the achievement and assessment of these competencies through a multifaceted approach. Specific learning objectives must be planned and repeated to allow for assessment as well as focused learning which can be recorded and tracked through the duration of a residency or fellowship training. Furthermore, it is important to recognize that skill degradation occurs over time if interval practice does not occur [4, 5]. Simulation-based practice cannot be a singular event, but requires revisiting on a regular basis with active curricula, given the evidence showing improved retention through interval training [6].

Arterial Access Cannulation

Arterial cannulation is performed to accurately monitor arterial blood pressure in real time for cardiothoracic and vascular procedures. Approximately eight million arterial catheters are placed each year [7]. The proper insertion of an arterial line requires repeated practice which can be facilitated through the use of a model or mannequin prior to performance on a live patient. This practice may limit the potential for known complications of the procedure including hemorrhage, thrombosis, or arterial dissection while decreasing potential patient discomfort [8].

The arterial cannulation simulators currently commercially available are composed of an artificial upper extremity with tubing inserted under the surface of simulated skin (Fig. 17.1). Arterial pulsations are generated either from a manually squeezed bulb or a cyclic pump. These models allow for multiple punctures but require replaceable tubing. Cost estimates vary from $500–900 depending primarily on the mechanism of pulse generation. While these models are beneficial in allowing for repetitive practice, they have some disadvantages. These models are stand-alone and cannot be easily integrated into a high-fidelity, simulation-based scenario without requiring suspension of disbelief on the part of participants. Repeated use results in significant wear and tear creating obvious entry markings which can detract from the practice of anatomical landmark-guided catheter placement.

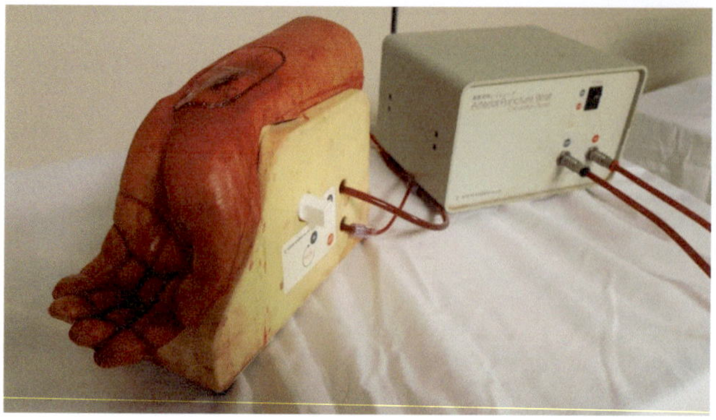

Fig. 17.1 The arterial cannulation simulator demonstrating a left upper extremity and corresponding pump which facilitates palpation of a pulsatile vessel in the radial artery

Central Venous Cannulation

Approximately five million central venous catheters (CVC) are placed annually in the United States [9]. CVCs have previously been placed blindly in patients using anatomical landmarks such as bony or muscular prominences and arterial pulsations. Studies have shown that anatomic variability accounts for an increased rate of known complications including hematoma, pneumothorax, and accidental arterial puncture [10]. Moreover, there is a negative correlation between the frequency of complications and operator experience with complication rates as high as 15% for those in the early stages of their training [11].

Over the past decade, the use of two-dimensional ultrasound (2D US) guidance has reduced the rate of mechanical complications and placement failure. Evidence has shown that 2D US-guided central line placement has been associated with decreases in punctures prior to successful cannulation, failed attempts, complications, and procedure duration [12, 13]. The Society of Cardiovascular Anesthesiologists (SCA) issued a statement designating 2D US guidance as the preferred method for CVC placement in both adults and children in elective situations and recommended consideration in emergency situations [14]. In addition, the Centers for Disease Control and Prevention (CDC) stated that US-guided CVC placement should be performed only by those who are properly trained and that efforts should be made to train those physicians who may be required to place a central line [15]. These factors, operator experience, and increased utilization of ultrasound guidance are clear indications for educational interventions using simulation-based training for CVC insertion.

Part task trainers for central venous access offer promising alternatives to bedside patient encounters. With this technology, trainees can practice sterile technique and master the manual dexterity involved with Seldinger technique, syringe manipulation, needle attachment, wire threading, dilation and catheter threading. In addition, cognitive components such as recognition of anatomic landmarks, familiarization with the contents of the central line kit, appropriate monitor placement, and vascular anatomy identification can also be achieved.

There are various simulation-based products commercially available to facilitate acquisition of the dexterity and skills required for CVC cannulation. Less expensive models have been created which significantly reduce the costs of training. These are equipped with compressible venous and more rigid arterial structures. While these models do not maintain ideal fidelity for patient anatomy, there is still great merit to their use. These lower-fidelity models can help familiarize the trainee with the use of ultrasound guidance and allow him/her to gain a greater understanding of the relationship between transducer frequency and depth of penetration to improve image resolution (Fig. 17.2). They also allow the trainee to facilitate needle placement and hand motion efficiency during the procedure.

More advanced mannequins allow the cannulation of internal jugular venous and subclavian venous sites in a more anatomically accurate model (Fig. 17.3). These models consist of tubing encased in a synthetic muscle and bony plate, sternal notch, and clavicular landmarks. The vasculature structures are created using bladders filled with artificial blood. The carotid artery can "pulsate" through the use of a manual pump. These models also allow for ultrasound guidance to facilitate a more realistic training experience.

Newer models have been designed to overcome the limitations of simpler mannequin-based designs allowing for a more "real-world" central venous cannulation experience. These models require simultaneous hand-eye coordination with concurrent interpretation of continuous physiologic data. By working with the full-size METI human patient simulators, the Louisville central line trainer simulates and coordinates physiologic output including central venous pressures and oxygen saturation. After CVC placement, left ventricular failure can be simulated with decreased contractility, increased left ventricular wedge pressure, and decreased cardiac output requiring institution of inotropic support and other supporting measures. In addition, this mannequin provides auditory output indicating patient discomfort or pain with catheter insertion as seen in CVC placement in the non-sedated patient.

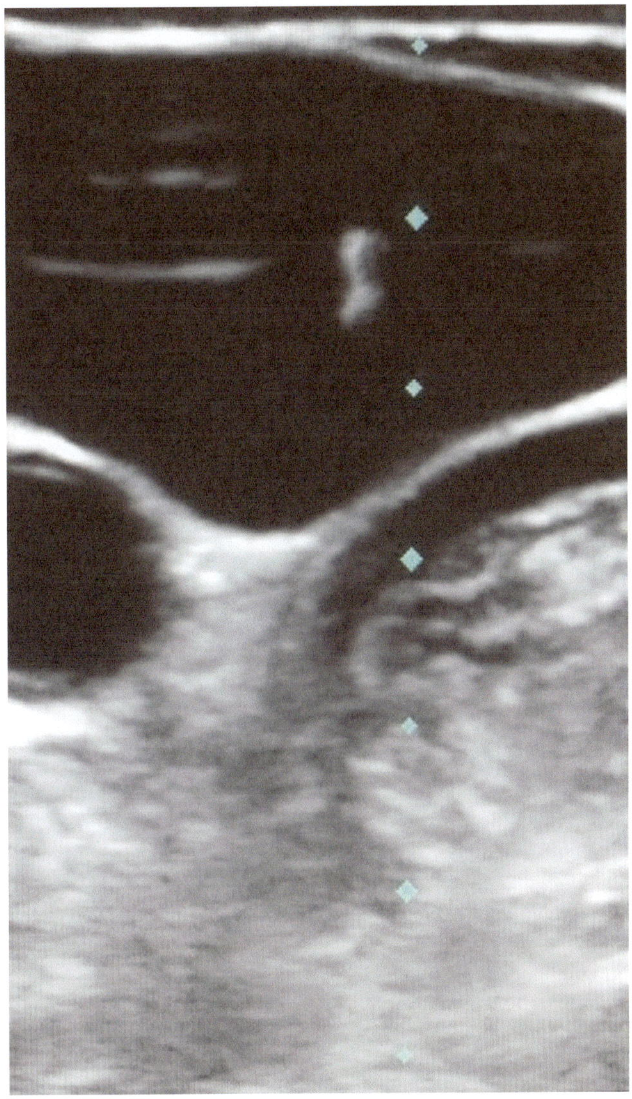

Fig. 17.2 Ultrasound image demonstrating placement of echogenic needle in compressible venous structure adjacent to more rigid arterial structure

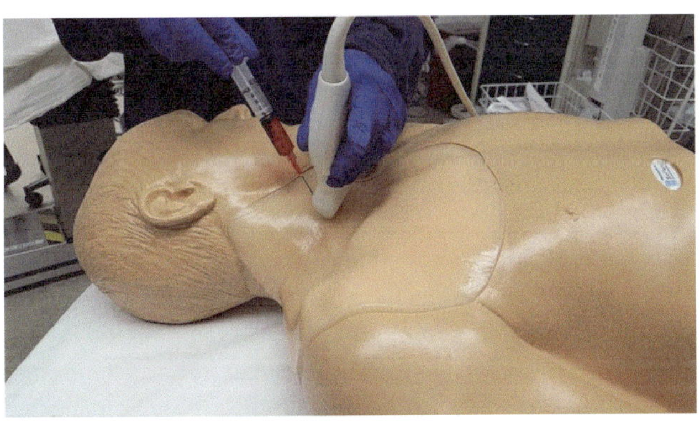

Fig. 17.3 Example of more advanced central line trainer which demonstrates a more anatomically correct model to facilitate practice of internal jugular or subclavian venous access using ultrasound guidance

Simulation-based training in central venous catheter insertion has been shown to improve performance in clinical practice. An observational cohort study of 103 residents in an intensive care unit demonstrated the beneficial effects of a simulation-based teaching program on resident skill. Simulator-trained residents were shown to have fewer needle passes, less arterial punctures, and a greater success rate at first cannulation compared to those receiving traditional didactic training. Those individuals who received simulation training also reported greater confidence in performance of the task [16]. Additional research has demonstrated decreased complication rates with central venous catheter insertion, reduced catheter-related bloodstream infections, and associated cost reductions following simulation-based training [17, 18].

Despite advantages of simulation-based education for CVC training in providing repetitive practice without risks to patient comfort or safety, major obstacles still exist for its widespread acceptance. Cost, limited space, ultrasound equipment availability, and a lack of trained teaching faculty can limit the implementation of this training model. There also remains a lack of clear recommendations for competency and proficiency training to establish the widespread implementation of US guidance in CVC placement.

Pulmonary Artery Cannulation

Cardiothoracic anesthesiologists must be capable of placing pulmonary artery catheters (PAC) and interpreting the hemodynamic information they can provide. PAC simulation can be easily accomplished using screen-based simulation tools that allow users to virtually insert the device and advance the catheter after balloon inflation (Fig. 17.4). This method allows users to simultaneously view electrocardiogram (ECG) and pulmonary artery pressure tracings during PAC placement. The trainee can advance the catheter by clicking distance arrows on the screen, and corresponding pressure waveforms are displayed as the catheter travels through the various chambers of the heart. Specific messages appear within correct technique such as excessive duration of balloon inflation or withdrawal of the catheter with an inflated balloon. In addition to normal physiology, various pathologic conditions such as acute myocardial infarction, pulmonary hypertension and mitral valve regurgitation can be depicted through associated changes in pressure waveforms. This low-cost software allows the trainee to master waveform recognition while practicing at his/her own pace.

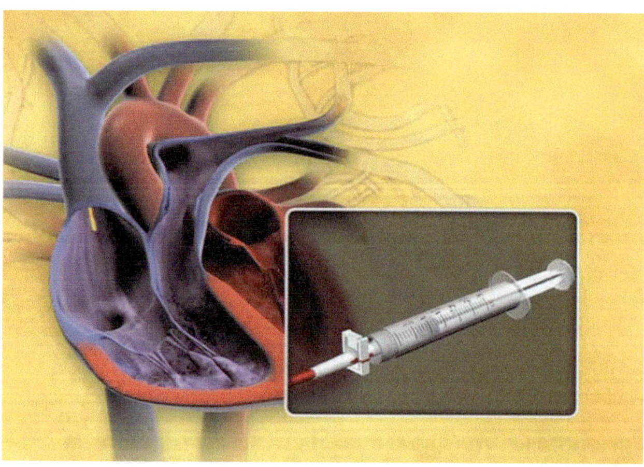

Fig. 17.4 Simulated computer-based pulmonary artery catheter (PAC) model that enables virtual advancement of this monitoring device into the pulmonary artery after inflation of the catheter balloon. Acknowledgment: Swan-Ganz pulmonary artery catheter; Edwards Lifesciences LLC, Irvine, CA

Other simulation-based models can be easily created allowing the trainee to *physically* place the PAC. By placing a large-lumen central venous catheter into a CVC trainer and simultaneously demonstrating the EKG and pulmonary artery pressure tracings on a computer monitor, the trainee can gain valuable experience in learning how to prep and drape the field for placement, understand how to prepare and troubleshoot pressure transducers, and experience the process of placing the PAC with enhanced fidelity.

Simulators for Bronchoscopy and Lung Isolation

With the evolution of minimally invasive and robotic heart surgery, there is a greater need for cardiac anesthesiologists to be facile in the use of fiber-optic bronchoscopy and techniques for lung isolation which are required to achieve optimal surgical exposure, facilitate gas exchange, and achieve differential lung ventilation [19]. Additional procedures that require the use of bronchoscopy include difficult airway management, diagnostic bronchoscopy, and pulmonary lavage. Given these indications and the infrequent need for fiber-optic bronchoscopy on an emergent basis, proficiency with bronchoscopy is a critical skill for the practicing cardiothoracic anesthesiologist.

Fiber-optic bronchoscopy requires both technical dexterity and a familiarity with bronchopulmonary anatomy. Hand-eye coordination is required to manipulate the scope to achieve maximal visualization and is achieved through repetitive practice. Furthermore, it is essential that the practitioner can recognize normal, variant, and pathologic anatomy.

There are many varieties of bronchoscopy simulators ranging from simple to complex with a range of cost, complexity, and educational utility. The simple models include easy to assemble box trainers which can be fashioned out of a cardboard box or a rigid box structure with an orifice [20]. This type of model improves endoscopic handling skills by teaching proper directional manipulation of the endoscope through a series of twists and turns as the trainee manipulates the fiber-optic bronchoscope through a custom-made obstacle course. Through this practice, the trainee can improve endoscopic manipulation skills and hand-eye coordination in a manner ideally transferable to the clinical arena. Using this model, Naik was able to demonstrate improved bronchoscopic performance in subjects after simulation-based training compared to learners receiving traditional training [21].These first-year anesthesiology residents receiving simulation-based training were also able to intubate more quickly and successfully, outperforming those who received didactic instruction. Although effective, these models meet limited learning objectives and lack incentive for practice given their absence of anatomic representation.

Virtual Bronchoscopy Simulators

Advanced computer hardware and software technologies have offered more realistic training environments through screen-based virtual reality (VR) simulator technology. AccuTouch by Immersion is a computerized virtual reality-simulated bronchoscopy product (Immersion Medical, Gaithersburg, Maryland) (Fig. 17.5). It consists of a flexible bronchoscope, a robotic interface with an orifice for entry, a monitor display, and a software which integrates user manipulation with a dynamic monitor display of anatomy to simulate clinical fiber-optic bronchoscopy. The operator can insert the bronchoscope into the interface coinciding with the appearance of an anatomically correct image on the screen of the airway as the scope is advanced. This anatomy is generated through data derived from the three-dimensional computer-generated model of the airway from the National Library of Medicine's Visible Human Project [22]. As the operator moves the bronchoscope further into the airway, images on the screen change in real time, corresponding to movements of the bronchoscope along the path of the virtual airway. This model is unique due to the haptic sensations the operator encounters as the scope is initially advanced into the oral opening associated with virtual patient responses such as rapid breathing and coughing. To simulate bronchoscopy for patients under general anesthesia, these features can be disabled.

This model contains four learning modules including an introduction to bronchoscopy, bronchoalveolar lavage, transbronchial needle aspiration, and difficult pediatric airway. Users can track performance, such as speed of passage through the airways, amount of local anesthestic used, and thoroughness of their bronchoscopic examination [23].

Bronchoscopy simulators have been shown to improve fiber-optic bronchoscopy skill and skill transfer in the clinical setting. Specifically research has shown that the use of this virtual reality simulator has led to significant improvements in the bronchoscopy skills of novices [24, 25]. Blum was able to demonstrate that novices trained with the virtual bronchoscopy simulator were able to perform intraoperative bronchoscopy more thoroughly than their counterparts who did not

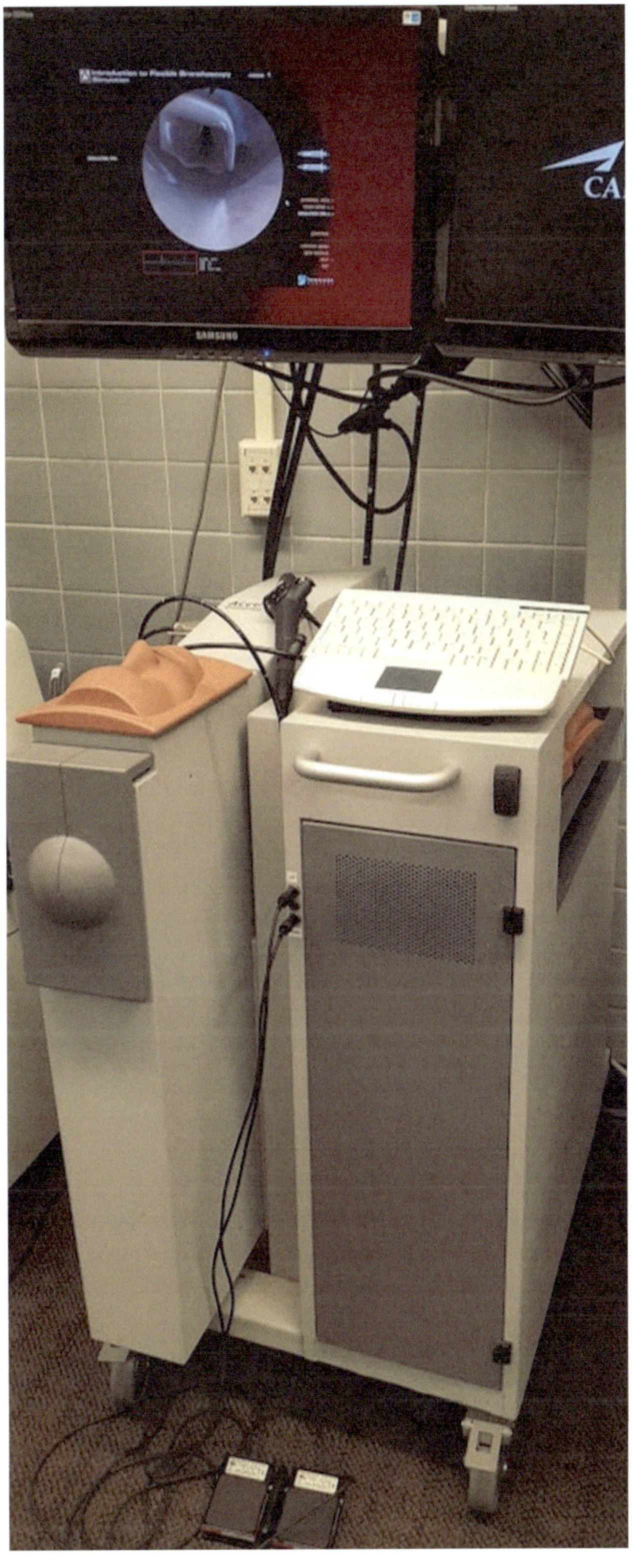

Fig. 17.5 A virtual reality bronchoscopy simulator (AccuTouch by Immersion Medical, Gaithersburg, Maryland) which consists of a flexible bronchoscope, a robotic interface with entry orifice, and a computer monitor with simulation software

receive training and possessed a comparable skill level when compared to more experienced residents. Colt et al. (2001) demonstrated that novice trainees practicing on a virtual trainer perform equal to or exceeded the expertise of skilled attending physicians with several years of experience [26]. In surgical training, the use of VR simulation with laparoscopic trainers was also shown to significantly improve the operative performance of residents versus their counterparts not trained with virtual reality simulation technology [27]. This research validates the transfer of procedural skill from VR to OR and sets the stage for more sophisticated uses of VR for assessment, training, error reduction, and certification.

Interestingly, not only do trainees who learn via simulation-based tools perform better in clinical situations, they also feel better and more confident in their abilities. Failor et al. studied 13 anesthesiology residents in a prospective observational trial to evaluate the effectiveness of the AirSim Bronchi simulator in teaching residents to manage complications of lung isolation [28]. The resident confidence scores in placing and managing double-lumen endotracheal tubes and bronchial blockers significantly increased after the simulation-based training.

While virtual bronchoscopy simulators can be an effective and novel training tool to improve training, efficiency, and ultimately patient safety, they are extremely expensive with a cost averaging $30,000. Moreover, there are currently no formal competency assessments for credentialing and no formal guidelines for assessment of bronchoscopy skills developed and universally accepted.

Transesophageal Echocardiography Simulators

Transesophageal echocardiography (TEE) is an essential skill for the cardiac anesthesiologist for diagnosis and monitoring of patient hemodynamics during both cardiac and noncardiac surgeries. Expert echocardiographic image acquisition requires repetitive practice and refinement of skills along with a high degree of manual dexterity.

Constraints to exposure during training due to limited time spent in the operating room, a variable number of relevant surgical cases, and lack of experienced and certified teaching faculty may limit perioperative TEE skill acquisition. Furthermore, given the nature of providing intraoperative care for a complex cardiac patient, skilled faculty can find it difficult to teach TEE skills while attending to patient care. Acquisition of skills for the new learner in TEE requires expert certified instructors, expensive equipment, and adequate time devoted to the performance and interpretation of the TEE images. Potential risks to the patient in terms of esophageal injury by an inexperienced operator also add ethical considerations in training.

Simulation-based TEE products can serve as ideal teaching tools for the cardiac anesthesiologist learning and practicing this complex skill [29]. Advanced computer hardware and software technologies have enabled realistic, simulation-based training through screen-based virtual reality technology. TEE simulators that show computer-controlled ultrasound images of an anatomically correct beating three-dimensional heart along with the image plane and location of the TEE probe tip have been developed for training in both transthoracic and transesophageal echocardiographies (Fig. 17.6). The Vimedix simulator by CAE Healthcare is an example of a TEE simulator that also incorporates a variety of pathological disease states including cardiac tamponade, mitral valve prolapse, aortic stenosis, and intracardiac masses. Screen images change appropriately as the trainee advances and manipulates the probe through the various planes of the echocardiographic exam. This system allows for an improved understanding of the scan planes as the heart model can be rotated and viewed from multiple perspectives.

Using these simulation-based technologies, trainees can practice TEE in a stress-free environment without the time constraints inherent in the operating room. Trainees' probe manipulation skills and clinical judgment can also be assessed [29]. Performance metrics are based on expert-acquired images of standard TEE views which are stored in the software. While training, the user is tasked with generating a view similar to these expert-acquired image combining their understanding of cardiac anatomy with their proficiency in probe manipulation. User-initiated probe movements made to generate images are tracked, assessed, and compared to past performances to obtain a comparative longitudinal evaluation of proficiency in image acquisition [30, 31].

There are few trials addressing the benefits of simulation-based echocardiographic training. Many incorporating echocardiographic simulators have involved small samples and have utilized computer-based assessment or self-evaluation

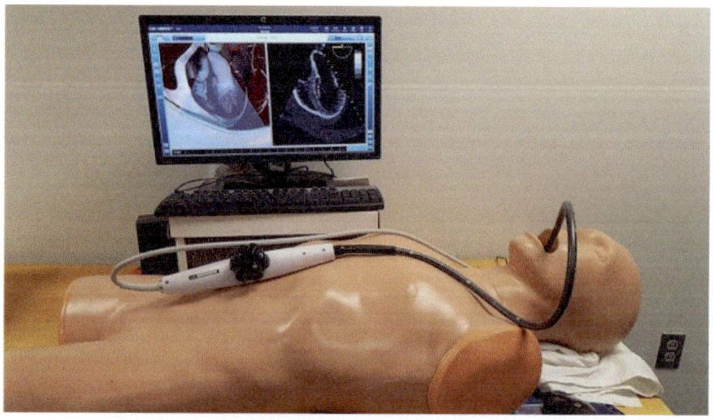

Fig. 17.6 The transesophageal echocardiography simulator is a valuable trainer for the cardiothoracic anesthesiologist to acquire the skills to diagnose and monitor the patient's hemodynamics during both cardiac and noncardiac surgeries

after simulation-based training [32–34]. One trial compared simulation-based training with traditional TEE teaching methods to determine transferability of simulation-based training methods to intraoperative TEE examination and image acquisition [35]. This research demonstrated an improved ability to obtain higher-quality images when performing standard views on a live anesthetized patient following training with a mannequin-based TEE simulator compared to a group receiving traditional didactic training. There is currently no data in a large prospective randomized trial to support the hypothesis that simulation-based TEE training improves patient outcomes or decreases the incidence of adverse events.

While TEE simulators have allowed trainees to gain valuable practice time without risk to actual patients, there is still room for improvement in its use as a standardized teaching tool. The high cost of these simulation tools may limit its use for many institutions.

Simulators for Management of Case-Specific Scenarios

There are specific screen-based simulation products for the training of cardiovascular anesthesia-specific case scenarios. Anesthesia simulator consultant (Anesoft, Issaquah, WA) allows trainees to manage scenarios such as mitral and aortic valve surgery, thoracic aortic dissection, carotid endarterectomy, and abdominal aortic aneurysm repair. These platforms are computer based (Windows and Macintosh) and focus on the cognitive skills involved in the management of the cardiothoracic or vascular procedure. The display includes dynamic electrocardiography, central venous and arterial pressure waveforms, pulse oximetry, end-tidal gas analysis, capnography, and pharmacologic infusions. Screen-displayed tabs are available to select patient monitors and administer medications. Appropriate physiologic changes occur with administration of pharmacologic agents initiated through on-screen tab selection. Available scenarios have complications embedded into their scripting with failure to take appropriate corrective action resulting in a negative outcome.

These screen-based simulators allow trainees to experience and manage a case prior to arriving to the operating room and may enable trainees to better manage complications when they occur [36]. For this reason, several residency programs have mandated this learning modality as a component of their training requirements [37].

History of Simulation in Cardiothoracic Anesthesiology

Mannequin-based simulators for cardiothoracic anesthesiology have been in existence for over 50 years. Resusci Anne marked the beginning of widespread use of simulation for medical training [38]. Created in the 1960s, this low-cost mannequin was designed by Asmund Laerdal, a Norwegian toy manufacturer [39]. Resusci Anne enabled training for mouth-to-mouth ventilation for resuscitation, a technique that was proven to be superior for return of spontaneous circulation (Fig. 17.7) [40, 41]. Further modifications with the addition of an internal spring attached to the chest wall enabled the practice of cardiac compressions during advanced cardiac life support (ACLS) as well as training for airway and breathing. Though of limited functionality, Resusci Anne remains a precursor to modern medical simulators and remains in use today.

The Harvey mannequin was first demonstrated in 1968 for use as a simulator of patient cardiovascular physiology (Fig. 17.8) [42, 43]. This mannequin displayed blood pressure, bilateral jugular venous pulse waveforms, arterial pulses, and precordial impulses. A wide spectrum of cardiac diseases could be simulated by varying blood pressure, respirations, pulses, and heart sounds.

Harvey has been used for training a wide variety of learners, including medical and nursing students, interns, residents, and licensed practitioners receiving continuing education. The efficacy of Harvey as a tool for instruction has been studied extensively. In one trial, fourth-year medical

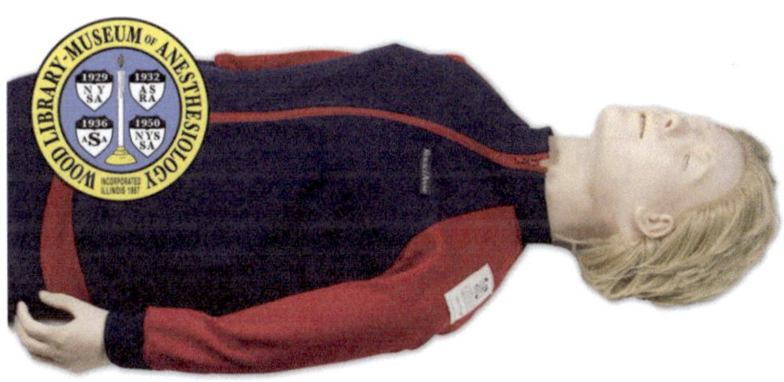

Fig. 17.7 The first mannequin, Resusci Anne, used for training in cardiopulmonary resuscitation, airway, and resuscitative skills. This low cost-effective training model is still used today. Image courtesy of the Wood Library-Museum of Anesthesiology, Schaumburg, Illinois

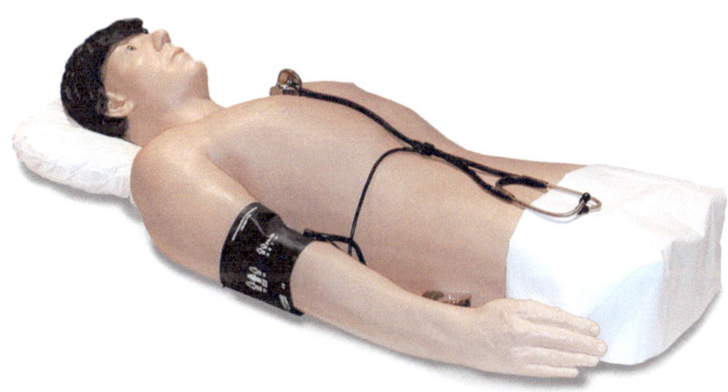

Fig. 17.8 Harvey, the cardiology mannequin, is a part task trainer for heart disease that teaches valuable clinical cardiac examination skills (image provided by Laerdal)

students trained with Harvey performed better on skill testing than their peers who interacted solely with patients [44]. In addition, students trained with Harvey showed increased confidence and ability to identify and interpret clinical findings at the bedside [45, 46]. Over the years, Harvey has evolved into a more comprehensive cardiopulmonary patient simulator with a curriculum that encompasses physical examination findings, laboratory data, and medical/surgical treatment.

More recent, high-fidelity mannequins with complex internal mechanics have the capability to present dynamic blood pressure, heart rate, breathing, respiratory sounds, heart sounds, as well as changes in pupil diameter and movements of extremities. These can display a wide variety of changes in vital signs and parameters involving the cardiorespiratory function and respiratory gas exchange in response to physiological or pharmacologic stimuli as seen in real patients. The use of these mannequin-based simulator models has provided an opportunity to practice patient care as a lone practitioner or as a member of a multidisciplinary team training in a realistic perioperative environment.

Life-Sized Mannequins

The newest life-sized simulators offer the most realistic training for full immersion into a clinical scenario. These include the Laerdal SimMan and the METI HPS which incorporate advanced internal mechanics with sophisticated software-controlled physiology that more accurately mimics the physiology of a real patient. The mannequins are driven by either a Windows-based PC platform (Laerdal) or both Windows and Apple (METI) with physiologic responses controlled by the operator or preprogramed as a response to the trainee actions (Fig. 17.9). Both models offer drug recognition software, Wi-Fi portability, and ultrasound capabilities for focused assessment with sonography for trauma (FAST). Monitor-displayed physiologic data includes pulse oximetry, capnography, electrocardiography, noninvasive blood pressure monitoring, and invasive central venous and arterial pressure waveforms.

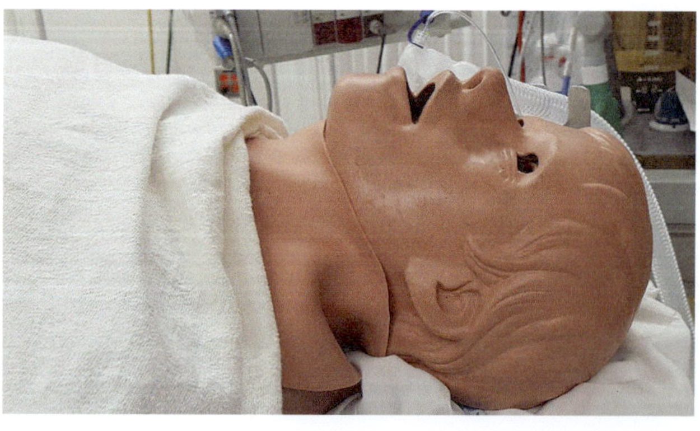

Fig. 17.9 Full-sized METI HPS mannequin offers realistic training for full immersion into clinical scenarios

Each model provides unique features to the simulationist engaged in cardiothoracic and cardiovascular anesthesiology instruction. The Laerdal SimMan contains a tracheobronchial tree that can support simple bronchoscopy and the insertion of double-lumen endotracheal tubes and bronchial blockers. However, anecdotal experience has demonstrated that left-sided double-lumen endotracheal tubes cannot be sufficiently accommodated to provide lung isolation due to a distal stenosis of the left main stem bronchus. Modifications can be made to accommodate this anatomic variation by changing the internal connector for the mannequin's left lung to safely accommodate a 35 French double-lumen endotracheal tube. Once placed, proper positioning of the double-lumen endotracheal tube can be verified by auscultations or fiber-optic bronchoscopy. The vital signs can then be adjusted to mimic physiologic response to lung isolation. Clinical situations such as hypoxia or bronchial obstruction can be simulated to teach the trainees the appropriate management of these conditions. Unfortunately, there will still be some suspension of disbelief on the part of the trainees who would expect a patient of average size to accommodate a larger double-lumen endotracheal tube for lung isolation.

The METI HPS model integrates software that produces vital signs output which closely mimics real patient physiology. Physiologic responses are produced through complex modeling in order that the mannequin appropriately responds to external stimuli such as administered medications, manual ventilation, and administration of oxygen. If the trainee performs an appropriate response to a clinical dilemma, the mannequin's condition will appropriately improve. However, given that physiologic responses with the METI HPS maintains a higher degree of fidelity through physiologic modeling as opposed to operator selection of specific vital sign output, extensive planning and testing for scenario development are required. The METI HPS also allows for the insertion of double-lumen endotracheal tubes; however, anatomic fidelity also ends at the bifurcation of the main stem bronchi, and mannequin adjustments need to be made to accommodate this method of ventilation and lung isolation. Furthermore, inaccuracies in the physiologic response to lung isolation need to be made through software adjustments to the capnography output or mechanical adjustment.

Given that physiologic parameters can be manipulated for both mannequins, a variety of anesthetic procedures specific to cardiovascular and thoracic anesthesia can be produced with a moderate degree of fidelity. Specific scenarios can be designed for multiple purposes: individual or team training, exposure to new anesthetic techniques, pilot testing for new systems to ensure efficacy and patient safety, addressing research questions regarding clinical behavior, and performance assessment.

Multidisciplinary Team Training

For many years, graduate medical educators and credentialing bodies had focused on technical skills and knowledge for training and evaluation of providers, with little appreciation of the importance of communication skills and performance as a member of medical professional teams. The contribution of human error and poor communication in adverse events, well known in the aviation industry, has also been shown to contribute to the majority of adverse outcomes in anesthesia administration, given the critical role of interpersonal and cognitive skills in delivering high-quality patient care [47, 48].

The benefits of simulation training for nontechnical skills, such as teamwork, leadership, and communication, have been established in both adult and pediatric critical care arenas [49]. Simulation training provides an engaging, high-fidelity learning environment that imitates the tasks, equipment, and environment encountered in the clinical setting of the cardiothoracic and vascular anesthesia environment (Fig. 17.10). As a safe environment for learning with no risk of patient harm, high-fidelity simulation-based team training allows for immediate feedback, maximizing learning. Given that many healthcare workers receive much of their clinical training as individuals with little training in teamwork, simulation-based training with well-scripted and realistic scenarios followed by a structured debrief can provide an education tool that delivers educational efficiency, curricular uniformity, and dynamic team-based interdisciplinary training [50]. It is essential to design scenarios with objectives focused on communication skills and teamwork for these sessions to be most effective [51]. Multiple investigators have described the use of mannequin-based high-fidelity simulation to enhance nontechnical skills, such as interdisciplinary teamwork and communication [52, 53]. This research shows participant find these experiences to be useful and would likely change their current clinical practice with regard to cognitive, social, and personal resource skills including situational awareness, decision-making, communication, teamwork, and leadership (Table 17.1).

High-Fidelity Simulation for Exposure

Simulation provides a safe way to expose trainees to high-acuity scenarios for patients undergoing cardiothoracic and vascular surgery. These simulated scenarios serve as a mechanism to address gaps in knowledge and better prepare trainees to respond quickly and appropriately when faced with critical clinical situations for the first time. Research has demonstrated the effectiveness of simulation-based training to improve physician performance in cardiac surgery, specifically during weaning from cardiopulmonary bypass [54]. Through the creation of standardized scenarios, simulation-based curricula can be easily reproduced and utilized by multiple educators intra- and interinstitutionally.

The importance of producing a realistic scenario that produces an immersive experience as participants interact with a mannequin that responds with appropriate physiology cannot be overemphasized. Additionally, making use of equipment similar to that which participants use in their standard clinical practice serves to maximize scenario fidelity and utility. Learners with the opportunity to engage in simulated clinical practice which achieves a high-degree of fidelity to setting, equipment, and patient physiology will

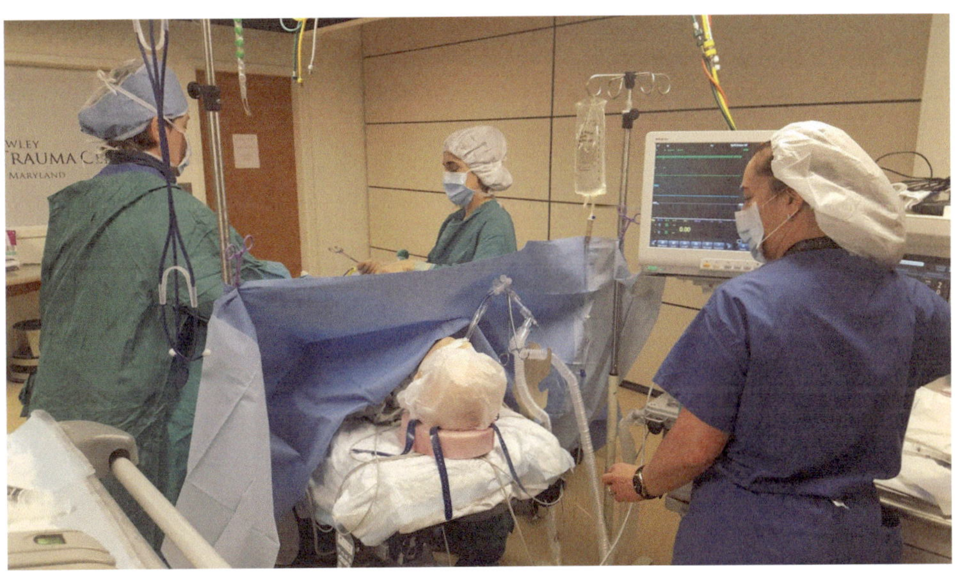

Fig. 17.10 Simulation training provides a multidisciplinary team training learning environment that replicates the tasks, equipment, and perioperative environment encountered in the real operating room environment. Here is a scene from a simulated one-lung ventilation course focused on the complications of lung separation

Table 17.1 An example of a multidisciplinary team training event for the cardiac surgical operative team with objectives identified and the appropriate actions of the scenario defined to achieve those objectives

Title: Emergent reinstitution of cardiopulmonary bypass after severe protamine reaction			
Audience: Cardiac anesthesiologists, cardiothoracic anesthesiology fellows, resident, and CRNA Cardiac surgery attending, cardiac surgery fellow, and residents Cardiac surgical technologists and certified surgical assistants and students Certified surgical technologists and certified surgical assistants and students Certified cardiovascular perfusionists and perfusion students Operating room registered nurses Anesthesia technicians			
Objectives: To allow the members of a specialized multidisciplinary team be exposed to an emergent intraoperative high-stake cardiac surgical scenario which allow them to practice their roles during the reestablishment of cardiopulmonary bypass after a protamine reaction			
Medical knowledge: Work through a differential diagnosis for intraoperative hypotension in the cardiac surgery patient. Understand the potential adverse reactions that can occur after administration of protamine			
Communication: Demonstrate situational awareness. Acknowledge and communicate the hypotensive state of the patient; respond appropriately to perform roles for emergent heparinization, recannulation, and subsequent initiation of cardiopulmonary bypass. Use elements of crew resource management and TEAMSTEPPS such as call backs, closed-loop communication to ensure patient safety			
Patient care: Treat patient for potential causes of hypotension. Recognize and respond to the patient's need for emergent reinstitution of cardiopulmonary bypass			
Professionalism: Demonstrate shared mental models, mutual respect, and principles of communication			
Case stem: A 67-year-old male with coronary artery disease has just undergone successful revascularization of his three-vessel disease with left internal mammary artery (LIMA) to left anterior descending coronary artery (LAD), saphenous vein graft (SVG) to obtuse marginal (OM), and SVG to right coronary artery (RCA). He has easily separated from bypass without the need for inotropic support. Protamine has been initiated to reverse the heparin			
Scenario setup: Cardiac operating room Patient supine and under general anesthesia with anesthesia machine and standard ASA monitors, right arterial line, 9.0 fr MAC catheter, and PAC in right internal jugular vein. Monitors include arterial BP, pulmonary artery pressures (PAP), central venous pressure (CVP), electrocardiography, and pulse oximetry Heart lung machine Cardiopulmonary bypass oxygenator and tubing circuit Patient mannequin with surgical drapes in place. Venous and arterial cannulae intact Mayo stand, back table, cardiac surgical instruments and supplies Blood cooler available			
State	**Patient status**	**Learner actions**	**Operator**
Baseline	Adult patient under general anesthesia on OR table with cardiac surgical team in appropriate positions. Surgical field exposed. BP 104/64; NSR at 84 bpm; RR 12; AC 500 cc tidal volume; 100% O2; PEEP 5; isoflurane 0.8; O2 sat 100%; Temp 36.5 degrees celcius; PAS/PAD 38/17; CVP 8	Patient safely weaned from bypass; surgeon requests protamine administration and begins venous decannulation	Baseline conditions
Anticoagulation reversal	VSS	Anesthesiologist initiates protamine administration per surgeon request Surgeon and assistant controlling bleeding	Normal blood pressure and vital signs
Decannulation	Removal arterial cannula	Surgeon inquires how much protamine administered and removes arterial cannulation.	Normal blood pressure and vital signs
Protamine reaction	Hypotensive BP 80–90 systolic, tachycardic to 110 PAS/PAD increase to 57/24	Anesthesiologist recognizes hypotension and treats with fluids, pressors. Lab studies; consider transfusion	Simulation of protamine reaction with decrease in BP and tachycardia, increasing PAS/PAD
Progressive hypotension despite treatment and ventricular fibrillation ensues	BP 40–50 systolic	Communication with surgeon regarding ongoing hemodynamic instability	Worsening protamine reaction

Table 17.1 (continued)

Reinitiation of CPB	Ventricular fibrillation – -start open cardiac massage	Surgeon: Decision for patient to be placed back on CPB. Perform open cardiac massage as needed Anesthesiologist: Full heparinization Surgery and assistant with surgical tech: recannulate right atrium and ascending aorta; de-air and proper connection of lines Anesthesia and perfusion: confirmation of adequate anticoagulation	Orpheus to simulate asystole and absence of blood pressure
Ending point – patient on CPB with therapeutic ACT	Patient blood flow and pressure stable; normal hemodynamics on CPB	Initiation of CPB	Orpheus blood pressure and EKG parameters altered to mimic normal CPB
Discussion points:			
Who first noticed that there was a change in the patient condition? Was everyone aware that there was an issue? How was the problem communicated to the rest of the operative team?			
What are your roles during emergency recannulation and initiation of cardiopulmonary bypass?			
What challenges did you face? Were there issues with communication? Was there special equipment needed? Was it immediately available? What special concerns are there for immediately instituting cardiopulmonary bypass?			
What could be done to mitigate these challenges?			
Did you encounter any safety issues? How can they be resolved if future problems occur?			
Learner feedback			
At the completion of the debriefing, learners complete an evaluation form to evaluate their simulation learning experience			

perform more quickly and confidently, while learning with dated equipment, low-fidelity environment, or nonrealistic patient physiology can frustrate participants engaged in exercises less relevant to their clinical practice.

Toward the goal of maximizing clinical fidelity, several cardiac and vascular simulated surgical models have been designed with biological tissues [55]. Specially preserved and prepared porcine heart models with artificial blood flow can be placed into an artificial mediastinum allowing cardiac surgical trainees to learn basic skills of cardiac cannulation, on- and off-pump coronary artery bypass, aortic valve replacement, and mitral valve replacement [56]. Through the use of an Orpheus cardiopulmonary bypass simulator (ULCO Technologies, Marrickville, Australia), consisting of a hydraulic pump and electronic interface run through proprietary software, cardiac surgeons, anesthesiologists, perfusionists, and nurses can engage in team-based practice [57]. A variety of adverse events such as air emboli, cannula displacement, power failure, and protamine reactions can be simulated in order to provide multidisciplinary teams an opportunity to engage in crisis management of events specific to their practice.

Robotic-assisted surgical systems are achieving wider use in a variety of cardiac surgical procedures including mitral valve repair, epicardial pacemaker lead placement, totally endoscopic coronary artery bypass (TECAB), transmyocardial revascularization, and resection of mediastinal masses [58–60]. Successful deployment of the da Vinci robot (Intuitive Surgical Inc., Sunnyvale, CA) for cardiac surgery has demonstrated a shortened bypass time, aortic cross-clamp time, and hospital length of stay [61]. However, the steep learning curve of robotic cardiac surgery remains a barrier to its widespread acceptance. Simulation for robotic cardiac surgery provides a haptic and interactive display in a three-dimensional virtual field giving learners an opportunity to encounter challenges, pitfalls, and methods for successfully managing potential complications [62]. These computer-assisted telemanipulators are burdened by their tremendous size, weight, and expense (about $1 million) while lacking tactile feedback for the surgeon [63].

High-Fidelity Simulation for Assessment

High-fidelity simulation provides an opportunity to assess the clinical performance of a trainee in a scheduled, structured, and standardized setting. Metrics for assessment can be developed with simple checklists for performance assessment and for establishing benchmarks of performance and competency expected of trainees prior to progression to independent practice. Selection of ideal simulation scenarios and targeting of the most relevant practice parameters are vital in providing assessments which reflect true ability [64]. For any given simulation scenario, content experts should determine which specific actions are most important for the trainee to display to proper management of the simulated event. These checklist-associated actions may be weighted or assessed based on order or timing. Evidence exists showing superiority of this method to assumption of competence based on training case volume or time requirements in surgical procedures [65, 66].

Challenges

While the costs of running a simulation center have been significantly reduced over the years, this resource still creates a large financial burden for any department. The main drivers of cost include high-fidelity mannequin-based systems and simulation personnel. Additionally, for simulation-based learning to be successfully and widely adopted, compensation for participating faculty must be better defined. Training of junior faculty as simulation educators can play a role in enhancing resident and medical student education while also providing an avenue for faculty development. Finally, while collaborative efforts with other disciplines create logistical difficulties, these efforts result in an enhanced experience for participants and relevance to the clinical setting [67].

Conclusion

As the field of cardiothoracic anesthesiology grows in complexity along with a reduction in resident training hours and clinical training exposure, medical simulation has provided a means to "fill the gap" in clinical education. Providers can learn to manage increasingly complex clinical scenarios and perform a variety of procedures allowing our specialty the ability to produce highly competent clinicians despite the challenges. While many simulation-based tools have shown educational efficacy through research aimed at their validation, even those not yet proven can offer a means to improve training, educational efficiency, and, ideally, improvements in patient safety.

References

1. Accreditation Council for Graduate Medical Education. Report of the work group on resident duty hours and the learning. Environment. June 11, 2002; http://www.acgme.org.
2. Stodel EJ, Wyand A, Crooks S, et al. Designing and implementing a competency based training program for anesthesiology residents at the University of Ottawa. Anesth Res and Pract. 2015; https://doi.org/10.1155/2015/713038.
3. Morgan PJ, Cleave-Hogg D. A worldwide survey of the use of simulation in anesthesia. Can J Anesthesia. 2002;49:659–62.
4. Wollard M, Whitfield R, Smith A, et al. Skill acquisition and retention in automated external defibrillator (AED) use and CPR by lay responders: a prospective study. Resuscitation. 2004;60:17–28.
5. Jenison EL, Gil KM, Lendvay TS, Guy MS. Robotic surgical skills: acquisition, maintenance, and degradation. JSLS. 2012;16:218–28.
6. Wayne DB, Butter J, Siddall VJ, et al. Mastery learning of advanced cardiac life support skills by internal medicine residents using simulation technology and deliberate practice. J Gen Intern Med. 2006;21(3):251–6.
7. Scheer B, Perel A, Pfeiffer UJ. Clinical review: complications and risk factors of peripheral arterial catheters used for haemodynamic monitoring in anaesthesia and intensive care medicine. Crit Care. 2002;6(3):199–204.
8. Burns SM, Chulay M. Essentials of critical care nursing pocket handbook. American Association of Critical Care Nurses (AACN). New York: McGraw-Hill Companies; 2006.
9. Denadai R, Toledo AP, Bernades DM, et al. Simulation based ultrasound guided central venous cannulation training program. Acta Cir Bras. 2014;29:1678–2674.
10. Abboud PA, Kendall JL. Ultrasound guidance for vascular access. Emerg Med Clin North Am. 2004;22(3):749–73.
11. McGee DC, Gould MK. Preventing complications of central venous catheterization. N Engl J Med. 2003;348:1123–33.
12. Lampert M, Bodenham AR, Pittiruti M, et al. International evidence-based recommendations on ultrasound-guided vascular access. Intensive Care Med. 2012;38(7):1105–17.
13. Dodge KL, Lynch CA, Moore CL, Biroscak BJ, et al. Use of ultrasound guidance improves central venous catheter insertion success rates among junior residents. J Ultrasound Med. 2012;31(10):1519–26.
14. Rupp SM, Apfelbaum JL, Blitt C, et al. American Society of Anesthesiologists Task Force on Central Venous Access. Practice guidelines for central venous access: a report by the American Society of Anesthesiologists Task Force on Central Venous Access. Anesthesiology. 2012;116(3):539–73.
15. O'Grady NP, Alexander M, Burns LA, et al. Healthcare Infection Control Practices Advisory Committee. Guidelines for the prevention of intravascular catheter-related infections. Am J Infect Control. 2011;39(4 Suppl 1):S1–34.
16. Barsuk JH, McGaghie WC, Cohen ER, et al. Simulation-based mastery learning reduces complications during central venous catheter insertion in a medical intensive care unit. Crit Care Med. 2009;37(10):2697–701.
17. Barsuk JH, Cohen ER, Feinglass J, et al. Use of simulation-based education to reduce catheter-related bloodstream infections. Arch Intern Med. 2009; Aug 10;169(15):1420–3.
18. Cohen ER, Feinglass J, Barsuk JH, et al. Cost savings from reduced catheter-related bloodstream infection after simulation-based education for residents in a medical intensive care unit. Simul Healthcare. 2010; Apr;5(2):98–102.
19. Bernstein WK, Walker A. Anesthetic issues for robotic cardiac surgery. Ann Card Anaesth. 2015;18:58–68.
20. Bainton CR. Models to facilitate the learning of fiberoptic technique. Int Anestheiol Clin. 1994;32:47–55.
21. Naik VN, Matsumoto ED, Houston PL, et al. Fiberoptic orotracheal intubation on anesthetized patients: do manipulation skills learned on simple model transfer into operating room? Anesthesiology. 2001;95:343–8.
22. Eason MP. Simulation devices in cardiothoracic and vascular anesthesia. Sem Cardiothor Vasc Anesth. 2015;9:309–23.
23. Schaefer JJ III. Simulators and difficult airway management skills. Ped Anesthesia. 2004;14:28–37.
24. Rowe R, Cohen RA. An evaluation of a virtual reality airway simulator. Anesth Analg. 2002;95:62–6.

25. Blum MG, Poers TW, Sundaresan S. Bronchoscopy simulator effectively prepares junior residents to competently perform basic clinical bronchoscopy. Ann Thorac Surg. 2004;78:287–91.
26. Colt HG, Crawford SW, Galbraith OIII. Virtual reality bronchoscopy simulation: a revolution in procedural training. Chest. 2001;120(4):1333–9.
27. Seymour NE, Gallagher AG, Roman SA, et al. Virtual reality training improves operating room performance: results of a randomized, double –blinded study. Ann Surg. 2002;236(4):458–63.
28. Failor E, Bowdle A, Jelacic C, Togashi K. High-fidelity simulation of lung isolation with double-lumen endotracheal tubes and bronchial blockers in anesthesiology resident training. J Cardiothorasc and VascAnesth. 2014;28(4):877–81.
29. Song H, Peng YG. Innovative transesophageal echocardiography training and competency assessment for Chinese anesthesiologists: role of transesophageal echocardiography simulation training. Curr Opin Anaesthesiol. 2012;25(6):686–91.
30. Shakil O, Mahmood F, Matyal R. Simulation in echocardiography: an ever-expanding frontier. J Cardiothorac Vasc Anesth. 2012;26(3):476–85.
31. Matyal R, Bose R, Warraich H, Shahul S, Ratcliff S, Panzica P, et al. Transthoracic echocardiographic simulator: normal and the abnormal. J Cardiothorac Vasc Anesth. 2011;25(1):177–81.
32. Bose RR, Matyal R, Warraich HJ, et al. Utility of a transesophageal echocardiographic simulator as a teaching tool. J Cardiothorac Vasc Anesth. 2011;25:212–5.
33. Weidenbach M, et al. EchoComTEE-A simulator for transesophageal echocardiography. Anaesthesia. 2007;62:347–53.
34. Neelankavil J, Howard-Quijano K, Hsieh TC, et al. Transthoracic echocardiography simulation is an efficient method to train anesthesiologists in basic transthoracic echocardiography skills. Anesth Analg. 2012;115:1042–51.
35. Ferrero NA, Bortsov AV, Arora H, et al. Simulator training enhances resident performance in transesophageal echocardiography. Anesthesiology. 2014;120:149–59.
36. Nyssen A, Larbuisson R, Janssens M, et al. A comparison of the training value of two types of anesthesia simulators: computer screen-based and mannequin-based simulators. Anesth Analg. 2002;94:1560–5.
37. Schwid HA. Graphical anesthesia simulators gain widespread use. APSF.org 1996; http://www.apsf.org/resource_center/newsletter/1996/fall/graphsim.htm.
38. Winchell SW, Safar P. Teaching and testing lay and paramedical personnel in cardiopulmonary resuscitation. Anesth Analg. 1966;45:441–9.
39. Grenvik A, Schaefer JJ. From Resusci-Anne to Sim Man: the evolution of simulators in medicine. Crit Care Med. 2004;32:556–7.
40. Safar P, Escarraga L, Elam J. A comparison of the mouth-to-mouth and mouth-to-airway methods of artificial respiration with the chest-pressure arm lift methods. N Engl J Med. 1958;258:671–7.
41. Safar P. Ventilatory efficacy of mouth-to-mouth artificial respiration. Airway obstruction during manual and mouth-to-mouth artificial respiration. JAMA. 1958;167:335–41.
42. Gordon MS. Cardiology patient simulator: development of an automated manikin to teach cardiovascular disease. Am J Cardiol. 1974;34:350–5.
43. Gordon MS, Ewy GA, Felner JM, et al. Teaching bedside cardiologic examination skills using "Harvey," the cardiology patient simulator. Med Clin North Am. 1980;64:305–13.
44. Cooper JB. Taqueti VR. A brief history of the development of mannequin simulators for clinical education and training. Qual Saf Health Care. 2004;13(suppl 1):11–8.
45. Ewy GA, Felner JM, Juul D, et al. Test of a cardiology patient simulator with students in fourth-year electives. J Med Educ. 1987;62:738–43.
46. Woolliscroft JO, Calhoun JG, Tenhaken JD, et al. Harvey: the impact of a cardiovascular teaching simulator on student skill acquisition. Med Teach. 1987;9:53–7.
47. Schwid HA, O'Donnell D. Anesthesiologists' management of simulated critical incidents. Anesthesiology. 1992;76(4):495–501.
48. Stocker M, Allen M, Pool N, et al. Impact of an embedded simulation team training program in a pediatric intensive care unit: a prospective, single-center, longitudinal study. Intensive Care Med. 2012;38:99–104.
49. Figueroa M. The role of simulation. SCCM. 2015;. Retrieved from: www.sccm.org/Communications/Critical-Connections/Archives/Pages/The-Role-of-Simulation-in-Promoting-Multidisciplinary-Teamwork.aspx
50. Trehan K, Kemp CD, Yang SC. Simulation in cardiothoracic surgical training: where do we stand? J Thorac Cardiovasc Surg. 2014;147:18–24.
51. McGaghie WC, Issenberg SB, Petusa ER, et al. A critical review of simulation-based medical education research 2003-2009. Med Educ. 2010;44:50–63.
52. Paige JT, Kozmenko V, Morgan B, et al. From the flight deck to the operating room: an initial pilot study of the feasibility and potential impact of true interdisciplinary team training using high-fidelity simulation. J Surg Educ. 2007;64(6):369–77.
53. Paige JT, Kozmenko V, Yang T, et al. High-fidelity, simulation-based, interdisciplinary operating room team training at the point of care. Surgery. 2009;145(2):138–46.
54. Bruppacher HR, Alam SK, LeBlanc VR, Latter D, Naik VN, Savoldelli GL, et al. Simulation-based training improves physicians' performance in patient care in high-stakes clinical setting of cardiac surgery. Anesthesiology. 2010;112:985–92.
55. Feins RH. Expert commentary: cardiothoracic surgical simulation. JTCVS. 2008;135(3):485–6.
56. Feins RH, Burkhart HM, Conte JV, et al. Simulation-based training in cardiac surgery. Ann Thorac Surg. 2016; pii: S0003-4975(16)30773-1. doi:https://doi.org/10.1016/j.athoracsur.2016.06.062.
57. Morris RW, Pybus DA. Orpheus cardiopulmonary bypass simulation system. JECT. 2007;39:228–33.
58. Mierdl S, Byhahn C, Dogan S, et al. Segmental wall motion abnormalities during telerobotic totally endoscopic coronary artery bypass grafting. Anesth Analg. 2002;94:774–80.
59. Yuh DD, Simon BA, Fernandez-Bustamente A, et al. Totally endoscopic robot-assisted transmyocardial revascularization. J Thorac Cardiovasc Surg. 2005;130:120–4.
60. Bodner J, Wykypiel H, Greiner A, et al. Early experience with robot-assisted surgery for mediastinal masses. Ann Thorac Surg. 2004;78:259–66.
61. Jones BA, Krueger S, Howell D, et al. Robotic mitral valve repair. Tex Heart Inst J. 2005;32:143–6.
62. Coste-Maniere E, Adhami L, Mourgues F, Carpentier A. Planning, simulation, and augmented reality for robotic cardiac procedures: the STARS system of the ChIR team. Semin Thorac Cardiovasc Surg. 2003;15:141–56.
63. Talamini MA, Hanly EJ. Technology in the operating suite. JAMA. 2005;293:863–6.
64. Boulet JR, Murray DJ. Simulation based assessment in anesthesiology: requirements for practical implementation. Anesthesiology. 2010;112:1041–52.
65. Seymour NE, Gallagher AG, Roman SA, et al. Virtual reality training improves operating room performance: results of a randomized, double-blinded study. Ann Surg. 2002;236:458–63.
66. Ahlberg G, Enochsson L, Gallagher AG, et al. Proficiency-based virtual reality training significantly reduces the error rate for residents during their first 10 laparoscopic cholecystectomies. Am J Surg. 2007;193:797–804.
67. Fann JI, Feins RH, Hicks GL, et al. Evaluation of simulation training in cardiothoracic surgery: the senior tour perspective. J Thorac Cardiovasc Surg. 2012;143:264–72.

Simulation in Obstetrics

18

Erik Clinton and Rebecca D. Minehart

Introduction

Acquiring technical skills and increasing the necessary competencies in obstetric anesthesiology can be challenging in modern medicine. An increasingly well-informed and well-educated patient population can influence trainees and staff, as more patients become active participants in their care and may express preferences for the experience level of providers performing procedures. Contributing to this is the fact that patients often present to the labor floor healthy and remain interactive and conscious during their hospital course. The anesthesiology clinician must be responsive to the stresses not only of their environment but also of the patients and their fetuses [1].

Historically, competence in medicine was assumed to be a time-based accomplishment where years of mentorship would allow for the natural development of skills. In modern medicine, ethical questions have been raised by the implication that patients can be harmed by the learners' participation in skill acquisition en route to competence [2]. Medical simulation in obstetric anesthesiology provides an opportunity for skill acquisition in an environment more conducive to learning and without the risks to real patients [2]. Healthcare simulation with deliberate practice has been shown to be superior to traditional clinical education in skill acquisition [3]. In this chapter, we will review simulation strategies aimed at helping the learner achieve competence in skills, teamwork, and attitudes. We will address some of the difficult situations and challenges associated with simulation in obstetric anesthesiology and explore the process for performing simulation.

E. Clinton (✉)
Department of Obstetrics and Gynecology, Massachusetts General Hospital, Boston, MA, USA

Harvard Medical School, Boston, MA, USA
e-mail: emclinton@mgh.harvard.edu

R. D. Minehart
Department of Anesthesia, Critical Care, and Pain Medicine, Massachusetts General Hospital, Boston, MA, USA

Harvard Medical School, Boston, MA, USA

Labor and Delivery Simulation

The variety of acuity and overlapping demands of the obstetric patient creates a complicated system of care. The care of one individual pregnant patient can span multiple professions, disciplines, work shifts, and hospital floors and care units. The coordination of care across these areas requires multiple handovers and physical transfer of equipment, personnel, and information [4]. In addition, the prompt coordination of care between multiple disciplines in an obstetric emergency requires recognition and communication of the needs of both mother and neonate for effective care [5, 6]. Coordinating care and communicating effectively in this environment in a way that supports safety require shifts from our social norms of communication. The patterns of speech between care providers may also differ, further complicating the coordination of care for a patient [7]. Interprofessional simulation can recreate realistic healthcare settings and challenges allowing participants to build teamwork skills in a complex environment without harmful patient consequences. Interprofessional simulation training in obstetrics has been shown to improve self-efficacy, team efficacy, and team functioning [8].

Skill Acquisition

While mentorship remains an important part of anesthesiology training and a key part of skill acquisition, competence is no longer deemed to be a time-based

B. Mahoney et al. (eds.), *Comprehensive Healthcare Simulation: Anesthesiology*, Comprehensive Healthcare Simulation,
https://doi.org/10.1007/978-3-030-26849-7_18

accomplishment. A modern view of competence allows for an objective measure of the skills, attitudes, and knowledge desired to practice medicine. Competency-based practice has been increasingly the focus of training both at the level of the resident and post-residency training; however, most direct observation assessment tools have not been validated [9].

The assessment of competence is complex, and, although it may lend itself well to the acquisition of technical skills, more research is needed to determine how these assessments can be applied to more nuanced skills. These include intraoperative blood pressure management, volume replacement in maternal hemorrhage, and management of postoperative complications. One area where competence assessment has been shown to be effective in the translation of skill acquisition is in neuraxial anesthetic techniques. This applies directly to obstetric anesthesia as neuraxial blocks are some of the most common procedures performed in the obstetric anesthesiology setting [2].

Throughout the world, numerous guides for neuraxial anesthesiology have emerged as these techniques have evolved rapidly over the last 20 years. There remains a more limited complement of assessment tools for establishing competence as it relates to acquired skills. One of the challenges faced in creating this system is that hand-motion efficiency analysis, although objective, is expensive [10]. The Delphi method is a structured process for collecting and filtering knowledge from a group of experts through a series of questionnaires and feedback. An example of a Delphi-distilled checklist for ultrasound-guided regional anesthesia can be seen in Box 18.1 [10].

Box 18.1. Assessment Checklist for Ultrasound-Guided Regional Anesthesia. Adapted from Cheung et al. [10] All tasks are scored either "not performed," "performed poorly," or "performed well."

1. Proper positioning of patient
2. Correct placement of ultrasound machine relative to patient to allow easy visualization of both
3. Choice of correct transducer
4. Correct depth, gain, and focal zone choices
5. Holds the probe appropriately (3 fingers holding the probe and 1 finger touching the patient)
6. Knowledge or confirmation of screen orientation (i.e., which side of probe corresponds to which side of screen)
7. Scanning of anatomy and proper identification of target
8. Use of Doppler to rule out vascular structures (if applicable)
9. Appropriate needle alignment
10. Maintenance of needle tip image during advancement of needle
11. Efficiency of regaining needle tip position (PART maneuver)
12. Recognition of proper nerve stimulation at appropriate levels (if nerve stimulation used)
13. Ensure that current is not <0.2 mA (if current is used)
14. Ask for initial aspiration to rule out intravascular injection
15. Visualization of needle tip before injection
16. Ask for 1- to 2-mL initial injection to rule out intraneural and intravascular injection
17. Ask patient or at least look for signs of pain/discomfort
18. Ask for proper aspiration every 5-mL increment injection
19. Recognition of proper needle tip position
20. Perform appropriate needle tip adjustments

There remains significant debate over the most effective way to teach epidural, spinal, and combined spinal-epidural skills as these are widely believed to be some of the most difficult anesthetic procedural skills to acquire. There is increasing evidence that the cost of the simulation device and the acquisition of skills may not be directly correlated [11]. Additionally, there is evidence to suggest that the novice learner's performance may be impeded by a complicated simulation system. The terms "low" and "high" fidelity are often used, but are not well defined by technology or cost, limiting the ability to compare models and apply previous research. Haptics often becomes a focus for creating an ideal model; however, evidence suggests that guided mental imagery may be as effective at helping novice learners acquire skills for epidural placement [12]. We have created a guide for partial task training in spinal anesthesia for novice learners (see Box 18.2). There are many types of partial task trainers [13] available for purchase for more realistic-appearing models (with varying capabilities for neuraxial ultrasound use or neuraxial anesthetic type), and there are published reports of homemade models using a potato, a banana or other fruits, and other materials, each with unique advantages to consider [14–18].

Box 18.2. Spinal Checklist Developed at Massachusetts General Hospital, Department of Anesthesia, Critical Care, and Pain Medicine [19]

1. Position the patient on the bed in the sitting or lateral position. Support their arms on a stand if sitting. Encourage posture with back flexion (curling forward).
2. Apply NIBP, SPO2, and ECG.
3. Consider oxygen and sedation if appropriate.
4. Gather equipment (spinal kit, spinal medications, special needles, sterile labeling supplies, and sterile gloves), bring trash receptacle nearby, turn on OR lights, and position to help you see the patient's back.
5. Put on hat and mask prior to opening kit; make sure all others in immediate area are similarly covered with hats and masks.
6. Remove the kit from the outer plastic container.
7. Open kit to create a sterile field.
8. Open sterile items like medications and needles onto the sterile field.
9. Open sterile gloves.
10. Take off rings, watches, or hand jewelry.
11. Perform hand hygiene with alcohol-based hand sanitizer.
12. Put on sterile gloves. You are now sterile.
13. Find the sterilizing equipment (e.g., Betadine or chlorhexidine), and leave other parts of the kit alone (e.g., leave plastic sheet on top of tray as a barrier).
14. If using Betadine, make a small tear in the package, and pour some into the tray.
    (a) Discard the remainder of the Betadine pouch into the trash.
    (b) Prep the back with Betadine (three times, with a spiral pattern, starting from the center of the back and working outward).
    (c) Allow the Betadine to dry (approximately 3 minutes).
    (d) Do not wipe off Betadine before it is dry—this negates its antiseptic effect. You may "blot" some when the Betadine is tacky.
15. If using chlorhexidine (new literature supports use as first line):
    (a) Activate applicator by squeezing the wings, and do not touch sponge applicator on unsterile area.
    (b) Allow the liquid to fill the sponge (depending on surface area covered, you may need two applicators—please check packaging for details).
    (c) Clean the back with at back-and-forth friction scrub for 30 seconds (repeat with appropriate numbers of applicators, as needed).
    (d) Allow the back to dry.
16. Place the fenestrated sterile drape over the lumbar site, making sure to keep your gloves sterile. We recommend using the sterile drape to protect your fingers from contamination (this is easier to show than to describe).
17. Discard any remaining prep supplies, keeping the prep from contaminating the rest of the kit.
18. Lift plastic cover off the rest of the spinal kit.
19. Find your local anesthesia (usually 1% lidocaine), open the ampoule, and draw up 3 ml. Attach the 25-g needle and label your syringe.
20. Find your spinal syringe, open the spinal anesthesia medication, and dose the syringe correctly (usually a 5-ml glass syringe with a frosted tip). Use a filter needle or filter straw to draw up any spinal medication. Label your spinal anesthetic syringe.
21. Find your spinal needle and your introducer needle, if using. Check the spinal needle and stylet to avoid equipment-related error.
22. If the prep is dry, proceed to locate the interspace on the patient's back (may be done through palpation or using neuraxial ultrasound).
23. Use the local anesthetic to anesthetize the skin by making a skin wheal and find relevant landmarks (like spinous processes).
24. Wait a few seconds for the local anesthetic to work and test the patient's level of numbness by touching the tip of any needle to the patient's back while asking, "Do you feel this as sharp?" Use more or wait longer if the patient is not yet numb, and repeat as necessary.
25. Use the introducer needle to establish the direction of your needle.
26. Pass the needle into the spinal space, redirecting on subsequent tries as needed.
27. Don't advance the needle without the stylet "snapped or locked" in place.
28. Remove the stylet after detecting a resistance change (occasionally felt as a "pop" or a "give").
29. Confirm CSF flow. If no CSF flow, replace stylet and advance further.
30. Attach spinal syringe, and confirm free flow of CSF using a small aspiration of the spinal syringe, looking for birefringence (if using hyperbaric medications).

31. Inject spinal medicine, and consider using test aspirations halfway and when finished.
32. Remove drape.
33. Move patient to the preferred position for spinal spread (usually supine, but sometimes this isn't helpful or is otherwise not needed)—see http://vam.anest.ufl.edu/simulations/spinalanesthesia.php for spinal anesthesia simulations (requires free account creation).
34. Take off gloves before touching monitors/equipment (dirty when CSF and blood have touched them).

In Situ Team-Based Simulation

In situ simulation in obstetric anesthesiology is simulation that occurs in the actual clinical environment. Interprofessional or interdisciplinary simulation training has been shown to increase provider comfort in managing obstetric emergencies [20]. Although most simulations involving the members of the obstetric anesthesiology team will occur on a labor and delivery unit, they can also occur anywhere where pregnant or postpartum patients receive care, such as in the emergency department, on the postpartum or antepartum units, or in the main operating room. In situ simulation may offer some advantages over center-based simulation, such as uncovering latent systems errors; however, there are also unique challenges when performing this type of simulation [21]. In situ team simulation training in obstetrics should be designed to maximize education without placing patients or participants at increased risk.

Challenges in *In situ* Obstetric Simulation

Coordinating the scheduling of space and of personnel can be uniquely challenging. Patient volume or acuity, or the need to use predesignated space, can increase the risk of cancelling in situ simulations. This risk is likely higher if the simulation participants are simultaneously responsible for direct patient care [21, 22]. The volume and acuity of patient care can vary dramatically throughout a 24-hour cycle, making planning and execution frustrating for the simulation faculty and its participants. In addition, the time and resources needed for setup, mobilizing equipment, and cleanup can easily exceed what most simulation teams have available. Planning appropriate timing and flexibility among the simulation staff can help alleviate some of these issues.

Another common challenge with in situ simulation is maintaining a safe learning environment for participants [22]. Participants are asked to take risks in the service of learning during any simulation, often with an audience of peers or co-workers. In performing at the edge of their social comfort and clinical expertise, all participants may benefit from the in situ environment, which may allow for more authentic practice. However, the participants are voluntarily placing themselves in vulnerable situations which may be more comfortable for them in a closed or remote simulation center than in a clinical environment [23]. In situ simulation may present barriers to engagement of learners because of fears about the perceptions of co-workers, nonparticipant staff, and patients in the immediate vicinity. Psychological safety is crucial for learning and only occurs when participants feel safe enough to express their true thoughts [24]. Often a labor floor is a closed unit in which patient and family members are freely moving around. In many instances, advertisement of the impending in situ simulation activity to all of these relevant groups can help alleviate these challenges.

The time pressures of in situ simulation are not unique to scenarios involving pregnant patients, but they can offer some unique challenges based on the unpredictability inherent to certain labor and delivery situations.

Here are some suggested strategies for in situ simulation team training in obstetrics:

1. Create a program that occurs at a consistent time. The potential problem of acuity, staffing, and simulation resources can be more accurately tracked and adjusted with consistency in time and space.
2. Schedule participants, rather than having spontaneous simulations. This helps ensure all members of the group are present.
3. Protect time for debriefing (see Chap. 4 for debriefing structure). Solidify the learning points and allow the participants to leave the simulation with an improved sense of the major takeaway lessons.
4. Limit participation in the simulation activity to only the personnel who have been scheduled. Spontaneous participants and observers can challenge the safe learning container and potentially create confusion in clinical coverage.
5. Notify patients, providers, and other L&D staff of the time, location, and staff involved in the medical simulation.
6. Use safety phrases, such as "this is a simulation" or "this is not a simulation" when mobilizing resources during the designated simulation activity times. This helps prevent confusion when real-life demands need attention.
7. Use staffing in the simulation that mimics the typical coverage of the labor and delivery unit.

Communication

Lapses in communication have been shown to contribute to medical errors [25]. Breakdowns in communication of the obstetrical team can lead to poor team performance and have been implicated as contributing to maternal death in emergencies, specifically situations of hemorrhage [26]. A comprehensive team training curriculum can help build familiarity among team members, and there is some evidence that team members' familiarity with each other may be associated with better care [27–29]. "Speaking up" can be defined as requesting clarification or explicitly challenging or correcting a task-relevant decision or procedure. Failure to speak up when team members do not feel empowered to share their ideas, or when their ideas are shared but they are dismissed outright by their colleagues, is a frequently cited form of communication lapse [30]. Fears related to retribution or appearing "wrong," professional courtesy and deference to hierarchy, excessive familiarity, or lack of familiarity can all be factors that contribute to ineffective speaking up [31]. Given that the driving motive for outward voice is the desire to help the team provide the best patient care possible, simulation team training in obstetrics may be a critical part of practicing these behaviors [32]. Mutual respect serves as a foundation for effective team communication by allowing providers to exchange information in a manner that develops mutual understanding and ultimately is more likely to lead to consensus and an action plan [33].

Creating a Program

Educational initiatives and simulation training in perinatal care have been shown to decrease malpractice claim activity [34]. The Risk Management Foundation of the Harvard Medical Institutions Incorporated (Controlled Risk Insurance Company, CRICO) provides malpractice insurance for the Harvard teaching institutions and has been instrumental in fostering initiatives to support interprofessional simulation activities. In the past two decades, one goal of theirs has been to focus on cyclical education and training of providers in high-risk specialtics. Obstetrics and anesthesiology have been two specialties targeted by these training initiatives, and, as a result, an increased number of interprofessional curricula have been developed between the Harvard Medical School-affiliated Departments of Anesthesia and the Departments of Obstetrics and Gynecology. At Massachusetts General Hospital, we have created a curriculum to allow combined interprofessional team simulation sessions to be incentivized. As part of the benefit of participating in team-based simulation sessions, the providers can receive malpractice insurance premium reductions as provided by the CRICO Risk Management Foundation of the Harvard Medical Institutions (see Chap. 9).

The curriculum for malpractice premium reduction at CRICO-insured hospitals occurs on a two-or three-year cycle. Obstetric providers alternate between a 1-hour simulation activity and a 4–6-hour simulation course annually. Anesthesiology and surgical providers have simulation requirements rotating on a 3-year cycle; the first year requirement is participation in a 4–6-hour simulation course, and the other 2 years have requirements for 1-hour "booster" educational activities, one of which must be an interprofessional simulation session. At MGH, our 1-hour simulation activity is typically scheduled in situ and consists of interprofessional and interdisciplinary simulation sessions between obstetric providers, anesthesia providers, and nursing staff. Examples of scenarios that have been used in this simulation activity are listed in Table 18.1.

Challenges with in situ simulation can lead to avoidance of simulation activities that require multiple teams, many participants, other departments, and nonprofessional staff that participate in healthcare situations. To minimize the challenges of in situ simulation, while maximizing the ability to coordinate more complicated simulation scenarios, some teams may choose to perform some simulation activities in a simulation center. At MGH under the CRICO malpractice premium reduction model, our 4.5-hour simulation course is interprofessional and conducted onsite in our MGH simulation center, known as the MGH Learning Laboratory. Participants are scheduled and are relieved of clinical duties during this time. The use of the onsite simulation center allows for a larger, more diverse group of providers to participate without the challenges of in situ team simulations and without the additional costs of outsourcing the educational activity to an outside simulation center. Examples of simulation scenarios and participating staff are included in Tables 18.2 and 18.3.

Table 18.1 Current MGH interprofessional team training curriculum

Potential simulation scenarios for interprofessional team training in obstetrics
Shoulder dystocia
High spinal
Anaphylaxis and difficult/surgical airway
Postpartum hemorrhage
Hypertensive emergency/eclampsia
Umbilical cord prolapse
Uterine rupture
Maternal cardiac arrest and perimortem Cesarean delivery
Hospital facility emergency (fire)
Abruption with the need for transfer of patient for Cesarean delivery
Trauma in pregnancy with visceral injuries

Table 18.2 Considerations for participants based on simulation scenarios

Obstetric simulation scenario	Participant groups
Massive hemorrhage/Cesarean Hysterectomy *Potential learning objectives: Massive transfusion protocols, use of newer hemorrhage therapies, team-based communication, decision to proceed with surgical care, team roles, and coordination*	Obstetricians, maternal fetal medicine Clinicians, anesthesia clinicians, neonatologists, gynecologic oncologists, certified nurse midwives, certified surgical technicians, obstetric nursing staff, operating room nursing staff, patient care coordinator, blood bank personnel, police and security, anesthesia technicians, intensivists
Maternal trauma *Potential learning objectives: Multi-team organization and shared leadership, coordination of resources when time is limited, dynamic prioritization of multiple crises, massive transfusion protocols and use of emergency release products, use of emergency equipment*	Obstetricians, maternal fetal medicine clinicians, anesthesia clinicians, trauma surgeons, neonatologists, certified nurse midwives, certified surgical technicians, obstetric nursing staff, operating room nursing staff, patient care coordinator, blood bank personnel, emergency department clinicians, anesthesia technicians, intensivists
Maternal cardiac arrest in the labor room due to amniotic fluid embolus *Potential learning objectives: Decision-making regarding arrest and care, coordinating multiple teams*	Obstetricians, maternal fetal medicine clinicians, anesthesia clinicians, neonatologists, certified nurse midwives, obstetric nursing staff, hospital cardiac arrest code team, cardiologists, other consultants
Active shooter on labor and delivery *Potential learning objectives: Ethical considerations for provider and patient safety, decision-making regarding an active shooter, latent vulnerabilities in locked units, challenging communication*	Obstetricians, maternal fetal medicine clinicians, anesthesia clinicians, neonatologists, certified nurse midwives, obstetric nursing staff, patient care coordinator, police and security, employee support staff (e.g., psychologists, psychiatrists, social workers)

Table 18.3 Simulation outline

Characters	Narrative	Vital signs	
High spinal 1. Patient (mannequin) 2. Primary RN 3. Primary MD Time 0:00–2.00 min	32 YO healthy G2P1 at 39 weeks in labor, s/p recent epidural placement	BP 110/60 HR 90 RR 20 SpO2 98% on room air	[ ] Engage patient [ ] Assess for pain or discomfort
II. Above, + Anesthesia Backup OB Second RN Resource nurse Time 2.00–4.00 minutes	Pt begins to feel anxious and is having troubled breathing	BP 100/60, dropping to BP 60s/40s over 2 minutes HR 110, drops to 45 over 2 minutes RR rises to 30 over 2 minutes SpO2 98%–88% Fetal late decelerations	[ ] Patient distress [ ] Call for help/backup [ ] Verbalize hypotension, hypoxemia [ ] Communicate critical event [ ] Emergency manual [ ] Exam and vital signs verbalization to group [ ] Shut off epidural pump [ ] Initiate treatment for hypotension, hypoxemia
III Above + Additional RN support Second anesthesia Second OB provider Any available additional help ——— Time 4.00–8.00 IV All team member Time 8.00–10.00	Patient unresponsive, unconscious Event pause and discuss situation (mini-debrief) to ensure proper treatment (optional) ——— Recovery with support	BP 55/30 HR 45, drops to 30 if not treated RR falls to 0 when SBP drops below 60 Sp02 88%, falls rapidly to 40% if not bag mask ventilated and then intubated Fetal HR prolonged deceleration ——— BP 90/60 HR 70 Fetal recovery with restitution of maternal vital signs	[ ] Support hypotension/anaphylaxis kit [ ] Ambu bag and ventilate [ ] Ventilation support/hypotension management with epinephrine infusion or other appropriate available alpha-/beta-agonists [ ] Communicate patient is unconscious (to team) [ ] Verbalize fetal intolerance of hypotension [ ] Establish event manager [ ] Communicate possible causes of loss of consciousness and initiate plan for immediate care [ ] Code cart, defibrillator [ ] Emergency manual ——— End scenario with resuscitation and plan for supportive/intensive care while spinal regresses

Debriefing in Obstetric Simulation

Debriefing is a critical part of the learning process in any obstetric simulation [35]. The details and rationale for debriefing can be found in Chap. 4. In relation to obstetric team training, there can be challenges in debriefing both in the in situ environment and in a simulation center. The need to return equipment and release personnel to their healthcare duties can lead to shortened or omitted debriefing which not only sacrifices significant learning opportunities but also can leave learners feeling frustrated, angry, and deceived or experiencing numerous negative emotions. This can have a negative impact on their subsequent patient care and the growth and support of a simulation program as outlined in Moore's Strategic Triangle (see Fig. 18.1).

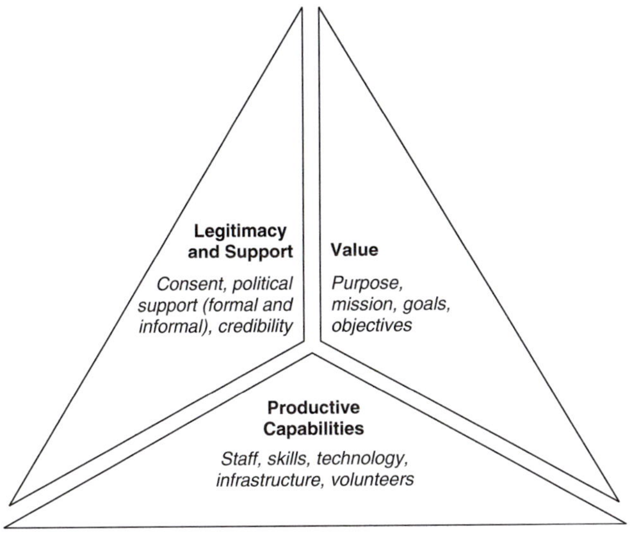

Fig. 18.1 Moore's strategic triangle

Co-debriefing can have many advantages over debriefing by a single facilitator. When debriefers represent different disciplines, such as obstetrics, nursing, and obstetric anesthesiology, they will naturally focus on different observations in the clinical scenario due to their unique training and backgrounds. They help engage learners of different role groups, who are similarly approaching clinical situations with different perspectives. Co-debriefers in obstetric team training can also help support each other in managing difficult debriefing situations should they arise, particularly in larger groups and interprofessional simulation activities [36] (Table 18.4).

Growing a Program

Plan-Do-Study-Act (PDSA) cycles can be used to improve the quality and safety of healthcare delivery. In medical simulation, PDSA cycles can be used for scenario development and in the planning and implementation of curricula and activities [37]. Although PDSA cycles offer a framework with which to start a simulation initiative, commitment and adherence to

Table 18.4 Sample obstetric scenario

Title: High spinal during Cesarean delivery		
Audience: Anesthesia resident		
Objectives:	*Medical knowledge:* Identify signs and symptoms of a high spinal anesthetic level	
	Patient care: Diagnosis and management of a high spinal anesthetic level	
	Communication: Utilize crew resource management skills to manage a clinical emergency	
Case stem: Ms. Jones is a 32-year-old, healthy, gravida 2, para 1parturient at 39 weeks of gestation in labor. Five minutes ago, she has had an epidural placed for labor analgesia		
Room setup: Labor room with patient in the left uterine displacement position following epidural placement. Epidural catheter present taped to the patient shoulder and an epidural medication infusion initiated		
The patient will have a noninvasive blood pressure cuff, pulse oximetry, and external fetal heart rate monitoring and tocometry present. A primary nurse and obstetrician serve as confederates		
State	**Patient status**	**Learner actions**
Baseline	Well appearing HR, 90; RR, 20; BP, 110/60; SpO2, 98% (RA); Category 1 FHT	The learner will introduce him/herself to the patient and care team Assess patient for pain or discomfort
Anxiety and dyspnea	Anxious appearing and dyspneic *(Over two minutes)* HR, 45; RR, 30; BP, 65/45; SpO2, 88% (RA) Late decelerations on FHT	Generate a differential diagnosis Communicate concern to the present team Call for help/backup care Discontinue epidural medication infusion Initiate supportive care for hypoxia/hypotension
Unresponsive	Unconscious/unresponsive *(If untreated over 2 minutes)* HR, 30; RR, 0; BP, 55/30; SpO2, 40%, prolonged deceleration on FHT	Support with positive pressure ventilation +/− endotracheal intubation Management of hypotension with epinephrine or other agents Communicate concerns with the team Recognize fetal intolerance and develop a plan for fetal support
Recovery	Unconscious/unresponsive *(after initiation of supportive care over 2 minutes)* HR, 70; RR, controlled; BP, 90/60; SpO2, 99%; FHT, recovery to baseline	Develop a plan for supportive/intensive care while spinal regresses
Discussion points: Differential diagnosis of acute hypoxemia and hypotension in the laboring patient, intrauterine fetal resuscitation, crew resource management on the labor and delivery unit		

cyclical assessment and change are difficult. One review article reported as little as 20% of the PDSA articles reported iterative cycles of change suggesting that learning from one cycle is often not used to inform future changes [37]. When applied to developing simulation programs and curricula, PDSA cycles should be applied rigorously to optimize improvements.

In developing a team-based obstetric simulation program, Moore's Strategic Triangle (Fig. 18.1) is often useful for deliberate growth and success. The model outlines a triad of interrelated concepts [38]. In developing an interdisciplinary obstetric team training program, "legitimacy" may constitute buy-in from division leaders, department chairs, and hospital executives. "Public value" in simulation curriculum development often relates to the education of providers, positive healthcare cultural changes, and improved patient safety. "Operational capabilities" may relate to creating or maintaining a simulation team, equipment, leadership training, and equipment. Investment in any individual portion of the triangle may fuel progress, and, conversely, weakening any portion of the triangle can have a profound negative impact on the overall success of a simulation program.

Kotter's eight-step model for change has been used to effectively promote practice changes in organizations, including the healthcare system [39, 40].Although this model can be useful in implementing change, determining the most crucial steps has proved to be challenging. There is evidence that not all steps are useful in initiating change in the healthcare setting, implying that some steps are more crucial in specific situations [41]. The use of Kotter's eight-step model should be tailored to local institutional culture and values, to meet the goals of your program's initiative (see Fig. 18.2) [42].

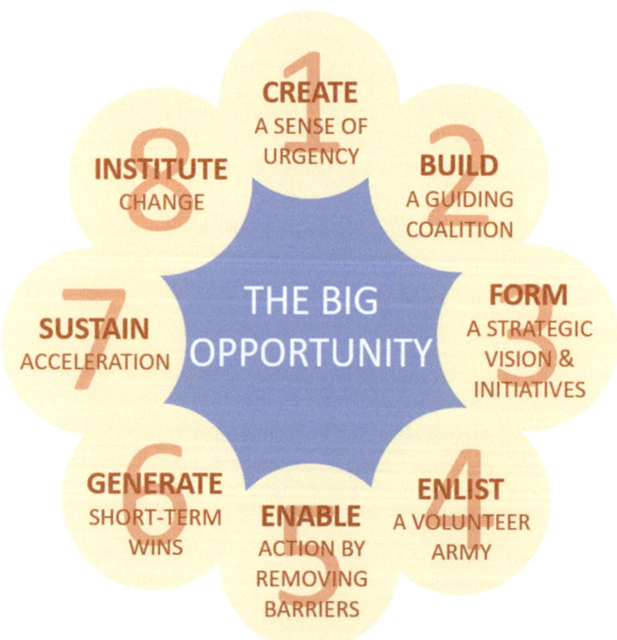
1 CREATE A SENSE OF URGENCY
2 BUILD A GUIDING COALITION
3 FORM A STRATEGIC VISION & INITIATIVES
4 ENLIST A VOLUNTEER ARMY
5 ENABLE ACTION BY REMOVING BARRIERS
6 GENERATE SHORT-TERM WINS
7 SUSTAIN ACCELERATION
8 INSTITUTE CHANGE
THE BIG OPPORTUNITY

Fig. 18.2 Kotter's eight-step model for implementing change [43]. (Adapted from Kotter (www.kotterinc.com))

Conclusion

Obstetric care is inherently team-based, and simulation provides enormous opportunity to not only practice rare situations but also to improve patient care through crisis resource management training, quality improvement initiatives, and creating a culture of respect and support. While challenges will continue to exist for implementing robust simulation initiatives uniformly on labor and delivery units, it is imperative to apply deliberate and time-tested models for sustained change.

References

1. Wenk M, Pöpping DM. Simulation for anesthesia in obstetrics. Best Pract ResClin Anaesth. 2015;29(1):81–6. https://doi.org/10.1016/j.bpa.2015.01.003.
2. Chin M, Lagasse RS. Assessment of competence: developing trends and ethical considerations. Curr Opin Anaesth. 2017;30(2):236–41. https://doi.org/10.1097/ACO.0000000000000431.
3. WC MG, Issenberg SB, Cohen ER, Barsuk JH, Wayne DB. Does simulation-based medical education with deliberate practice yield better results than traditional clinical education? A meta-analytic comparative review of the evidence. Acad Med. 2011;86(6):706–11. https://doi.org/10.1097/ACM.0b013e318217e119.
4. Austin N, Goldhaber-Fiebert S, Daniels K, Arafeh J, Grenon V, Welle D, Lipman S. Building comprehensive strategies for obstetric safety: simulation drills and communication. Anesth Analg. 2016;123(5):1181–90. https://doi.org/10.1213/ANE.0000000000001601.
5. Daniels K, Lipman S, Harney K, Arafeh J, Druzin M. Use of simulation based team training for obstetric crises in resident education. Simul Healthc. 2008;3(3):154–60. https://doi.org/10.1097/SIH.0b013e31818187d9.
6. Eason M, Olsen ME. High spinal in an obstetric patient: a simulated emergency. Simul Healthc. 2009;4(3):179–83. https://doi.org/10.1097/SIH.0b013e31819543e8.
7. Minehart RD, Pian-Smith MCM, Walzer TB, Gardner R, Rudolph JW, Simon R, Raemer DB. Speaking across the drapes: communication strategies of anesthesiologists and obstetricians during a simulated maternal crisis. Simul Healthc. 2012;7(3):166–70. https://doi.org/10.1097/SIH.0b013e31824e73fb.
8. Egenberg S, Øian P, Eggebø TM, Arsenovic MG, Bru LE. Changes in self-efficacy, collective efficacy and patient outcome following interprofessional simulation training on postpartum haemorrhage. J Clin Nurs. 2017;26(19–20):3174–87. https://doi.org/10.1111/jocn.13666.
9. Blum RH, Boulet JR, Cooper JB, Muret-Wagstaff SL. Simulation-based assessment to identify critical gaps in safe anesthesia resident performance. Anesthesiology. 2014;120(1):129–41. https://doi.org/10.1097/ALN.0000000000000055.
10. Cheung JJ, Chen EW, Darani R, McCartney CJL, Dubrowski A, Awad IT. The creation of an objective assessment tool for ultrasound-guided regional anesthesia using the Delphi method. Reg Anesth Pain Med. 2012;37(3):329–33. https://doi.org/10.1097/AAP.0b013e318246f63c.
11. Friedman Z, Siddiqui N, Katznelson R, Devito I, Bould MD, Naik V. Clinical impact of epidural anesthesia simulation on short- and long-term learning curve: high- versus low-fidelity model training. Reg Anesth Pain Med. 2009;34(3):229–32. https://doi.org/10.1097/AAP.0b013e3181a34345.
12. Lim G, Krohner RG, Metro DG, Rosario BL, Jeong JH, Sakai T. Low-fidelity haptic simulation versus mental imagery training for epidural anesthesia technical achievement in novice

anesthesiology residents: a randomized comparative study. Anesth Analg. 2016;122(5):1516–23. https://doi.org/10.1213/ANE.0000000000001260.
13. Vaughan N, Dubey VN, Wee MYK, Isaacs R. A review of epidural simulators: where are we today? Med Eng Phys. 2013;35(9):1235–50. https://doi.org/10.1016/j.medengphy.2013.03.003.
14. Moens Y, Lehmann H. The 'Epibox': a simple tool to train epidural injection technique in small animals. Vet Anaesth Analg. 2017;44(3):690–1. https://doi.org/10.1016/j.vaa.2016.06.010.
15. Leighton B. A greengrocer's model of the epidural space. Anesthesiology. 1989;70(2):368–9.
16. Paw HGW. A trainer for identification of the epidural space. Anaesthesia. 1995;50(10):914. https://doi.org/10.1111/j.1365-2044.1995.tb05871.x.
17. Tuckey J. The epidural potato! Anaesthesia. 1998;53(12):1232. https://doi.org/10.1046/j.1365-2044.1998.0716h.x.
18. van den Berg AA, Liao D. Teaching neuraxial analgesia: identification of loss of resistance (epidural) and intrathecal (spinal) placement of needles—avoid "making a lemon" of yourself. Anesth Analg. 2013;117(2):533–4. https://doi.org/10.1213/ANE.0b013e318296b956.
19. Charnin J, Kamdar BB, Minehart RD. Steps for placing a spinal anesthetic. Department of Anesthesia, Critical Care and Pain Medicine, Massachusetts General Hospital, last revised 11/8/2018.
20. Lutgendorf MA, Spalding C, Drake E, Spence D, Heaton JO, Morocco KV. Multidisciplinary in situ simulation-based training as a postpartum hemorrhage quality improvement project. Military Med. 2017;182(3):e1762–6. https://doi.org/10.7205/MILMED-D-16-00030.
21. Bajaj K, Minors A, Walker K, Meguerdichian M, Patterson M. "No-go considerations" for in situ simulation safety. Simul Healthc. 2018;13(3):221–4. https://doi.org/10.1097/SIH.0000000000000301.
22. Patterson MD, Blike GT, Nadkarni VM. In situ simulation: challenges and results. In: Henriksen K, Battles JB, Keyes MA, Grady ML, editors. Advances in patient safety: new directions and alternative approaches (Vol 3: Performance and tools). Agency for Healthcare Research and Quality (US): Rockville; 2008.
23. Rudolph JW, Raemer DB, Simon R. Establishing a safe container for learning in simulation: the role of the presimulation briefing. Simul Healthc. 2014;9(6):339–49. https://doi.org/10.1097/SIH.0000000000000047.
24. Palaganas JC, Fey M, Simon R. Structured debriefing in simulation-based education. AACN Adv Crit Care. 2016;27(1):78–85. https://doi.org/10.4037/aacnacc2016328.
25. Arbous MS, Grobbee DE, van Kleef JW, de Lange JJ, Spoormans HH, Touw P, Werner FM, Meursing AE. Mortality associated with anaesthesia: a qualitative analysis to identify risk factors. Anaesthesia. 2001;56(12):1141–53.
26. Jacobs PJ. Using high-fidelity simulation and video-assisted debriefing to enhance obstetrical hemorrhage mock code training. J Nurses Prof Dev. 2017;33(5):234–9. https://doi.org/10.1097/NND.0000000000000387.
27. Joshi K, Hernandez J, Martinez J, AbdelFattah K, Gardner AK. Should they stay or should they go now? Exploring the impact of team familiarity on interprofessional team training outcomes. Am J Surg. 2018;215(2):243–9. https://doi.org/10.1016/j.amjsurg.2017.08.048.
28. Kurmann A, Keller S, Tschan-Semmer F, Seelandt J, Semmer NK, Candinas D, Beldi G. Impact of team familiarity in the operating room on surgical complications. World J Surg. 2014;38(12):3047–52. https://doi.org/10.1007/s00268-014-2680-2.
29. Finnesgard EJ, Pandian TK, Kendrick ML, Farley DR. Do not break up the surgical team! Familiarity and expertise affect operative time in complex surgery. Am J Surg. 2018;215(3):447–9. https://doi.org/10.1016/j.amjsurg.2017.11.013.
30. Kolbe M, Burtscher MJ, Wacker J, Grande B, Nohynkova R, Manser T, Spahn DR, Grote G. Speaking up is related to better team performance in simulated anesthesia inductions: an observational study. Anesth Analg. 2012;115(5):1099–108. https://doi.org/10.1213/ANE.0b013e318269cd32.
31. Raemer DB, Kolbe M, Minehart RD, Rudolph JW, Pian-Smith MC. Improving anesthesiologists' ability to speak up in the operating room: a randomized controlled experiment of a simulation-based intervention and a qualitative analysis of hurdles and enablers. Acad Med. 2016;91(4):530–9. https://doi.org/10.1097/ACM.0000000000001033.
32. Okuyama A, Wagner C, Bijnen B. Speaking up for patient safety by hospital-based health care professionals: a literature review. BMC Health Serv Res. 2014;14(1):61. https://doi.org/10.1186/1472-6963-14-61.
33. Klipfel JM, Carolan BJ, Brytowski N, Mitchell CA, Gettman MT, Jacobson TM. Patient safety improvement through in situ simulation interdisciplinary team training. Urol Nurs. 2014;34(1):8.
34. Riley W, Meredith LW, Price R, Miller KK, Begun JW, McCullough M, Davis S. Decreasing malpractice claims by reducing preventable perinatal harm. Health Serv Res. 2016;51:2453–71. https://doi.org/10.1111/1475-6773.12551.
35. Rudolph JW, Simon R, Dufresne RL, Raemer DB. There no such thing as "nonjudgmental" debriefing: a theory and method for debriefing with good judgment. Simul Healthc. 2006;1(1):49–55.
36. Cheng A, Palaganas J, Eppich W, Rudolph J, Robinson T, Grant V. Co-debriefing for simulation-based education: a primer for facilitators. Simul Healthc. 2015;10(2):69–75. https://doi.org/10.1097/SIH.0000000000000077.
37. Taylor MJ, McNicholas C, Nicolay C, Darzi A, Bell D, Reed JE. Systematic review of the application of the plan-do-study-act method to improve quality in healthcare. BMJ Qual Saf. 2014;23(4):290–8. https://doi.org/10.1136/bmjqs-2013-001862.
38. Moore M, Khagram S. On creating public value: what business might learn from government about strategic management. Corporate Social Responsibility Initiative Working Paper No. 3. Cambridge, MA: John F. Kennedy School of Government, Harvard University; 2004.
39. Ellsbury DL, Clark RH, Ursprung R, Handler DL, Dodd ED, Spitzer AR. A multifaceted approach to improving outcomes in the NICU: the Pediatrix 100 000 babies campaign. Pediatrics. 2016; 137(4): e20150389–e20150389. https://doi.org/10.1542/peds.2015-0389.
40. Small A, Gist D, Souza D, Dalton J, Magny-Normilus C, David D. Using Kotter's change model for implementing bedside handoff: a quality improvement project. J Nurs Care Qual. 2016;31(4):304–9. https://doi.org/10.1097/NCQ.0000000000000212.
41. Chappell S, Pescud M, Waterworth P, Shilton T, Roche D, Ledger M, Slevin T, Rosenberg M. Exploring the process of implementing healthy workplace initiatives: mapping to Kotter's Leading Change model. J Occup Environ Med. 2016;58(10):e341–8. https://doi.org/10.1097/JOM.0000000000000854.
42. Baloh J, Zhu X, Ward MM. Implementing team huddles in small rural hospitals: how does the Kotter model of change apply? J Nurs Manag. 2018;26(5):571–8. https://doi.org/10.1111/jonm.12584.
43. Kotter JP. Leading change: why transformation efforts fail. Harv Bus Rev. 1995;73:59–67.

Suggested Reading

Palaganas JC, Epps C, Raemer DB. A history of simulation-enhanced interprofessional education. J Interprof Care. 2014;28(2):110–5. https://doi.org/10.3109/13561820.2013.869198.

Navedo A, Pawlowski J, Cooper JB. Multidisciplinary and interprofessional simulation in anesthesia. Int Anesth Clin. 2015;53(4):115–33. https://doi.org/10.1097/AIA.0000000000000077.

Simulation in Interdisciplinary Pain Medicine

19

Jesse T. Hochkeppel and Jordan L. Newmark

Introduction

The creation of any interdisciplinary pain medicine curriculum requires the identification of goals and objectives relevant to the learner. This applies to simulation and immersive learning techniques as well. A well-rounded approach to the learner targets three key aspects of interdisciplinary pain care: (i) high-quality interactions with patients and the team of care providers, (ii) acquisition of interventional skills, and (iii) well-coordinated crisis management. Developing these three areas requires interweaving fundamentals of basic knowledge, teamwork, professionalism, and procedural skills. Current simulation-based modalities available for use are wide ranging and include anatomical models or cadavers, tasks trainers, mannequins, standardized patients (SPs), computer-based modules, high-fidelity simulation (HFS) laboratories, or combinations of multiple modalities.

There are unique considerations that must be taken into account when developing simulation curriculum for interdisciplinary pain medicine. This includes the varied educational backgrounds of pain learners, as they may come from differing specialty backgrounds, including and not limited to anesthesiology, physical medicine and rehabilitation, neurology, and psychiatry. Another consideration is related to scheduling. Simulation can be an expensive teaching modality, not only to produce but in terms of lost clinical revenues during the training sessions. Lastly, it remains unclear as to the most reliable manner in which simulation should be utilized in teaching interdisciplinary pain care. These considerations necessitate an honest evaluation of efficiency and potential results when developing a simulation-based pain curriculum.

Pain simulation curricula and methods vary widely within the primary literature. This chapter will present an overview of the literature and describe present and future uses of simulation for interdisciplinary pain medicine teaching.

Patient Interaction Simulations

Direct patient interaction accounts for the majority of a chronic pain provider's professional time. These interactions not only involve the patients but can also include their family members, caretakers, and other healthcare providers. These discussions can involve challenging situations such as delivering bad news, discussing end-of-life care and goals, or managing combative behaviors [1]. Furthermore, chronic pain states are sometimes associated with mental health concerns which must also be appreciated and managed. Restrictions on the amount of time that clinicians can spend with their patients make it more challenging to optimize these interactions. Engaging in these sometimes difficult pain-related clinical discussions with clarity, efficiency, and empathy requires training and practice [2].

Despite the recognized challenges inherent to interactions with pain patients, there is currently no formalized education or training requirements surrounding these situations beyond random exposure. In a survey of 171 fellows in pediatric oncology and critical care, the exposure to role-play and simulation for difficult conversations was only 20% and 13%, respectively. This study advocated that simulation training can help prepare practitioners for difficult conversations [3].

J. T. Hochkeppel
Interventional Pain Management, Connecticut Pain Care/OrthoConnecticut, Danbury, CT, USA

J. L. Newmark (✉)
Department of Anesthesiology, Division of Pain Medicine, Alameda Health System, Oakland, CA, USA

Department of Anesthesiology, Perioperative & Pain Medicine, Stanford University School of Medicine, Palo Alto, CA, USA
e-mail: jnewmark@stanford.edu

B. Mahoney et al. (eds.), *Comprehensive Healthcare Simulation: Anesthesiology*, Comprehensive Healthcare Simulation,
https://doi.org/10.1007/978-3-030-26849-7_19

Furthermore, using simulated patient actors (SPs) for exposure to challenging conversations has the added benefit of reinforcing basic history-taking, physical examination, and communication skills.

Standardized Patients

The use of SPs for training with difficult conversations is directly applicable to pain medicine practitioners (see Fig. 19.1). A review of recent studies in this space provides sample scenarios and templates that can be utilized when building a simulated encounter with an SP for pain medicine [1]. These same studies demonstrate the importance of the debriefing process to augment the learning experience [1]. Learners self-reported improved confidence in handling difficult conversations after undergoing the training [1]. Separately, an interdisciplinary group from the University of Kentucky has developed a 2-hour Structured Clinical Instruction Module (SCIM) to teach clinical and interpersonal skills, referred to as the Cancer Pain SCIM. Eight workstations allow for multiple SP interactions, including opportunities to obtain patient history and physical examination and practice communication skills about analgesic treatment options, physical therapy considerations, cancer pain syndromes, and radiotherapy [4]. Although this course was focused on third year medical students, it provides a comprehensive template for a structured, high-yield intervention that can be adapted for pain practitioners of various educational levels and sub-specialties.

The value of SPs has been demonstrated for high-stakes assessment of pain medicine practitioners and trainees via Objective Structured Clinical Examinations (OSCEs). Pain-related OSCEs have been published and can help assess the ability of participants to engage in difficult pain-related clinical conversations, such as those related to palliative care [5, 6]. Interestingly, multiple studies have shown a poor correlation between empathy scores that were self-reported vs those reported by SPs, using the Jefferson Scale of Empathy [5, 6]. These examples support the utility of SPs for assessment in pain medicine training, while acknowledging how complex assessments of personal qualities, such as empathy, can be.

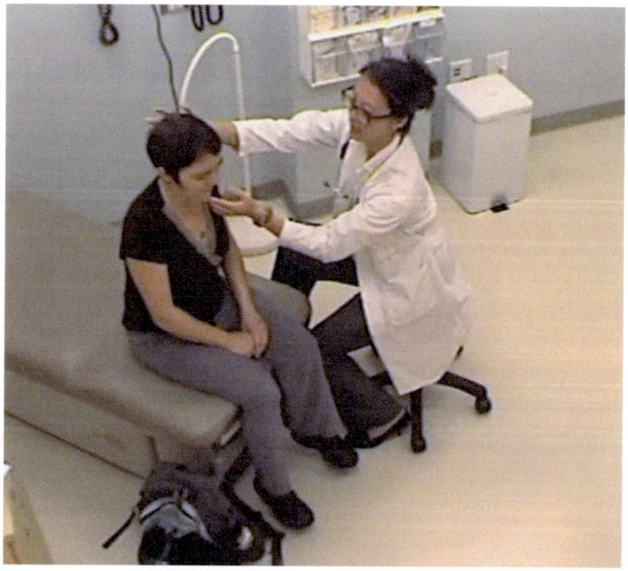

Fig. 19.1 SP-based pain simulation

Virtual Patients

Virtual patients (VPs) are computer and/or Internet-based patients, which are becoming increasingly popular as a simulation alternative to SPs. Once developed, VP-based programming is associated with lower operational costs, is more standardized, and eliminates the need for coaching and preparation of SPs. VP programming has the advantage of providing participant access at any time and thus can be used as part of an ongoing curriculum, as opposed to a scheduled workshop model [7]. The use of VPs in computer-based modules has varying formats, ranging from low-fidelity 2-D animation and text to high-fidelity video replication of real patient encounters [8].

Evidence in the current literature supports an important role for VPs in clinical training. Triola et al. evaluated the use of VPs as compared to SPs as part of a continuing medical education (CME) course for primary care physicians. There were no performance differences in clinical skills following the course between the two groups, suggesting a meaningful role for VPs in ongoing clinical training when compared to SPs [9]. Haglund et al. identified a gap in formal education about physician-patient interactions for neurosurgical trainees. To address this need, a formalized web-based module was created utilizing VPs with video examples of SP interactions for modeling various behaviors. These modules were incorporated into a neurosurgical "boot camp" training program, with participants self-reporting improved confidence and skill in patient communication [10].

VPs are also utilized to train practitioners with clinical assessment and to understand the patient factors that impact clinical decision-making. The VP modules incorporate facial imaging software to replicate different levels of pain expression [11]. Modifiable VP demographics such as age, sex, ethnicity, occupation, and economic status have been shown to impact clinical decision-making. There was further analysis comparing varied types of practitioners, as well as comparing treatment options [11–14]. In this provocative way, programming with VPs not only provides opportunities for practice but can generate data with which to frame reflection about bias and decision-making.

Interventional Skill-Based Simulation

Pain-related interventional skills are an essential aspect of training in pain medicine. The ethical dilemma of allowing a novice practitioner to learn and develop skills on real patients has been well documented [15]. Other than obvious patient care and safety factors inherent in this dilemma, learner considerations such as additional, prolonged radiation exposure should also be considered [16]. The benefits of procedure-based simulation training have been described in many arenas such as general surgery, neurosurgery, anesthesiology, critical care, robotic procedures, and endovascular image-guided interventions [17, 18]. Simulation can accelerate skill acquisition through repetitive and diverse exposure that may not be readily available, by chance, with real patients.

Utilizing simulation for interventional skills training requires an understanding of learner skill acquisition [19]. The component skills required to perform interventional pain procedures include a familiarity with anatomy, needle-driving technique, ultrasound guidance, fluoroscopic imaging, and open surgical techniques. The following discussion focuses on the current and potential future simulation modalities that can be utilized to teach these important skills.

Pain-Related Anatomy

A complete understanding of anatomy underlies safe and effective performance of interventional pain procedures. The two main simulation formats for learning relevant anatomy are reproduced physical anatomical models and computer-based anatomy programs. Basic anatomical models are easily accessible and are typically cost-efficient. These models range from very basic reproductions of anatomical structures to those with a high degree of realism. Commonly used pain-related modeled structures include the spine, musculoskeletal system, peripheral and central nervous system, and skull. Recently, high-fidelity reproductions have utilized 3-D printing technology based on real patient computed tomography (CT) images [20]. Low-fidelity anatomical models are most efficient as a task trainer for novice learners which allow for manipulation of needles and other interventional devices.

Interactive, computer-based, anatomical programs have the advantage of being accessed remotely at any time and utilized independently by the learner. One published study evaluated a virtual spine-based imaging platform for novice learners performing neuraxial, ultrasound-guided procedures [21]. They found that independent utilization of this program for 2 weeks prior to clinical performance enhanced structure identification and procedural acumen [21]. Further development of such computer-based simulation programs to include fluoroscopic imaging focusing on pain interventions could be of great benefit to practitioners in the field of pain medicine.

Needle-Driving Technique

Safe and effective needle driving is an essential technique for pain-related interventional procedures. Without simulation modalities, training is limited to clinical practice, which is less efficient and does not allow for repetitive, deliberate practice. To accelerate the learning process, Chen and colleagues explored the utility of a 30-minute session on a M43B lumbar puncture simulator for improving resident comfort and skill with needle driving. They demonstrated increased comfort and accuracy in needle driving among the participants when performing a similar procedure immediately following their training session [22]. Although this study served to validate a "warm-up" methodology for needle driving, the utility of such practice has potential benefit beyond this research paradigm.

Ultrasound

The use of ultrasound guidance is rapidly growing in the field of interventional pain medicine. This trend lies in the ability for ultrasound to provide real-time visualization of needle placement, visualization of critical anatomical structures, and sparing of radiation exposure to the patient and provider. A recent survey that was sent to 97 US and 4 Canadian chronic pain fellowship programs, with 31 programs responding, revealed 84% of programs were training their fellows in ultrasound-based techniques [23].

This escalation in use led to the release of a joint recommendation regarding education and training in ultrasound-guided pain procedures by the American Society of Regional Anesthesia and Pain Medicine, the European Society of Regional Anaethesia and Pain Therapy, and the Asian Australasian Federation of Pain Societies. With regard to fellowship-level training specifically, the recommendations suggest pre-studying web-based content, using oneself or colleagues to learn ultrasound scanning techniques and utilizing task trainers and cadavers for needle driving [24].

Given that cadavers are not always easily accessible, phantom technology is the most widely used application for nonhuman ultrasound training. The Blue Phantom (CAE Healthcare, Seattle, WA) is made with elastomeric rubber that provides tactile feedback while also preventing needle track marks from repeated use [25]. Some potential drawbacks of this modality include its high cost and a low-background echogenicity which makes target identification easier than in vivo.

Certainly these trainers have value for initial practice of procedures associated with a higher-risk profile. A recently published curriculum utilizes phantom technology for training of ultrasound-guided intercostal nerve blocks and stellate ganglion blocks in both novice and expert practitioners [26]. The results indicate improved performance and safety after participation in the programming [26]. Another report explored the role of tele-simulation for remote training on high-fidelity ultrasound simulators [27]. Tele-simulation enhances access to remote learners, enabling greater exposure to pain-related simulation training [27].

Fluoroscopy-Guided Interventional Procedures

Fluoroscopic imaging is the hallmark of many interventional pain procedures and a technique with which many novice practitioners have limited experience. At present, simulation of fluoroscopy for pain medicine procedures is limited. There is promise for development in the future, as high-fidelity fluoroscopy simulators are being developed and utilized in other fields, such as urology for training in percutaneous renal procedures [16].

Considerations for future development could include computer-based programs dedicated to pain-related fluoroscopy, as well as a high-fidelity virtual reality (VR) simulation that would enable interaction with a patient, operating room table, C-arm, and corresponding imaging. Another area for development is the use of fluoroscopically compatible mannequins (see Fig. 19.2) [28]. Using these mannequins in a procedure or operating room with a C-arm would enable high-fidelity simulation of imaging but could be limited by factors such as cost, space resources, and radiation exposure.

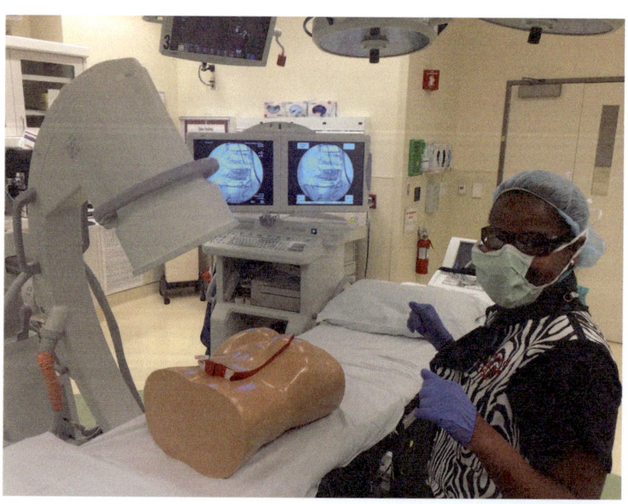

Fig. 19.2 Fluoroscopic, lumbar spine task trainer

Percutaneous Procedures

The majority of interventional pain procedures are performed percutaneously, with targets including peripheral nerves, joints and bursa, sympathetic ganglions, neuraxial structures, and other pain-related anatomic targets. Most procedures are performed in a procedure suite with concomitant use of imaging modalities. A very effective method for the simulation of such procedures includes utilizing part task trainers and part SP or VR [19].

Task trainers enable simulation of percutaneous procedures such as neuraxial and ultrasound-guided nerve blocks. Although they are not computer-driven, the proprioceptive feedback and anatomic accuracy enable a higher degree of fidelity that are beneficial in training for less complex procedures [29]. A task trainer with even greater utility in pain medicine is the AR 315 Adam Rouilly Pain Relief Manikin (see Fig. 19.3). It is fluoroscopy- and ultrasound-compatible. It can be used for a wide range of procedures including cervical and lumbar facet joint blocks, trigeminal ganglion blocks, epidurals at all levels, lumbar sympathetic blocks, celiac and superior hypogastric nerve plexus blocks, and sacroiliac joint injections [28]. Many studies have shown that less expensive and lower-fidelity task trainers can be just as effective [30]. Such low-fidelity part task trainers can be "homemade" by placing radiopaque paint on an inexpensive anatomical model and then immersing it in a homemade plastic cast, gelatin mold, or memory foam pillow. Lerman and colleagues have described such a model for cervical epidural injections [31]. A potential limitation of this study is that there is no evaluation of skill transfer to live patients or clinical decision-making, where enhanced fidelity may prove beneficial [31].

High-fidelity VR simulators present theoretical benefit for training pain practitioners in procedural skills, but their use is limited by availability and costs. The first haptic (tactile feedback) epidural simulator with computer control was developed in 1996 by Stredney et al. [28]. Since that time, VR simulators combining haptics with imaging derived from various sources have continued to develop. One example is the Common Platform Medical Skills Trainer (CPMST) from Touch of Life Technologies, which provides an immersive, high-fidelity environment for performing ultrasound-guided nerve blocks. Medical Simulation Corporation's (MSC) SimSuite neurostimulation simulator is another novel VR modality that uniquely employs virtual fluoroscopy for 3-D tracking of the needle, C-arm manipulation, programmable complications, and pain-mapping options that enable skill training for spinal cord stimulator (SCS) placement. Creation of high-fidelity environments for interventional skill training involving simulated procedural suites with a functioning operation table and control panel, integrated C-arm, and VR simulation has been described in the literature and utilized in multiple specialties [32].

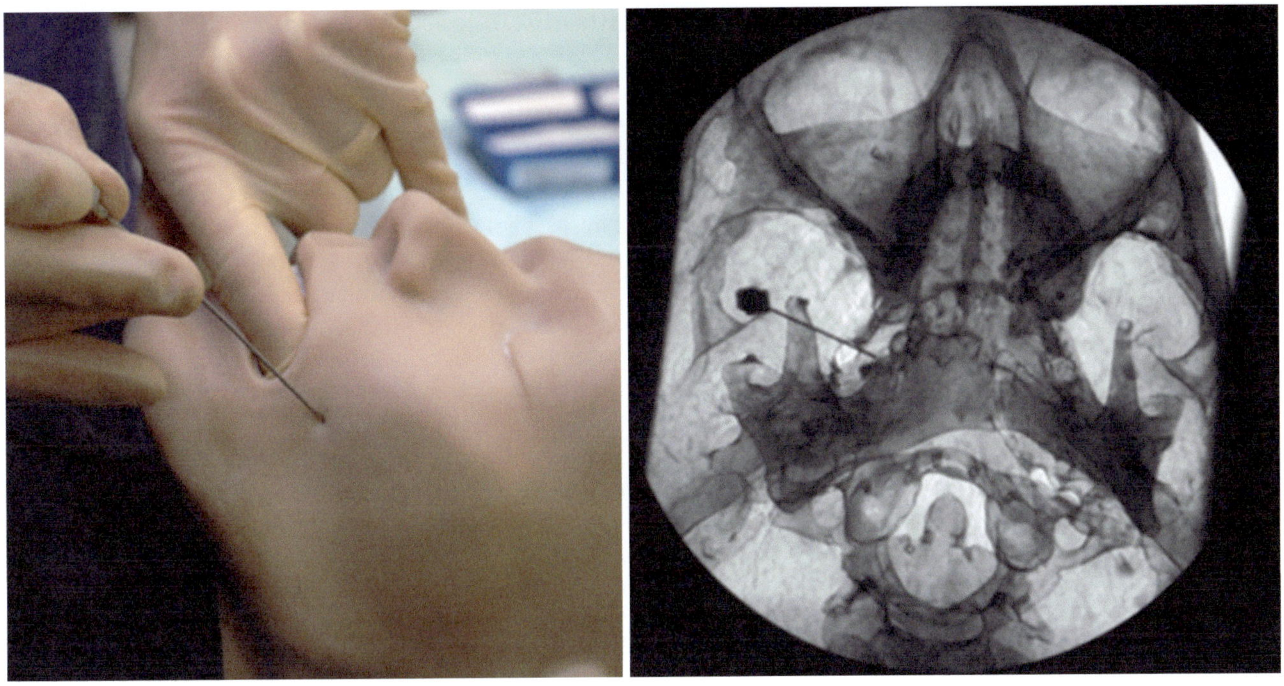

Fig. 19.3 AR351 Adam Rouilly Pain Relief Manikin

Open Surgical Procedures

Open surgical procedures for pain management are becoming more common. The most common open surgical procedures include implantation of spinal cord stimulators and intrathecal drug delivery systems. These procedures are referred to collectively as neuromodulation. With continuous development of neuromodulation technology and techniques, the need for open procedural skill attainment will increase in the future. An inherent challenge exists in training practitioners on a chance-based exposure model, as access to these procedures is distributed unevenly throughout pain medicine practices and training programs [33]. Simulation offers unique advantages to meet this training need [15].

Currently, the most common simulation programming for neuromodulation skills training exists in the form of cadaver labs and surgical skills workshops. This is fitting, as many chronic pain practitioners come from nonsurgical training backgrounds. Thus, development of surgical skills such as suturing and identification of surgical equipment should be included when developing a curriculum. Pig skin-based models are commonly used for developing suture skills and have the advantage of realism (similar to human skin), low cost, and easy accessibility [34]. VR simulators for laparoscopic suturing skills have proven beneficial for skills training, whereas VR for open suturing techniques is less well established with only prototypes described in the literature [35]. To acquire the remaining surgical skills needed for neuromodulation, such as making skin incision, tunneling subcutaneous leads/catheters, and creating implant pockets, cadaver labs remain the most sound modality. Unfortunately, this is a limited resource that is most amenable to occasional workshops, rather than ongoing skills development.

Crisis Resource Training

Critical events in the practice of pain medicine are rare, but there is always the potential for acute complications and emergencies from the various procedures. Pain medicine clinicians train in different medical specialties, with a range of knowledge, skills, and abilities to manage crisis events. Most pain medicine fellowship training programs and hospitals which credential practicing pain clinicians require BLS and ACLS certification. Additionally, ACGME-approved pain medicine programs require training in basic airway management and placement of intravenous access. Simulation modalities are often used as a platform to train pain clinicians in crisis management [36–39]. Furthermore, adverse outcomes have been shown to have a significant emotional impact on the clinicians involved [40]. Simulation and debriefings may help to mitigate this for clinicians as well.

An emerging body of literature has developed regarding curriculum development for the management of serious adverse events in pain medicine. Brenner et al. describe a pain medicine curriculum focusing on three components:

managing an acute crisis, ethical decision-making during an acute event, and managing medical errors. Utilizing a hybrid HFS model composed of computer-controlled mannequins, standardized healthcare providers, and SPs, they performed 15 pilot courses between the years 2004 and 2010. They reported that 66 out of 68 participants rated the course as "excellent" and recommended instituting a curriculum with pain medicine fellows participating twice at 6-month intervals [41].

Hoelzer and colleagues describe similar HFS curriculum development for pain medicine training. They focused on two types of simulations: managing adverse events and engaging in difficult conversations. In both cases, the goals of the simulation were to teach critical skills such as event recognition, teamwork, ACLS algorithms, communication skills, and resource management [1]. Simulated scenarios include anaphylaxis, seizure following stellate ganglion block, respiratory arrest from an intrathecal pump refill complication, serotonin syndrome from interaction of an opioid with a tricyclic antidepressant, a hypertensive emergency, pneumothorax after intercostal nerve block, hypoxia following sedation administration, and hypotension following a celiac plexus block. Of note, both Brenner et al. and Hoelzer et al. highlighted the importance of the debriefing in these scenarios. These two examples of utilizing a hybrid HFS model to teach crisis management to pain medicine clinicians can serve as a framework or curriculum template for future training.

Interdisciplinary Team Training

Ideal management of chronic pain includes the collaborative efforts of interdisciplinary teams. This includes, but is not limited to, pain physicians and other specialists, advanced practice providers, nurses, medical assistants, pain psychologists, physical and occupational therapists, and administrative staff. The entire team contributes to positive outcomes and also may be negatively impacted by critical events. Studies performed on medical errors in team environments cited such factors as poor teamwork, lack of communication, impaired decision-making from stress, equipment availability, production pressures, and fear of expressing opinions as examples of barriers to appropriate management [42]. These events have been shown to impact team members emotionally, on a personal and professional level, for an extended period of time [43] (Table 19.1).

Addressing critical event management with an interdisciplinary team approach is a well-established model for HFS [43]. Specifically for pain medicine, two important areas include handling difficult patients and managing emergencies. Since multiple members of the team interact with each patient, these scenarios lend themselves to training with interdisciplinary teams [2]. Brenner et al. noted the importance of involving the entire treatment team in their critical event scenarios. They noted that the debriefing sessions had richer conversation topics when an interdisciplinary team

Table 19.1 An example of an interventional pain medicine scenario with learning objectives and associated performance metrics

Title: Decompensation during stellate ganglion block [41]			
Learners: Pain medicine fellows, anesthesiology residents			
Objectives:			
Medical knowledge: Recognize potential complications during stellate ganglion block			
Patient care: Treat physiological derangements during stellate ganglion block			
Communication: Discuss clinical situation with colleagues in the procedure area, and delegate tasks with closed-loop communication methodology			
Case stem: The patient is an otherwise healthy middle-aged individual with upper extremity complex regional pain syndrome (CRPS). The plan is to perform a stellate ganglion via landmark approach. The patient takes no medications and has no allergies, prior anesthetic complications, nor relevant family history. The patient is having the procedure performed by a junior trainee under the supervision of the participant. The junior trainee abruptly performs the procedure before the learner can appropriately supervise the block. The learner must then manage patient decompensation from an apparent complication of the block			
Room setup: Procedure area (OR, PACU, or related monitored setting) with patient in supine position on a stretcher or OR table. Patient is covered in drapes except for the neck which is exposed. Patient will have O2 via nasal cannula and a single IV with normal saline running. Monitoring is ongoing and includes EKG, BP cuff, and continuous pulse oximetry. A crash cart will be within the procedure area with airway equipment, induction drugs, cardiovascular medications, intralipid, and cardiac defibrillator. A mayo stand is at the head of the bed with a spinal nerve block tray with local anesthetics and local needle for skin wheal, 25 g 3.5-inch spinal needle for the block, and bupivacaine and decadron for block medications			
State	**Patient status**	**Learner actions**	
Baseline	Awake, alert, responsive, and oriented x3 VS are WNL (HR 60-NSR; RR9, BP 120/82, SpO2 100% on NC)	Learner accepts handoff from RN and junior trainee regarding patient's position, prep/drape completed, informed consent signed, and ready to undergo stellate ganglion block	If learner does not introduce themselves within 60–90 seconds, RN in procedure area will initiate and complete the introductions

Table 19.1 (continued)

Stellate block procedure	The RN in the room will pull learner aside room the patient to ask a question as a distraction technique. During this time the junior trainee will perform the stellate ganglion block in an unsupervised fashion and inform the learner that the procedure is now completed VS are similar except slightly higher HR and BP from injection-related pain (HR 85-NSR; RR 9, BP 133/89, SpO2 100% on NC)	Learner inquires with junior trainee about how procedure was performed and what medications were given	
Respiratory arrest and loss of consciousness	Respiratory effort stops, and patient becomes unresponsive to commands or painful stimuli (e.g., sternal rub) VS demonstrate decompensation (HR 39-SB w/PVCs, RR 0, BP 70/35, SpO2 81%)	Learner generates differential diagnosis for respiratory failure. Without airway intervention vital signs continue to decline Learner is expected to assist with ventilation via bag mask, LMA, or endotracheal intubation. Learner should also consider cardiovascular medications (e.g., epinephrine atropine) When assigning tasks, learner uses closed-loop communication.	If learner does not observe the clinical decline, the RN and junior trainee ask the learner why the vital signs are changing
Stabilizes	With airway management and cardiovascular medications, VS improve (HR 94 NSR, RR as generated by the learner, BP 135/90, SpO2 98%)	Learner articulates ddx, anticipates further clinical challenges and disposition for the patient	
Debriefing and discussion points:			
DDx for respiratory arrest during stellate ganglion block (intrathecal injection with high spinal, pneumothorax, intravascular injection of anesthetics, direct airway injury).			
What clinical signs and/or symptoms would help solidify the diagnosis?			
Why and how did this patient decompensate? What is the appropriate treatment for this, as well as the appropriate aftercare setting?			
Was the RN and/or junior trainee in the procedure area aware of the patient's clinical status?			
How could the RN and/or junior trainee have assisted with the resuscitation? And what effective communication techniques could have been used for assigning them treatment tasks?			
Overall, what do you perceive went well, and what could have been done better?			
References: [41]. Brenner GJ et al. *Anesth Analg*. 2013 Jan;116(1):107–10			

was present, when compared to only one provider type [41]. Such simulations using the hybrid HFS model with a deliberate focus on interdisciplinary debriefing have the potential to improve teamwork and communication, empower team members, educate about emergency protocols, and facilitate "stress inoculations" where subsequent real emergencies need not be debilitating.

Conclusion

The use of simulation for pain medicine training can enrich the learning environment, allow development of specific skills, enhance exposure to various key pain-related events, promote teamwork, and improve communication skills. In particular, simulation can target specific challenging aspects of patient interactions, interventional skills, and crisis management. By utilizing hybrid scenarios that combine multiple simulation modalities, an engaging and immersive pain-related learning experience can be created. The presence of experienced educators and a dedicated debriefing session are key to the value of pain-related simulation experiences.

References

1. Hoelzer BC, Moeschler SM, Seamans DP. Using simulation and standardized patients to teach vital skills to pain medicine fellows. Pain Med. 2015;16(4):680–91.
2. Marken PA, Zimmerman C, Kennedy C, Schremmer R, Smith KV. Human simulators and standardized patients to teach difficult conversations to interprofessional health care teams. Am J Pharm Educ [Internet]. 2010 [cited 2016 Sep 14];74(7). Available

from: https://www-ncbi-nlm-nih-gov.laneproxy.stanford.edu/pmc/articles/PMC2972514/.
3. Kersun L, Gyi L, Morrison WE. Training in difficult conversations: a national survey of pediatric hematology–oncology and pediatric critical care physicians. J Palliat Med. 2009;12(6):525–30.
4. Plymale MA, Sloan PA, Johnson M, LaFountain P, Snapp J, Sloan DA. Cancer pain education: the use of a structured clinical instruction module to enhance learning among medical students. J Pain Symptom Manage. 2000;20(1):4–11.
5. Parikh PP, Brown R, White M, Markert RJ, Eustace R, Tchorz K. Simulation-based end-of-life care training during surgical clerkship: assessment of skills and perceptions. J Surg Res. 2015;196(2):258–63.
6. Grosseman S, Novack DH, Duke P, Mennin S, Rosenzweig S, Davis TJ, et al. Residents' and standardized patients' perspectives on empathy: issues of agreement. Patient Educ Couns. 2014;96(1):22–8.
7. Leung JYC, Critchley LAH, Yung ALK, Kumta SM. Evidence of virtual patients as a facilitative learning tool on an anesthesia course. Adv Health Sci Educ. 2014;20(4):885–901.
8. Critchley L, Leung JY, Kumta SM, Yung AL. Introduction of virtual patients onto a final year anesthesia course: Hong Kong experience. Adv Med Educ Pract. 2011:71.
9. Triola M, Feldman H, Kalet AL, Zabar S, Kachur EK, Gillespie C, et al. A randomized trial of teaching clinical skills using virtual and live standardized patients. J Gen Intern Med. 2006;21(5):424–9.
10. Haglund MM, Rudd M, Nagler A, Prose NS. Difficult conversations: a national course for neurosurgery residents in physician-patient communication. J Surg Educ. 2015;72(3):394–401.
11. Boissoneault J, Mundt JM, Bartley EJ, Wandner LD, Hirsh AT, Robinson ME. Assessment of the influence of demographic and professional characteristics on health care providers' pain management decisions using virtual humans. J Dent Educ. 2016;80(5):578–87.
12. Wandner LD, Heft MW, Lok BC, Hirsh AT, George SZ, Horgas AL, et al. The impact of patients' gender, race, and age on health care professionals' pain management decisions: an online survey using virtual human technology. Int J Nurs Stud. 2014;51(5):726–33.
13. Hirsh AT, Hollingshead NA, Bair MJ, Matthias MS, Kroenke K. Preferences, experience, and attitudes in the management of chronic pain and depression: a comparison of physicians and medical students. Clin J Pain. 2014;30(9):766–74.
14. Hollingshead NA, Meints S, Middleton SK, Free CA, Hirsh AT. Examining influential factors in providers' chronic pain treatment decisions: a comparison of physicians and medical students. BMC Med Educ [Internet]. 2015 [cited 2016 Sep 12];15(1). Available from: http://www.biomedcentral.com/1472-6920/15/164.
15. The Use of Computers for Perioperative Simulation in Anesthesia, Critical Care, and Pain Medicine – ClinicalKey [Internet]. [cited 2016 Sep 13]. Available from: https://www-clinicalkey-com.ezproxy.stanford.edu/#!/content/playContent/1-s2.0-S1932227511000437?returnurl=null&referrer=null.
16. Veneziano D, Smith A, Reihsen T, Speich J, Sweet RM. The SimPORTAL fluoro-less C-arm trainer: an innovative device for percutaneous kidney access. J Endourol. 2014;29(2):240–5.
17. Niazi AU, Peng PW, Ho M, Tiwari A, Chan VW. The future of regional anesthesia education: lessons learned from the surgical specialty. Can J Anesth Can Anesth. 2016;63(8):966–72.
18. Edrich T, Seethala RR, Olenchock BA, Mizuguchi AK, Rivero JM, Beutler SS, et al. Providing initial transthoracic echocardiography training for anesthesiologists: simulator training is not inferior to live training. J Cardiothorac Vasc Anesth. 2014;28(1):49–53.
19. Grantcharov TP, Reznick RK. Teaching procedural skills. BMJ. 2008;336(7653):1129–31.
20. Javan R, Bansal M, Tangestanipoor AA. Prototype hybrid gypsum-based 3-dimensional printed training model for computed tomography-guided spinal pain management. J Comput Assist Tomogr. 2016;40(4):626–31.
21. Niazi AU, Tait G, Carvalho JCA, Chan VW. The use of an online three-dimensional model improves performance in ultrasound scanning of the spine: a randomized trial. Can J Anesth Can Anesth. 2013;60(5):458–64.
22. Chen H, Kim R, Perret D, Hata J, Rinehart J, Chang E. Improving trainee competency and comfort level with needle driving using simulation training. Pain Med. 2016;17(4):670–4.
23. Conway JA, Adhikary SD, Giampetro D, Stolzenberg D. A Survey of Ultrasound Training in U.S. and Canadian Chronic Pain Fellowship Programs. Pain Med. 2015;16(10):1923–9.
24. Narouze SN, Provenzano D, Peng P, Eichenberger U, Lee SC, Nicholls B, et al. The American Society of Regional Anesthesia and Pain Medicine, the European Society of Regional Anaesthesia and Pain Therapy, and the Asian Australasian Federation of Pain Societies Joint Committee Recommendations for Education and Training in Ultrasound-Guided Interventional Pain Procedures. Reg Anesth Pain Med. 2012;37(6):657–64.
25. Kim YH. Ultrasound phantoms to protect patients from novices. Korean J Pain. 2016;29(2):73.
26. Brascher A-K, Blunk JA, Bauer K, Feldmann R, Benrath J. Comprehensive curriculum for phantom-based training of ultrasound-guided intercostal nerve and stellate ganglion blocks. Pain Med. 2014;15(10):1647–56.
27. Burckett-St.Laurent DA, Cunningham MS, Abbas S, Chan VW, Okrainec A, Niazi AU. Teaching ultrasound-guided regional anesthesia remotely: a feasibility study. Acta Anaesthesiol Scand. 2016;60(7):995–1002.
28. Vaughan N, Dubey VN, Wee MYK, Isaacs R. A review of epidural simulators: where are we today? Med Eng Phys. 2013;35(9):1235–50.
29. Siddiqui NT, Arzola C, Ahmed I, Davies S, Carvalho JCA. Low-fidelity simulation improves mastery of the aseptic technique for labour epidurals: an observational study. Can J Anesth Can Anesth. 2014;61(8):710–6.
30. Gonzalez-Cota A, Chiravuri S, Stansfield RB, Brummett CM, Hamstra SJ. The effect of bench model fidelity on fluoroscopy-guided transforaminal epidural injection training: a randomized control study. Reg Anesth Pain Med. 2013;38(2):155–60.
31. Lerman IR, Souzdalnitski D, Narouze S. A low-cost, durable, combined ultrasound and fluoroscopic phantom for cervical transforaminal injections. Reg Anesth Pain Med. 2012;37(3):344–8.
32. Lonn L, Edmond JJ, Marco J, Kearney PP, Gallagher AG. Virtual reality simulation training in a high-fidelity procedure suite: operator appraisal. J Vasc Interv Radiol. 2012;23(10):1361–1366.e2.
33. Johnson T. Counterbalancing clinical supervision and independent practice: case studies in learning thoracic epidural catheter insertion. Br J Anaesth. 2010;105(6):772–6.
34. DiMaggio PJ, Waer AL, Desmarais TJ, Sozanski J, Timmerman H, Lopez JA, et al. The use of a lightly preserved cadaver and full thickness pig skin to teach technical skills on the surgery clerkship—a response to the economic pressures facing academic medicine today. Am J Surg. 2010;200(1):162–6.
35. Choi K-S, Chan S-H, Pang W-M. Virtual suturing simulation based on commodity physics engine for medical learning. J Med Syst. 2010;36(3):1781–93.
36. Gaba DM, DeAnda A. A comprehensive anesthesia simulation environment: re-creating the operating room for research and training. Anesthesiology. 1988;69(3):387–94.
37. Blum RH, Raemer DB, Carroll JS, Sunder N, Felstein DM, Cooper JB. Crisis resource management training for an anaesthesia faculty: a new approach to continuing education. Med Educ. 2004;38(1):45–55.
38. Small SD, Wuerz RC, Simon R, Shapiro N, Conn A, Setnik G. Demonstration of high-fidelity simulation team training for

emergency medicine. Acad Emerg Med Off J Soc Acad Emerg Med. 1999;6(4):312–23.

39. Stevens L-M, Cooper JB, Raemer DB, Schneider RC, Frankel AS, Berry WR, et al. Educational program in crisis management for cardiac surgery teams including high realism simulation. J Thorac Cardiovasc Surg. 2012;144(1):17–24.
40. Aasland OG, Førde R. Impact of feeling responsible for adverse events on doctors' personal and professional lives: the importance of being open to criticism from colleagues. Qual Saf Health Care. 2005;14(1):13–7.
41. Brenner GJ, Nemark JL, Raemer D. Curriculum and cases for pain medicine crisis resource management education. Anesth Analg. 2013;116(1):107–10.
42. Sexton JB, Thomas EJ, Helmreich RL. Error, stress, and teamwork in medicine and aviation: cross sectional surveys. BMJ. 2000;320(7237):745.
43. Bognár A, Barach P, Johnson JK, Duncan RC, Birnbach D, Woods D, et al. Errors and the burden of errors: attitudes, perceptions, and the culture of safety in pediatric cardiac surgical teams. Ann Thorac Surg. 2008;85(4):1374–81.

Simulation in Critical Care Medicine

20

David L. Schreibman and Wendy K. Bernstein

Introduction

Critical care medicine is defined as the provision of complex care where critical illness or injury acutely impairs one or more vital organ systems with a high probability of imminent life-threatening deterioration in the patient's condition. This care occurs in a unit where the delivery of this medical care requires complex decisions, plans of care, technology, and procedures to assess, manipulate, and support this vital organ failure in a multidisciplinary environment. Anesthesiology has a deep involvement in the evolution of critical care medicine culminating in its being recognized by the American Board of Anesthesiology in 1986 as an area of specialty where physicians work in concert with various specialists on the patient care team in the intensive care unit (ICU) to utilize recognized skills that are vital to the support of the multi-system injuries [1]. Over the years, critical care medicine has become more protocol driven with a large number of complex technical procedures required to be performed by highly trained clinicians.

Training of critical care physicians includes not only the understanding of the complex pathophysiology of critical disease and mastering of procedural skills but also the ability to prioritize tasks, make quick decisions in a time-sensitive environment, assess and evaluate a myriad of clinical data, and work effectively as members of a multidisciplinary critical care team during stressful periods when patients are acutely unstable. Anesthesiologists in the critical care unit, like in the operating rooms, do not function in a vacuum. There are physicians of various specialties that have unique training and communication skills that must work together in the intensive care unit environment. Besides the obvious physician/nurse corroboration, many other professionals are involved in the care of the same patients. These may include but not limited to pharmacists, respiratory therapists, physical therapists, occupational therapists, speech-language pathologists, nutritionists, nursing assistants, social workers, and case managers. The use of multidisciplinary care teams in this high-risk stressful environment has been shown to improve patient care and decrease mortality in a critical care unit [2, 3].

The clinical experience provided in a residency or fellowship program remains unchallenged as the foundation for specialty training, but assuring that all trainees get adequate exposure to multiple clinical situations remains a logistic challenge for all training programs [4]. Critical care medicine in real-life situations creates a poor context for learning due to the uncertainty of a patient's response, confounding variables and simultaneous processes occurring, and the stress resulting from the urgent response required [5]. Little didactic teaching can occur in the midst of a crisis, and learners are often moved to the observer role as more experienced clinicians take over. The mere acquisition of knowledge is insufficient as it is now necessary to have proficiency in the required clinical skills, be them technical or nontechnical in nature. The classical tradition of bedside teaching involving "see one, do one, teach one" is no longer an accepted practice as there is a limited opportunity to assess available patients and specific clinical situations associated with a limited number of work hours to experience all possible encountered scenarios.

By its very nature, critical care medicine lends itself to the use of simulation as a primary educational modality. Simulation-based education complements but cannot replace education involving real patients and genuine settings. Simulation has been applied to the acquisition of routine skills, critical event training, and competency assessment, to promote learning and practicing a wide variety of high-risk scenarios and master the necessary relevant clinical skills without risk to the patient. Patient-based training often

D. L. Schreibman (✉)
Department of Anesthesiology, University of Maryland School of Medicine, University of Maryland Medical Center, Baltimore, MA, USA
e-mail: dschreibman@som.umaryland.edu

W. K. Bernstein
Division of Cardiac Anesthesiology, Department of Anesthesiology and Perioperative Medicine, University of Rochester Medical Center, Rochester, MN, USA

B. Mahoney et al. (eds.), *Comprehensive Healthcare Simulation: Anesthesiology*, Comprehensive Healthcare Simulation,
https://doi.org/10.1007/978-3-030-26849-7_20

leads to varying quality and consistency of the educational goal, but simulation allows medical learners to gain education through repetition of well-defined controlled clinical scenarios, including uncommon events, and work through difficult situations without compromising actual patient care [6]. Simulated patient care scenarios allow training in unit-specific protocols, checklists, competencies, and procedures necessary to be performed leading to improved utilization of technology, support of high-risk clinical decision-making, and the development of effective critical care multidisciplinary teams. Simulation training promotes self-directed adult active learning as opposed to passive learning, and its repetitive nature allows clinicians to hone their skills with the overall experience being sustained with deliberate practice over time. Training of this nature leads not only to individual educational gains but overall unit quality assurance and safety measure improvement. An advantage of simulation education is that familiarity or comfort with the simulation environment does not appear to have a significant effect upon a clinician's performance. Training utilizing high-fidelity simulation enhances the participants' engagement in the exercise leading to quicker response times, less deviation from accepted guidelines, and performing better in handling crisis situations when compared to standard practice [7].

Types of Simulation

As described in earlier chapters of this book, simulation is an interactive educational technique that replicates real life allowing healthcare professionals to immerse themselves in experiential learning. Medical simulations aim to imitate real patients, anatomic regions, or clinical tasks to mirror the real-life circumstances in which medical services are rendered [8]. Types of simulators that are particularly valuable in critical care medical education are standardized patients, partial task trainers, computer-based programs with or without virtual reality, and high-fidelity patient simulation.

Standardized Patients

As described in Chap. 10, standardized patients are actors who are trained to portray a specific patient or person in a consistent stereotypical fashion. Critical care professionals require excellent communication skills, interpersonal skills, and professionalism to effectively interact with their patients, their families, and other professionals within the high-stress critical care environment. We have utilized standardized patients in place of the usual high-fidelity mannequin to display different clinical conditions and allow a more realistic interaction between the patient and the critical care professional. Standardized patients may also be employed to create interactions between professionals and patient's families to discuss difficult clinical conditions including devastating disease, medical error, or death. Lastly standardized patients may be employed to simulate communication with other professionals in healthcare team members regarding discussions related to clinical care to enhance communication skills, professionalism, and conflict resolution. The incorporation of standardized patients into scenarios is an effective modality to assure that the clinical competencies such as communication, professionalism, and system-based practice are taught, evaluated, and perfected [9].

Partial Task Trainer Simulation

As outlined in Chap. 11, partial task trainers are life-size models of various body parts designed to teach specialized skills utilizing anatomical models that reinforce hand-eye coordination for the specific technical skill. Clinical skill acquisition and competency is an integral part of critical care medicine utilization of simulation-based training. Simulation allows clinicians to practice and hone their skills in required procedures to allow them to practice independently. Critical care procedures that are amenable to partial task trainer simulation include central [10] and arterial vascular access, airway management and endotracheal intubation [11], thoracostomy tube insertion, bronchoscopy, thoracentesis [12], paracentesis, pericardiocentesis, and percutaneous tracheostomy. A multifaceted learning strategy incorporating computer-based learning, task trainers, and high-fidelity simulation provides the necessary conceptual and technical fundamentals of the procedures to allow for the performance in the critical care unit on patients [13]. The use of simulation allows for the acquisition of visual and spatial skills necessary for the repetitive practice of the defined procedural techniques allowing for risk-free deliberate practice away from the bedside. Simulator-trained residents performing central line insertion display clinical skill acquisition, showing increased self-confidence and less needle passes when performing the actual procedure [14] which ultimately produces fewer central line infections and decreased lengths of stay, making the cost savings from the quality improvement far exceed the cost of the educational intervention [10]. Any deviation from the expected execution of a skill on a simulator from reality must be made clear to the learner to avoid negative transfer effects incurred by learning "shortcuts" of the simulated environment [15].

Computer Program-Based or Virtual Reality Simulation

Computer program-based simulation is useful in the critical care environment where patient symptoms and data are displayed permitting diagnostic and therapeutic interventions to be discerned and evaluated. Screen-based computer simulations incorporate models of pathophysiology of critical care disease to present clinical situations, such as certification programs in advanced cardiac life support (ACLS) or basic life support (BLS) training utilized by the American Heart Association. This type of computer training allows the trainee to independently evaluate and manage a clinical scenario by interacting with a simulated patient utilizing various monitoring equipment and diagnostic studies to make treatment decisions and observing the effects of their actions. Traditional ACLS training has been shown to be less effective than focused deliberate practice utilizing simulation-based training that improves adherence to accepted guidelines and overall quality of resuscitation [16].

Virtual reality computer simulations utilize a three-dimensional image and virtual equipment such as an ultrasound or bronchoscope (i.e., SonoSim® and EndoVR™, respectively) to illustrate how the equipment's use complements clinical situations in a realistic clinical environment. The use of bronchoscopy in critical care medicine requires both acquired manual dexterity and a thorough understanding of bronchopulmonary anatomy to care for patients. Advanced bronchoscopy trainers provide a realistic exposure to utilizing a replica bronchoscope with haptic feedback and state-of-the-art virtual reality graphics to impart realistic clinical situations on an on-call basis. The use of computer-based simulation programs allows the learner to independently review knowledge and practice skills as required to improve overall retention. Instruction and practice utilizing bronchoscopy simulators allow novice users to attain advanced technical skills similar to that achieved through years of clinical experience [17].

Ultrasound's most basic function in critical care has been its utilization in gaining access to central and arterial catheterization and guiding invasive procedures such as thoracentesis, paracentesis, pericardiocentesis, and chest tube placement that leads to fewer complications [18]. There has been a rapid increase in the use of point-of-care ultrasonography (POCUS) as one of the most versatile diagnostic modalities in critical care for assessing the cardiovascular, pulmonary, and abdominal systems. POCUS is used as an adjunct to clinical examination to provide a rapid accurate noninvasive assessment to assist in resuscitation and stabilization of an unstable patient. Critical care ultrasonography is typically oriented toward complex disease states rather than single organs requiring an accurate and timely transversal approach to multiple systems rather than a comprehensive examination of the single anatomical region done in other specialties [19]. It has been used for supplementing physical examination in both assessing hemodynamics via transthoracic echocardiography and diagnosis of acute pathological states utilizing non-cardiac ultrasound. Critical care ultrasound course improves acquired skills in ultrasound knowledge, imagery acquisition, pathological image interpretation, and comfort with ultrasound techniques that persists for 3 months and leads to increased ultrasound use in clinical practice [20]. Transthoracic ultrasound has been useful in assessing volume status by evaluating inferior vena cava (IVC) diameter and associated ventricular function or diagnosing pulmonary pathology (i.e., pleural effusion or pneumothorax). Critical care physicians can continuously practice on computer-based virtual reality ultrasound equipment to prevent natural decay of infrequently performed competencies and to keep pace with continuous development of technology and procedures [19].

Transthoracic echocardiography (TTE) and transesophageal echocardiography (TEE) are gaining popularity in critical care to assess cardiac anatomy and function, hemodynamic parameters, and inotropic support titration. The standard transthoracic views required to perform a focused examination are parasternal long-axis, parasternal short-axis, apical four-chamber, and subcostal four-chamber, and IVC views allow a quick assessment of cardiac function in the ICU. Computer simulation has evolved to correlate three-dimensional anatomic cuts to TTE and TEE views. Focused TTE simulation training leads to an improved ability to efficiently acquire higher-quality images and better identify cardiac anatomic structures [21] allowing intensivists with minimal training to assess left ventricular (LV) function with reasonable accuracy [22]. Competency requirements for image acquisition and interpretation has been outlined for ultrasonography and echocardiography, but there remains no consensus on how the education, training, and evaluation of the competencies should be achieved [23, 24].

High-Fidelity Patient Simulation

As discussed in Chap. 11, the use of high-fidelity patient simulators allows multidisciplinary teams of critical care providers to gain experience managing patients in an ICU environment. Learning is improved by setting the simulator within a realistic clinical environment with appropriate resources such as monitors, equipment, and staff [25]. We create a critical care environment that as closely as possible resembles the intensive care unit that the participants work in by placing the monitors and ventilators in similar locations relative to the bed, create supply carts that resemble those used on the unit, and try to group the personnel participants that are usually available when critical events occur in the unit (Fig. 20.1). The mannequin enables clinicians to perform invasive procedures such as tracheal intubation, vascular access, and cardiopulmonary resuscitation (CPR) and defibrillation. In creating scenarios, we require that participants must actually perform the task that is required to be done besides simply vocalizing a need for it. If a clinician desires intravenous access or invasive monitors, instead of "allowing" a line, we have created mannequin accesso-

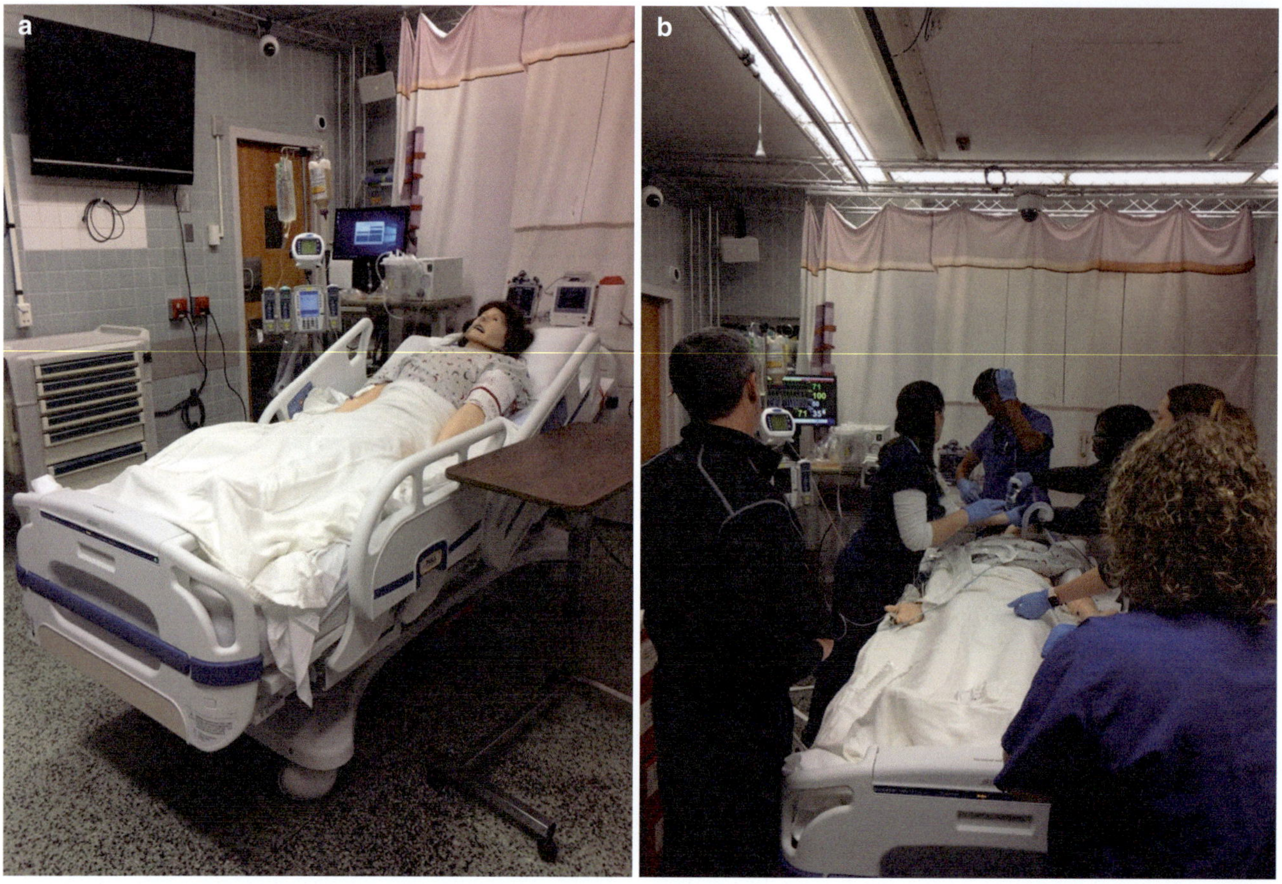

Fig. 20.1 The environmental factor in critical care simulation. (**a**) Shows the room with all the equipment including an ICU room supply cart, monitor, patient, table, O2, and suction. In the hallway are crash (code) cart, ventilator, intubation box, videoscopic laryngoscope, and anesthesia stat bag (which contains various airway management equipment for intubation and/or invasive airway management). (**b**) Shows how the bare room becomes a bustling critical care unit during an acute event

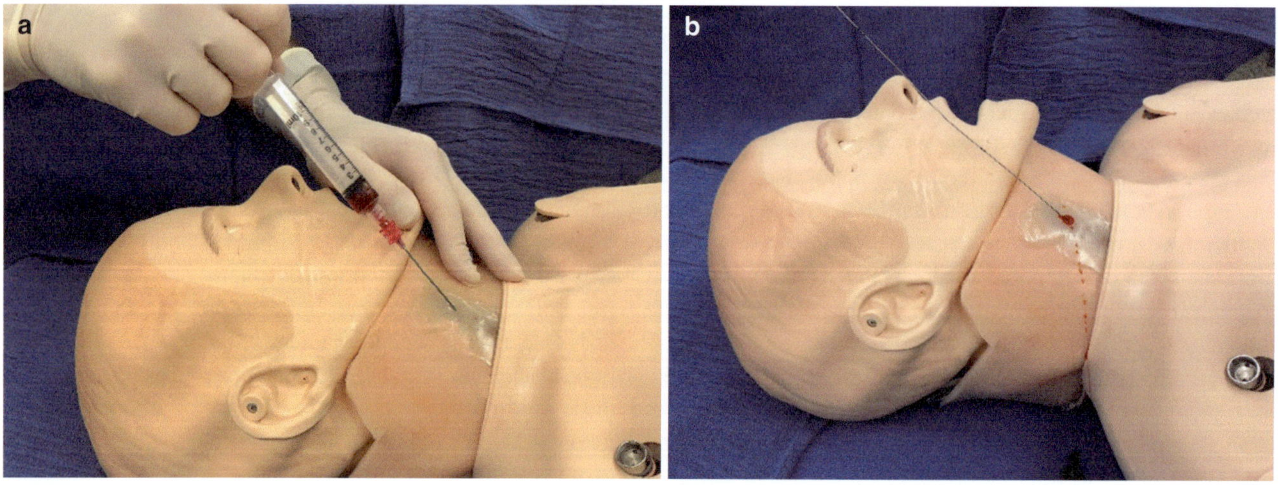

Fig. 20.2 Enhancing reality in simulation. To enhance realism and understand constraint on manpower and time, we utilized the central line insertion accessory to the mannequin to allow insertion of central lines during a scenario. The accessory allows ultrasound guidance and is accessed with a Seldinger technique

ries that allow the performance of that technical skill. This allows the participants to feel the actual constraints that the task puts on the team in both manpower and time. The central line accessory allows ultrasound guidance and can be accessed with a Seldinger technique (Fig. 20.2). It is essential that physiologic changes that occur in the clinical scenario be clearly and accurately reproduced so that learner is not distracted from the primary objectives of the scenario.

For example, high airway pressures occurring in the small "lungs" of these mannequins are often misinterpreted by the learners as a physiologic change that wasn't intended to occur in the scenario. "In situ" simulation in the actual critical care unit has been implemented where we substitute a high-fidelity mannequin or standardized patient for an actual patient. Anesthesiologists trained on a high-fidelity simulator have been shown to respond more quickly, deviate less from accepted guidelines, and perform better in handling crisis situations [7].

Improving Patient Safety in Critical Care Through Simulation

Training on technical skills alone is insufficient to achieve maximum safety [26]. Patients who are critically ill are subjected to multiple interventions and longer hospital stays and are more likely to suffer serious injury as a result of medical mistakes [27]. Common errors that may occur in a critical care environment include drug administration errors, failures in communication, and insufficient monitoring, which are not related primarily to clinical knowledge or technical skills but rather to other nontechnical problems [28]. Ineffective teamwork that encompasses poor communication, and lack of shared goals, situational awareness, role clarity, leadership, coordination, mutual respect, and post-event debriefings, has been linked to such adverse patient outcomes as nosocomial infection, adverse drug events, and increased risk-adjusted mortality [29]. A clinical team's performance involves a dynamic interaction between multiple people with heterogeneous backgrounds, disciplines, knowledge, skills, and attitudes. Deficiencies in nontechnical skills can increase the chance of error which in turn can increase the chance of an adverse event, whereas good nontechnical skills (situational awareness, decision-making, team working and leadership, and task management) can reduce the likelihood of error [30]. The use of crisis resource management (CRM) techniques adapted from the airline industry has long been advocated for use by anesthesiologists to promote a team approach to patient care and safety in the critical care unit. Gaba identifies leadership, problem-solving, situational awareness, communication skills, and resource management as key aspects of effective CRM [31]. Critically ill patients are vulnerable to iatrogenic injury because of the severity and instability of their illness and their frequent need for high-risk interventions and medications. Iatrogenic injuries are most common during treatments and procedures, ordering or administration of medications, errors associated with communication or reporting clinical information, and failure to follow prescribed protocols [32]. The critical care environment's multidisciplinary interactions of varied professional expertise benefit from the use of simulation techniques that encourage CRM. Critical care physicians appear more satisfied with physician-nurse collaboration after simulation training, whereas nurses report that their input is not well received and they find it difficult to speak up and provide their opinions on critical decisions [33]. Critical care simulation training for multidisciplinary teams leads to more cohesive interaction allowing healthcare providers to learn how to better communicate and value the contributions of each member of the team leading to increased collegiality and cohesiveness [34]. It must be noted that care in an intensive care environment unfortunately differs from performance in an airline cockpit. Within the intensive care unit teams, clinical judgments, rather than simple protocols, allow multidisciplinary teams to perform a diverse range of hands-on, problem-solving, and monitoring tasks on multiple patients at the same time making team and task skills more essential for avoiding or managing emergency situations [35]. Working as members of a team in critical care units is an important way to optimize patient outcomes during clinical crises. Although few healthcare workers receive training in teamwork, they work cohesively in the ICU despite having different clinical disciplines that have traditionally trained separately. Using simulation-based training, significant improvement in measures of teamwork, particularly leadership, team coordination, and communication has been observed, and retention of these skills was supported by participants 3 months later [36]. As daily scheduling leads to different personnel being present at varying times, it behooves us to utilize these training resources to promote a cohesive team atmosphere no matter the available personnel.

The Committee on Quality of Health Care in America believes that healthcare organizations should establish team training programs for personnel in critical care areas using proven methods such as crew resource management techniques employed in aviation, including simulation. People make fewer errors when they work in teams. When processes are planned and standardized, each member knows his or her responsibilities as well as those of teammates, and members "look out" for one another, noticing errors before they cause an accident. In an effective interdisciplinary team, members come to trust one another's judgments and attend to one another's safety concerns [37]. Clearly to prepare for the unexpected, staff in many high-reliability organizations are trained intensively in drills and simulations. Simulation is especially important where the unusual events are dangerous or where practicing within the real system is impossible or too costly.

The *TeamSTEPPS®* [38] (Team Strategies and Tools to Enhance Performance and Patient Safety) program was developed by the Agency for Healthcare Research and Quality and the US Department of Defense to maximize medical teamwork and lead to the improvement in the quality, safety, and cost-effectiveness of healthcare delivery. The four key principles of the program involve leadership, situational monitoring, mutual support, and communication.

Communication, the process by which information is clearly and accurately exchanged among team members, emphasizes the importance of the "callout" and "checkback." "Callout" communicates important or critical information that informs all team members simultaneously and allows them to anticipate the next steps and directing responsibility to a specific individual to carry out the task, and "checkback" is the use of closed-loop communication to ensure that information is conveyed clearly to a responsible provider and is understood. Research has shown that TeamSTEPPS® leads to an increase in desirable teamwork and safety attitudes, as well as increased communication, teamwork behaviors, clinical process, compliance, efficiency, and overall performance in a variety of medical settings. In an ICU setting, staff experience a positive perception of team performance and communication openness, but continued behavior reinforcement is necessary to maintain continuous process improvement [39].

Besides individual learning and team performance, simulation education may be utilized to improve system functionality in specific clinical entities. The principal use for simulation is to provide learners with an opportunity for deliberate practice where they can make mistakes in a safe environment, learn from those mistakes, and achieve proficiency by attaining predefined benchmarks [40]. The complexity of critical care offers a unique opportunity to create new ways to improve the quality of care and patient safety. It is paramount that we identify areas of improvement, create methods for improving clinical outcomes, and assess ways to analyze and measure the clinical effectiveness of those changes. Checklists, protocols, and handoffs are strategies utilized to improve the quality of care in an ICU [41]. A checklist is a list of essential action items or criteria arranged in a systematic manner allowing the verification of completion of a task without necessarily leading users to a specific conclusion, which is important for guarding against cognitive biases [42]. A protocol involves the detailed plan for a treatment or procedure with mandatory items for completion leading to a predetermined outcome. Handoffs are the transfer of information, responsibility, and authority for a patient during transition of care, which may include a change in providers from various services, change of shift, or change of floor or unit.

The ultimate goal of checklists is the reduction of error by leading to improvement in compliance with best practice, especially during stressful periods. The use of a simple bedside checklist has been shown to decrease the incidence of catheter-related bloodstream infections [43] and assist in the assessment of patients suitability for weaning from mechanical ventilation [44] and the use of a daily goal checklist to better understand the goal of care for that day [45]. Our hospital instituted an Emergency Management of the Surgically Altered Airway Project to educate staff regarding the difference between tracheostomy and laryngectomy and created signage (Fig. 20.3) to indicate the type of altered airway the patient has to foster a systematic approach to the emergency care of a displaced or dislodged surgically altered airway. The project was intended to ensure that staff have knowledge in the care of the altered airway, the proper equipment was available at bedside in case of emergencies, and a cognitive aid in the form of a management algorithm for the use in the case of a displaced airway was immediately available. A high-fidelity scenario was created to further educate ICU staff in the care of a displaced tracheostomy (Table 20.1) The scenario identified problems that were not initially

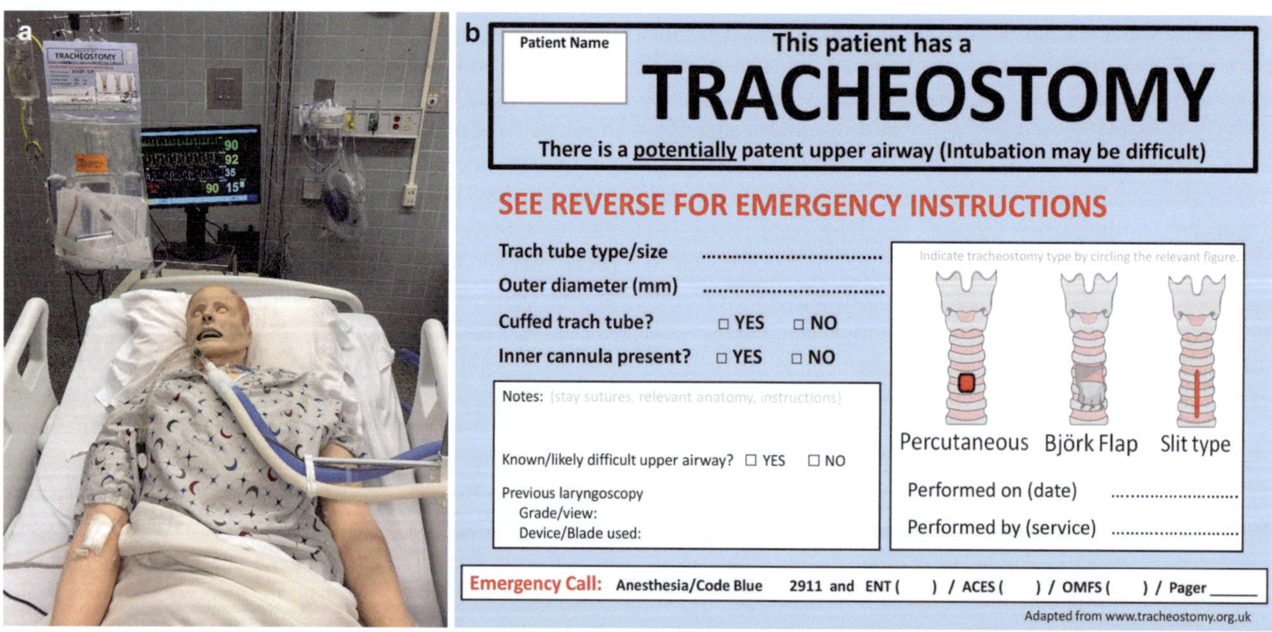

Fig. 20.3 Emergency management of the surgically altered airway scenario. (**a**) Room setup with tracheostomy sign displayed above ICU bed and patient with tracheostomy attached to ventilator. (**b**) Tracheostomy signage used in the ICU that identifies a patient with a surgically altered airway and immediate availability of pertinent facts. (**c**) Backside of each sign displaying emergency algorithm for management of surgically altered airway

c

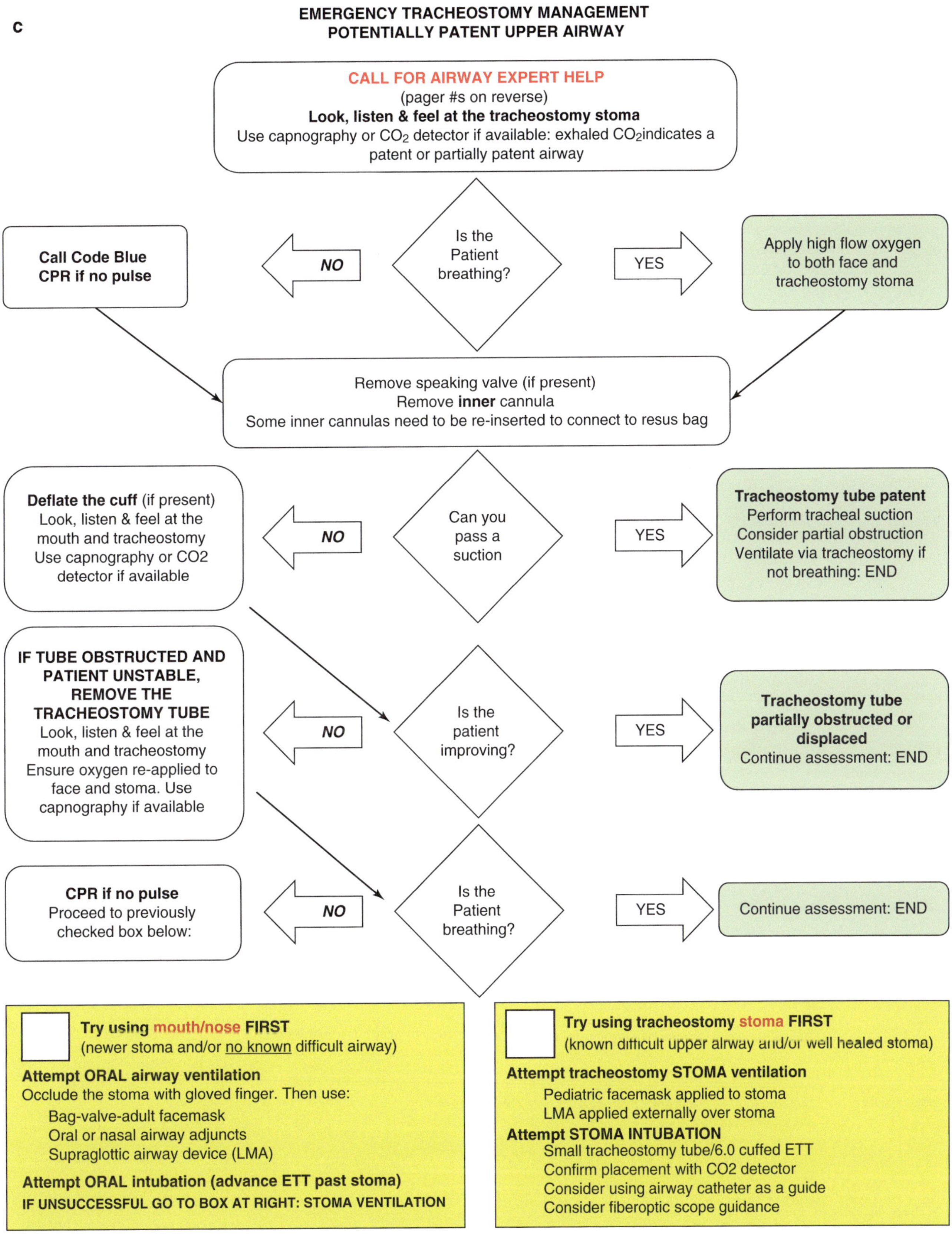

Fig. 20.3 (continued)

Table 20.1 An example of a multidisciplinary scenario of a critical care acute event with instituted signage and associated checklist cognitive aid

Title: Alternate Airways Safety Project: blocked or displaced tracheostomy scenario

Audience: ICU provider (fellow, nurse practitioner), anesthesiology resident, ICU nurse, respiratory therapist

Objective

Medical knowledge: Identify understanding of the Alternate Airways Safety Project - specifically care of a displaced advanced airway and the use of the associated cognitive aid checklist

Patient care: Management of the blocked or displaced fresh tracheostomy in a critical care patient

Communication: Utilize CRM and TeamSTEPPS approaches to the management of a critical airway issue

Case stem: Mr. Robert Giardano is a 55-year-old male transferred from an outside hospital with 4 days of decreased level of consciousness eventually requiring intubation. PMH: hypertension, hyperlipidemia. Pt received a tracheostomy 2 days ago. You are in his room and the ventilator begins to alarm for increased airway pressure. On examination, there is a small amount of blood around tracheostomy stoma. There are stay sutures taped to the patient's neck

Room setup: Intensive care unit room with patient with tracheostomy in bed connected to the ventilator. Pt has a 20G IV in his L arm connected to IV fluid administered through a pump. He has an EKG, blood pressure cuff, pulse oximeter, and end tidal CO_2 monitoring attached. On the IV pole next to the bed, there is the designated "Tracheostomy" sign and attached supply package. In the hallway is the arrest (code) cart and the emergency airway box. The anesthesia resident has a stat bag (which contains various airway management equipment for intubation and/or invasive airway management) and videolaryngoscope

State	Vital signs	Patient action/triggers	Expected participant response
High airway pressure Ventilator alarming	BP 140/60 HR 70 O2 sat 94%	ET CO2 absent Increased inspiratory pressure Pt is not breathing	Examine patient Look, listen, feel at stoma Auscultate chest Note bloody secretions Change FiO2 to 100% Call respiratory therapist
Decreasing O2 saturation	BP 160/90 HR 60 O2 sat 88%	Respiratory therapist present Note vital sign changes Decreased airway compliance/ increased resistance – resistance to bagging No chest rise	Communication Attempt to bag-valve-mask 100% FiO2 Auscultate chest Call for help Advanced provider Anesthesiology Surgical service
Diagnosis	BP 160/90 HR 50 with ectopyO2 sat 85%	Advanced provider present Decreasing O2 saturation Unable to pass suction catheter Decreased airway compliance/ increased resistance No spontaneous breathing No ETCO2	Communication Pass suction catheter Change inner cannula Repass suction catheter Deflate the cuff Check ET CO2 Remove tracheostomy
Therapy	BP 100/60 HR 40 O2 sat 80%	Anesthesiologist present Decreasing O2 saturation Unable to pass suction catheter Decreased airway compliance/ increased resistance No spontaneous breathing No ETCO2	Communication Bag ventilate with face mask Occlude stoma with gloved finger Bag ventilate stoma Pediatric facemask applied to stoma LMA applied externally over stoma
Obtain airway	(Vitals) BP 60/40 HR 30 O2 sat 70%	Decreased airway compliance/ increased resistance No spontaneous breathing (+) ETCO2 after successful securing of airway	Intubation Oral – occlude stoma Stoma – with small ETT/ tracheostomy via direct visualization of trachea using: Stay sutures Airway catheter Fiber-optic scope guidance
Deterioration	Main stem intubation/pneumothorax/ pneumomediastinum/subcutaneous emphysema	Desaturation (+) ETCO2 R sided breath sounds	Auscultate chest Check capnography Order CXR
	Cardiac arrest BP 0/0 (40/20 with chest compressions) HR 30 (PEA) O2 sat 0%	PEA	Identify no pulse CPR Epinephrine 1 mg q3–5 minutes Continue attempts to ventilate and secure airway Auscultate chest Monitor capnography
Stabilization	Successful securing airway BP 160/80 P 90 O2 saturation increase to 100%	ROSC if PEA Improved O2 saturations and HR if airway secured without PEA	Secure airway Attach to ventilator Order CXR

Table 20.2 An example of a multidisciplinary team training event for reinforcement of the utilization of an established guideline

Title: Diagnosing and therapy of a patient with sepsis utilizing the International Guidelines for Management of Sepsis and Septic Shock 2016

Audience: Critical care physicians (fellow, resident), critical care advanced practice providers, ICU nurses, respiratory therapist, pharmacist

Objective – medical knowledge: To allow the members of a multidisciplinary critical care team to engage in the diagnosis and management of a complex patient utilizing early goal-directed therapy in severe sepsis and septic shock

Patient care: Sepsis is a medical emergency caused by an overwhelming immune response to infection that requires immediate treatment and resuscitation. Identify septic shock and begin Surviving Sepsis Protocol to treat underlying infection and maximize organ perfusion. Empiric broad-spectrum IV antibiotics will be initiated, and specific anatomic diagnosis of infection requiring emergent source control will be identified or excluded as rapidly as possible. Resuscitation from sepsis-induced hypoperfusion will be initiated to maintain a MAP >65 mmHg utilizing frequent reassessment of hemodynamic status. After using crystalloids, norepinephrine should be initiated along with adding vasopressin or epinephrine to reach target MAP

Communication: Demonstrate situational awareness. Acknowledge and communicate the hypotensive/hypoxic state of the patient. Identify necessary personnel to quickly and properly diagnose and initiate therapy to patient. Demonstrate shared mental models, mutual respect, and principles of communication utilizing elements of crew resource management and TeamSTEPPS such as callbacks and closed-loop communication to ensure patient safety

Case stem: Fred Mertz is a 67-year-old 95 kg male with hypertension, hyperlipidemia, and diabetes admitted directly from a rehabilitation facility 1 week after a right total hip replacement for altered mental status and "inflamed" painful right hip. He was admitted directly to the ICU by the operating surgeon

Room setup: Intensive care unit room with patient in bed moaning. Pt has a 20G IV in his L arm connected to IV fluid administered with crystalloid infusing at 100 ml/hr through a pump and 3 L O_2 via nasal cannula. He has an EKG, blood pressure cuff, and pulse oximeter monitoring attached. In the hallway is the arrest (code) cart and the emergency airway box. The anesthesia resident has a stat bag (which contains various airway management equipment for intubation and/or invasive airway management) and videolaryngoscope

State	Vital signs	Patient action/triggers	Expected participant response
Baseline	BP 90/45 HR 115 O2 sat 91% RR: 30	Pt moaning unresponsive Red inflamed R hip Rhonchi respirations	Assess patient Place monitors Initiate admission orders Draw labs Call necessary personnel Advanced practice provider Respiratory therapist
Initial actions	BP 80/40 HR 120 O2 sat 88% RR: 30 T 38.5 deg C	Neuro unchanged Increasing hypovolemia with hypotension/ tachycardia/tachypnea until interventions	Check VS including Temp Increase FiO2 delivery Increase IV fluid rate Call physician
Sepsis diagnosis	BP 70/40 HR 125 O2 sat 85% RR: 35	Neuro unchanged Increasing hypovolemia with hypotension/ tachycardia/tachypnea until interventions	Obtain labs – BMP, CBC, Coags, Lactate Draw cultures – blood, sputum, urine Place Foley catheter
Initiate Surviving Sepsis Protocol	BP 75/35 P 125 O2 sat 93% RR 35 T 38.5 deg C	Targets MAP >65 mmHg HR <90 Lactate <4mMol RR <20 SaO2 > 92% Hct >7	Place arterial line Place central line Consider intubation Initiate mechanical ventilation <6 ml/kg volume Send ABG/VBG Administer 1 L crystalloid Begin empiric broad spectrum antibiotics
Result of actions		Adjust BP/P according to fluid administration/ inotrope dose (MAP >65) Adjust O2 sat according FiO2/mechanical ventilation (O2 sat >92%)	Administer 30 ml/kg crystalloid Assessment of volume status POCUS, CVP, urine output, ScvO2, pulse pressure variation, lactate clearance Consider inotrope norepinephrine, then vasopressin (0.03 U/min), epinephrine Consider hydrocortisone Contact orthopedics for source control
Endpoint	MAP >65 HR <100 ScvO2 > 70 O2 sat >92%	Hemodynamic stability Adequate ventilation/oxygenation	IV fluids running at designated rate Inotropes infusing Antibiotics started Mechanical ventilation established

anticipated when the program was introduced: essential equipment was not available in an emergency as it was readily removed from the enclosed package and not replaced, the algorithm was rarely employed as it was not emphasized as an important component of the signage to be used as a cognitive aid in an emergency, and practitioners at all levels were reticent to remove the tracheostomy in an emergency especially if it was sutured in place.

Protocols have the potential to minimize errors and improve patient safety and outcomes by minimizing inconsistencies in the care of similar patients by the myriad critical care providers [46]. Protocols are not the all-inconclusive one size fits all but assists care providers to manage the basic complex disease leading to better organized care avoiding unnecessary tests and unneeded therapies while maximizing resource utilization and decreasing overall healthcare costs [46]. The use of guidelines in critical care medicine has been introduced allowing for the utilization of consistent evidence-based practice. Protocols such as "Surviving Sepsis Campaign: International Guidelines for Management of Sepsis and Septic Shock: 2016" [47] and "Mechanical Ventilation in Adult Patients with Acute Respiratory Distress Syndrome" [48] lead to a favorable process of care by minimizing inconsistencies and highlighting the potential to decrease medical errors and the likelihood of injury, increase patient safety, and improve patient outcomes [46]. Protocols rehearsed in simulation scenarios allow multidisciplinary participants to better integrate and perform their responsibilities in a specific clinical event. A critical care scenario was created in the diagnosis and therapy of a patient with septic shock, which utilizes the Surviving Sepsis Guidelines (Table 20.2). Performance improvement programs related to compliance to the Surviving Sepsis Protocol lead to reductions in mortality especially when initiated early [49]. The utilization of this type of scenario enables participants to enact the important components of the guidelines and showcases the importance of early goal-directed therapy leading to a significant mortality reduction [50]. Participants in simulation training can immediately see the consequences of their decisions and resultant actions. Errors can be allowed to occur and reach a conclusion, whereas in real life, supervising clinicians would have to intervene to prevent patient injury [51]. Compliance with evidenced-based clinical practice guidelines is often poor due to access to such guidelines at point of care; inability to modify them based on variability of patient population and physiology, being viewed as limitation to clinical judgment and decision autonomy related to personal clinical experience; and availability of an overwhelming number of checklists [42].

Transitions of care occur frequently in the critical care environment with every handoff, providing an opportunity for errors in communication, making standardized handoffs a priority to improve patient safety. Successful handoffs are accomplished through management of barriers to effective communication such as time pressure, patient acuity, and competing priorities [52]. The use of simulation has proven effective in improving handoff performance, especially related to interpersonal verbal skills, as opposed to actual physical behaviors (i.e., checking ventilator settings or monitors) [53]. The use of a specific standardized template (i.e., SBAR [54], iPASS [55]) is employed to improve communication in handoffs, providing structured succinct information that minimizes the risk of deletions of critical information delivered in a hard stop situation designed to limit interruption or distraction between providers [56]. The utilization of a simulation-based training program for standardization of handoffs led to an improvement in communication behaviors using interpersonal verbal skills; however, it did not change actual physical behaviors such as checking of monitors or ventilators [53]. The use of simulation to practice and actively participate in the employment of patient safety maneuvers such as checklists, protocols, and handoffs allows for the analysis of the process while not interfering with actual patient care. Reflective debriefing after the simulation sessions allows the evaluation of the process' effectiveness, identifies opportunities for improvement, and explored the relevance of incorporation of the necessary behavioral changes into future personal practice. As critical care teams become more familiar with our high-fidelity simulation environment, the more pronounced the important nontechnical aspects of their performance become. The initial quiet team going about their responsibilities under the direction of the deeply involved leader has become a more vocal environment with clear concise direction from an identifiable leader who is more adept at allowing other team members to perform their assigned roles, with interactive team members discussing important care decisions and clear callback of completed responsibilities with the assumption that these improvements are carried over into daily clinical responsibilities.

Advantages of Simulation in Critical Care (Table 20.3)

There are many advantages to simulation training in the critical care environment. Critical care has long depended on the classic apprentice-style training. The classic critical care educational setting of rounds and prepared lectures lead to passive acquisition of knowledge that is not readily retrieved in the intensive care environment under high-stress situations. This often is insufficient as basic fundamental critical care opportunities may not occur during a trainee's rotation, leading to potential educational deficiencies. Education

Table 20.3 Advantages of simulation training

1.	Provides a risk-free environment for the patient and trainees where errors can be played out to their conclusion
2.	Unlimited exposure to a wide variety of scenarios including complicated, rare, and/or important clinical events
3.	Ability to create and plan for training opportunities rather than awaiting clinical situation
4.	Recreates concise repetitive scenarios that incrementally improve trainee performance by providing reproducible standardized educational experiences
5.	Promotes clinical and nontechnical skills acquisition and encourages deliberate practice with clinical problems that complement clinical experiences
6.	Adapts to accommodate multiple learning strategies
7.	Allows the use of specific ICU equipment with available personnel
8.	Permits flexible scheduling of training in an era of reduced resident work hours
9.	Provides immediate feedback to trainees allowing for introspection and reflection
10.	Scenario performance recordings facilitate review and feedback
11.	Opportunity for crisis resource management/team training that provides increased safety

Adapted from Refs. [5, 57, 69]

in critical care is challenging due to complexities of care being provided, vast medical knowledge required for management, and need for rapid decision-making potentially with multiple patients concomitantly. Simulation affords the trainee the opportunity to learn high-risk emergency events, even uncommon ones, presented in an uninterrupted concentrated method that allows for the assessment of the presenting symptoms under time and logistic pressures, and fosters critical thinking to solve the presented clinical entities, priority setting to provide appropriate interventions in a timely fashion, management of the response to various treatment modalities, and evaluation of the clinical outcomes predicated on the trainee's decision-making skills which all work to create an environment that allows clinicians to experience a real event for the purpose of practice, learning, evaluation, and testing or to gain understanding of systems or human actions [57]. These scenarios can be defined with goal-oriented clinical experiences that are standardized to be repetitive of content and interactive learning [58]. Training via high-fidelity simulation enhances the participants' engagement in an exercise leading to quicker response times, less deviation from accepted guidelines, and better performance in handling crises when compared to standard practice [7]. Using simulation in the critical care environment allows for improving team performance in the workplace through familiarity with equipment, personnel, care plans, and situations. Critical care systems can be evaluated, uncovering ways to practice and improve existing care when local system errors are revealed. Simulation allows participants to learn about the environment in which they work and the processes in place from various clinical perspectives. Latent safety threats (LSTs) in medicine are defined as system-based threats to patient safety that can materialize at any time, previously unrecognized by healthcare providers resulting from conditions such as time pressure, understaffing, fatigue, inadequate equipment and experience, inadequate supervision, and miscommunication precipitating errors in violations. Simulation training allows for the identification of LSTs, deliberate practice of teamwork and communication skills, and provides multiple opportunities to improve patient safety [59].

How to Set Up a Well-Defined Scenario (Table 20.4)

The first step in creating a clinical scenario is to identify the critical care unit's educational needs. Scenario creation can be based upon a critical event that has occurred, new or existing protocols (such as sepsis and handoffs), a common event or disease entity that occurs frequently, or an obvious unit educational or competency need that requires practice. The next step requires defining the objective of the simulation scenario. Examples include the diagnosis of the condition and initiation of therapy, technical procedural tasks that the staff must apply, effective team interactions, or the adherence to the unit protocols or standards. After determining the existing knowledge base of the participants, the expected educational goals of the participants in the scenario can be defined. These outcomes can be technical, clinical, team training, emotional or a specific message that needs to be conveyed. Simulations should be designed to allow for leadership or hierarchical organization, situational awareness, structured communication techniques including closed-loop communication and handoffs, shared mental model, team member expertise, and interdependence that functions to further unit interpersonal communication and performance (see Chap. 3 for more details).

It is important to define the necessary physical environment (i.e., ICU, mannequin, monitors, and personnel), the patient encompassing realistic pathology and physiology, the equipment and supplies available to the participants, as well as a description of the patient's present state when the scenario begins. To create a realistic environment for learning in simulation, the participants are advised to adhere to a simple rule that mimics reality – "if you don't do it – it wasn't done." It is not sufficient to simply vocalize an aspect of care; medication must actually be given and procedures performed. The participants should have a period of time to become accustomed to their surroundings and the patient. It is important to keep the clinical scenarios simple involving one or two clinical event stimuli within a short time to keep

Table 20.4 Creating a well-defined ICU simulation scenario

1. Identify critical care educational need
Critical event that occurred
Existing protocols, i.e., sepsis, handoff
"Common" event – clinical disease entities
Fill an obvious unit educational need – area for practice
Crisis resource management, TeamSTEPPS®
2. Define the objective
Diagnosis of condition and initiation of therapy
Technical procedural tasks
Effective team interactions
Adherence to unit protocol or standards
3. Define learning outcomes – what are the expected educational goals
Define existing knowledge of participants
What is to be learned from scenario
Technical
Clinical
Team Training
Emotional
Specific message
4. Create a realistic environment for learning
Imitation of actual events – realistic pathology/physiology
Critical care environment – Mannequin, equipment, monitors
Rules of simulation
If you don't do it – it isn't done
What happens here – stays here
Keep it simple
One or two clinical event stimuli within a short time period
Allow multiple possible solutions to successful conclusion
5. Create a storyboard of the scenario
Define stimulus to action
Delineate expected progression of events
Critical event to be diagnosed – ways to enhance identification
Endpoint of scenario
6. Debriefing
Open ended discussion – "How did it go?"
Identification of problem encountered and plan for treating
Reflect on actions – experiential learning
Relate actions to everyday practice
Team coordination for more effective management
7. Learner assessment of simulation exercise
Recognition of objectives
Identification of activity's value to daily responsibilities
Strengths of exercise
Areas of improvement
8. Assess influence of activity on quality of care
Does it impact clinical care – learners utilize learning objectives
Can utilize
Self-assessment
Questionnaires
Group discussion
Direct observation
Performance audits

the participants engaged. As the participants interact with the patient simulator, specific triggers occur that are clinical events that precipitate the scenario and require specific essential actions and behaviors of the participants. These events can be an alteration in the patient's status, the discovery of a new clinical change, an environmental modification, or a circumstance precipitated by a participant (confederate). Often a confederate, an associate with insight related to the scenario, may be utilized to impart information or initiate an action that should instigate further actions by members of the scenario clinical team. This creates the crux of the scenario where there is a new set of circumstances, new data to be assessed, or other changes that require the learner to respond in a desired way. As the participants proceed, it is important to have a clear clinical endpoint that adheres to the teaching points related to an actual patient event, new procedure, protocol, or evidence-based practice. The best scenarios are those in which actions by the participants are met by a clinically correct response of the environment or patient simulator (i.e., administration of atropine leads to persistent tachycardia) and not preprogrammed to occur as if it is a simple ACLS scenario. This appears to make the scenario more realistic and provide greater opportunities for success. The ultimate goal of the created scenario is that the behavior of the clinical team determines a realistic successful conclusion to the clinical scenario. If scenarios are well-crafted, trainees will be engaged, gain experience, and develop accurate mental models on how to respond to similar situations faced on the job (transfer of training), gaining higher confidence levels when responding to similar situations, improving memory recall leading to better and quicker decision-making [60]. Debriefing is an integral part of any experiential-learning simulation technique (see also Chap. 4). Feedback of one's performance is the single most important feature of simulation-based medical education as it slows the decay of acquired skills and allows learners to self-assess and monitor their progress toward skill acquisition and maintenance [61]. The purpose of debriefing is to reinforce experiential learning by reviewing the participants' understanding of what occurred and allow them to reflect on how this scenario relates to real-life critical care situations. Participants should feel safe to voice their opinions without judgment from others in the scenario group, and it should be made clear that all discussions that occur remain confidential to that specific group – "what happens here – stays here." Elements of a successful debriefing include creating a friendly atmosphere; utilizing open-ended questions; facilitating self-reflection, positive reinforcement, and open discussions on management aspects; pointing out underlying principles that lead to misconceptions/errors; using cognitive aids; showing alternatives; stressing that everybody makes mistakes; concentrating on a few key learning points; and emphasizing the positive aspects [62]. It is important to allow all members of the critical care multidisciplinary team to clarify their roles and responsibilities in the scenario. Debriefing feedback should allow for initial self-assessment, utilization of the self-assessment to provide both positive and corrective feedback, and then create an action plan for improvement. This approach allows for incorporation of the trainee's perspective, avoids judgment, and promotes self-reflection. It is essential that the debriefing provide a clear understanding of crucial errors that can perpetuate medical mistakes and undermine patient safety when the trainee returns to the real clinical environment [63]. Simulation debriefing should create a safe environment for students so that they feel comfortable discussing mistakes. Discussing students' emotional involvement during simulation allows them to confront possible uncomfortable occurrences and deal with them in a controlled and safe setting to allow them to become more confident in their professional practice and develop strategies for dealing with these feelings during real patient situations [64]. There may be benefit to debrief real-life critical events as it allows participants to better reflect with immediate feedback [65]. After completion of a simulation scenario, it is important to get the participants' evaluations of the exercises. Evaluation should include the recognition and achievement of objectives and identification of the scenarios' value to daily responsibilities, strengths of the scenario, and areas for improvement.

It is impossible to recreate the critical care environment and atmosphere exactly in simulation. The major dissatisfiers for simulation participants have been the unfamiliarity with the simulation environment and the artificial nature of the mannequin. There are often complaints regarding the room and supplies that do not match "my ICU" (particularly if the simulation environment is held not in situ but in another location) and the response to the ongoing situation does not match the amount or quality of help they expect. It is common for participants to voice the opinion that the mannequin does not act exactly like its human counterpart. That opinion usually becomes moot when the scenario is ongoing and the vital signs and environmental changes become more synonymous with the mannequin. Another problem encountered in the simulation exercises is that the participants become fixated looking for a specific problem that occurs that it is not intended as part of the scenario. It is often necessary to use distractors (signals not related to the actual scenario) to discourage participants from becoming fixated on unintended specific events. Familiarity or comfort with the simulation environment fortunately does not appear to have a significant effect on performance. Increased realism achieved by performing simulation-based training in a recreated intensive care environment or in situ simulation that occurs in the critical care unit allows participants to utilize their own environment and equipment and allows for deliberate practice around procedures and protocols that are specific and relevant to that team [66]. After simulation training has been utilized, it is recommended that you assess the influence of the activity on the quality of care in the intensive care unit and includes assessing whether the simulation training impacted clinical care and whether the learners utilized the learning objectives that were imparted. Methods to assess the utility of simulation training are self-assessment, questionnaire, group discussion, direct observation, and performance audits.

The key element to the successful utilization of simulation is that the simulations themselves become integrated throughout the entire critical care curriculum so that deliberate practice will allow practitioners to acquire expertise over time. Knowledge alone is insufficient to successfully implement protocols as teamwork and communication abilities are also required [67]. Communication and teamwork errors can be difficult to identify and correct during actual clinical events. Deliberate practice and not solely experience in clinical settings is the key to the development of medical clinical competence [61].

Conclusion

The application of simulation training to critical care medicine affords a type of learning that cannot be replicated in didactic presentations such as lectures, rounds, and discussions. Simulation training leads to better clinician education, technical skill development, crisis resource management and teamwork training, and evaluation of unit clinical performance and processes [68]. Simulation should not totally replace traditional real-life teaching methods but should serve as an appropriate complement to allow trainees to ascertain how to provide best care practices for the critically ill patient. Through the use of simulation technology, real-life critical care scenarios and environments can lead to trainees who use higher analytical skills to complete tasks and result in improvement in long-term performance, reduced response time, and increased adherence to the evidence-based standard care practices.

References

1. Hanson CW 3rd, Durbin CG Jr, Maccioli GA, et al. The anesthesiologist in critical care medicine: past, present, and future. Anesthesiology. 2001;95:781–8.
2. Kim MM, Barnato AE, Angus DC, Fleisher LA, Kahn JM. The effect of multidisciplinary care teams on intensive care unit mortality. Arch Intern Med. 2010;170:369–76.
3. Baggs JG, Schmitt MH, Mushlin AI, et al. Association between nurse-physician collaboration and patient outcomes in three intensive care units. Crit Care Med. 1999;27:1991–8.
4. Murray DJ. Clinical simulation: technical novelty or innovation in education. Anesthesiology. 1998;89:1–2.
5. Hammond J. Simulation in critical care and trauma education and training. Curr Opin Crit Care. 2004;10:325–9.
6. Cooke JM, Larsen J, Hamstra SJ, Andreatta PB. Simulation enhances resident confidence in critical care and procedural skills. Fam Med. 2008;40:165–7.

7. Chopra V, Gesink BJ, de Jong J, Bovill JG, Spierdijk J, Brand R. Does training on an anaesthesia simulator lead to improvement in performance? Br J Anaesth. 1994;73:293–7.
8. Scalese RJ, Obeso VT, Issenberg SB. Simulation technology for skills training and competency assessment in medical education. J Gen Intern Med. 2008;23(Suppl 1):46–9.
9. Levine AI, Swartz MH. Standardized patients: the "other" simulation. J Crit Care. 2008;23:179–84.
10. Cohen ER, Feinglass J, Barsuk JH, et al. Cost savings from reduced catheter-related bloodstream infection after simulation-based education for residents in a medical intensive care unit. Simul Healthcare: J Soc Simul Healthcare. 2010;5:98–102.
11. Nishisaki A, Nguyen J, Colborn S, et al. Evaluation of multidisciplinary simulation training on clinical performance and team behavior during tracheal intubation procedures in a pediatric intensive care unit. Pediatric Crit Care Med: J Soc Crit Care Med World Feder Pediatric Intens Crit Care Soc. 2011;12:406–14.
12. Wayne DB, Barsuk JH, O'Leary KJ, Fudala MJ, McGaghie WC. Mastery learning of thoracentesis skills by internal medicine residents using simulation technology and deliberate practice. J Hosp Med. 2008;3:48–54.
13. Lammers RL, Davenport M, Korley F, et al. Teaching and assessing procedural skills using simulation: metrics and methodology. Acad Emerg Med Off J Soc Acad Emerg Med. 2008;15:1079–87.
14. Barsuk JH, McGaghie WC, Cohen ER, Balachandran JS, Wayne DB. Use of simulation-based mastery learning to improve the quality of central venous catheter placement in a medical intensive care unit. J Hosp Med. 2009;4:397–403.
15. Maran NJ, Glavin RJ. Low- to high-fidelity simulation - a continuum of medical education? Med Educ. 2003;37(Suppl 1):22–8.
16. Wayne DB, Didwania A, Feinglass J, Fudala MJ, Barsuk JH, McGaghie WC. Simulation-based education improves quality of care during cardiac arrest team responses at an academic teaching hospital: a case-control study. Chest. 2008;133:56–61.
17. Colt HG, Crawford SW, Galbraith O 3rd. Virtual reality bronchoscopy simulation: a revolution in procedural training. Chest. 2001;120:1333–9.
18. Mercaldi CJ, Lanes SF. Ultrasound guidance decreases complications and improves the cost of care among patients undergoing thoracentesis and paracentesis. Chest. 2013;143:532–8.
19. Neri L, Storti E, Lichtenstein D. Toward an ultrasound curriculum for critical care medicine. Crit Care Med. 2007;35:S290–304.
20. Dinh VA, Giri PC, Rathinavel I, et al. Impact of a 2-day critical care ultrasound course during fellowship training: a pilot study. Crit Care Res Prac. 2015;2015:675041.
21. Neelankavil J, Howard-Quijano K, Hsieh TC, et al. Transthoracic echocardiography simulation is an efficient method to train anesthesiologists in basic transthoracic echocardiography skills. Anesth Analg. 2012;115:1042–51.
22. Melamed R, Sprenkle MD, Ulstad VK, Herzog CA, Leatherman JW. Assessment of left ventricular function by intensivists using hand-held echocardiography. Chest. 2009;135:1416–20.
23. Frankel HL, Kirkpatrick AW, Elbarbary M, et al. Guidelines for the appropriate use of bedside general and cardiac ultrasonography in the evaluation of critically ill patients-part I: general ultrasonography. Crit Care Med. 2015;43:2479–502.
24. Levitov A, Frankel HL, Blaivas M, et al. Guidelines for the appropriate use of bedside general and cardiac ultrasonography in the evaluation of critically ill patients-part II: cardiac ultrasonography. Crit Care Med. 2016;44:1206–27.
25. Gaba DM, DeAnda A. A comprehensive anesthesia simulation environment: re-creating the operating room for research and training. Anesthesiology. 1988;69:387–94.
26. Gaba DM. Structural and organizational issues in patient safety: a comparison of health care to other high-hazard industries. Calif Manag Rev. 2000;43:83–102.
27. Weingart NS, Wilson RM, Gibberd RW, Harrison B. Epidemiology of medical error. BMJ. 2000;320:774–7.
28. Fletcher G, Flin R, McGeorge P, Glavin R, Maran N, Anaesthetists PR. Non-Technical Skills (ANTS): evaluation of a behavioural marker system. Br J Anaesth. 2003;90:580–8.
29. McGaghie WC, Issenberg SB, Petrusa ER, Scalese RJ. A critical review of simulation-based medical education research: 2003–2009. Med Educ. 2010;44:50–63.
30. Flin R, Patey R, Glavin R, Maran N. Anaesthetists' non-technical skills. Br J Anaesth. 2010;105:38–44.
31. Gaba DM, Fish KJ, Howard SK. Crisis management in anesthesia. New York: Churchill Livingstone; 1994.
32. Rothschild JM, Landrigan CP, Cronin JW, et al. The critical care safety study: the incidence and nature of adverse events and serious medical errors in intensive care. Crit Care Med. 2005;33:1694–700.
33. Thomas EJ, Sexton JB, Helmreich RL. Discrepant attitudes about teamwork among critical care nurses and physicians. Crit Care Med. 2003;31:956–9.
34. Enhancing nurse-physician collaboration using pediatric simulation. J Contin Educ Nurs. 2015;46:243.
35. Reader TW, Flin R, Cuthbertson BH. Team leadership in the intensive care unit: the perspective of specialists. Crit Care Med. 2011;39:1683–91.
36. Frengley RW, Weller JM, Torrie J, et al. The effect of a simulation-based training intervention on the performance of established critical care unit teams. Crit Care Med. 2011;39:2605–11.
37. Kohn LT, Corrigan JM, Donaldson MS, editors. To err is human: building a safer health system. Washington (DC); 2000.
38. https://www.ahrq.gov/teamstepps/instructor/index.html.
39. Mayer CM, Cluff L, Lin WT, et al. Evaluating efforts to optimize TeamSTEPPS implementation in surgical and pediatric intensive care units. Jt Comm J Qual Patient Saf. 2011;37:365–74.
40. Aggarwal R, Mytton OT, Derbrew M, et al. Training and simulation for patient safety. Qual Saf Health Care. 2010;19(Suppl 2):i34–43.
41. Bauman KA, Hyzy RC. ICU 2020: five interventions to revolutionize quality of care in the ICU. J Intensive Care Med. 2014;29:13–21.
42. Hales BM, Pronovost PJ. The checklist--a tool for error management and performance improvement. J Crit Care. 2006;21:231–5.
43. Berenholtz SM, Pronovost PJ, Lipsett PA, et al. Eliminating catheter-related bloodstream infections in the intensive care unit. Crit Care Med. 2004;32:2014–20.
44. Walsh TS, Dodds S, McArdle F. Evaluation of simple criteria to predict successful weaning from mechanical ventilation in intensive care patients. Br J Anaesth. 2004;92:793–9.
45. Pronovost P, Berenholtz S, Dorman T, Lipsett PA, Simmonds T, Haraden C. Improving communication in the ICU using daily goals. J Crit Care. 2003;18:71–5.
46. Chang SY, Sevransky J, Martin GS. Protocols in the management of critical illness. Crit Care. 2012;16:306.
47. Rhodes A, Evans LE, Alhazzani W, et al. Surviving sepsis campaign: international guidelines for management of sepsis and septic shock: 2016. Crit Care Med. 2017;45:486–552.
48. Fan E, Del Sorbo L, Goligher EC, et al. An Official American Thoracic Society/European Society of Intensive Care Medicine/Society of Critical Care Medicine Clinical Practice Guideline: Mechanical Ventilation in Adult Patients with Acute Respiratory Distress Syndrome. Am J Respir Crit Care Med. 2017;195:1253–63.
49. Gu WJ, Wang F, Bakker J, Tang L, Liu JC. The effect of goal-directed therapy on mortality in patients with sepsis - earlier is better: a meta-analysis of randomized controlled trials. Crit Care. 2014;18:570.
50. Nguyen HB, Jaehne AK, Jayaprakash N, et al. Early goal-directed therapy in severe sepsis and septic shock: insights and comparisons to ProCESS, ProMISe, and ARISE. Crit Care. 2016;20:160.
51. Gaba DM. Anaesthesiology as a model for patient safety in health care. BMJ: Br Med J. 2000;320:785.

52. Slagle JM, Kuntz A, France D, Speroff T, Madbouly A, Weinger MB. Simulation training for rapid assessment and improved teamwork-lessons learned from a project evaluating clinical handoffs. Proceedings of the Human Factors and Ergonomics Society Annual Meeting. 2007;51:668–72.
53. Berkenstadt H, Haviv Y, Tuval A, et al. Improving handoff communications in critical care: utilizing simulation-based training toward process improvement in managing patient risk. Chest. 2008;134:158–62.
54. Eberhardt S. Improve handoff communication with SBAR. Nursing. 2014;44:17–20.
55. Starmer AJ, Spector ND, Srivastava R, Allen AD, Landrigan CP, Sectish TC. I-pass, a mnemonic to standardize verbal handoffs. Pediatrics. 2012;129:201–4.
56. Dunlap E, Talley D, Silverman D, et al. 1105: Improving patient safety with a formalized postoperative handoff in the ICU. Crit Care Med. 2016;44(12):Supplement:352.
57. Eppich WJ, Adler MD, McGaghie WC. Emergency and critical care pediatrics: use of medical simulation for training in acute pediatric emergencies. Curr Opin Pediatr. 2006;18:266–71.
58. Steadman RH, Coates WC, Huang YM, et al. Simulation-based training is superior to problem-based learning for the acquisition of critical assessment and management skills. Crit Care Med. 2006;34:151–7.
59. Patterson MD, Geis GL, Falcone RA, LeMaster T, Wears RL. In situ simulation: detection of safety threats and teamwork training in a high risk emergency department. BMJ Qual Safety. 2013;22:468–77.
60. Salas E, Wilson KA, Burke CS, Priest HA. Using simulation-based training to improve patient safety: what does it take? Jt Comm J Qual Patient Saf. 2005;31:363–71.
61. Issenberg SB, McGaghie WC, Petrusa ER, Lee Gordon D, Scalese RJ. Features and uses of high-fidelity medical simulations that lead to effective learning: a BEME systematic review. Med Teach. 2005;27:10–28.
62. Rall M, Manser T, Howard SK. Key elements of debriefing for simulator training. Eur J Anaesthesiol. 2000;17:516–7.
63. Rudolph JW, Simon R, Dufresne RL, Raemer DB. There's no such thing as "nonjudgmental" debriefing: a theory and method for debriefing with good judgment. Simul Healthcare: J Soc Simul Healthcare. 2006;1:49–55.
64. Henneman EA, Cunningham H. Using clinical simulation to teach patient safety in an acute/critical care nursing course. Nurse Educ. 2005;30:172–7.
65. Savoldelli GL, Naik VN, Park J, Joo HS, Chow R, Hamstra SJ. Value of debriefing during simulated crisis management: oral versus video-assisted oral feedback. Anesthesiology. 2006;105:279–85.
66. Allan CK, Thiagarajan RR, Beke D, et al. Simulation-based training delivered directly to the pediatric cardiac intensive care unit engenders preparedness, comfort, and decreased anxiety among multidisciplinary resuscitation teams. J Thorac Cardiovasc Surg. 2010;140:646–52.
67. Mah JW, Bingham K, Dobkin ED, et al. Mannequin simulation identifies common surgical intensive care unit teamwork errors long after introduction of sepsis guidelines. Simul Healthcare: J Soc Simul Healthcare. 2009;4:193–9.
68. Lighthall GK, Barr J. The use of clinical simulation systems to train critical care physicians. J Intensive Care Med. 2007;22:257–69.
69. Grenvik A, Schaefer JJ, DeVita MA, Rogers P. New aspects on critical care medicine training. Curr Opin Crit Care. 2004;10:233–7.

21 Simulation in Regional Anesthesia

Amanda H. Kumar and Ankeet D. Udani

Abbreviations

ACGME	Accreditation Council for Graduate Medical Education
ASRA	American Society of Regional Anesthesia and Pain Medicine
AV	Atrioventricular
CAD	Coronary artery disease
CNS	Central nervous system
CPR	Cardiopulmonary resuscitation
EKG	Electrocardiogram
ESRA	European Society of Regional Anaesthesia and Pain Therapy
IV	Intravenous catheter
LAST	Local anesthetic systemic toxicity
OSCE	Objective structured clinical examinations

Introduction

Given the growing role of simulation within medical education and anesthesia training, as the scope of regional anesthesia practice continues to expand, so too must that of medical simulation in order to provide trainees with a means of practice and trial. This comes at a time of increasing requirements for simulation-based medical education in anesthesia training. Within the context of Accreditation Council for Graduate Medical Education (ACGME) yearly requirements for resident participation in simulated clinical experiences [1] and the American Board of Anesthesiology (ABA) recommendations for a simulation component for its Maintenance of Certification in Anesthesiology [2], the American Society of Regional Anesthesia and Pain Medicine (ASRA) and the European Society of Regional Anaesthesia and Pain Therapy (ESRA) Joint Committee acknowledge the expanding scope of ultrasound-guided regional anesthesia and encourage practitioners, both trainees and physicians already in practice, to utilize simulation-based programs to hone skills [3].

While the demand for simulation in regional anesthesia appears to be increasing, the validation of various modes of simulation training for regional anesthesia is still emerging. One trial showed that trainees achieve competency in regional anesthesia procedures at different learning curves, with an estimate that novices may require 28 supervised trials of a particular block with feedback in order to achieve competency in ultrasound-guided needle visualization [4].

Regional anesthesia requires meticulous skill and precision given the aim of depositing local anesthetic in close proximity to vital structures, such as blood vessels, pleura, and organs, while avoiding direct injection into nerves themselves. Sites et al. showed that one common error observed in inexperienced anesthesia trainees during simulation was advancing the needle without accurate needle visualization resulting in excessive depth of penetration which can result in iatrogenic injury in the clinical setting [5]. Simulation in regional anesthesia can allow the opportunity for hands-on experience in an environment that eliminates potential harm to patients during the process of learning while allowing for repetition of procedural skills and immediate feedback. The simulated environment also provides an opportunity for exposure to clinical events that many trainees will not experience during their training due to their rare incidence (i.e., local anesthetic systemic toxicity, wrong-sided block, etc.).

A. H. Kumar (✉) · A. D. Udani
Department of Anesthesiology, Duke University Medical Center, Durham, NC, USA
e-mail: Amanda.Kumar@duke.edu; Ankeet.Udani@duke.edu

B. Mahoney et al. (eds.), *Comprehensive Healthcare Simulation: Anesthesiology*, Comprehensive Healthcare Simulation,
https://doi.org/10.1007/978-3-030-26849-7_21

Part Task Trainers and Skill Acquisition

Successful regional anesthetic blocks rely upon the appropriate distribution of local anesthetic around target nerve structures. The use of ultrasound guidance has allowed for direct visualization of nerves and surrounding anatomic structures as well as both direct and indirect visualization of local anesthetic spread [6]. Proficiency in regional anesthesia not only relies upon sound knowledge of sonoanatomy but also a mastery of the art of needling. Needling requires hand-eye coordination for manipulation of the ultrasound transducer to achieve an optimal image of the target while simultaneously advancing the needle in a dynamic setting.

Part task training through the use of simulators allows students to practice hand-eye coordination. Resident anesthesiologists who received a 1-hour simulation training session on needling using low-fidelity, inorganic part task trainers were more successful than a control group receiving no simulation, as measured by clinical block success on real patients [7]. Another randomized trial assigned anesthesia residents to receive simulation-based deliberate practice teaching on a task trainer or to a base curriculum without simulation to learn how to perform subarachnoid blocks [8]. Performance scores as evaluated by a task checklist improved in the group receiving simulation-based training, though there was no difference between groups in time to perform a subarachnoid block in real patients. Both studies, despite their limitations, support that exposure to simulation-based practice in a low-fidelity setting can result in improved regional anesthesia performance.

Anesthesia residents utilizing an agar model showed a dose-dependent improvement with faster performance and less technical flaws for students who received 2 hours of simulation as compared to those that received only 1 hour or no simulation training [9]. One group calculated a mathematical model of the learning curve for novice ultrasound users showing that inexperienced ultrasound users can improve their hand-eye coordination to find a target nerve after five subsequent trials using a simple phantom model [10]. These trials lend support to the assertion that simulation can improve block efficiency, a key skill for clinical practice.

Given the monetary, clinical, and administrative demands on teaching institutions, resource allocation can often be a concern when introducing a simulation curriculum. A study of resident anesthesiologists learning to place epidural catheters utilizing either low-fidelity or high-fidelity models showed similar performance scores, revealing that lower-fidelity models which are more cost-effective may yield comparable efficacy [11]. In fact, a comparison of three different low-cost phantom models showed that novice residents had decreased number of errors and decreased time to task completion with each additional practice attempt in simulation regardless of the type of simulator [12].

There are many simulation tools in use for part task training for ultrasound-guided regional anesthesia based on the needs of the learner and the available resources. Inorganic materials, also called phantom models, both anatomic and nonanatomic, are commercially available and reusable; however, these models often lack realistic tactile sensation and haptic feedback and do not allow for injection of liquid solutions (Figs. 21.1 and 21.2). Advantageously, inorganic models can be created from common operating room

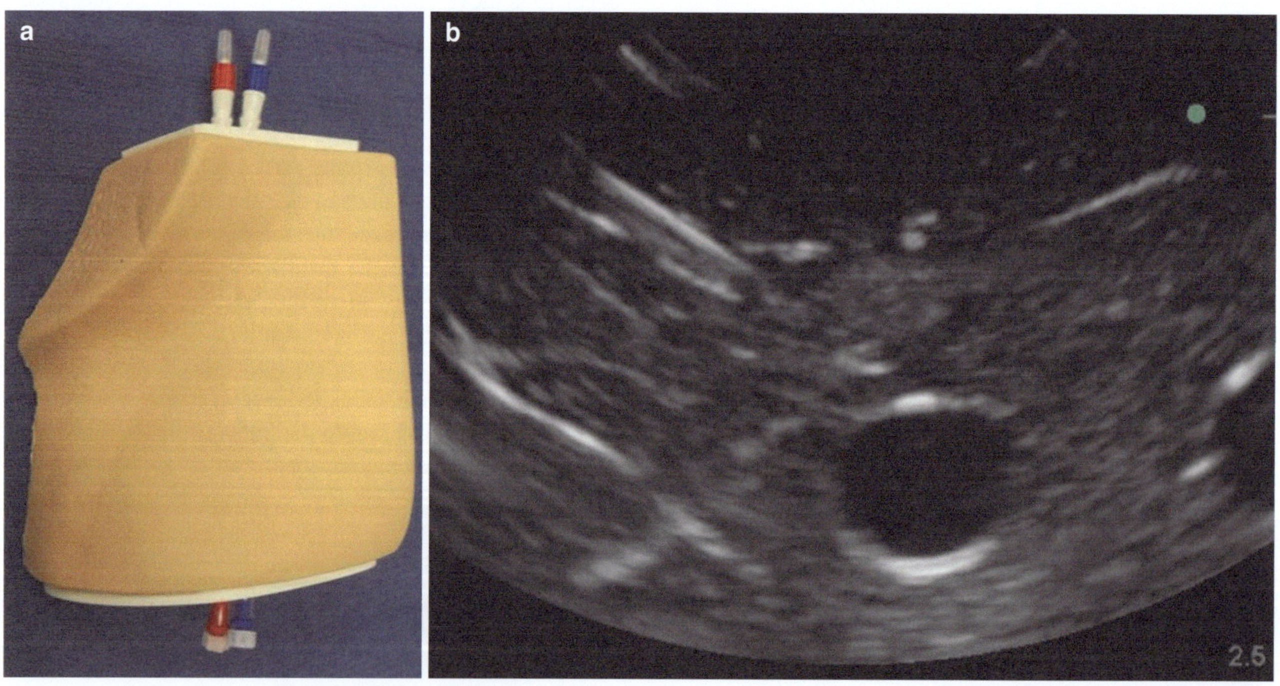

Fig. 21.1 Inorganic anatomic phantom model (**a**) with sample sonogram (**b**) for ultrasound-guided regional anesthesia part task simulation

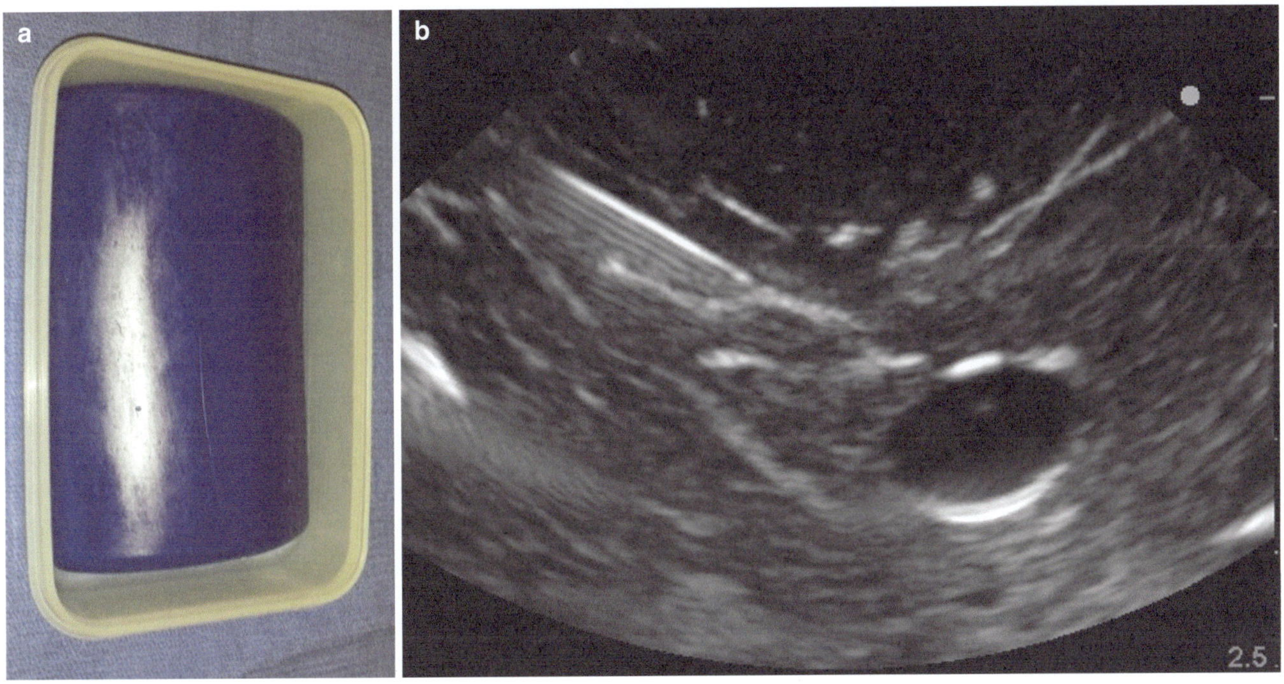

Fig. 21.2 Inorganic nonanatomic agar phantom model (**a**) with sample sonogram (**b**) for ultrasound-guided regional anesthesia part task simulation

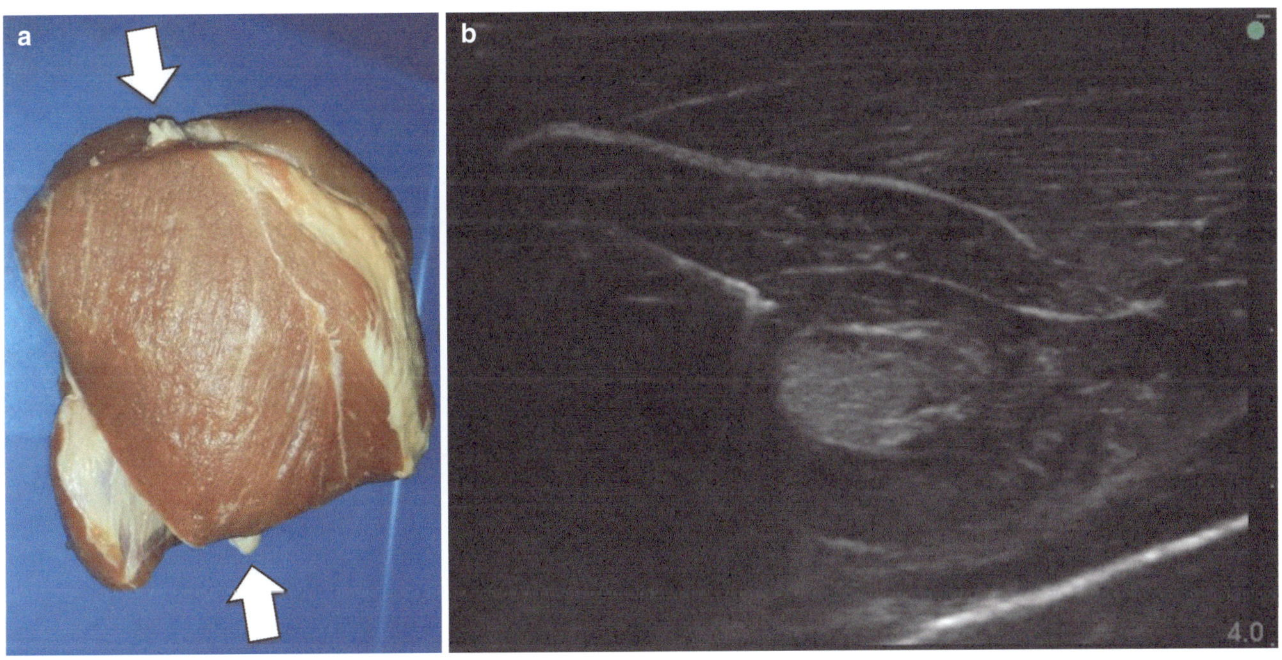

Fig. 21.3 Organic phantom using porcine meat specimen (**a**) with sample sonogram (**b**) for ultrasound-guided regional anesthesia part task simulation. Bovine tendon inserted to represent target "nerve" (indicated by arrows)

materials [13]. Sonoanatomic inorganic models have the additional advantage of mimicking real anatomy, allowing for enhanced learning [14]. These models may be ideal for teaching procedural steps, probe placement, target identification, and needle alignment.

In addition to inorganic part task trainers, organic models can provide similar training and repetition for procedural techniques (Fig. 21.3). Currently utilized organic models include bovine muscle, pork loin, pig shoulder, and turkey breast. These organic phantom models provide more realistic tactile feedback and allow for injection of solutions (and even catheter placement); however, they are often perishable and must be replaced after each training session.

There are, however, further limitations to the use of phantom model technology in addition to those mentioned previously. Needle visibility relies on the relative echogenicity of the needle and the material surrounding the needle. For example, gelatin phantoms have very low background echogenicity, making needle visibility easy, which could lead to false confidence with regard to needling skill.

Cadaveric phantoms are also in use, with unembalmed cadavers providing the medium most similar to live human tissue. These models demonstrate the most realistic static and dynamic anatomy, preserving natural anatomy with extremity movement [15]. However, use of cadavers may be limited by abnormal vascular anatomy as cadaveric vessels are often collapsed [16].

Other novel part task trainer designs include virtual reality and robot-assisted models. Virtual reality models utilize magnetic resonance imaging to create a flexible and dynamic learning environment to perform virtual nerve blocks [17]. Three-dimensional virtual reality animations have been shown to improve understanding of anatomical and technical principles related to peripheral nerve blocks in moderately experienced practitioners [18]. Morse et al. showed that a robot-assisted technique in simulation led to more consistent blocks with a faster learning curve compared to the traditional manual technique [19].

High-Fidelity Simulation for Exposure

High-fidelity simulation immerses the student into a realistic clinical environment. While procedural competency may be included as an educational goal, management of the patient and the simulated clinical environment (i.e., block area, operating room, preoperative clinic, etc.) can be incorporated as well. In these more complex simulated environments, rare and critical situations can be presented to learners. Many regional anesthesiologists may complete their training without seeing critical events such as local anesthetic systemic toxicity (LAST). However, it is essential that expert practitioners are able to promptly diagnose and treat these life-threatening conditions. Utilization of high-fidelity simulation to provide exposure to uncommon and critical events can result in a meaningful and positive impact on overall patient care. One sample scenario is shown in Table 21.1.

The scope of practice of the regional anesthesiologist extends well beyond nerve blocks. High-fidelity simulation allows for students and practitioners to continually practice and work toward competency in crisis resource management, refining both nontechnical and technical skills. Though in its germinal stage, scenarios include difficult patient interactions (i.e., demented elderly patient with hip fracture), rare events, team management, and more.

Table 21.1 A sample regional anesthesia simulation scenario

Title:	Popliteal and saphenous peripheral nerve blocks with LAST		
Audience:	Anesthesia trainees, anesthesiologists		
Objectives:	Medical knowledge	List five possible complications of peripheral nerve blocks Demonstrate medical management of LAST	
	Patient care	Demonstrate proper performance of popliteal and saphenous peripheral nerve blocks	
	Communication	Apply crisis resource management key points; communicate effectively using closed loops	
	Professionalism	Apply crisis resource management key points; establish role clarity and designate leadership	
Case stem:	Mrs. Smith is a 74-year-old 45 kg female with a history of coronary artery disease (CAD) status post percutaneous coronary intervention a decade ago on aspirin, ischemic cardiomyopathy with ejection fraction 30%, atrial fibrillation on procainamide, hypertension, and poorly controlled type 2 diabetes mellitus, who is presenting for debridement of a gangrenous foot and leg wound. Given her significant comorbidities, the surgical and anesthesia teams have decided to proceed with a surgical regional block. The learner has been instructed to place the appropriate block		
Scenario Setup:	Regional block area with patient laying supine in gurney Block cart with regional anesthesia supplies and emergency drugs available Equipment for single-shot peripheral nerve blocks on top of cart (e.g., Pajunk needle with two 20 mL syringes of 0.5% bupivacaine) Monitors available but not attached to patient		
State:	**Patient status:**	**Learner actions:**	**Response:**
Pre-op	Patient comfortable on gurney	Choose appropriate block Choose appropriate local anesthetic and dose Consent patient Apply monitors, provide supplemental oxygen, ensure running intravenous catheter (IV)	–

Table 21.1 (continued)

Block	Patient positioned for block HR 70, NSR, RR 10, BP 120/70, SpO_2 100% on 2L NC, T 36.5	Perform pre-block timeout Perform selected blocks using ultrasound guidance and phantom model	If learner does not choose adequate blocks, patient will complain of discomfort in appropriate distribution
Post-block	Patient resting comfortably, drowsy, good block onset HR 80, NSR, RR 8, BP 140/90, SpO_2 97% on 2L NC	Ensure patient monitored by another anesthesiologist or nurse after block placement	Learner called away to speak on phone in another room regarding a floor patient
Seizure	Patient becomes agitated then has seizure HR 110, ST, RR 3, BP 170/100, SpO_2 92% on 2L NC	Call for help Support oxygenation with 100% FiO_2 and ventilation Give benzodiazepine to stop seizure	If benzodiazepine given within 2 minutes, saturation stabilizes If no benzodiazepine given within 2 minutes, patient SpO_2 drops to 79% and requires intubation
Hypotension	Patient becomes unresponsive, bradycardic, hypotensive, and develops a wide complex QRS on electrocardiogram (EKG) HR 40, SB, RR 10, BP 80/50, SpO_2 96% on FM	Provide cardiovascular support with IV fluids and vasopressors Intubate Start intralipid	If learner starts intralipid within 5 minutes, go to stabilizes If learner does not start intralipid within 5 minutes, go to code
Code	Patient develops ventricular fibrillation	Call for code team Start cardiopulmonary resuscitation (CPR) Give intralipid Give low-dose epinephrine Consider cardiopulmonary bypass	After five rounds of CPR, if intralipid and low-dose epinephrine given, go to stabilizes
Stabilizes	Patient is intubated HR 90, NSR, BP 100/70, SpO_2 96%	Discuss differential diagnosis and LAST with surgeon and team	Surgeon asks what happened
Discussion points:	What are appropriate maximum doses of local anesthetics? Note that if learner used appropriate volume of 0.5% bupivacaine, can rationalize that it was syringe swap for 3% mepivacaine Why is it imperative to stop the seizure activity? Leads to hypercarbia and acidosis which can worsen toxicity What is the ideal agent to stop seizures? Benzodiazepines. Avoid propofol in patients with cardiovascular instability. Propofol will not serve as a lipid sink in LAST What is the correct intralipid dose? Bolus 1.5 mL/kg of 20% intralipid, can repeat bolus 1–2 times for persistent cardiovascular collapse. Start infusion at 0.25–0.5 mL/kg/min, and continue for at least 10 minutes after attaining circulatory stability. Intralipid should be dosed to ideal body weight. Recommended upper limit is 10 mL/kg in first 30 minutes. Note that severe CAD can impair efficacy of intralipid What medications should be avoided in LAST? Calcium channel blockers, beta blockers, local anesthetics, vasopressin, phenytoin. ACLS/code drug doses need to be reduced: $<$ 1 mcg/kg/dose of epinephrine What are the classic symptoms of LAST? Symptoms can be variable. Neurologic symptoms include tinnitus, dizziness, blurred vision, circumoral numbness, metallic taste, central nervous system (CNS) depression, and coma. Cardiovascular symptoms include prolonged PR interval, widened QRS, sinus bradycardia, atrioventricular (AV) block, asystole, and ventricular arrhythmias. Patients are often initially tachycardic and hypertensive but then develop bradycardia and hypotension What is the incidence of LAST? Approximately 1 in 1000 [20] How do we minimize the risk of LAST? Have a clear understanding of toxic dose limits and give lower doses, aspirate prior to each dose, give in incremental doses. Always monitor patients for at least 30 minutes after blocks How can we improve systems-based practice? Always have emergency equipment available, and know where the intralipid is kept		

As the use of ultrasound guidance in the practice of regional anesthesia is a relatively recent innovation, there is a great need for comprehensive training for both current anesthesia trainees and physicians who may have completed their training prior to the use of current technology and are still in practice. Anesthesiologists and anesthesia trainees who viewed an educational video and participated in a computer-based interactive simulation subsequently showed improved knowledge of ultrasound anatomy as assessed by a written test and had greater confidence compared to those who viewed a sham video [21]. However there was no improvement in hands-on ultrasound-guided live-model scanning or localization of the nerve target, implying that computer-based simulation can be helpful for imparting explicit knowledge but that other modalities are needed to improve hands-on ultrasound procedural skills. Another study showed that student nurse anesthetists who were provided with electronic training via CD-ROM and human simulation showed better scanning performance compared to those who received a single teaching modality [22]. Overall, evidence for the effectiveness of simulation in regional anesthesia training is still limited due to a lack of comparative effectiveness [23].

Simulation for Assessment

In the educational setting, simulation allows for assessment in a consistent, reproducible manner. This provides an advantage over the clinical setting where no two patients or circumstances are exactly alike. Several studies have utilized regional anesthesia skill assessment tools to measure performance [21, 22]. Residents of all levels improved their performance after implementation of a comprehensive curriculum that included anatomy workshops, live model scanning, simulation of complex scenarios using high-fidelity mannequins, and other non-traditional didactics based on objective structured clinical examinations (OSCE) [24].

Simulation can also be used to improve poor technique recognized by formative assessment tools. Sites et al. identified five quality-compromising patterns of behavior in performing regional anesthesia blocks [25]. Their work suggests that practice in the simulated environment can then be targeted to focus on consistent needle imaging, ensuring appropriate spread of local anesthetic, appreciating intramuscular needle tip location, reducing unintentional probe movement, and confirming correct "sidedness" of the ultrasound probe.

There is ongoing work in creating validated simulation-based scenarios to provide summative assessments of trainees. The Israeli Board Examination Committee in Anesthesiology has made strides in incorporating an OSCE component of their national board examination, which includes a regional anesthesia scenario that requires that the trainee demonstrates competence with regard to relevant surface anatomy, needle insertion location, needle direction, and dosage of local anesthetics [26]. A standardized patient then demonstrates various procedure-induced complications prompting the trainee to respond to the critical event. Similar modes of assessment may soon be introduced into other institutions and accreditation committees. At this time, based on current literature and practice, simulation instructors still express caution to ensure safeguards are in place prior to widespread use of simulation for student summative assessments [27].

Multidisciplinary Team Training

Simulation-based instructional courses teaching ultrasound-guided nerve blocks to non-anesthesiologist physicians have been shown to increase familiarity and comfort level with performing regional anesthetic techniques. Courses also increase these physicians' intent to use nerve blocks as adjuncts to pain control [28]. However, effects seem short-lived with no significant impact beyond 1 month after course completion. This suggests the need for ongoing or maintenance of training for physicians from all specialties managing acute pain. This may serve to broaden the scope of regional anesthesia to other subspecialty areas allowing for better patient-centered multimodal treatment of perioperative pain.

The management of the patient in the perioperative setting is no single provider's responsibility. Effective responses to crises and complex events require cohesive teamwork from all members of the medical staff including physicians, trainees, nurses, and technicians. High-fidelity simulated clinical scenarios allow for teams to practice crisis management and problem-solve in a multidisciplinary manner. Multidisciplinary team-based debriefings can improve clinical performance, ethical decision-making, and interpersonal communication [29].

Using the Simulated Environment for Testing

The simulated clinical environment and simulated patient have been used to critically evaluate novel approaches to performance of peripheral nerve blocks. Again, this is due to the reproducibility and consistency provided in comparison to the clinical environment. New medical devices have been evaluated through the use of simulation including needle insertion guides, non-Luer connectors, and echogenic needles and catheters [30–34]. Innovative regional techniques, such as the "air test" for localization of the tip of a perineural catheter and the "hand-on-syringe" technique that allows a single operator to perform a block without assistance, have also been critically evaluated through use of simulation [35–37].

Simulation has also played a key role in further development of crisis resource management tools specific to the field of regional anesthesia. Neal et al. evaluated the use of the ASRA checklist for management of local anesthetic systemic toxicity [38]. In their simulated environment, anesthesia trainees who used the ASRA checklist completed more critical steps in the management of LAST compared to trainees who did not use the checklist. The trainees were also shown to have greater knowledge retention on evaluation 2 months later.

Conclusion

Simulation technology in the field of regional anesthesia has shown great promise with ongoing research in the validation of simulation education methods, analysis of novel techniques and devices, and creation and implementation of multidisciplinary team training curricula. The unique value of simulation-based education in regional anesthesia lies in its ability to provide students with a means of training that avoids harm to patients while allowing repetitive practice, exposure to rare events, and immediate feedback. The simulated environment allows adequate time for debriefing and open conversations, which may not be possible or appropriate in a busy clinical practice. When developing a simulation-based curriculum, one must consider the potential downsides to the use of simulation technology in regional anesthesia. A simulation-based curriculum can require a large investment in equipment as well as both educators' and trainees' time. There are several solutions to these potential limitations such as the use of low-cost part task trainer models which can still achieve the basic objectives of the simulated learning exercise. Results to date are encouraging and supportive, showing a multitude of benefits despite these limitations.

References

1. ACGME. ACGME program requirements for graduate medical education in anesthesiology. 2015 Feb [cited 2016 July 25]. Available from: https://www.acgme.org/Portals/0/PFAssets/ProgramRequirements/040_anesthesiology_2016.pdf.
2. The American Board of Anesthesiology. Simulation Education: American Society of Anesthesiologists. [cited 2016 July 25]. Available from: http://www.theaba.org/MOCA/About-MOCA-2-0.
3. Sites BD, Chan VW, Neal JM, Weller R, Grau T, Koscielniak-Nielsen ZJ, et al. The American Society of Regional Anethesia and Pain Medicine and the European Society of Regional Anaesthesia and Pain Therapy Joint Committee Recommendations for education and training in ultrasound-guided regional anesthesia. Reg Anesth Pain Med. 2010;35:S74–80.
4. Barrington MJ, Wong DM, Slater B, Ivanusic JJ, Ovens M. Ultrasound-guided regional anesthesia: how much practice do novices require before achieving competency in ultrasound needle visualization using a cadaver model. Reg Anesth Pain Med. 2012;37(3):334–9.
5. Sites BD, Gallagher JD, Cravero J, Lundberg J, Blike G. The learning curve associated with a simulated ultrasound-guided interventional task by inexperienced anesthesia residents. Reg Anesth Pain Med. 2004;29(6):544–8.
6. Marhofer P, Greher M, Kapral S. Ultrasound guidance in regional anaesthesia. Br J Anaesth. 2005;94(1):7–17.
7. Niazi AU, Haldipur N, Prasad AG, Chan VW. Ultrasound-guided regional anesthesia performance in the early learning period: effect of simulation training. Reg Anesth Pain Med. 2012;37(1):51–4.
8. Udani AD, Macario A, Nandagopal K, Tanaka MA, Tanaka PP. Simulation-based mastery learning with deliberate practice improves clinical performance in spinal anesthesia. Anesthesiol Res Pract. 2014;2014:659160.
9. Baranauskas MB, Margarido CB, Panossian C, Silva ED. Simulation of ultrasound-guided peripheral nerve block: learning curve of CET-SMA/HSL anesthesiology residents. Rev Bras Anestesiol. 2008;58(2):106–11.
10. Kim SC, Hauser S, Staniek A, Weber S. Learning curve of medical students in ultrasound-guided simulated nerve block. J Anesth. 2014;28(1):76–80.
11. Friedman Z, Siddiqui N, Katznelson R, Devito I, Bould MD, Naik V. Clinical impact of epidural anesthesia simulation on short- and long-term learning curve: high- versus low-fidelity model training. Reg Anesth Pain Med. 2009;34(3):229–32.
12. Liu Y, Glass NL, Glover CD, Power RW, Watcha MF. Comparison of the development of performance skills in ultrasound-guided regional anesthesia simulations with different phantom models. Simul Healthc. 2013;8(6):368–75.
13. Liu Y, Glass NL, Power RW. Technical communication: new teaching model for practicing ultrasound-guided regional anesthesia techniques: no perishable food products! Anesth Analg. 2010;110(4):1233–5.
14. Rosenberg AD, Popovic J, Albert DB, Altman RA, Marshall MH, Sommer RM, et al. Three partial-task simulators for teaching ultrasound-guided regional anesthesia. Reg Anesth Pain Med. 2012;37(1):106–10.
15. Kessler J, Moriggl B, Grau T. Ultrasound-guided regional anesthesia: learning with an optimized cadaver model. Surg Radiol Anat. 2014;36(4):383–92.
16. Hocking G, Hebard S, Mitchell CH. A review of the benefits and pitfalls of phantoms in ultrasound-guided regional anesthesia. Reg Anesth Pain Med. 2011;36(2):162–70.
17. Grottke O, Ntouba A, Ullrich S, Liao W, Fried E, Prescher A, et al. Virtual reality-based simulator for training in regional anaesthesia. Br J Anaesth. 2009;103(4):594–600.
18. Lim MW, Burt G, Rutter SV. Use of three-dimensional animation for regional anaesthesia teaching: application to interscalene brachial plexus blockade. Br J Anaesth. 2005;94(3):372–7.
19. Morse J, Terrasini N, Wehbe M, Philippona C, Zaouter C, Cyr S, et al. Comparison of success rates, learning curves, and inter-subject performance variability of robot-assisted and manual ultrasound-guided nerve block needle guidance in simulation. Br J Anaesth. 2014;112(6):1092–7.
20. Mulroy MF. Systemic toxicity and cardiotoxicity from local anesthetics: incidence and preventive measures. Reg Anesth Pain Med. 2002;27(6):556–61.
21. Woodworth GE, Chen EM, Horn JL, Aziz MF. Efficacy of computer-based video and simulation in ultrasound-guided regional anesthesia training. J Clin Anesth. 2014;26(3):212–21.
22. Gasko J, Johnson A, Sherner J, Craig J, Gegel B, Burgert J, et al. Effects of using simulation versus CD-ROM in the performance of ultrasound-guided regional anesthesia. AANA J. 2012;80(4):S56–S9.
23. Udani AD, Kim TE, Howard SK, Mariano ER. Simulation in teaching regional anesthesia: current perspectives. Local Reg Anesth. 2015;8:33–43.
24. Garcia-Tomas V, Schwengel D, Ouanes JP, Hall S, Hanna MN. Improved residents' knowledge after an advanced regional anesthesia education program. MEJ Anesth. 2014;22(4):419–27.
25. Sites BD, Spence BC, Gallagher JD, Wiley CW, Bertrand ML, Blike GT. Characterizing novice behavior associated with learning ultrasound-guided peripheral regional anesthesia. Reg Anesth Pain Med. 2007;32(2):107–15.
26. Berkenstadt H, Ziv A, Gafni N, Sidi A. Incorporating simulation-based objective structured clinical examination into the Israeli National Board Examination in Anesthesiology. Anesth Analg. 2006;102(3):853–8.
27. Wen LY, Gaba DM, Udani AD. Summative assessments using simulation requires safeguards. Anesth Analg. 2017;124(1):369.

28. Bretholz A, Doan Q, Cheng A, Lauder G. A presurvey and postsurvey of a web- and simulation-based course of ultrasound-guided nerve blocks for pediatric emergency medicine. Pediatr Emerg Care. 2012;28(6):506–9.
29. Brenner GJ, Newmark JL, Raemer D. Curriculum and cases for pain medicine crisis resource management education. Anesth Analg. 2013;116(1):107–10.
30. Whittaker S, Lethbridge G, Kim C, Keon Cohen Z, Ng I. An ultrasound needle insertion guide in a porcine phantom model. Anaesthesia. 2013;68(8):826–9.
31. Gupta RK, Lane J, Allen B, Shi Y, Schildcrout JS. Improving needle visualization by novice residents during an in-plane ultrasound nerve block simulation using an in-plane multiangle needle guide. Pain Med. 2013;14:1600–7.
32. Cook TM, Payne S, Skryabina E, Hurford D, Clow E, Georgiou A. A simulation-based evaluation of two proposed alternatives to Luer devices for use in neuraxial anaesthesia. Anaesthesia. 2010;65(11):1069–79.
33. Kilicaslan A, Topal A, Tavlan A, Erol A, Otelcioglu S. Differences in tip visibility and nerve block parameters between two echogenic needles during a simulation study with inexperienced anesthesia trainees. J Anesth. 2014;28(3):460–2.
34. Mariano ER, Yun RD, Kim TE, Carvalho B. Application of echogenic technology for catheters used in ultrasound-guided continuous peripheral nerve blocks. J Ultrasound Med. 2014;33(5):905–11.
35. Johns J, Harrison TK, Steffel L, Howard SK, Kim TE, Kou A, et al. A pilot in vitro evaluation of the "air test" for perineural catheter tip localization by a novice regional anesthesiologist. J Ultrasound Med. 2014;33(12):2197–200.
36. Kan JM, Harrison TK, Kim TE, Howard SK, Kou A, Mariano ER. An in vitro study to evaluate the utility of the "air test" to infer perineural catheter tip location. J Ultrasound Med. 2013;32:529–33.
37. Johnson B, Herring A, Stone M, Nagdev A. Performance accuracy of hand-on-needle versus hand-on-syringe technique for ultrasound-guided regional anesthesia simulation for emergency medicine residents. West J Emerg Med. 2014;15(6):641–6.
38. Neal JM, Hsiung RL, Mulroy MF, Halpern BB, Dragnich AD, Slee AE. ASRA checklist improves trainee performance during a simulated episode of local anesthetic systemic toxicity. Reg Anesth Pain Med. 2012;37(1):8–15.

Simulation in Orthotopic Liver Transplantation

22

Alan Julius Sim, Jeron Zerillo, Daniel Katz, Sang Kim, and Bryan Hill

Abbreviations

ABA	American Board of Anesthesiology
ACGME	Accreditation Council for Graduate Medical Education
ACRM	Anesthesia Crisis Resource Management
CA-1	Clinical Anesthesia Year 1
CA-2	Clinical Anesthesia Year 2
CA-3	Clinical Anesthesia Year 3
CPR	Cardiopulmonary resuscitation
CRM	Crisis resource management
ECG	Electrocardiography
GRS	Global rating scale
HFS	High-fidelity simulation
ICU	Intensive care unit
IV	Intravenous
MDT	Multidisciplinary team training
NBME	National Board of Medical Examiners
OPTN	Organ Procurement and Transplantation Network
OR	Operating room
PACU	Post Anesthesia Care Unit
TeamSTEPPS	Team Strategies and Tools to Enhance Performance and Patient Safety
UNOS	United Network for Organ Sharing

A. J. Sim (✉) · J. Zerillo · D. Katz
Department of Anesthesiology, Perioperative and Pain Medicine, Icahn School of Medicine at Mount Sinai, New York, NY, USA
e-mail: alan.sim@mountsinai.org; jeron.zerillo@mountsinai.org; daniel.katz@mountsinai.org

S. Kim
Department of Anesthesiology, Critical Care & Pain Management, Hospital for Special Surgery, New York, NY, USA
e-mail: sang.kim@mountsinai.org

B. Hill
Department of Anesthesiology, The Ohio State University Wexner Medical Center, Columbus, OH, USA
e-mail: bryan.hill@mountsinai.org

Introduction

Perioperative care for patients undergoing orthotopic liver transplantation (OLT) provides a variety of challenges for both the anesthesiologist and surgical team. The surgical procedure itself is a multifarious one involving meticulous dissection to remove the diseased native liver, numerous vascular and biliary anastomoses, and periods of significant hemodynamic instability secondary to blood, fluid, and electrolyte shifts [1]. In addition, patients with end-stage liver disease (ESLD) have a deranged physiology resulting in serious hemodynamic, hemostatic, and metabolic consequences [1–3]. This resultant anesthetic management can be taxing for the anesthesiologist's technical and tactical abilities. Transfusion of a large quantity of blood products, maintenance of homeostasis, interoperative critical care, and effective communication during critical surgical periods such as the anhepatic phase and reperfusion require experienced judgement, knowledge, and interdisciplinary collaboration.

Development of expertise in caring for patients undergoing OLT remains based primarily on direct experience and involvement at a relatively limited number of institutions in which clinical volume permits exposure conducive to such specialization and training. Although the number of transplant centers has increased, this has served to decrease the average number of transplants performed per institution with a wide degree of interinstitutional variablity [4]. This creates an extremely heterogeneous transplant experience between anesthesiology resident trainees across institutions. Despite the complexity of anesthetic management, given the sporadic and limited exposure to liver transplantation, anesthesiology training programs are not required by the American Board of Anesthesiologists (ABA) or Accreditation Council of Graduate Medical Education (ACGME) to expose residents to such cases [5]. The use of live-patient simulation, high-fidelity simulation, and part-task trainers can help to create a more homogenous training experience across anesthesiology residency training programs [6]. The goals of such simulation-based training would be twofold: the development of relevant

B. Mahoney et al. (eds.), *Comprehensive Healthcare Simulation: Anesthesiology*, Comprehensive Healthcare Simulation,
https://doi.org/10.1007/978-3-030-26849-7_22

technical skills such as advanced arterial and venous access, point-of-care ultrasound (POCUS) techniques, and basic transesophageal echocardiography (TEE) and the honing of cognitive and clinical skills for the management of critical issues encountered during OLT while developing the pattern recognition which flows from experience to identify common intraoperative problems and treat them effectively. In this chapter, we will describe the role of simulation in teaching and assessing the necessary skills to provide anesthetic management for orthotopic liver transplantation and function effectively as a member of the liver transplantation perioperative team.

Part-Task Trainers and Skill Acquisition

Orthotopic liver transplantation (OLT) submits the patient to tremendous surgical trespass. Combined with the physiology of ESLD, the anesthesiologist must be prepared for intraoperative hypotension and hemodynamic instability resulting from blood loss and large fluid shifts encountered during drainage of ascites, significant hemorrhage, and cross-caval clamping during the anhepatic phase. As a result, the anesthesiologist must be facile in technical skills such as placement of large-bore peripheral access, central venous access, and invasive monitoring including arterial and pulmonary artery catheters. They must also be proficient in basic point-of care ultrasound technique, whether to guide placement of invasive arterial or central access or to perform transesophageal echocardiography to assess hemodynamic status and guide fluid resuscitation.

Several characteristics unique to the ESLD patient population and OLT can provide challenges to healthcare trainees still mastering technical procedures utilized in clinical care (Table 22.1). There are several part-task trainers that can facilitate the attainment of expertise or ensure maintenance of skills in the seasoned provider.

ESLD produces unique changes both physiologic and anatomic in patients undergoing surgery due to cirrhosis and increased portal hypertension. These patients suffer from ascites, increased abdominal girth, and esophageal varices. In addition, given the rare and unplanned nature of most transplantation procedures, the patient may not have fasted appropriately prior to surgery leading to significant risk of pulmonary aspiration. Splenomegaly-induced platelet sequestration, portal hypertension, dilated splanchnic vasculature, fluid overload, and severe coagulopathy render the patient at risk for hematoma formation and profuse bleeding during central and peripheral line placement. Induction of anesthesia, endotracheal intubation, placement of central venous, and invasive monitoring must all be performed skillfully and expeditiously in order to decrease cold ischemic organ time. Risk of needle stick injury in caring for patients with hepatitis C or concurrent HIV further heightens the importance of mastery of such techniques, a mastery that can be facilitated through work in the simulation lab where these procedures can be learned in a setting that is safe for both the patient and the healthcare provider.

Table 22.1 Skills and considerations for ESLD patients for OLT

Type of skill	Considerations in ESLD patients for OLT
Airway	Full stomach due to abdominal ascites and NPO status Coagulopathy and friable mucosa leading to blood in the oropharynx Decreased functional residual capacity leading to rapid oxygen desaturation Patients with nonalcoholic steatohepatitis (NASH) may have increased body mass index and a non-reassuring airway
Ventilation management	Increased peak airway pressures due to ascites or placement of surgical retractors Hepatopulmonary syndrome Hydrothorax due to ascites
Intravenous access	Coagulopathy may lead to hematoma formation Increased portal pressures and fluid overload may increase bleeding during line placement Large bore access required for rapid infusion systems
Central line placement and invasive monitors	Risk of bleeding and hemothorax Multiple neck catheters may be required for hemodialysis or veno-veno bypass Ultrasound-guided placement for access decreases risk of arterial puncture and multiple punctures in coagulopathic patients
Resuscitation	Familiarity with rapid infusion systems Familiarity with doses for various vasopressor infusions Management of hyperkalemia Team coordination during ACLS and CPR Transthoracic and transesophageal echocardiography for diagnosis and treatment of hemodynamic instability
Regional anesthesia techniques	Familiarization with ultrasound-guided truncal blocks such as rectus sheath blocks and transverse abdominal planus blocks for hepatobiliary surgery

Familiarity with rapid fluid infusion systems, veno-veno bypass, and massive transfusion practices is essential for one to be successful in the resuscitation of patients during transplant surgery. Hypovolemic and hyperkalemic cardiopulmonary arrests are not uncommon during liver transplantation surgery, and maintenance of the anesthesiologist's proficiency in advanced cardiac life support and coordination of care can be practiced, honed, and maintained with repetitive scenarios and drills in the simulation lab.

Although regional anesthetic techniques for postoperative pain management in OLT are rarely utilized, such narcotic sparing techniques may be beneficial in enhancing recovery or facilitating early extubation after OLT. Truncal blocks such as the rectus sheath and transverse abdominal planus blocks have been shown to be effective in liver resection and hepatobiliary surgery and could be incorporated into any anesthetic for major abdominal cases.

Part-task trainers can be utilized in the training of practitioners in the acquisition and mastery of the skills mentioned above. Although low fidelity and unable to fully replicate real-life patients, they provide a basis for skill acquisition in an isolated, risk-free environment allowing learners to develop speed and proper technique through repetitive drills with educator feedback.

Part-Task Trainers

Vascular Access: Central Line Placement and Arterial Line Catheterization

Due to the anesthetic complexity and advanced techniques necessary in OLT, the majority of anesthesia trainees will not be exposed to such cases until the completion of at least 1 year of clinical anesthesiology training. Despite their prior experience in the placement of central venous lines and arterial catheters, the goals of part-task simulation in preparation for OLT will likely exceed past exposure. These goals include an understanding of vascular access for veno-veno bypass or continuous veno-veno hemofiltration, the anatomic options for line placement and their associated risks, and unique risks in the coagulopathic patient. Emphasis is placed on preparation of the procedure tray, patient preparation, ultrasound-guided identification of landmarks, and confirmation of correct catheter position.

Generally, vascular access part-task trainers are designed as fluid-filled phantoms which may or may not allow for ultrasound-guided visualization. Some may be integrated with mannequins to provide a sense of anatomic landmarks and more realistic placement. Visual confirmation of access may be provided through the use of dyed fluid or echogenic imaging on ultrasound. Several models are specific for venous or arterial access through utilization of a pump or motor to simulate pulsatile flow providing visual (i.e., compressibility vs. pulsatility on ultrasound) or tactile feedback. Tactile fidelity in imitation of the skin can vary depending on the material used for the vascular access phantom. These trainers, in conjunction with a simulated environment incorporating standard operating room equipment, can be used to identify extra or redundant steps to increase speed and efficiency while decreasing the risk for line-associated infection or practitioner needlestick.

Transesophageal and Transthoracic Echocardiography Simulators

The use of transesophageal echocardiography in OLT is increasing as a means to monitor and guide fluid therapy or to diagnose catastrophic critical pathology such as cardiac tamponade, pulmonary artery embolism, air embolism, and right heart failure. Given the known risks of pulmonary artery catheterization, TEE can provide a relatively safer alternative to invasive pressure monitoring in OLT, but its use is limited by barriers such as training, specialization, and certification in basic TEE for non-cardiac.

Virtual reality part-task training simulators in TEE and TTE can serve as a method for gaining experience without reliance on surgical or clinical volume or the frequency of relevant pathologies in patients. They allow for instructor- or software-provided feedback as real-time graphic representation of the anatomy is obtained with image quality dependent upon probe placement and rotation. This simulated learning experience allows learners an opportunity to develop the psychomotor skills necessary to obtain useful echocardiographic imaging prior to implementation during OLT. Many commercially available TEE and TTE simulators provide both normal and pathological scenarios that can be accessed to better simulate specific disease states seen in OLT such as pulmonary hypertension, pulmonary embolus, and right heart strain. Through their use, the time required to obtain competency can potentially be shortened and training standardized.

High-Fidelity Simulation for Orthotopic Liver Transplantation

Expertise in management of end-stage liver disease patients undergoing OLT can only be obtained through real-life clinical exposure. A recent study demonstrated that the quantity of anesthesia provider experience is significantly associated with OLT outcomes [7]. However, with the unequal distribution of liver transplantations performed across transplant centers nationwide, anesthesiology providers necessarily receive uneven OLT training and exposure. As the number of liver transplant centers continues to grow, this further serves to dilute exposure seen at both less active and busier centers. In 2015, the 20 highest volume transplant centers averaged 136 liver transplantation procedures per year, while the other 119 centers averaged only 37. Given this variability, it is not surprising that only 26% of anesthesiology residents participated in structured OLT-related education according to a 2013 survey [8]. Training programs, even in active transplant centers, may find it difficult to standardize training and exposure to these highly complex cases. Aggerwal et al. examined a day-long educational course employing a combination of mannequin-based simulation with didactic sessions. Another group presented a series of porcine model-based simulations of liver transplantation designed to improve anesthesia provider performance by demonstrating the physiologic changes that occur during OLT [9]. Both of these groups demonstrated enhanced performance after the training sessions as measured by cognitive and task performance metrics obtained prior to and after the simulation-based learning experience. Exposure to simulation-based scenarios can help standardize curricula while strengthening trainees' medical knowledge, clinical aptitude, and confidence when confronted with the management of OLT.

An effective high-fidelity simulation-based curriculum for exposure to OLT would include an accurate representation of clinical events that would provide the learner with a better understanding of the natural progression of liver transplantation. This would ideally enhance practitioner pattern recognition of common problems in order to allow them to better anticipate and respond to complex events which may occur during the procedure. For example, the pre-anhepatic or dissection phase is fraught with significant periods of hypotension due to drainage of ascites, blood loss, and hypocalcemia, whereas the reperfusion phase is commonly marked by hypotension due to hyperkalemia, pulmonary embolus, or graft nonfunction. These clinical states occur with widely differing patterns in presentation such that the practitioner must be able to interpret variable signs and symptoms to come to the correct diagnosis and treatment. A sample scenario can be seen in Table 22.2.

Such a scenario would serve to highlight common perioperative problems while providing a general introduction to liver transplantation. It can also serve as a means to reduce the heterogeneity in exposure to OLT that comes with the

Table 22.2 Liver transplant anesthesiology scenario

Room setup	High-fidelity mannequin Anesthesia backstand with common OR setup Anesthesia machine High-fidelity monitor (EKG, blood pressure, CVP, ABP, PAP, SPO2, ETCO2, temp) Rapid infusion system TEE probe/machine Ultrasound Surgical tray with instruments Central line introducer kit
Actors needed	Patient, circulating nurse, transplant surgeon, and anesthesiologist
Case stem	A 50-year-old male with a history of alcoholic cirrhosis and end-stage liver disease presents for orthotopic liver transplantation. His history is significant for multiple episodes of spontaneous bacterial peritonitis and ascites. Lab values reflect anemia, thrombocytopenia, and a MELD score > 30
Progression of scenario	The participant must care for this critically ill patient in the perioperative setting. After completing an appropriate preoperative evaluation and review of labs and studies, they proceed with induction and each stage of the transplant: Pre-anhepatic, test clamp, total vascular isolation and anhepatic phase, reperfusion, and post-reperfusion phase. Each phase is marked by commonly seen problems during that phase (e.g., massive blood loss during pre-anhepatic, severe hypotension on IVC cross-clamp, hypocalcemia during anhepatic phase, hyperkalemia/acidosis on reperfusion)
Resolution	Scenario will progress based on initiation/failure of treatment by the participant. Failure of treatment may result in cardiopulmonary arrest and death
Learning objectives for debriefing	Review with facilitators prior to the pre-briefing: 1. What information can be gained by the preoperative evaluation to better prepare for the case? (a) Signs of portal hypertension? (b) Possible difficult dissection and significant blood loss? (c) Pretreatment with products? 2. What problems can be anticipated with induction of anesthesia? 3. What invasive monitoring or lines need to be placed prior to or after induction? 4. What are the common reasons for intraoperative hypotension during the pre-anhepatic phase? 5. What laboratory data should be monitored, and what parameters can be corrected? (a) Interpretation of POC testing such as thromboelastography (b) What resources are available through the perfusionist or the blood bank? 6. What is the role of the test clamp in assessing fluid status prior to the anhepatic phase? (a) What blood pressure would be appropriate before proceeding? (b) Should veno-veno bypass be initiated? 7. What special conditions arise from the anhepatic state? (a) Hypocalcemia (b) Hypocoagulability (c) Decreased cardiac output and venous return on clamp 8. What can be done to reduce the risk of hyperkalemic cardiac arrest? 9. Was appropriate help requested? (a) If so, what? (b) Did the practitioner direct the resources effectively? 10. What were the barriers to communication within the case? (a) Unfamiliarity with case resources (b) Anxiety with difficult surgeon

erratic occurrence of transplantation procedures while providing an opportunity to gain a baseline of knowledge and experience necessary to manage these patients effectively.

One potentially promising (yet unstudied) teaching modality for OLT training and exposure is the "serious game." Serious games are interactive, screen-based digital applications created for the purpose of imparting knowledge or skills which leverage the self-motivating elements of video games [10]. The use of serious games in healthcare education has been growing steadily [11]. Investigators have designed and successfully used serious games to improve central venous catheter technique and safety [12, 13], teach emergency management skills [14] and situational awareness [15], enhance medical decision-making [16, 17], and even refine ultrasound skills for interventional radiologists [18].

At the Human Emulation, Education, Evaluation Lab for Patient Safety and Professional Study (HELPS) center at the Icahn School of Medicine at Mount Sinai (ISMMS) Hospital, we have developed our own serious game. The "OLT Trainer" was designed using the GameSalad® platform, a low-cost system that is able to publish games and applications in multiple formats including HTML, IOS®, and Android®. We designed the game to fit the iPad® interface as each our residents receives an iPad® through their departmental education fund. The game is designed as a linear, chronologically based clinical course through which the player performs a preoperative assessment, manages the patient through the intraoperative period, and concludes with disposition to the intensive care unit (Table 22.3 and Fig. 22.1). The player begins with a credit bank that they can "spend" to obtain various "assets" (seen in Fig. 22.1) which include a wide array of preoperative tests, invasive line options, acquisition and transfusion of blood products, or the performance of intraoperative tests or medication administration. If the player's performance falls outside of the standard of care (e.g., unnecessary testing) or leaves the patient in a critical state (e.g., hypotensive or severely anemic), credits are continually deducted over time (a discussion of how such scoring elements were determined follows below). If at any point the player reaches 0 credits, the game ends with the presentation of a feedback screen wherein they can see critical actions for which points were awarded or deducted (e.g., appropriate transfusion, failing to defibrillate). The player may then opt to either start over or return to the last screen with the credit total they had prior to beginning that stage in an attempt to address the errors. There is no limit to the number of times the scenario can be reattempted. Likewise, once the game is completed, the player may replay the scenario with a new bank of credits and attempt to complete the game with more credits with each subsequent iteration.

The nature of OLT lends itself well to serious gaming education initiatives. For example, there is inherent variability in the liver transplantation exposure for residents over the course of their training, even at high-volume centers. The uneven distribution of cases creates a challenge for the training of residents who often have a limited exposure to the specialty delimited by discrete, month-long rotations. A serious game can diminish experiential variability, thus providing all trainees with a similar baseline level of education and exposure by guaranteeing they will have an opportunity to manage the simulated case. The game can also be used to harness a reverse (flipped) classroom approach [19], whereby the focus of learning is shifted from the traditional instructor (attending anesthesiologist) to the learner. In this pedagogical model, the learner masters the core content independently prior to the traditional didactic or clinical session with an instructor occurs and can tailor the curriculum to fit their educational needs by utilizing all available educational materials. Classroom/didactic/operating room teaching time is then spent on applying the already acquired core knowledge and addressing more advanced topics.

Table 22.3 Stages of OLT serious game (flowsheet)

Stage	Content
Case selection	
Preop assessment	Medical history
	Surgical history
	Physical examination
	Laboratory and invasive testing
	Assessment quiz
	Feedback
Induction	Planning of pre-induction monitors
	Preoxygenation
	Utilization of rapid sequence induction
	Induction steps mini-game
Vascular access	Venous access type, gauge, and location
	Arterial access type, gauge, and location
	Feedback
Pulmonary artery catheter (PAC)	Stages of "floating" a PAC
	Assessment of pulmonary hypertension
	Feedback
Perfusion needs	Option to obtain rapid infuser
	Option to obtain cell salvage
	Feedback
Timeout	Surgical timeout
Dissection phase	Drainage of ascites
	Large-volume blood loss
	Feedback
Pre-anhepatic and anhepatic phase	Management of test clamp hemodynamics
	Management of anhepatic physiology
	Feedback
Reperfusion	Preparation for reperfusion
	Management of volume and electrolytes during reperfusion
	Feedback
Summary	Case 1 summary
	Credit total

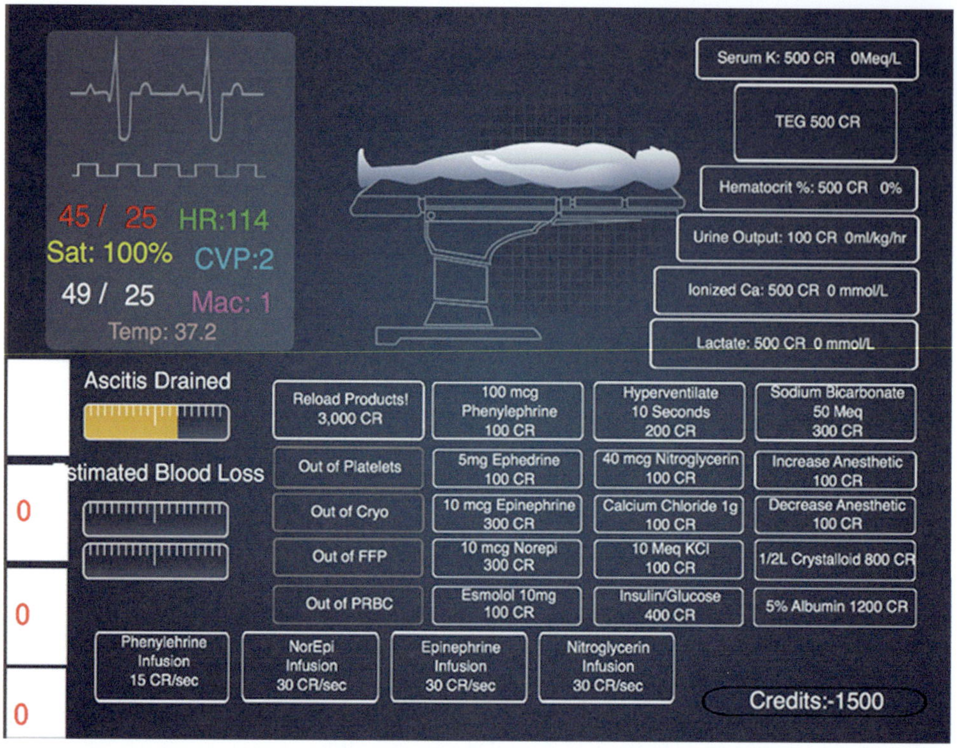

Fig. 22.1 Screenshot of liver transplant game

Such pedagogical models have proven effective in various medical education initiatives [20–23]. Serious gaming can supplement clinical learning in this manner when the learning during clinical exposure may be low for a variety of reasons. For example, following an overnight OLT when trainees are fatigued, a serious game can be utilized the next day after sleeping to solidify what was encountered in the operating room. This can provide a strategy to educators when confronted with current literature on fatigue demonstrating decreased learning and memory of anesthesiology residents after night shift work [24]. Having complete, unfettered access to a tablet-based OLT game allows users to both obtain and maintain pertinent knowledge. In addition to these potential benefits, the ISMMS HELPS center found that utilization of the game was very high following its introduction and required no concerted effort on the part of educators to encourage student participation.

The OLT game can also serve as a warm-up tool to refresh knowledge and technique prior to a case, particularly for practitioners with limited exposure at low-volume centers. Studies of the effect of simulation as a method for warm-up before surgical procedures have found improved performance in the operating room [25, 26]. Additionally, given the often significant period between the coordination of an orthotopic liver transplantation and the time at which it occurs, trainees could reorient themselves to critical elements of the procedure through use of serious games while awaiting the arrival of the donor organ and recipient.

Combined with standard high-fidelity simulation and clinical experience, use of a serious game can enrich the liver transplantation curriculum and training for residents and improve performance while also facilitating the retraining and retaining of skill among experienced practitioners.

High-Fidelity Simulation for Assessment

High-fidelity simulation offers the ability to reinforce pattern recognition and provide experiential exposure to common critical episodes which occur during liver transplantation. It can serve as an adjunct to real-life clinical experience or serve as a tool for primary exposure; however, its utility as a substitute for clinical exposure is debatable and requires further study. Nguyen et al. explored the impact of a liver transplantation exposure through a formal clinical rotation on residents' ability to respond to simulated crises such as hyperkalemic cardiac arrest in a high-fidelity simulation [27]. Their data suggested that residents with exposure and experience in the anesthetic care during a liver transplantation subsequently respond faster to a simulated hyperkalemic crisis than those without clinical exposure.

Although liver transplantation anesthesia care can be taught in a simulation-based setting, clinical exposure to liver transplantation anesthesia care may have a positive effect on the development of a trainee's aptitude in crisis resource management. Hyperkalemic crisis, massive hemorrhage, and hemodynamic instability are common occurrences during liver transplant but also can occur during routine anesthesia care. It would seem reasonable to expect that all anesthesia providers are able to effectively manage these events. Nguyen et al.'s findings support the use of simulation-based assessment of clinical skills for evaluating anesthesia resident performance during an intraoperative crisis related to liver transplantation.

All US residency training programs have been directed by the ACGME to document residents' skill progression during their residency through the assessment and reporting of various competency-based milestones. The ability to respond and manage crisis situations in the operating room in a timely manner is essential for any competent anesthesiology practitioner and is reflected in milestones identified and described by the ACGME. High-fidelity simulation can be used to objectively assess these abilities in clinical practice [28]. For example, a standardized score based on the focused preoperative evaluation of an ESLD patient undergoing OLT (Table 22.4) can better elucidate a resident's clinical judgement and critical thinking skills based on the information they receive during the simulated preoperative examination. Such simulations can be reviewed, debriefed, and analyzed for differences in clinical practice based on a resident's training level. These can serve as valuable tools to assess milestone progression over the course of anesthesiology residency training.

Table 22.4 Example of a preoperative liver transplant simulation scenario and scoring

Case stem	50-year-old alcoholic cirrhotic presenting for OLT
Scoring sheet	
Checklist scoring:	**Preoperative assessment** Introduce self Complete and targeted medical history Complete and targeted physical exam Assess for encephalopathy (PSE) Previous diagnosis? Active confusion Encephalopathy meds Assess for portal hypertension Varices? Hx of esophageal bleed? Ascites? Frequency of drainage? Assess for signs of difficult dissection History of upper/mid-abdominal surgery History of bacterial peritonitis (SBP) Assess for tumor Assess for aspiration risk Assess renal function *Labs* CBC CMP PT/PTT, platelets, easy bruising/bleeding Type and cross and blood products available Determine types of blood products required to start Determine and order other drugs/fluids 5% albumin DDAVP *Imaging* TTE or stress test, exercise tolerance (METs) ECG If elevated pulmonary artery pressure, right heart cath/if questionable cardiopulmonary reserve, stress testing, RVSP
	Total score out of 10

Multidisciplinary Team Training

Care for patients undergoing or being evaluated for liver transplant has always required a multidisciplinary team (MDT) model. Providers from a variety of fields are involved including hepatologists, nephrologists, infectious disease specialists, social care workers, transplant coordinators, surgeons, anesthesiologists, and intensivists. This creates multiple points in which coordinated teamwork and communication between varied fields must take place in order to ensure optimal care. Throughout the perioperative course of the OLT patient, from preoperative optimization to postoperative complications, simulation can play a role in improving communication and resource management during critical periods.

Sample Scenario

Below is an example of a simulation scenario (Tables 22.5 and 22.6) designed to improve communication and situational awareness involving multiple healthcare workers of varied training background. A structured plan focuses the group on the performance of specific skills and goals dur-

Table 22.5 Simulation scenario toolkit

Objectives	1. Establish situational awareness and systematic response during transplant emergencies 2. Improve perioperative staff performance of initial management steps during a transplant emergency 3. Promote an increased comfort level of perioperative staff during posttransplant emergencies 4. Encourage better communication between support staff and physicians
Critical actions to be performed by participant	1. Recognize hypotension with ventilation changes on spirometry 2. Initiate ACLS 3. Attain the code cart. *Note the time taken to bring cart in room* 4. Attach defibrillator pads. *Note the time taken to place pads* 5. Recognize pneumothorax post-central line placement. *Note the time taken to recognize PTX* 6. Perform needle decompression 7. Communicate with CT surgery 8. Initiate massive transfusion protocol. *Note the time taken to obtain blood products* 9 *Utilization of closed-loop communication*

Table 22.6 Scenario development tool

Scenario background	Patient presents for OLT. "Dr. A," attending anesthesiologist, is starting the case with a clinical anesthesia year 3 (CA-3) resident. The induction is uneventful, and the central line is placed. Soon after, bradycardia, hypotension, and increased peak pressures begin	
Progression	Ventilation becomes difficult, and the oxygen saturation rapidly falls from 98% to 88%. There is now significant hypotension and bradycardia with a decrease in end-tidal CO_2	
Primary survey	Airway: Endotracheal tube in place Breathing: Immobile right chest, unilateral excursion	
Secondary survey	Head, ear, eye, nose, throat exam: Eyes closed Cardiovascular: No pulses palpable Lungs: No breath sounds auscultated on right Extremities: Cool, pale	
Labs	Hct initially 30 now 22	
Radiology	None	
EKG	Bradycardia with progression to asystole and eventual ventricular fibrillation	
Case chronology of events		
Scenario status	*Patient status*	*Actions to be performed by participants*
Initial induction and intubation	Hemodynamically stable	Nurse charting, scrub tech, and nurse beginning to count
Suturing central line	Desaturation and increased peak airway pressures	Attempts to listen to right and left breath sounds, surgeon at bedside, nurse calling out for help
Patient progresses to cardiac arrest	Asystole	Nurse getting code cart, scrub tech initiating compressions, ultrasound of chest shows pneumothorax
	Pulseless ventricular tachycardia	New intravenous access established, needle decompression reveals pneumohemothorax

ing the exercise. Depending on the participant makeup, case content, and skills targeted, these exercises can range from simple to complex.

This simple scenario includes a core of participants (surgeon, circulating nurse, scrub technician, anesthesia resident, anesthesia attending) and can be expanded to include a perfusionist, cardiothoracic surgery resident, or additional responders if help is called for. The focus should be on team training and communication during a crisis.

Curriculum Development and Resources

Creating a curriculum for trainees in liver transplant anesthesiology can be daunting. Several factors that can potentially limit or enhance resident training include case volume, faculty specialization, educational resources, and time. Regulatory bodies such as the ACGME, UNOS, and OPTN provide some limited guidance on required trainee time and exposure for evidence of sufficient expertise. Currently, liver transplant anesthesiology is not recognized as a subspecialty by the ACGME. At several centers in which clinical volume is significant, anesthesia residents may participate in a liver transplant rotation in order to gain clinical experience. However, the ACGME does require that each resident must demonstrate competency in anesthetic management of complex, immediately life-threatening pathology of at least 20 patients. This may include patients undergoing open or endovascular procedures on major vessels, including carotid, intrathoracic, intraabdominal, or peripheral vascular. While exposure to orthotopic liver transplantation is not specifically required by the ACGME, management of such cases clearly meets the definition of complex and immediately life-threatening pathology.

UNOS/OPTN requires that liver transplantation programs shall designate a director of liver transplant anesthesia with expertise in the perioperative care of patients undergoing liver transplantation and can serve as a faculty advisor to other members of the team. The director of liver transplant anesthesia must be a diplomate of the American Board of Anesthesiology (or hold equivalent foreign certification) and should meet one of the following criteria:

(a) Fellowship training in a Critical Care Medicine, Cardiac Anesthesiology, or Liver Transplant Fellowship that includes the perioperative care of at least ten liver transplant recipients.
(b) Experience in the perioperative care of at least 20 liver transplant recipients in the operating room within the last 5 years not including experience acquired during postgraduate (residency) training [29].

The foundation for a robust curriculum and in any liver transplant anesthesia rotation lies in direct exposure to liver transplantation and hepatobiliary procedures. This exposure would ideally involve supervision by faculty proficient in the management of liver transplantation through a formal fellowship or experience in the care of over 20 patients undergoing OLT as a faculty anesthesiologist. However, resident duty hours limitations provide an opportunity to supplement sporadic clinical education through alternative methods including lectures, reading material, and simulation. The current curriculum at the Icahn School Of Medicine at Mount Sinai Department of Anesthesiology involves a single mannequin-based, high-fidelity simulation performed at the initiation of the resident liver transplant rotation. One week prior to the rotation, residents are provided with access to a library of contemporary liver transplant literature and are encouraged to gain familiarity with the material prior to clinical exposure. A mannequin-based simulation session (Table 22.2) is provided for each resident participant and lasts for 1 hour inclusive of a post-scenario debrief. The rotating resident is taken through each stage of the operation, preoperative assessment to ICU disposition, by two instructors, both the member of the liver transplant anesthesia team and the simulation education team. Each simulation scenario is followed by a standardized debrief in which feedback is provided based on resident performance and framed by the specific practices utilized by the liver transplant anesthesia team at the Icahn School of Medicine at Mount Sinai, a quaternary care center that performs over 110 liver transplants per year.

Conclusion

Simulation can serve to provide consistency and quality in training for liver transplantation anesthesia, a field with inherent challenge complexity and exposure for the anesthesiologist in training. The acquisition of several procedural skills necessary to provide safe and effective care can be facilitated by part-task trainers in a safe and reproducible environment. Transesophageal and transthoracic echocardiography simulation technology can provide significant exposure to assist in recognition of life-threatening pathology which may occur during a liver transplantation. High-fidelity simulation or serious games representative of common events seen during liver transplantation such as hyperkalemia, massive hemorrhage, and cardiopulmonary arrest allow exposure and assessment of trainees' abilities and milestones attainment. Simulation can also provide a platform for the development of communication and teamwork between multiple disciplines caring for the liver transplant. Finally, simulation can provide solutions to the challenges inherent in the creation of a robust clinical liver transplant curriculum by providing a standardized environment despite limited resources.

References

1. Hall TH, Dhir A. Anesthesia for liver transplantation. Semin Cardiothorac Vasc Anesth. 2013;17(3):180–94. https://doi.org/10.1177/1089253213481115.
2. Schumann R, Mandell MS, Mercaldo N, et al. Anesthesia for liver transplantation in United States academic centers: intraoperative practice. J Clin Anesth. 2013;25(7):542–50. https://doi.org/10.1016/j.jclinane.2013.04.017.
3. Steadman RH. Anesthesia for liver transplant surgery. Anesthesiol Clin North America. 2004;22(4):687–711. https://doi.org/10.1016/j.atc.2004.06.009.
4. Organ Procurement and Transplantation Network. OPTN: Organ Procurement and Transplantation Network. 2015. http://optn.transplant.hrsa.gov/latestData/rptData.
5. American Board of Anesthesiology. Residency program requirements. Available at: https://www.acgme.org/acgmeweb/tabid/128/ProgramandInstitutionalAccreditation/HospitalBasedSpecialties/Anesthesiology.aspx. Accessed 1 Dec 2016.
6. Aggarwal S, Bane BC, Boucek CD, Planinsic RM, Lutz JW, Metro DG. Simulation: a teaching tool for liver transplantation anesthesiology. Clin Transpl. 2012;26(4):564–70. https://doi.org/10.1111/j.1399-0012.2011.01570.x.
7. Hofer I, Spivack J, Yaport M, et al. Association between anesthesiologist experience and mortality after orthotopic liver transplantation. Liver Transpl. 2015;21(1):89–95. https://doi.org/10.1002/lt.24014.
8. Mandell MS, Pomfret EA, Steadman R, et al. Director of anesthesiology for liver transplantation: existing practices and recommendations by the United Network for Organ Sharing. Liver Transpl. 2013;19(4):425–30. https://doi.org/10.1002/lt.23610.
9. Martín-Cancho MF, Calles C, Celdrán D, Sánchez-Margallo FM. Experimental training in anaesthesia management during hepatic transplant. Med Educ. 2011;45(11):1147. https://doi.org/10.1111/j.1365-2923.2011.04121.x.
10. Bergeron B. Developing serious games. Hingham: Charles River Media; 2006.
11. Wang R, DeMaria S, Goldberg A, Katz D. A systematic review of serious games in training health care professionals. Simul Healthc. 2016;11(1):41–51. https://doi.org/10.1097/SIH.0000000000000118.
12. Dong Y, Suri HS, Cook DA, et al. Simulation-based objective assessment discerns clinical proficiency in central line placement: a construct validation. Chest. 2010;137(5):1050–6. https://doi.org/10.1378/chest.09-1451.
13. Katz D, Goldberg A, Khanal P, Kahol K, DeMaria S. Using serious gaming to improve the safety of central venous catheter placement: a post-mortem analysis. IJGCMS. 2015;6(4):34–45.
14. Dankbaar MEW, Roozeboom MB, Oprins EAPB, et al. Preparing residents effectively in emergency skills training with a serious game. Simul Healthc. 2016; https://doi.org/10.1097/SIH.0000000000000194.
15. Graafland M, Bemelman WA, Schijven MP. Appraisal of face and content validity of a serious game improving situational awareness in surgical training. J Laparoendosc Adv Surg Tech A. 2015;25(1):43–9. https://doi.org/10.1089/lap.2014.0043.
16. Lagro J, van de Pol MHJ, Laan A, Huijbregts-Verheyden FJ, Fluit LCR, Olde Rikkert MGM. A randomized controlled trial on teaching geriatric medical decision making and cost consciousness with the serious game GeriatriX. J Am Med Dir Assoc. 2014;15(12):957.e1–6. https://doi.org/10.1016/j.jamda.2014.04.011.
17. Diehl LA, Souza RM, Alves JB, et al. InsuOnline, a serious game to teach insulin therapy to primary care physicians: design of the game and a randomized controlled trial for educational validation. JMIR Res Protoc. 2013;2(1):e5. https://doi.org/10.2196/resprot.2431.
18. Chan W-Y, Qin J, Chui Y-P, Heng P-A. A serious game for learning ultrasound-guided needle placement skills. IEEE Trans Inf Technol Biomed. 2012;16(6):1032–42. https://doi.org/10.1109/TITB.2012.2204406.
19. Prober CG, Heath C. Lecture halls without lectures–a proposal for medical education. N Engl J Med. 2012;366(18):1657–9. https://doi.org/10.1056/NEJMp1202451.
20. Bonnes SL, Ratelle JT, Halvorsen AJ, et al. Flipping the quality improvement classroom in residency education. Acad Med. 2016;92:101. https://doi.org/10.1097/ACM.0000000000001412.
21. Lew EK. Creating a contemporary clerkship curriculum: the flipped classroom model in emergency medicine. Int J Emerg Med. 2016;9(1):25. https://doi.org/10.1186/s12245-016-0123-6.
22. Morton DA, Colbert-Getz JM. Measuring the impact of the flipped anatomy classroom: the importance of categorizing an assessment by Bloom's taxonomy. Anat Sci Educ. 2016;10:170. https://doi.org/10.1002/ase.1635.
23. Rose E, Claudius I, Tabatabai R, Kearl L, Behar S, Jhun P. The flipped classroom in emergency medicine using online videos with interpolated questions. J Emerg Med. 2016;51(3):284–291.e1. https://doi.org/10.1016/j.jemermed.2016.05.033.

24. Chang LC, Mahoney JJ, Raty SR, Ortiz J, Apodaca S, De La Garza R. Neurocognitive effects following an overnight call shift on faculty anesthesiologists. Acta Anaesthesiol Scand. 2013;57(8):1051–7. https://doi.org/10.1111/aas.12120.
25. Calatayud D, Arora S, Aggarwal R, et al. Warm-up in a virtual reality environment improves performance in the operating room. Ann Surg. 2010;251(6):1181–5. https://doi.org/10.1097/SLA.0b013e3181deb630.
26. Chen CCG, Green IC, Colbert-Getz JM, et al. Warm-up on a simulator improves residents' performance in laparoscopic surgery: a randomized trial. Int Urogynecol J. 2013;24(10):1615–22. https://doi.org/10.1007/s00192-013-2066-2.
27. Nguyen D, Gurvitz-Gambrel S, Sloan PA, et al. The impact of exposure to liver transplantation anesthesia on the ability to treat intraoperative hyperkalemia: a simulation experience. Int Surg. 2015;100(4):672–7. https://doi.org/10.9738/INTSURG-D-14-00279.1.
28. Schwid HA, Rooke GA, Carline J, Steadman RH, Murray WB, Olympio M, et al. Evaluation of anesthesia residents using mannequin-based simulation: a multi-institutional study. Anesthesiology. 2002;97(6):1434–44.
29. Organ Procurement and Transplantation Network. Attachment I to Appendix B of the OPTN bylaws. http://optn.transplant.hrsa.gov/policiesandBylaws2/bylaws/OPTNByLaws/pdfs/bylaw_162.pdf. Accessed Dec 2012.

Simulation in Trauma/Advanced Cardiac Life Support

23

Cesar Padilla and Michaela Kristina Farber

Introduction

The goals of anesthesiology simulation training for trauma and advanced cardiac life support (ACLS) are to facilitate proficiency in the performance of specific required tasks through part-task training modalities, replicate real-life scenarios using high-fidelity simulation, and enhance both individual and team performance. Simulation of trauma/ACLS allows multidisciplinary teams to practice the coordination and communication skills required for management of low-frequency, high-acuity events. The focus of this chapter is on each of these components and their relevance to trauma and ACLS resuscitation training for the anesthesiologist.

Part-Task Trainers and Skill Acquisition

Part-task training focuses on dividing a complex task into components and intensive focus on those individual components. Part-task procedures such as placement of a chest tube in a mannequin or inserting an intravenous line in an artificial limb are relevant to trauma/ACLS. Benefits over higher-fidelity simulation include lower cost, portability of equipment, and emphasis on development of muscle and eye coordination for required procedural skills [1]. Restriction of resident work hours by the Accreditation Council for Graduate Medical Education (ACGME) raises legitimate concern about a decrease in procedural experience among young physicians. There is an increasingly perceived lack of procedural skills and patient management skills among newly trained physicians by departmental leaders [2]. Part-task simulation allows residents to practice procedural techniques in a safe setting with feedback about motor skill acquisition [3]. While part-task simulation training has proven effective for improving procedural skills among colorectal surgery residents, procedural skills are not yet measured or assessed for certification [4]. Part-task training may gain further emphasis in training programs, as procedural skill assessment is increasingly advocated.

Acquiring task proficiency requires a complex set of behavioral modifications. Motor skill acquisition occurs through the following three steps: cognition, integration, and automation [5]. Cognition involves the understanding of the task, integration involves coordinating mechanical skills, and automation involves performing the task with speed and efficiency [5]. The transfer of performance skills from part-task simulation, or low-fidelity models to higher-fidelity models, has been well documented. Therefore, it is helpful to create a foundation for trauma/ACLS training using part-task simulators to ameliorate the stress and variability of performing an unfamiliar procedure during an emergency situation. Simulation courses integrating part-task trauma/ACLS skills such as endotracheal intubation, cricothyroidotomy, and intravenous access with full simulations have been shown to increase medical student confidence when performing these tasks [3]. Part-task training for anesthesiology skills in trauma/ACLS includes endotracheal intubation, cricothyroidotomy, central and peripheral line placement, and chest compressions [6].

Endotracheal Intubation

Endotracheal intubation during ACLS or trauma situations is essential for airway protection and provision of adequate ventilation. Intubation during an emergency requires baseline proficiency. An airway-specific part-task trainer (Laerdal Airway Management Trainer; Fig. 23.1) has been utilized to evaluate force applied to the epiglottis, number of attempts required for intubation, time to intubation, and appropriate

C. Padilla
Anesthesiology and Pain Management, Cleveland Clinic, Pepper Pike, OH, USA

M. K. Farber (✉)
Department of Anesthesiology, Perioperative, and Pain Medicine, Brigham and Women's Hospital, Boston, MA, USA

Harvard Medical School, Boston, MA, USA
e-mail: mfarber@bwh.harvard.edu

B. Mahoney et al. (eds.), *Comprehensive Healthcare Simulation: Anesthesiology*, Comprehensive Healthcare Simulation,
https://doi.org/10.1007/978-3-030-26849-7_23

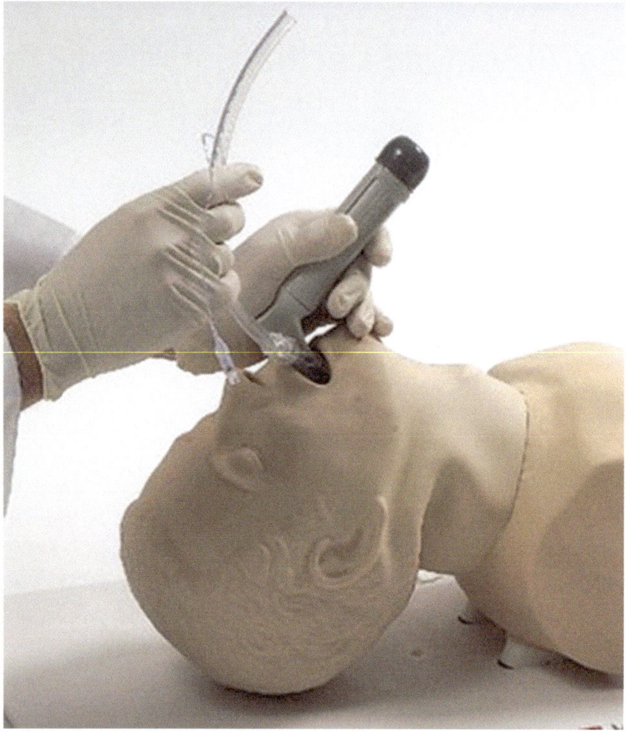

Fig. 23.1 Laerdal Airway Management Trainer. (Photo courtesy of Laerdal Medical. All rights reserved. www.laerdal.com)

hand position on the laryngoscope among healthcare providers [7]. Teaching laryngoscopy skills using a video laryngoscope may be more effective than traditional teaching with a standard laryngoscope. Those taught using a video laryngoscope for training and then subjected to simulated normal airway (Laerdal Airway Manager) and difficult airway (Sim Man) conditions required fewer attempts and repositioning maneuvers and had more confidence and improved knowledge of airway anatomy [8]. Furthermore, the use of video laryngoscopy for real-time airway establishment during ACLS chest compressions has been suggested to facilitate endotracheal intubation with shorter interruption of chest compressions. The goal is to fully secure the airway without interrupting chest compressions or with a brief pause of less than 5 seconds [9]. Mannequin studies comparing tools for airway establishment in trauma/ACLS situations may not translate to real-life situations. A randomized crossover mannequin study evaluating hands-off time for intubation showed no benefit of the video laryngoscope under easy intubating conditions, by experienced providers [10]. Further studies may demonstrate utility of the video laryngoscope during trauma/ACLS situations, particularly for difficult airways and providers with less airway experience. Furthermore, video laryngoscopy was superior to direct laryngoscopy for achieving intubation with no interruption in chest compressions in real patients in the emergency department [11]. These discrepancies likely reflect the various factors that influence emergency intubation in real circumstances; impaired visualization of the airway by blood, vomit, debris or secretions, anatomic challenges, patient positioning, and distractions such as noise level may make laryngoscopy in real trauma/ACLS situations more difficult [12].

Airway compromise is a leading cause of death in trauma patients, and immediate cricothyroidotomy in cases of failed ventilation or intubation can be lifesaving. Fewer than 1% of trauma patients require this maneuver, limiting exposure to, and practice of, this procedure. Part-task training for emergency airway access facilitates knowledge of anatomic landmarks and surgical dexterity. Detailed instructions for creation of affordable, low-fidelity cricothyroidotomy simulators are available [13].

Vascular Access

Obtaining vascular access in an unstable patient can be challenging. Simulation training for different approaches has been described. In situations such as upper thoracic trauma where superior vena cava flow may be disrupted, vascular access below the diaphragm is paramount to ensure flow via the inferior vena cava [14]. Obtaining access in the lower extremity is a challenging and unfamiliar task for untrained personnel. Advanced life trauma support (ATLS), a sub-segment of the American College of Surgeons, recommends placement of two large-bore intravenous lines (16 gauge or larger) in a patient with suspected of hemorrhagic shock or with serious injuries [14].

Intravenous access may be challenging in patients with hemodynamic collapse or certain injuries such as burns or fractures. A systematic review evaluated the impact of simulation training and outcomes for central venous catheter placement and found greater success and fewer attempts in groups exposed to simulation training for this procedure [15]. The established safety and efficacy of ultrasound-assisted central venous catheter insertion also highlights

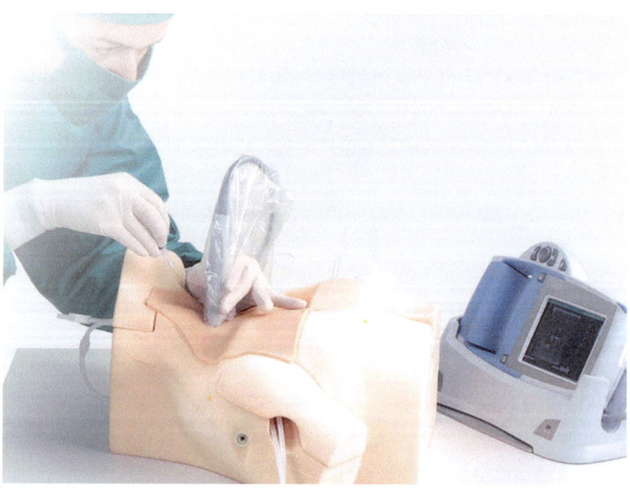

Fig. 23.2 CVC Insertion Simulator2 for central venous access placement by Kyoto Kagaku LTD. (Photo courtesy of Kyoto Kagaku, Ltd. (www.kyotokagaku.com))

the importance of establishing competency among medical trainees with ultrasound-based techniques [16] (Fig. 23.2).

An alternative approach to obtaining access is by the intraosseous (intramedullary) approach, which can be lifesaving for vascular administration of resuscitation medications when peripheral access is delayed or impossible. A part-task simulator, the Stat Adult ALS Manikin with intraosseous Leg Trainer (Simulaids, Saugerties, NY), has been used to compare success rates of three devices that establish intraosseous access by paramedics [17]. Use of two different intraosseous access devices in real patients in the emergency room yielded equal success [18]. As this approach gains popularity, task training simulation teaching will be important, to ensure proper use and safety of intraosseous access during trauma and ACLS.

Chest Compressions

The first CPR mannequin defined the paradigm for part-task simulation in medicine. Resusci-Annie™ was developed in 1960, after Drs. Elam and Safar first demonstrated that mouth-to-mouth ventilation provided adequate oxygenation and elimination of carbon dioxide [19]. Dr. Safar commissioned a toymaker, Asmund Laerdal, to create the first lifelike CPR mannequin. While this mannequin lacks haptic feedback of higher fidelity simulators, it continues to be a powerful tool for assessment of part-task performance and skill acquisition. Today's Resusci-Annie, the Resusci Anne® QCPR (Laerdal Medical, Orpington, UK; Fig. 23.3) measures chest compression depth and rate using a displacement sensor, with a recording system.

Continuous evaluation and immediate improvement of chest compressions during CPR continue to be a major focus in ACLS simulation part-task training. Pozner and colleagues demonstrated that CPR feedback improved the quality of chest compressions [20]. Smartphone applications with a built-in accelerometer assist in CPR training with chest compression feedback [21]. The quality of chest compressions during CPR by medical students was similar when comparing human feedback by a second rescuer to a mechanized audiovisual device (HeartStart MRx with Q-CPR technology) [22]. The deterioration of chest compression quality with transport of a patient in a simulated maternal cardiac arrest study was demonstrated using the part-task CPR mannequin; interruptions in CPR were observed in 92% of cases in which transport was performed during CPR, compared to 7% in the stationary group, with demonstrated deficiencies in adequate depth of compressions, hand placement on the sternum, and allowance for elastic recoil [23]. CPR is a physically strenuous task, and rescuer performance declines quickly over time. A part-task simulator scenario of CPR administration compared three CPR feedback technologies (PocketCPR, CPRmeter, and iPhone app Pocket PCR) to CPR without feedback and found that effective compressions were not improved by any CPR feedback device and that the devices may cause substantial delay in CPR initiation [24]. With continued advances in technology using smartphone and other integrated technology, part-task training with CPR mannequins will continue to play a central role for validating this technology and for enhancing the performance of physicians integrating these new modalities.

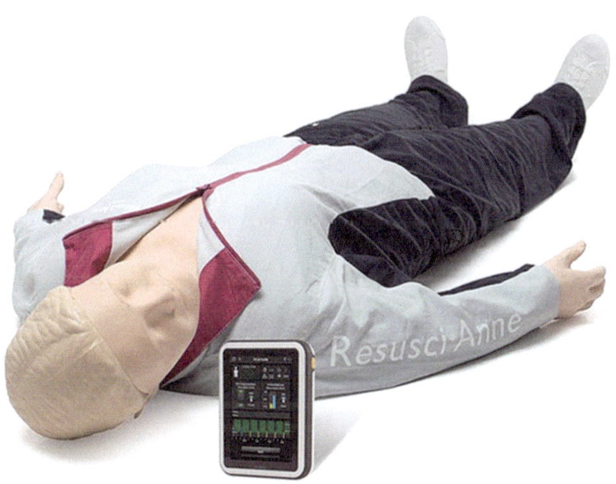

Fig. 23.3 The Resusci Anne® QCPR adult CPR training mannequin with sensor to indicate correct hand placement, ventilation system with chest wall rise, and wired connectivity to SimPad SkillReporter or Resusci Ann Wireless SkillReporter software. (Photo courtesy of Laerdal Medical. All rights reserved. www.laerdal.com)

High-Fidelity Simulation for Exposure

Advanced Cardiac Life Support

High-fidelity simulation for advanced cardiac life support (ACLS) training has significantly improved in quality and technology in the past 20 years [25–27]. High-fidelity simulation, which is defined as an object or experience resembling a real-world object or scenario, has been extensively studied using ACLS and trauma scenarios. While part-task simulation focuses on acquiring the necessary skill to accomplish a specific task, high-fidelity training focuses on the overall experience of the trainee with an emphasis on teamwork, interpersonal skills, and clinical decision-making. Participants who underwent high-fidelity simulation training for ACLS achieved higher scores in skill, cognitive knowledge, and competency compared to a low-fidelity simulation group [28]. Third-year medical students exposed to a high-fidelity simulation curriculum on ACLS management tasks reported increased preparedness, comfort level, and ability to be in charge of a code as team leader compared to those exposed to a traditional curriculum [29]. It is unclear whether high-fidelity simulation during medical school increases clinical competency in residency. However, Wayne and colleagues demonstrated that medical residents exposed to high-fidelity ACLS scenarios had enhanced clinical performance after simulation training and achieved higher ACLS knowledge base scores compared to those who completed the American Heart Association ACLS provider course [30].

Trauma

The use of high-fidelity simulation to expose medical providers to trauma resuscitation training is worthwhile, as the rate of avoidable death after injury has been reported as high as 25% [31]. The implementation of trauma protocols has been shown to decrease the rate of preventable deaths based on large population-based models [32]. Team training through simulated trauma scenarios has also been shown to improve teamwork and interpersonal communication [30].

The use of simple mannequins compared to standardized patients for trauma team training has been compared [31]. Participants reported high educational quality with both modalities and equal credibility and sense of realism in scenarios that utilized a mannequin compared to a standardized patient. Although study participants favored scenarios in which standardized patients were used, both modalities were effective for fulfilling educational goals of leadership, cooperation, and communication. This study underscores the value of using mannequins to achieve high-impact team training through simulation.

Trauma and ACLS resuscitations are characterized by low-frequency, high-acuity events. The unpredictable nature of such events can evoke stress, and the importance of a unified, multidisciplinary team approach to management cannot be overstated. Simulation-based team training sessions improved mannequin survivability in high-fidelity trauma scenarios among healthcare team consisting of nurses, physicians, and respiratory therapists [33]. The authors of this study emphasized the benefit of simulation training toward the goal of

Table 23.1 Sample trauma/ACLS scenario

Title: Loss of consciousness after motor vehicle accident		
Audience: Anesthesia resident		
Objectives:	*Medical knowledge:* Identify signs and symptoms of an unstable trauma patient	
	Patient care: Diagnosis and management of cardiac arrest after trauma	
	Communication: Utilize crew resource management skills to manage a trauma emergency	
Case stem: Mr. Smith is a 41-year-old man who sustained a motor vehicle accident. Blunt liver trauma is suspected		
Room setup: Emergency room bay with patient supine on a stretcher. He was in a motor vehicle accident		
The patient will have a noninvasive blood pressure cuff, pulse oximetry, and EKG electrodes in place. An IV bag is hanging and primed but not yet placed. An emergency room nurse and physician serve as confederates. The patient is a Resusci Anne® QCPR adult CPR training mannequin with sensor to indicate correct hand placement, ventilation system with chest wall rise, and wired connectivity to SimPad SkillReporter software		
State	**Patient status**	**Learner actions**
Baseline	Otherwise healthy, acutely injured patient with slight somnolence HR, 112; RR, 20; BP, 89/40; SpO2, 94% (RA) A focused assessment with ultrasonography for trauma (FAST) exam reveals free fluid in the RUQ	The learner will introduce himself/herself to the patient and care team Assess patient orientation and level of consciousness Prioritize rapid IV placement and fluid administration Prioritize calling for a massive transfusion protocol (MTP)
Anxious and agitated	The IV is attempted twice without success Anxious appearing and agitated (over 1 minutes) HR, 131; RR, 30; BP, 65/45; SpO2, 90% (RA)	Generate a differential diagnosis Communicate concerns to the present team Call for help/backup care (surgical team) Prepare for possible intraosseous access Initiate supportive care for hypoxia/hypotension
Unresponsive	Unconscious ETCO2 10 mmHg	Recognize pulseless electrical activity (PEA) and initiate ACLS Adequate chest compression frequency and depth, ventilation, IV or IO access Epinephrine 1 mg IV or IO Initiation of MTP Communicate concerns with the team; review the 5Hs and 5Ts for etiology. ANTS system situational awareness
Recovery	Regains consciousness with ACLS and early resuscitation (after initiation of supportive care over 2 minutes) HR, 110; RR, 15; BP, 90/60; SpO2, 99%	Develop a plan for supportive/intensive care and transport while the operating room team is notified
Discussion points: Differential diagnosis of cardiac arrest after acute trauma; establishing rapid IV or IO access and activation of MTP; appropriate ACLS maneuvers; crew resource management in the ED for identifying surgical emergency patients		

overall efficiency of the crisis team, focusing on communication and functionality of the team rather than individual skills and contributions. See Table 23.1 for a sample scenario.

High-Fidelity Simulation for Assessment

Assessment of anesthesia performance during high-fidelity simulation of ACLS and trauma scenarios has become increasingly sophisticated. Gaba and colleagues demonstrated good inter-rater reliability and feasibility through the separate measurement of technical and behavioral performance of videotaped cardiac arrest and malignant hyperthermia scenarios using a specific, point-based checklist system [34]. The nontechnical performance in this study was scored in two separate time periods, before and after the critical event. Furthermore, timing for nontechnical scoring was specified to improve inter-rater reliability. This more refined scoring method was used by Mudumbai and colleagues [35]. A global rating system has been advocated over a checklist-based method for scoring the complex performance of trauma/ACLS in high-fidelity simulated scenarios. A global rating scale utilizing three categories of performance, knowledge, behavior, and overall performance, was found to have good inter-rater reliability for evaluation of anesthesiologist performance during cardiac arrest and other critical medical situations [36]. Interest in how simulation scores relate to other measures of ability has intensified with the American Board of Anesthesiology (ABA) initiation of simulation-based training as part of the Practice Performance Improvement and Assessment component for the Maintenance of Certification in Anesthesiology (MOCA). The validity of scores may be best when multiple scenarios are scored, using multiple observations, different patient encounters, and evaluation of both nontechnical and technical skills [37]. The performance of graduating anesthesiology residents was evaluated in multiple short scenarios and one long scenario, based on technical skills (using a set of key clinical actions) and nontechnical skills (using a validated scoring system, ANTS) [35]. This comprehensive study found moderate correlation between simulation scores and other markers of ability, including USMLE scores, ABA in-training examination scores, and faculty and nursing global ranking scores.

Multidisciplinary Team Training

Effective, multidisciplinary teamwork and communication are key for management of critical clinical events. In situ simulation may be the optimal approach for team training in the true clinical environment. In an observational study of a level 1 trauma center emergency department, team performance was measured at baseline and then after exposure to didactic sessions and in situ trauma simulation drills [38]. While the program improved teamwork and communication, the effect was not sustained after the drills were stopped. Thus re-exposure of multidisciplinary teams to in situ drills are required to prevent degradation of teamwork skills; the frequency with which retraining is needed has not yet been determined.

Defining the role of each team member during crisis management has the potential to improve team performance. The evaluation of a cognitive aid for role definition (CARD) used among 16 interprofessional operating room teams during in situ simulation of cardiac arrest found no significant differences in team performance with or without CARD use [39].

Communication among team members may hold greater relevance, in conjunction with each team member having a defined role during crisis management. Verbalizing situation assessments during a crisis in order to coordinate task management with the least time spent on task delegation and an emphasis on task performance may yield better team coordination [40]. Two-person anesthesiology teams managing a high-fidelity simulation of malignant hyperthermia had the lowest performance scores when a shared plan was not verbalized to the rest of the team [40]. A high-fidelity simulation study of communication between care providers (anesthesiologists and obstetricians) during maternal crisis management demonstrated a shortcoming in both the anesthesiologists' inquiry of the obstetricians' plan and in the formation of a jointly managed clinical plan [41]. Strategies to overcome deficient communication patterns that are identified between providers may be incorporated into both content development and debriefing of simulated crisis scenarios.

Curriculum Development and Resources

Assessment of Technical Skills

A scoring system for 12 simulated intraoperative scenarios can be utilized to distinguish skills of more experienced anesthesiologists from residents in early training [42].

Mudumbai and colleagues suggest multiple short scenarios using high-fidelity simulation to evaluate technical skills [35]. The appendix to this chapter provides key actions that can be used for short simulation scenarios such as acute hemorrhage, tension pneumothorax, and unstable ventricular tachycardia, all of which are pertinent to trauma/ACLS.

Assessment of Nontechnical Skills

The most widely accepted and validated scoring system for nontechnical performance in simulation for anesthesiologists is the Anaesthetists' Non-Technical Skills (ANTS) system developed by Fletcher and colleagues [43]. The ANTS system defines categories of teamwork, situational awareness, task management, and decision-making using a 4-point Likert scale and can be applied at specific time points within a simulation to avoid the issue of variable performance over time [34]. This application of the ANTS system with specific nontechnical elements measured at specific time points is described by Mudumbai and colleagues (Appendix C) [35].

Doumouras and colleagues described and evaluated a pilot of trauma team training curriculum focusing on nontechnical performance [44]. Deficiencies in trauma resuscitation often result from ineffective team leadership, nonstandardized communication among team members, lack of situational awareness, or inappropriate prioritization. The described curriculum emphasizes these components. A nontechnical skills scale for trauma (T-NOTECHS) enables teaching and assessment of teamwork skills during multidisciplinary trauma resuscitation and has been validated for clinical grading of nontechnical skills during simulated trauma scenarios [45].

Conclusion

The ability for anesthesiologists to perform critical tasks effectively, to recognize a crisis situation, and to coordinate a multidisciplinary response team with effective communication and technical performance requires a great deal of skill and practice. Anesthesiologists have limited exposure to low-frequency, high-acuity events such as unstable trauma or cardiac arrest. Low- and high-fidelity simulation will continue to serve as meaningful mechanisms of training and exposure of anesthesiologists to these situations, for optimization of personal and team-related performance.

References

1. Stirling ER, Lewis TL, Ferran NA. Surgical skills simulation in trauma and orthopaedic training. J Orthop Surg Res. 2014;9:126.
2. Crosson FJ, Leu J, Roemer BM, Ross MN. Gaps in residency training should be addressed to better prepare doctors for a twenty-first-century delivery system. Health Aff (Millwood). 2011;30:2142–8.
3. Shukla A, Kline D, Cherian A, et al. A simulation course on lifesaving techniques for third-year medical students. Simul Healthc. 2007;2:11–5.
4. de Montbrun SL, Roberts PL, Lowry AC, et al. A novel approach to assessing technical competence of colorectal surgery residents: the development and evaluation of the Colorectal Objective Structured Assessment of Technical Skill (COSATS). Ann Surg. 2013;258:1001–6.
5. Reznick RK, MacRae H. Teaching surgical skills--changes in the wind. N Engl J Med. 2006;355:2664–9.
6. Sahu S, Lata I. Simulation in resuscitation teaching and training, an evidence based practice review. J Emerg Trauma Shock. 2010;3:378–84.
7. Garcia J, Coste A, Tavares W, Nuno N, Lachapelle K. Assessment of competency during orotracheal intubation in medical simulation. Br J Anaesth. 2015;115:302–7.
8. Low D, Healy D, Rasburn N. The use of the BERCI DCI video laryngoscope for teaching novices direct laryngoscopy and tracheal intubation. Anaesthesia. 2008;63:195–201.
9. Berg RA, Hemphill R, Abella BS, et al. Part 5: adult basic life support: 2010 American Heart Association guidelines for cardiopulmonary resuscitation and emergency cardiovascular care. Circulation. 2010;122:S685–705.
10. Schuerner P, Grande B, Piegeler T, et al. Hands-off time for endotracheal intubation during CPR is not altered by the use of the C-MAC video-laryngoscope compared to conventional direct laryngoscopy. A randomized crossover manikin study. PLoS One. 2016;11:e0155997.
11. Kim JW, Park SO, Lee KR, et al. Video laryngoscopy vs. direct laryngoscopy: which should be chosen for endotracheal intubation during cardiopulmonary resuscitation? A prospective randomized controlled study of experienced intubators. Resuscitation. 2016;105:196–202.
12. Helm M, Hossfeld B, Schafer S, Hoitz J, Lampl L. Factors influencing emergency intubation in the pre-hospital setting – a multicentre study in the German Helicopter Emergency Medical Service. Br J Anaesth. 2006;96:67–71.
13. Pettineo CM, Vozenilek JA, Wang E, Flaherty J, Kharasch M, Aitchison P. Simulated emergency department procedures with minimal monetary investment: cricothyrotomy simulator. Simul Healthc. 2009;4:60–4.
14. Bourgeois SL Jr. Central venous access techniques. Atlas Oral Maxillofac Surg Clin North Am. 2015;23:137–45.
15. Madenci AL, Solis CV, de Moya MA. Central venous access by trainees: a systematic review and meta-analysis of the use of simulation to improve success rate on patients. Simul Healthc. 2014;9:7–14.
16. Ball RD, Scouras NE, Orebaugh S, Wilde J, Sakai T. Randomized, prospective, observational simulation study comparing residents' needle-guided vs free-hand ultrasound techniques for central venous catheter access. Br J Anaesth. 2012;108:72–9.
17. Kurowski A, Timler D, Evrin T, Szarpak L. Comparison of 3 different intraosseous access devices for adult during resuscitation. Randomized crossover manikin study. Am J Emerg Med. 2014;32:1490–3.
18. Leidel BA, Kirchhoff C, Braunstein V, Bogner V, Biberthaler P, Kanz KG. Comparison of two intraosseous access devices in adult patients under resuscitation in the emergency department: a prospective, randomized study. Resuscitation. 2010;81:994–9.
19. Cooper JB, Taqueti VR. A brief history of the development of mannequin simulators for clinical education and training. Qual Saf Health Care. 2004;13(Suppl 1):i11–8.
20. Pozner CN, Almozlino A, Elmer J, Poole S, McNamara D, Barash D. Cardiopulmonary resuscitation feedback improves the quality of chest compression provided by hospital health care professionals. Am J Emerg Med. 2011;29:618–25.
21. Song Y, Oh J, Chee Y. A new chest compression depth feedback algorithm for high-quality CPR based on smartphone. Telemed J E Health. 2015;21:36–41.
22. Pavo N, Goliasch G, Nierscher FJ, et al. Short structured feedback training is equivalent to a mechanical feedback device in two-rescuer BLS: a randomised simulation study. Scand J Trauma Resusc Emerg Med. 2016;24:70.
23. Lipman SS, Wong JY, Arafeh J, Cohen SE, Carvalho B. Transport decreases the quality of cardiopulmonary resuscitation during simulated maternal cardiac arrest. Anesth Analg. 2013;116:162–7.
24. Zapletal B, Greif R, Stumpf D, et al. Comparing three CPR feedback devices and standard BLS in a single rescuer scenario: a randomised simulation study. Resuscitation. 2014;85:560–6.

25. Conlon LW, Rodgers DL, Shofer FS, Lipschik GY. Impact of levels of simulation fidelity on training of interns in ACLS. Hosp Pract (1995). 2014;42:135–41.
26. Adams AJ, Wasson EA, Admire JR, et al. A comparison of teaching modalities and fidelity of simulation levels in teaching resuscitation scenarios. J Surg Educ. 2015;72:778–85.
27. O'Brien G, Haughton A, Flanagan B. Interns' perceptions of performance and confidence in participating in and managing simulated and real cardiac arrest situations. Med Teach. 2001;23:389–95.
28. Rodgers DL, Securro S Jr, Pauley RD. The effect of high-fidelity simulation on educational outcomes in an advanced cardiovascular life support course. Simul Healthc. 2009;4:200–6.
29. Ko PY, Scott JM, Mihai A, Grant WD. Comparison of a modified longitudinal simulation-based advanced cardiovascular life support to a traditional advanced cardiovascular life support curriculum in third-year medical students. Teach Learn Med. 2011;23:324–30.
30. Wayne DB, Butter J, Siddall VJ, et al. Mastery learning of advanced cardiac life support skills by internal medicine residents using simulation technology and deliberate practice. J Gen Intern Med. 2006;21:251–6.
31. Wisborg T, Brattebo G, Brinchmann-Hansen A, Hansen KS. Mannequin or standardized patient: participants' assessment of two training modalities in trauma team simulation. Scand J Trauma Resusc Emerg Med. 2009;17:59.
32. Esposito TJ, Sanddal TL, Reynolds SA, Sanddal ND. Effect of a voluntary trauma system on preventable death and inappropriate care in a rural state. J Trauma. 2003;54:663–9. discussion 9–70.
33. DeVita MA, Schaefer J, Lutz J, Wang H, Dongilli T. Improving medical emergency team (MET) performance using a novel curriculum and a computerized human patient simulator. Qual Saf Health Care. 2005;14:326–31.
34. Gaba DM, Howard SK, Flanagan B, Smith BE, Fish KJ, Botney R. Assessment of clinical performance during simulated crises using both technical and behavioral ratings. Anesthesiology. 1998;89:8–18.
35. Mudumbai SC, Gaba DM, Boulet JR, Howard SK, Davies MF. External validation of simulation-based assessments with other performance measures of third-year anesthesiology residents. Simul Healthc. 2012;7:73–80.
36. Weller JM, Bloch M, Young S, et al. Evaluation of high fidelity patient simulator in assessment of performance of anaesthetists. Br J Anaesth. 2003;90:43–7.
37. Kogan JR, Holmboe ES, Hauer KE. Tools for direct observation and assessment of clinical skills of medical trainees: a systematic review. JAMA. 2009;302:1316–26.
38. Miller D, Crandall C, Washington C 3rd, McLaughlin S. Improving teamwork and communication in trauma care through in situ simulations. Acad Emerg Med. 2012;19:608–12.
39. Renna TD, Crooks S, Pigford AA, et al. Cognitive Aids for Role Definition (CARD) to improve interprofessional team crisis resource management: an exploratory study. J Interprof Care. 2016;30:582–90.
40. Manser T, Harrison TK, Gaba DM, Howard SK. Coordination patterns related to high clinical performance in a simulated anesthetic crisis. Anesth Analg. 2009;108:1606–15.
41. Minehart RD, Pian-Smith MC, Walzer TB, et al. Speaking across the drapes: communication strategies of anesthesiologists and obstetricians during a simulated maternal crisis. Simul Healthc. 2012;7:166–70.
42. Murray DJ, Boulet JR, Avidan M, et al. Performance of residents and anesthesiologists in a simulation-based skill assessment. Anesthesiology. 2007;107:705–13.
43. Fletcher G, Flin R, McGeorge P, Glavin R, Maran N, Patey R. Anaesthetists' Non-Technical Skills (ANTS): evaluation of a behavioural marker system. Br J Anaesth. 2003;90:580–8.
44. Doumouras AG, Keshet I, Nathens AB, Ahmed N, Hicks CM. Trauma Non-Technical Training (TNT-2): the development, piloting and multilevel assessment of a simulation-based, interprofessional curriculum for team-based trauma resuscitation. Can J Surg. 2014;57:354–5.
45. Steinemann S, Berg B, DiTullio A, et al. Assessing teamwork in the trauma bay: introduction of a modified "NOTECHS" scale for trauma. Am J Surg. 2012;203:69–75.

24 Simulation in Otolaryngology and Airway Procedures

Christine Lan Mai, Maricela Schnur, and Adam I. Levine

Introduction

The field of anesthesiology has become increasingly sub-specialized, with unique challenges that demand high-quality teaching and training. Advancements in technology have ensured higher standards for patient safety, quality, and efficiency within the traditional operating room and in remote sites. While many surgical environments benefit from a collegial team dynamic, the characteristics of the otolaryngologic environment require a unique interdisciplinary collaboration for optimal patient outcomes [1]. Anesthesiologists and otolaryngologists work quite literally side by side and share overlapping concerns and physical space. Patients undergoing head and neck surgery can also be at high risk for potentially devastating events if the airway anatomy is distorted from pathologic conditions or previous surgical interventions. Therefore, both specialties benefit from a shared comprehensive understanding of each other's practice.

Most of the current ear, nose, and throat (ENT) simulation education literature is focused on improvement of procedural skills or sub-specialty training, either for the surgeon or anesthesia provider alone [2, 3]. Clearly, this is not sufficient for prevention or management of high-stress situations where crisis resource management and interdisciplinary communication skills can affect patient outcomes. High-quality ENT anesthesia simulation should provide several things to clinicians including (1) deliberate practice of procedural skills and/or (2) familiarization with equipment and their failure modes, (3) management of basic and critical events associated with ENT patients and surgery, (4) interdisciplinary crisis resource management skills during head and neck surgery including decision-making under pressure and delegation of roles, and (5) debriefing, reflection, and valuable feedback [3]. In this chapter we will review the current simulation technology and describe ways to incorporate them into an educational experience to enrich technical and nontechnical skills. Finally, we will conclude with a completely developed scenario of an airway fire and list other examples of scenario stems that can be used for anesthesiology training or developed to include multidisciplinary training with our surgical and nursing colleagues.

Review of Procedural Airway Devices

Although basic and advanced airway management is ubiquitous for the training of all anesthesiologists, ENT anesthesia (with its patient population and specific surgical procedures) requires proficiency of both noninvasive and invasive techniques. An assortment of devices can be utilized based on the characteristics of each technology and the clinical lessons that are desired [4]. Simulation devices are divided into two broad categories, partial-task trainers and whole-task trainers. Partial-task trainers are models designed to allow participants to practice clinical skills and tasks; many are simple devices designed for learning or practicing specific procedures (e.g., mask ventilation, laryngoscopy, needle cricothyrotomy). Others are sophisticated devices that are coupled with computer and robotic interfaces, which can enhance the physical and virtual aspects of the simulators for practicing more complex procedures (e.g., bronchoscopy and endoscopy). These devices are useful

C. L. Mai (✉)
Department of Anesthesia, Critical Care and Pain Medicine, Massachusetts General Hospital, Boston, MA, USA

Harvard Medical School, Boston, MA, USA
e-mail: CMAI1@mgh.harvard.edu

M. Schnur
Interventional Pain Management, St. Luke's, Duluth, MN, USA

Department of Anesthesiology, Perioperative and Pain Medicine, Department of Otolaryngology, and Pharmacological Sciences, Icahn School of Medicine at Mount Sinai, New York City, NY, USA

A. I. Levine
Department of Anesthesiology, Perioperative and Pain Medicine, Department of Otolaryngology, and Pharmacological Sciences, Icahn School of Medicine at Mount Sinai, New York City, NY, USA

B. Mahoney et al. (eds.), *Comprehensive Healthcare Simulation: Anesthesiology*, Comprehensive Healthcare Simulation,
https://doi.org/10.1007/978-3-030-26849-7_24

for training in procedural skills, independent of a specific clinical situation. For example, cricothyrotomy training on a partial-task simulator allows for practice of the procedure, regardless of the clinical setting or indication (e.g., airway loss, angioedema, burns, obstructing mass, or hemorrhage). Partial-task trainers can also be a building block for a more sophisticated simulation with gradations of clinical context and complexity. Paring down a task to only the essential aspects may facilitate learning for a novice. The ability to simplify and manipulate the learning environment through simulation can decrease the likelihood that learners will feel overwhelmed and increase their chances for success [5]. Of note, partial-task trainers are typically not intended to, or capable of, turning a novice into an expert. The purpose of these devices is to provide a substrate on which learners can build their skills. The use of partial-task trainers in a multimodality immersive simulation environment can thus be conducive for coaching and deliberate practice [6].

Human patient simulators (HPS), such as the Laerdal SimMan® CAE HPS® or SimBaby (Laerdal Medical, Stavanger, Norway), are whole-task trainers which exhibit vital signs, variable airway features (e.g., tongue swelling and laryngospasm), breathing patterns and sounds (e.g., retractions to illustrate upper airway obstruction, breath sounds [wheezing], and pneumothorax), cardiovascular features (e.g., heart sounds and peripheral pulses [diminished or absent]), and other relevant clinical findings (e.g., abdominal sounds and distension and fontanelle bulging) [4]. Incorporated into a simulated clinical setting outfitted with biomedical equipment and teams of healthcare providers, these mannequins can provide a high degree of clinical authenticity and realism to facilitate participants' engagement. In the next sections, we will review some different types of simulation technologies that are used to design airway scenarios. For further details, we refer you to Chap. 11 "Mannequin-Based Simulators and Partial-Task Trainers" in this book.

Partial-Task Trainers: Airway Trainers

Airway task trainers were developed in the early 1970s and were among the first partial-task trainers available for medical skills training [7]. Live animals (e.g., cats, ferrets, rabbits, pigs) have traditionally served as airway task trainers; however, costs and ethical considerations limit the practicality of this approach [8, 9]. In addition to animal models, synthetic bench models as well as human cadaveric models have been used for surgical simulations of tracheostomy placement and cricothyrotomy procedures [2]. Today, a variety of virtual reality simulators and mannequin airway devices are available to help understand airway anatomy and to facilitate practicing airway management and technical skills. These models are particularly useful for teaching basic airway skills (e.g., mask ventilation, supraglottic airway placement), invasive and rare procedures (e.g., emergency cricothyrotomy), complex psychomotor skills requiring repetitive training (e.g., awake fiberoptic intubation), or those that are relatively simple but create increased anxiety for either the learner or the patient and their family (e.g., neonatal intubation). Airway task trainers such as the Laerdal adult airway mannequin allow for practice of proper mask ventilation, as well as placement of an oral airway, endotracheal tube, or an LMA (Fig. 24.1). These partial-task trainers frequently are equipped with anatomical landmarks such as the sternum, cricoid cartilage, and substernal notch. Of note, the Laerdal mannequins SimMan® 3G and Junior, but not the Pedi models, can be used for airway training.

In addition to the standard airway partial-task trainers, there are airway trainers that include inflatable bladders to simulate a difficult airway [5]. Using these models, one can simulate a difficult-to-ventilate, difficult-to-intubate situation where an awake fiberoptic intubation or needle cricothyrotomy must be undertaken. Even in the absence of electronics, some models include sophisticated features such as limited neck flexion, manually inflatable tongue and posterior pharynx, or a smaller mouth opening to simulate

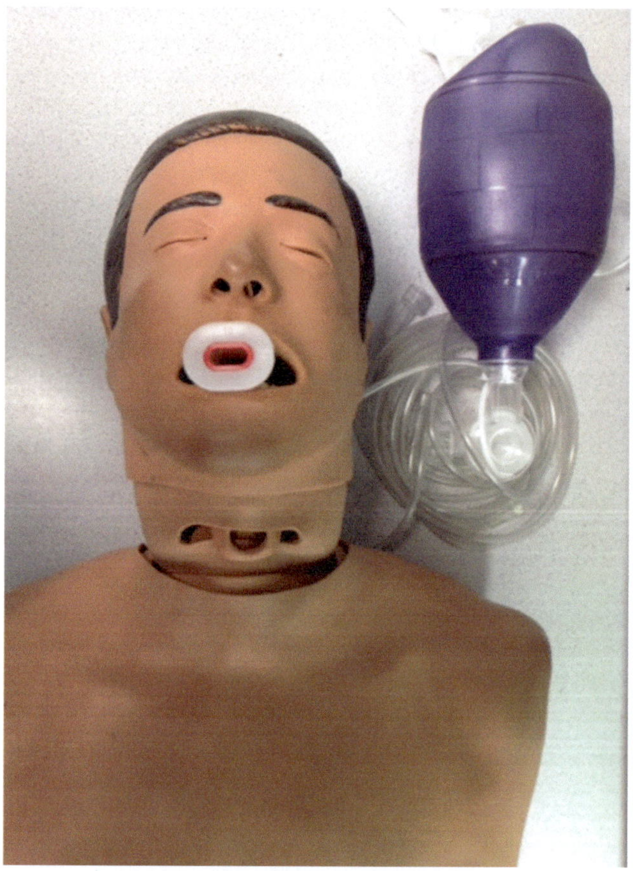

Fig. 24.1 An airway partial-task trainer

a difficult airway [8]. In certain models, high-fidelity electronics have been added to remotely control the degree of airway difficulty. For example, the tongue can be inflated in real time to mimic airway swelling, the vocal cords can be clamped to mimic laryngospasm, and the simulator can produce stridorous sounds suggestive of airway obstruction [8].

Advantages of airway task trainers include the ability for learners to practice a skill in a variety of patient sizes and as many times as possible without potentially causing harm to an actual patient. Coaching by the instructor and deliberate practice on behalf of the learner allows the opportunity for sharing valuable feedback in a safe learning environment [6]. Direct laryngoscopy and video laryngoscopy for endotracheal tube placement are difficult skills for a novice to master. With the aid of airway task trainers, studies have found that new learners can master these challenging skills with proficiency [7, 10]. In their 2014 systematic review of the literature on teaching airway management using simulation technology, Kennedy et al. found that when compared to no intervention, simulation training was associated with improved outcomes for knowledge and skills, but not for behavior or patient outcomes [10]. In comparison to non-simulation interventions, simulation training was associated with increased learner satisfaction, improved skills, and patient outcomes, but not knowledge [10]. Some of the reasons for these findings could be that the fidelity of the simulation models could contribute to the learner's experience. For example, disadvantages such as the rigid plasticity and lack of secretions in the mannequin head compared to the malleable soft tissues of a human airway may add a level of complexity for the novel learner to manipulate the airway. However, some ways to mitigate this limitation is to add silicone sprays, simulated mucous, and commercially available blood, and emesis may help facilitate placement of airway devices and increase fidelity [11].

Bronchoscopy Devices

Visualizing and securing the airway using flexible bronchoscopy are an essential skill for an anesthesiologist as they encounter challenging airways on a frequent basis. Although video laryngoscopes have decreased the number of bronchoscope intubations performed by trainees, bronchoscopy still remains the gold standard for difficult airway management [12]. Thus, simulation training in bronchoscopy is more imperative than ever because this skill is practiced less often in the clinical setting. Bronchoscope airway trainers such as the GI-BRONCH Mentor™ (3D Systems, Littleton, CO, USA) are important tools that allow learners to practice how to correctly hold and maneuver the scope prior to clinical patient care. Several devices currently exist and vary in their cost as well as ability to simulate real life situations.

First, and most cost effective, are homemade mazes or models that simulate twists and turns that the novice can utilize for psychomotor training [12]. These can be made with corrugated tubing for a simple homemade model. Alternatively, commercially manufactured static fiberoptic task trainers can be purchased. It is worth noting that no difference in psychomotor training has been associated with more complex models versus those that are simple [12].

With constantly improving technology, there has been an increase in "virtual" bronchoscope trainers, which utilize a stationary oral cavity with a corresponding bronchoscope controller and screen-based airway (Fig. 24.2). These bronchoscopes are used not only in anesthesia training but can also be utilized by surgical staff for endoscopy training. These devices are useful in that they can track progress as well as demonstrate a wide range of scenarios such as masses occluding the airway or copious secretions. Although endotracheal tubes cannot be placed with these devices to simulate the entire task of flexible bronchoscopy and subsequent intubation, Samuelson and colleagues have reported that novice anesthesiology residents demonstrated improved psychomotor skills in performing bronchoscopy on actual patients shortly after a short training session with a virtual bronchoscope trainer [13].

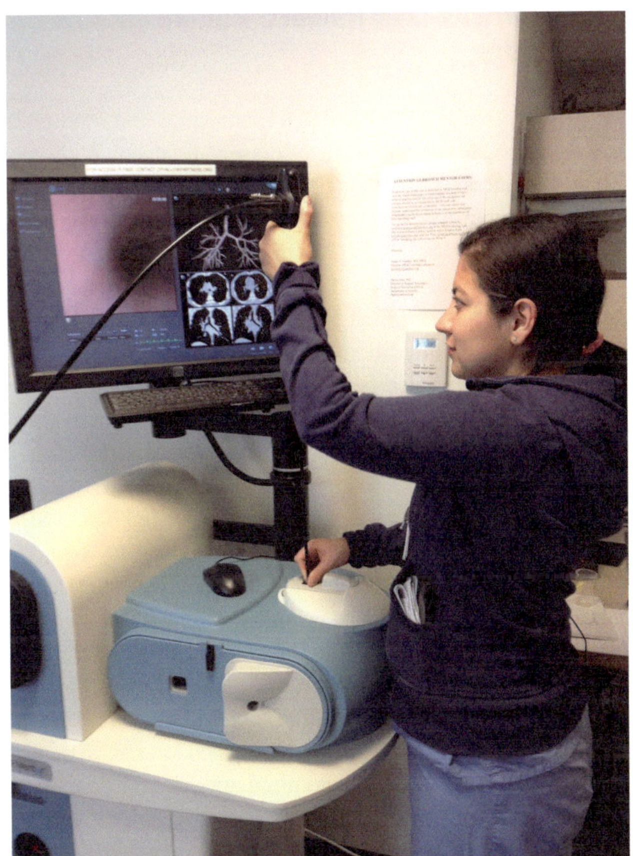

Fig. 24.2 A trainee practicing on a virtual bronchoscopy task trainer

Invasive and Surgical Airways

In addition to being used for the insertion of endotracheal tubes and laryngeal mask airways, partial-task trainers can also be used to facilitate surgical airway practice. For example, inserting and securing a tracheostomy device can be practiced on a mannequin model with a permanent hole drilled into the hollow neck [7]. In addition, animal models such as porcine tracheas have been utilized to simulate the adult airway, and rabbit tracheas have been utilized to simulate percutaneous cricothyrotomy in pediatric patients [8, 9]. Although performing a cricothyrotomy is part of the difficult airway algorithm, the 4th National Audit Project of the Royal College of Anaesthetists and the Difficult Airway Society (NAP4) demonstrated that there was a high failure rate of anesthesiologists performing this procedure during real airway emergencies. The recommendation was that anesthesiologists should avoid doing the procedure, but in reality the need for opportunities to practice to proficiency should have also been suggested [14]. Commercial head and neck task trainers are available for practicing cricothyrotomy insertion. Studies have analyzed the speed, efficacy, and retention of skills using these commercial models [15, 16].

Whole Airway Task Trainers: Human Patient Simulators

A full-scale patient simulator is a mannequin that represents the entire body typically made of plastic and metal, without a bony skeletal frame. Although popularized in the 1990s, the first mannequin-based simulator (SimOne) was developed at the University of Southern California in the 1960s for medical education and training [17]. Using SimOne, anesthesiology residents developed airway skills more quickly than those training in a traditional manner. Adult full-scale simulators became commercially available in the early 1990s. In 1999, the first high-fidelity pediatric simulator was introduced. The METI PediaSIM (CAE Healthcare, Sarasota, FL) represented a child between 5 and 7 years of age. By 2005, two infant simulators became available: the METI BabySIM and the Laerdal SimBaby (Laerdal Medical, Stavanger, Norway). These models exhibited standard vital signs and variable airway features (e.g., tongue swelling and laryngospasm), breathing patterns and sounds (e.g., retractions to illustrate upper airway obstruction, breath sounds [wheezing], and pneumothorax), cardiovascular features (e.g., heart sounds and peripheral pulses [diminished or absent]), and other clinical signs (e.g., abdominal sounds and distension and fontanelle bulging). Although sophisticated, the educational benefits of the additional airway anatomy fidelity of these devices have been brought into question [18–20]. The use of HPS enables learners to combine knowledge they have gained utilizing partial-task trainers with clinical case scenarios. Several studies have shown that these whole-task airway trainers can be utilized for teaching emergency operating room scenarios in novice anesthesia learners [21, 22].

Use of Multimodality Simulation for Immersive Interprofessional Team Training

Interprofessional education (IPE) occurs when two or more healthcare professions learn about, from, and with each other to enable effective collaboration and improved health outcomes [23]. One of the main goals of IPE is to create a highly trained, cohesive workforce that is ready to work with a team-oriented approach to provide patient-centered care [24]. In ENT anesthesia training, the incorporation of interprofessional learning between the anesthesiologist and otolaryngologist is particularly important because it promotes collaborative practice and interaction between the two professions. Immersive simulations can incorporate standardized patients (live actors), simulated patients (mannequins), and hybrid simulators to provide an appropriate level of realism and fidelity to engage the learners. When creating these interprofessional simulations, it is important to have representation from anesthesiology, surgery, and nursing simulation educators in order to create a learning environment that benefits a multidisciplinary team. For effective interprofessional team training, the simulation scenario and the debriefing must meet the needs of all participants in the program and engage all professional role groups. In order to meet the needs of the different groups, the goals and objectives must be clear and relevant to all parties [24].

The use of simulation in IPE training has been found to be a highly effective, low-risk model for enabling learners to not only enhance their clinical skills but also enhance nontechnical, crisis resource management skills (i.e., communication, team dynamics, and leadership) which are essential to patient safety [25, 26]. Errors in healthcare systems have been attributed to poor communication, increased dependence on technology, limited manpower, and other human factors [27]. These human factors may be highlighted in simulation clinical scenarios that emphasize the need for awareness of social interactions, effective communication, and situational stressors that affect a high-functioning team [24]. TeamSTEPPS ® (http://teamstepps.ahrq.gov/) is one example of an evidence-based system that was created to improve communication and teamwork skills among healthcare providers. Therefore, immersive simulation with participants from different professional backgrounds can provide opportunities for interdisciplinary reflection that provides insight into the other disciplines' focus and concerns that might not otherwise occur if the professions trained separately. In the next sections, we will review the use of simulation technology to create multidisciplinary team training skills and clinical scenarios.

Putting It All Together

Use of Part-Task Trainers for Interprofessional Team Training

As discussed previously, there is a variety of commercially available airway partial-tasks trainers that can be utilized for individual subspecialty training. However, these devices can be incorporated in interprofessional skills training labs to enrich the shared experiences of the anesthesiology and otolaryngology learners. Examples of airway skills that may require both anesthesiology and otolaryngology involvement include management of aspirated foreign bodies, control of epistaxis, and the managment of the difficult airway requiring a surgical intervention. In order to create a foreign body in the airway model, a foreign object such as a toy marble or food substance can be inserted into the oropharynx or trachea of a mannequin head to create an exercise whereby both anesthesiology and otolaryngology trainees must practice handling and managing the airway. Both specialties can practice manipulating the airway with appropriate instruments and coordinating the care during this simulated airway crisis [28]. Management of epistaxis can be another example where both the anesthesiologist and ENT surgeon must collaborate to manage the airway. By using a nasal cannula glued to the inside of a mannequin's nose, a facilitator can control the flow of "blood" through the tubing to simulate bleeding [8, 29]. Although there are several commercially available tracheostomy partial-task trainers that are capable of simulating the "can't ventilate, can't intubate" scenario, most of these mannequins are utilized by anesthesiology and surgery residency programs to train their learners in separate silos. A novel approach would be to combine airway training sessions for both anesthesiology and surgery residents, to facilitate shared reflection and a shared appreciation of the nuances of the difficult airway from both sides of the curtain. Some of these mannequins have cervical landmarks whereby insertion of a scalpel blade through the skin can cause bleeding, resistance, and edema [30]. Since an anesthesiology trainee would not normally be making this incision, having co-learning sessions with a surgical resident could provide an opportunity for discussion and reflection on how the actions of one role group can directly impact the tasks and challenges of the other.

ENT Clinical Scenarios for In Situ Interprofessional Team Training and System Improvement

Interprofessional teamwork training can help identify latent errors and mitigate threats to patient safety. In situ simulations that are physically integrated in the clinical workplace can provide a powerful method to uncover systems-based problems, workflow disruptions, system integration errors, and challenges to introducing new devices. For example, a case scenario involving transportation of a patient with a fresh tracheostomy from the operating room to the intensive care unit can provide interdisciplinary teaching points for both anesthesiology, nursing, and otolaryngology learners. At Cincinnati's Children's Hospital Medical Center, Patterson demonstrated that emergency department in situ simulations revealed latent system errors at a rate that was seven times that of simulation center-based interdisciplinary simulation [31]. At Johns Hopkins, an interdisciplinary difficult airway response team was developed to manage hospital-wide airway emergencies, and in situ simulation proved to be an invaluable tool to test the system, identify defects in resources and processes, and develop improvement strategies [32]. Faculty at Boston Children's Hospital use an in situ high-fidelity simulation course to teach teamwork, crisis resource management, and decision-making of high-risk, low-frequency airway emergencies to a team of otolaryngology residents, anesthesia trainees, and operating room nurses [33].

Although in situ simulation is a powerful tool for training and system interrogation and improvement, the technique is not without its concerns, difficulties and risks. When used, actual clinical resources such as operating rooms and emergency room bays are occupied and thus off-limits for actual patient care. Hence the timing and implementation of the training sessions must be carefully designed and scheduled so as to not compromise actual patient care. In addition, if used to probe the effectiveness of a system environment, one would want to use as many items from the actual clinical environment as possible. Invariably, simulated and "simulation-only" items such as medications, intravenous fluids and blood products, and devices will need to be used. Although it was unclear how these items were introduced into the clinical environment, in 2014, the New York Department of Health sent a warning to report that two patients were infused with "simulation-only" intravenous fluid resulting in sepsis and disseminated intravascular coagulopathy [34]. Therefore, it is critical that "simulation-only" items are clearly marked and are catalogued and removed from the actual patient care spaces.

In the next sections, we will discuss clinical scenarios where immersive team training simulations can be designed for anesthesiology, ENT, and nursing learners.

Airway Fire Simulation

Every year airway fires affect hundreds of patients and have the potential to lead to significant patient morbidity and even mortality [35]. A large portion of the airway fires occurs in patients receiving ear, nose, and throat surgery as many of these procedures are near the airway and can involve the use of lasers and electrocautery units. The American Society of Anesthesiologists updated their practice guidelines for operating room fires in 1993 and recommended with category

B evidence the use of operating room fire drills which they define as a formal and periodic rehearsal of the operating room teams' planned response to a fire [36]. Simulation can provide operating room staff with training regarding proper operating room procedures in the occurrence of one of these rare events [37] (Table 24.1). When designing an airway fire scenario, key features of the "fire triad" or "fire triangle" need to be defined such as (1) oxidizers, (2) ignition sources, and (3) fuel [35–37]. Learning points include identifying factors that increase the risk of a fire, including surgical use of laser or electric cautery near an oxidizer source, utilization of alcohol skin prep with inadequate drying time, and requirements of high FiO2 in a procedure involving the head and neck. Risk reduction factors include identifying the fire risk during a surgical time out, avoiding high FiO2, eliminating oxidizer pooling, avoiding moistened towels near potential ignition sources, and using laser-resistant endotracheal tubes which should be discussed in the debriefing. In addition, management steps both intraoperatively and postoperatively should be included in the debriefing [37].

Post-tonsillectomy Hemorrhage Simulation

Post-tonsillectomy hemorrhage (PTH) is a serious, albeit infrequent, complication occurring in approximately 5% of all tonsillectomies performed [38]. Two types of PTH exist, primary and secondary. Primary bleeding refers to hemorrhage which occurs within the first 24 hours following surgery, while secondary bleeding refers to hemorrhage occurring several days following a tonsillectomy and is generally due to disruption of clot [39–41]. Many studies have been undertaken to discover patient and procedure risk factors which can predict these postoperative bleeds. Although not all aspects which contribute to PTH have been elucidated, several factors that do not affect PTH are surgical technique used, NSAID use, or the utilization of perioperative antibiotics [40]. Conversely, patients older than 11 years old, those with chronic tonsillitis or history of ADHD, and patients with lower socioeconomic status have been found to be at increased risk for PTH [40].

PTH is considered to be an airway emergency, and if the airway is edematous and bloody, it presents challenges for both the surgeon and anesthetist. Potential outcomes of PTH can be life-threatening and include hematemesis, aspiration, airway edema, and even hypovolemia [41]. Team training simulations can prepare both anesthesiologists and ENT surgeons for this infrequent yet potentially disastrous scenario (Table 24.2).

For more examples of ENT clinical scenarios, we refer to Table 24.3.

Table 24.1 An example of an airway fire scenario with objectives identified and the actions of the learner specifically tailored to achieve those objectives [36–38]

Title: Airway fire
Audience: Anesthesia residents, CRNA, SRNA, otolaryngology residents
Objectives – medical knowledge: 1. Recognize the signs of airway fire 2. Identify the components of the "fire triad" 3. Describe the management of an airway fire 4. Once the airway is reestablished, arrange an appropriate postoperative management plan for a patient who has suffered an airway injury
Patient care: Recognize and manage an airway fire in the simulated operating room setting
Communication: Demonstrate appropriate leadership and communication skills with operating room personnel during the airway fire, such as maintaining constant communication with the surgeon and circulating nurse before, during, and after the fire
Case stem: Ms. Jones is a 25-year-old female with moderate obstructive sleep apnea who is scheduled for a tonsillectomy and adenoidectomy Past medical history significant for occasional smoker with mild asthma on albuterol inhaler as needed Past surgical history: No surgeries before current admission Allergies: None known Weight 60 kg; height 160 cm Vital signs: blood pressure 115/60; heart rate 70; respiratory rate 12; temperature 36.5 °C; SpO_2 100% RA The patient has been induced with general anesthesia and successfully intubated with a 7.0 endotracheal tube, taped at 21 cm at the lip Intraoperative ventilator settings: mode, volume control; tidal volume 500 mL; positive end-expiratory pressure, 5 cmH_2O; FiO_2 1.0
Room setup: Full environment-simulated operating room with anesthesia machine, operating table, surgical drapes, mayo stand, and surgical instruments An anesthesia machine with induction drugs and airway equipment is available Mannequin simulator in which airway can be entered surgically Mannequin is in supine position with 7.0 ETT (blacken ETT tip with indelible marker to appear charred), single IV with running saline, ECG, pulse oximeter, and BP cuff The bed is turned away from the anesthesia machine at 180° where an ENT surgeon will be standing at the head of the bed Portable smoke machine Audio clip of smoke/fire alarm (optional) Surgical kit: 6.0 reinforced ETT, 6.0 Shiley-style tracheostomy kit, scissors, Yankauer suction, umbilical tape, or commercial ETT securing device

Table 24.1 (continued)

State	Patient status	Anesthesiology learner actions	Surgical learner actions
Baseline	General anesthesia, intubated, mechanically ventilated HR 90, NSR; RR 10; BP 110/80; Sat 100%	After handoff, introduces himself to surgeon and circulating nurse, checks IV, monitors, and drugs	Introduces himself to anesthesia provider
Beginning of surgery	Surgeon announces he is cauterizing in the airway to remove tonsils and maintain hemostasis HR 110, ST, RR 10; BP 120/90; Sat 100%	Learner should identify FiO_2 1.0 and decrease the FiO_2 to <0.5 (ideally <0.3)	Learner should communicate with anesthesia provider about lowering the FiO_2
Airway fire initiated	Surgeon announces he sees smoke in the airway Confederate in the room could turn on the portable smoke machine HR 120, ST, RR 10; BP 130/95; Sat 95%	Learner should recognize airway fire Identify and announce to surgeon and nurse about the airway fire Stop the oxygen source Communicate with the surgeon to flood the field Remove the ETT	Learner should recognize airway fire Communication with anesthesia and nursing personnel Flood the surgical field with saline Remove the ETT
Deterioration	If reintubation is attempted, the airway occluder and tongue-swelling functions are enabled making laryngoscopy unsuccessful, mask ventilation difficult, and necessitating surgical tracheostomy by the surgeon to establish a definitive airway HR 130, ST; RR 20; BP 150/98; Sat 88%	Learner should communicate to the surgeon the difficult nature of the airway and advocate for a surgical airway Discussion about starting steroid administration Support the airway with either an LMA or facemask ventilation while the surgeon is performing the tracheostomy	Learner should recognize a surgical airway is needed and initiate tracheostomy. Discussion about bronchoscopic airway evaluation is also warranted
Airway stabilization	The surgeon completes the tracheostomy and the circuit is attached to the Shiley trach. The saturation improves HR 90, SR; RR 12; BP 120/80; at 98%	The learner should have a discussion with the surgeon about the postoperative plan including ICU admission, steroid administration, the need for a bronchoscopic examination of the airway, and discussion with family about the patient's status	The learner should have a discussion with the anesthesiologist about the postoperative plan including ICU admission, steroid administration, the need for a bronchoscopic examination of the airway, and discussion with family about the patient's status

Discussion points:

1. Discuss fire triad sources and common examples found in operating room
2. Identify factors that make certain cases high risk
3. Discuss strategies for risk reduction utilizing ASA practice guidelines
4. Discuss the management of airway fires according to ASA practice guidelines
5. As OR tables are commonly rotated 180 degrees in ENT surgeries, discuss what role each member will play in the management plan if an airway fire were to occur
6. Locate nearest CO2 fire extinguisher, and review PASS acronym (point, aim, squeeze and sweep)
7. Discuss the potential of a surgical airway following an airway fire and location of equipment in room
8. Discuss a postoperative management plan for a patient with an airway burn

Table 24.2 An example of a post-tonsillectomy hemorrhage scenario [39–41]

Title: Post-tonsillectomy hemorrhage

Audience: Anesthesia residents, CRNA, SRNA, otolaryngology residents

Objectives – medical knowledge:

1. Recognize the type of PTH
2. Describe factors which increase the risk for a PTH
3. Describe the intraoperative management of PTH
4. Create an appropriate plan for extubation and postoperative management

Patient care: Appropriately care for a patient with a post-tonsillectomy hemorrhage in the simulated operating room setting

Communication: Demonstrate appropriate leadership and communication skills with operating room personnel during the PTH such as maintaining constant communication with the surgeon, asking for additional personnel when appropriate

(continued)

Table 24.2 (continued)

Case stem: J.P. is a 12-year-old male with a history of recurrent tonsillitis and obstructive sleep apnea now s/p tonsillectomy and adenoidectomy. After approximately 2 hours in the PACU, the patient begins to vomit frank blood and is emergently taken back to the operating room
Past medical history significant for eczema
Past surgical history: Tympanostomy tubes
Allergies: Penicillin-hives
Weight 50 kg; height 140 cm
Vital signs: blood pressure 95/47; heart rate 110; respiratory rate 20; temperature 36.5 °C; SpO_2 100% RA

Room setup:
Full environment-simulated operating room with anesthesia machine, operating table, surgical drapes, mayo stand, and surgical instruments
An anesthesia machine with induction drugs including both non-depolarizing and depolarizing muscle relaxants and airway equipment is available
Mannequin simulator in which airway can be altered to simulate swelling
Mannequin in supine position with single IV with running saline, ECG, pulse oximeter, and BP cuff
Mannequin is simulated to appear crying with blood around the mouth
The head of the bed is toward the anesthesia machine
Surgical kit: 6.0 reinforced ETT, 6.0 Shiley-style tracheostomy kit, scissors, Yankauer suction, umbilical tape, or commercial ETT securing device

ecBaseline	Patient status	Anesthesiology learner actions	Surgical learner actions
Pre-induction	Tachypnic HR 120, tachycardic; RR 20; BP 90/52; Sat 100%	Checks IV, monitors, suction and drugs Begins to pre-oxygenate patient Asks for additional items if needed and introduced themselves to the operating room staff	Introduces themselves to anesthesia provider
Induction	Surgeon announces urgency of case. Mentions significant blood loss HR 125, ST, RR 10; BP 88/48; Sat 100%	Learner should identify correct drugs for RSI and have appropriate amount of pre-drawn atropine in case of bradycardia Suction and bougie should be positioned close	Offers to perform cricoid pressure Ensures equipment for an emergency airway is nearby
Deterioration	HR 40, SB, RR 0; BP 75/32; Sat 85% During intubation the patient begins to deteriorate with bradycardia and subsequent hypotension ensuing Airway should appear edematous with an experience user obtaining a grade 3 view using direct laryngoscopy	Learner should first attempt direct laryngoscopy with an appropriately sized ETT. If this fails they should then utilize bougie and call for video laryngoscope and/or difficult airway cart Identify and announce to the surgical staff that the patient has an edematous airway Appropriately utilize bougie or videolaryngoscope for intubation	Surgical learner should know criteria for initiating CPR on patient
Extubation:	Patient should be stable with the procedure occurring without complication HR 95, sinus; RR 20; BP 117/93; Sat 98%	Learner should communicate to the surgeon the plan to extubate patient with head up and awake Patient should receive full nausea prophylaxis Postoperative analgesia should be discussed	Learner should recognize the need to have patient fully awake with all airway reflexes despite the potential for coughing Clotting deficiencies should be suggested prior to extubation
Postoperative care:	The surgeon initiates a discussion about caring for patient in a PICU setting HR 90, SR; RR 12; BP 120/80; Sat 98%	The learner should have a discussion with the surgeon about the postoperative care plan including PICU admission, steroid administration, and postoperative analgesia plan	The learner should have a discussion with the anesthesiologist about the postoperative care plan including PICU admission, steroid administration, and postoperative analgesia plan Surgical learner should announce plan to talk with patients' family following conclusion of procedure

Discussion points:
1. Discuss the difference between primary and secondary hemorrhage following a tonsillectomy as well as potential causes
2. Identify risk factors for PTH
3. Discuss common complications related to PTH
4. Discuss anesthetic and surgical techniques to prevent complications
5. As pediatric patients have specific fluid management, discuss resuscitation with both fluid and blood.

Table 24.3 More examples of ENT case scenarios

I. Postoperative airway bleed
1. Immediate or delayed bleed after tonsillectomy in a 12-year-old 2. A 45-year-old female is stridorous in the PACU after a thyroidectomy 3. A 78-year-old male status post-total laryngectomy and tracheostomy presents with sentinel bleed and presumed trachea-innominate fistula
II. Angioedema
A 48-year-old morbidly obese patient with a history of hypertensive crisis presents with angioedema after lisinopril was added to her therapeutic regiment
III. Foreign body aspiration
A 5-year-old with retractions and stridor presents for emergent panendoscopy
IV. Patients with tracheostomy
1. A 68-year-old status post-glossectomy, free flap, and tracheostomy (with a Jackson trach) 3 years ago, now presents for an upper GI endoscopy 2. A 83-year-old ventilator-dependent female with an acute pneumonia status post-total laryngectomy 8 months ago, whose tracheostomy has now fallen out during suctioning 3. A 58-year-old male status post-TORS and neck dissection and tracheostomy 1 hour ago, whose trach was dislodged during suctioning
V. Patient with a drug-eluding stent for a cochlear implant
1. A 73-year-old male with a history of hypertension type 2 diabetes and coronary artery disease status post multiple drug eluting stents (most recently 3 months ago) off clopidogrel and aspirin 2. The same patient now 13 months s/p last drug eluting stent off aspirin 3. The same patient as above s/p cochlear implant with a change of mental status in the PACU about to be discharged (acute coronary syndrome that progress from non-ST to elevated ST myocardial infarction, to ventricular tachycardia-ventricular fibrillation, to return of spontaneous circulation) 4. The same patient as above awaiting for cath lab intervention, and his son is irate because they knew their father would not have wanted to be on a "machine"
VI. Jet ventilation
A 37-year-old female with idiopathic subglottic stenosis for laryngoscopy and possible tracheal dilation or resection (jet ventilation, lasers, apneic techniques)

Conclusion

In conclusion, ENT anesthesia is a unique subspecialty that requires the development and maintenance of outstanding technical skills. Because of the proximity of the airway to the surgical site and the shared considerations with our surgical colleagues, nontechnical skills are critical to develop and maintain. Team training simulations can be an effective adjunct to the training of the individual anesthesiologist's technical skills with airway management. Interdisciplinary team simulations provide a rich environment for surgical, nursing, and anesthesia learners to practice communication and team performance, as well as to probe the effectiveness of resources in an attempt to improve the system in which we work.

References

1. Levine A, DeMaria S, Govindaraj S. Anesthesiology and otolaryngology. Chapter 1: working side by side: the important relationship between anesthesiologists and otolaryngologists. 1st ed. New York: Springer; 2013.
2. Musbahi O, Aydin A, Omran YA, Skilbeck CJ, Ahmed K. Current status of simulation in otolaryngology: a systematic review. J Surg Ed. 2017;74(2):2013–215.
3. Park CS. Simulation and quality improvement in anesthesiology. Anesthesiol Clin. 2011;29(1):13–28. Epub 2010 Dec 16.
4. Schaefer JJ. Simulators and difficult airway management skills. Paediatr Anaesth. 2004;14(1):28–37.
5. Torsher L, Craigo P. The comprehensive textbook of healthcare simulation. Chapter 17: simulation in anesthesiology. New York: Springer; 2014.
6. Ericsson KA. Deliberate practice and acquisition of expert performance: a general overview. Acad Emerg Med. 2008;15(11):988–94.
7. Howells TH, Emery FM, Twentyman JE. Endotracheal intubation training using a simulator. An evaluation of the Laerdal adult intubation model in the teaching of endotracheal intubation. Br J Anaesth. 1973;45:400–2.
8. White ML, Ades A, Shefrin AE, Kost S. Comprehensive healthcare simulation: pediatrics. Chapter 11. Task and procedural skills training. Switzerland: Springer International Publishing; 2016.
9. Frommer M, Graf BM, Kwok P, Metterlein T, Sinner B, et al. Emergency cricothyrotomy in infants—evaluation of a novel device in an animal model. Paediatr Anaesth. 2011;21:104–9.
10. Kennedy CC, Cannon EK, Warner DO, Cook DA. Advanced airway management simulation training in medical education: a systematic review and meta-analysis. Crit Care Med. 2014;42:169–78.
11. Merica BJ. Medical moulage: how to make your simulations come alive. Philadelphia: F.A. Davis Company; 2012. (Chapter 3: Blood, p32–43; Chapter 7: Drainage and Secretions, p 74–81; Chapter 27: Vomit, p. 32–43).
12. Yang D, Wei YK, Xue FS, Deng XM, Zhi J. Simulation-based airway management training: application and looking forward. J Anesth. 2016;30(2):284–9.
13. Samuelson ST, Burnett G, Sim AJ, et al. Simulation as a set-up for technical proficiency: can a virtual warm-up improve live fibre-optic intubation? Br J Anaesth. 2016;116(3):398–404.
14. RCoA, DAS. NAP 4 (airway complications).; 2012.
15. Deransy R, Dupont H, Duwat A, Hubert V, Mahjoub Y, et al. Effect of simulation training on compliance with difficult airway management algorithms, technical ability, and stills retention for emergency cricothyrotomy. Anesthesiology. 2014;120:999–1008.
16. Boet S, Borges BC, Bould MD, Chandra D, Joo HS, Naik VN, Riem N, Siu LW, et al. Complex procedural skills are retained for a minimum of 1 year after a single high-fidelity simulation training session. Br J Anaesth. 2011;107:533–9.
17. Rall M, Gaba DM. Patient simulators. In: Miller RD, editor. Miller's anesthesia. 6th ed. Philadelphia: Elsevier; 2005. p. 30–78.
18. Schebesta K, Hüpfl M, Rössler B, Ringl H, Müller MP, Kimberger O. Degrees of reality: airway anatomy of high-fidelity human patient simulators and airway trainers. Anesthesiology. 2012;116(6):1204–9.
19. Schebesta K, Spreitzgrabner G, Hörner E, Hüpfl M, Kimberger O, Rössler B. Validity and fidelity of the upper airway in two high-fidelity patient simulators. Minerva Anestesiol. 2015;81(1):12–8.
20. Schebesta K, Hüpfl M, Ringl H, Machata AM, Chiari A, Kimberger O. A comparison of paediatric airway anatomy with the SimBaby high-fidelity patient simulator. Resuscitation. 2011;82(4):468–72.
21. Schwid HA, Rooke GA, Carline J, Steadman RH, Murray WB, Olympio M, Tarver S, Steckner K, Wetstone S. Anesthesia Simulator Research Consortium. Evaluation of anesthesia residents

using mannequin-based simulation: a multi-institutional study. Anesthesiology. 2002;97(6):1434–44.
22. Murray DJ, Boulet JR, Avidan M, Kras JF, Henrichs B, Woodhouse J, Evers AS. Performance of residents and anesthesiologists in a simulation-based skill assessment. Anesthesiology. 2007;107(5):705–13.
23. Freeth D, Hammick M, Reeves S, Koppel I, Barr H. Effective interprofessional education: development, delivery and evaluation. Oxford: Blackwell Publishing; 2005.
24. O'Brien RP, Mould J. Interprofessional education, Manual of simulation in healthcare: Oxford University Press; 2016.
25. Bradley P, Postlethwaite K. Setting up a clinical skills learning facility. Med Educ. 2003;37(1):6–13.
26. Robertson J, Bandali K. Bridging the gap: enhancing interprofessional education using simulation. J Interprof Care. 2008;22(5):499–508.
27. Institute of Medicine. Crossing the quality chasm: a new health system for the 21st century. Washington, DC: National Academy Press; 2001.
28. Deutsch ES. High-fidelity patient simulation manikins to facilitate aerodigestive endoscopy training. Arch Otolaryngol Head Neck Surg. 2008;134:625–9.
29. Deutsh ES, Javia LR. The comprehensive textbook of healthcare simulation. Chapter 13: simulation in otolaryngology. New York: Springer; 2013.
30. John B, Suri I, Hillermann C, Mendonca C. Comparison of cricothyroidotomy on manikin vs. simulator: a randomized cross-over study. Anaesthesia. 2007;62(10):1029–32.
31. Patterson MD, Geis GL Falcone RA, et al. In situ simulation: detection of safety threats and teamwork training in a high risk emergency department. BMJ Qual Saf. 2013;22:468–77.
32. Mark LJ, Herzer KR, Cover R, et al. Difficult airway response team: a novel quality improvement program for managing hospital-wide airway emergencies. Anesth Analg. 2015;121:127–39.
33. Volk MS, Ward J, Irias N, Navedo A, Pollart J, Weinstock PH. Using medical simulation to teach crisis resource management and decision-making skills to otolaryngology housestaff. Otolaryngol Head Neck Surg. 2011;145(1):35–42.
34. https://apps.health.ny.gov/pub/ctrldocs/alrtview/postings/Notification_17915.pdf. Website accessed 4-13-2017.
35. Mullen L, Byrd D. Using simulation training to improve perioperative patient safety. AORN J. 2013;97(4):419–27.
36. Apfelbaum JL, Caplan RA, Barker SJ, Connis RT, Cowles C, Ehrenwerth J, et al. Practice advisory for the prevention and management of operating room fires: an updated report by the American Society of Anesthesiologists Task Force on Operating Room Fires. Anesthesiology. 2013;118(2):271–90.
37. DeMaria S Jr, Schwartz AS, Narine V, Yang S, Levine AI. Management of Intraoperative Airway Fire. Simul Healthc. 2011;6:360–3.
38. Roger ML, Nickalls RW, Brackenbury ET, Salama FD, Beattie MGH, Perks AG. Airway fire during tracheostomy: prevention strategies for surgeons and anaesthetists. Ann R Coll Surg Engl. 2001;83:376–80.
39. Lane JC, Dworkin-Valenti J, Chiodo L, Haupert M. Postoperative tonsillectomy bleeding complications in children: a comparison of three surgical techniques. Int J Pediatr Otorhinolaryngol. 2016;88:184–8.
40. Spektor Z, Saint-Victor S, Kay DJ, Mandell DL. Risk factors for pediatric post-tonsillectomy hemorrhage. Int J Pediatr Otorhinolaryngol. 2016;84:151–5.
41. Fields RG, Gencorelli FJ, Litman RS. Anesthetic management of the pediatric bleeding tonsil. Paediatr Anaesth. 2010;20(11):982–6.

Simulation in Neuroanesthesia

25

Michelle Lee Humeidan, Rashmi Vandse, and January Kim

Abbreviations

AH	Autonomic hyperreflexia
ACLS	Advanced cardiac life support
BP	Blood pressure
CN	Cranial nerves
CVP	Central venous pressure
ECG	Electrocardiogram
$EtCO_2$	End-tidal carbon dioxide
HTN	Hypertension
ICP	Intracranial pressure
IV	Intravenous
MAC	Monitored anesthesia care
NAD	No apparent distress
NSR	Normal sinus rhythm
PEA	Pulseless electrical activity
PERRL	Pupils equal, round, reactive to light
RRR	Regular rate and rhythm
RSI	Rapid sequence induction
SSEP	Somatosensory-evoked potentials
VAE	Venous air embolism

Introduction

Neurosurgical cases can encompass a wide range of perioperative complications and require care of patients with profound physiologic disturbances. Neurological cases can also present with several complications. Medical emergencies require sole focus on patient care, not allowing significant teaching opportunities. However, anesthesiologists must be well-versed on how to handle neurosurgical and neurological emergencies, and simulation-based learning provides a safe environment to experience and practice managing these emergency situations. Simulation-based learning in neuroanesthesia can be a powerful educational experience, fostering success in the operating room by offering a safe environment for learners to experience and manage complex and serious scenarios. It is especially important now because of the current shortfall of teaching anesthesiologists [1]. Residency, and even fellowship training in anesthesia for brain and spine surgery, varies greatly across hospitals and training programs. For these reasons, simulation should be recognized as a valuable tool for the preparation of anesthesiologists to care for neurosurgical and neurological patients, allowing learners to practice management of the unique anesthetic concerns for these patients, with additional opportunity to gain experience with difficult, uncommon clinical situations.

Presently, formal coursework that focuses solely on neuroanesthesia simulation is primarily available internationally. NeuroSim, The Neuroanaesthesia Simulation Course, is offered in Cambridge and Sussex and "provides experience in managing perioperative emergencies and clinical dilemmas in neurosurgical patients" by utilizing high-fidelity mannequin simulation. Participants work under the faculty of neuroanesthetists, neurosurgeons, and intensivists to manage scenarios with the simulator. Then, the participants partake in the facilitator-style debrief which includes relevant information about physiology, pharmacology, and clinical management. The scenarios that are presented in this course are streamlined with the neuroanesthesia curriculum and the revalidation continuing professional development matrix of the Royal College of Anaesthetists. NeuroSim states that because their course links knowledge with a concrete experience, it may make it easier to recall information when compared to reading a textbook. Oxford University's One

M. L. Humeidan (✉)
Department of Anesthesiology, The Ohio State University Wexner Medical Center, Columbus, OH, USA
e-mail: Michelle.Humeidan@osumc.edu

R. Vandse
Department of Anesthesiology, Loma Linda University Medical Center, Loma Linda, CA, USA

J. Kim
Institute of Behavioral Medicine Research, The Ohio State University Wexner Medical Center, Columbus, OH, USA

B. Mahoney et al. (eds.), *Comprehensive Healthcare Simulation: Anesthesiology*, Comprehensive Healthcare Simulation,
https://doi.org/10.1007/978-3-030-26849-7_25

Brain Neuroanaesthesia Simulation Course in England and Macquarie University's Neuroanaesthsia Simulation Course in Australia are similar courses [2].

Although courses that specifically focus on neuroanesthesia simulation are primarily available abroad, several anesthesiology residency programs in the United States such as The Ohio State University; University of California, San Diego; University of California, Los Angeles; and Stony Brook University include simulation in their neuroanesthesia curriculum. University of California, San Diego, includes simulation in their instructional and/or assessment methods in several of their educational objectives such as discussing neurophysiology, anesthetic neuropharmacology, cerebral pathophysiology, management of recurrent clinical issues, and specific neurosurgical procedures [3]. Simulation has emerged as such a valuable component of anesthesiology training and education that the American Board of Anesthesiology implemented its use in the Maintenance of Certification in Anesthesiology Program (MOCA), and it is being considered as a new component of primary board certification [4].

Simulation-based education in neuroanesthesia allows learners to experience success and commit errors without putting patients in danger. This experience, combined with the constructive feedback that learners receive from their instructors, can improve their ability to manage cases in real life. Another benefit to neuroanesthesia simulation is that it offers a safe environment for learners to manage rare scenarios that they might not otherwise see in their training. Because these scenarios can have serious consequences if not managed appropriately, it is crucial that resident physicians are comfortable dealing with them. Simulation-based learning also allows for more individualized learning as learners proceed at their own pace with less dependence on instructors [1]. In this chapter we present three simulation cases (venous air embolism (VAE), intracranial aneurysm, and autonomic hyperreflexia) using a high-fidelity mannequin. With growing acclaim, simulation may become a standard in teaching neuroanesthesia.

Scenario 1: Venous Air Embolism

The objective of this simulation is for the participant to take a thoughtful, systematic approach to the patient who develops acute air embolism under general anesthesia (Tables 25.1 and 25.2). Although this is a rare situation, it is one that needs to be quickly recognized. The scenario is designed to

Table 25.1 Setup for Scenario 1: venous air embolism

Monitors available to participant	Additional required equipment	Audiovisual equipment needed	Supporting files
Code cart with pacing/ defibrillation pads	Anesthesia machine that has passed the check out with circuit and $EtCO_2$ tubing extensions	Speakers for precordial Doppler sound file (normal and mill-wheel murmur)	Patient preoperative report
Five-lead electrocardiogram (ECG) monitoring	Airway equipment (laryngoscope and blades, endotracheal tubes, empty 10-mL syringe)	Computer or smart board with images and sounds for debriefing lecture	Debriefing lecture on VAE
Noninvasive blood pressure cuff, a-line (if requested)	Two prepared 1000 mL intravenous fluid bags on blood infusion lines		Recent manuscript about VAE to distribute to participants
Pulse-oximetry, capnography	Pharmacologic agents available upon request: propofol, etomidate, ketamine, succinylcholine, vecuronium, midazolam, fentanyl, atropine, ephedrine, phenylephrine, epinephrine, norepinephrine, vasopressin, neostigmine, glycopyrrolate, metoprolol, esmolol, dexmedetomidine, nitroprusside, mannitol, remifentanil		MP3 of precordial Doppler (Mill Wheel, murmur)
Temperature probe	Yankauer suction		
CVP (if requested)	Record keeping material (computer or paper)		
Precordial Doppler (if requested, mocked-up device)	Foley catheter –w/100 cc yellow urine		
	Audio recording of precordial Doppler		
	Anesthesia circuit and $EtCO_2$ sample line extensions		
	Pumps for continuous delivery of intravenous (IV) anesthetics		
	Mocked-up SSEP monitoring with wires		
	Central line (right internal jugular) that can aspirate both air and blood (50 mL)		
	Surgical instrumentation and draping to mock up a neurosurgery case		

Table 25.2 Scenario 1: venous air embolism

Title: Venous air embolism

Audience: Anesthesia resident, patient, surgeon, circulating nurse/scrub technician

Objectives-medical knowledge: Describe the pathophysiology of venous air embolism; describe methods to monitor for this condition; demonstrate treatment steps for venous air embolism

Patient care: Management of venous air embolism in a patient with posterior fossa brain tumor. Manage induction, intubation, and emergence for this patient

Communication: Utilize crew resource management skills to successfully manage an intraoperative emergency

Case stem: TC is a 60-year-old male presenting for resection of a posterior fossa brain tumor. He has experienced ataxia and vertigo for 2 weeks, and MRI yesterday showed aforementioned tumor. He has a past medical history significant only for mild hypertension and type II insulin-dependent diabetes. He has no history of anesthetic complications. Your job is to come up with a plan for induction, intubation, and emergence for this patient. Patient has been NPO for 10 hours. You may ask additional questions

Scenario setup: (see Table 25.1)

Patient will have 18 g IV in the right hand. He will have ECG, BP cuff, pulse oximeter, and temperature probe

An anesthesia machine will be 180 degrees from patient's head with induction drugs and airway equipment available

State	**Patient status**	**Learner actions**	
Baseline	Awake, alert, responds slowly, blown left pupil HR 88, NSR; RR 12, BP 125/80, Sat 98%, $EtCO_2$ present, CVP 5, T 37	Develop a plan for smooth induction, intubation with head of the bed away while maintaining intracranial pressure (ICP). Learner should obtain a second set of hands (second learner) to assist. Communicate positioning/monitoring concerns with the surgeon, and obtain additional access and monitoring (invasive arterial monitoring, CVP, precordial Doppler)	If learner successfully intubates, go to maintenance
Maintenance of anesthesia	Anesthetized, paralyzed, mechanically ventilated HR 95, sinus tachycardia; RR ventilator, BP 107/54, Sat 98% on 40%, $EtCO_2$ 30, CVP 5 over 1 min, T 37	Following intubation the surgeon will ask for head up approximately 30 degrees. Patient will be undergoing SSEP monitoring. If high (>0.7 minimum alveolar concentration of volatile agent is used), the learner will be informed that the signal is poor. He may ask for dexmedetomidine, propofol or remifentanil infusions. Surgeon will notify learner prior to entering the dura. Learner should adjust anesthetic technique to maintain cerebral perfusion and allow for SSEP monitoring	When surgeon makes dural incision, go to venous air embolism
Venous air embolism	Anesthetized, paralyzed, mechanically ventilated. "Mill-wheel murmur" audible on precordial Doppler (if available). Decompensation to this state will occur quickly (over about 30 seconds) HR 120, sinus tachycardia; RR ventilator, BP 107/54, Sat 94% on 40%, $EtCO_2$ 20, CVP 10, T 37	The surgeon will continue with surgery unless asked to stop. Communicate with surgeon regarding possible VAE. Call for help. Increase FiO_2–1.0, flood the field, aspirate from CVP if available, head down position, B/L jugular venous compression, and administer inotropes to support BP	If learner chooses proper intervention, go to recovery If learner chooses improper intervention, go to further deterioration
Further deterioration	Anesthetized, paralyzed, mechanically ventilated HR 130, Sinus tachycardia with ST depression; RR ventilator, BP 65/32, Sat 85% on 100%, $EtCO_2$ 15, CVP 22, T 37	Further deterioration will occur over the next 1 minute. Surgeon will notice deterioration and stop operating Failure to address will result in PEA and the scenario will end	If learner chooses proper intervention, go to recovery If learner chooses improper intervention, go to PEA
Recovery	Anesthetized, paralyzed, mechanically ventilated HR 95, Sinus tachycardia; RR ventilator, BP 107/54, Sat 98% on 40%, $EtCO_2$ 30, CVP 5, T 37	Patient will be undergoing SSEP monitoring. If high (>0.7 MAC of volatile agent is used), the learner will be informed that the signal is poor. He may ask for dexmedetomidine, propofol, or remifentanil infusions. Learner should adjust anesthetic technique to maintain cerebral perfusion and allow for SSEP monitoring	End scenario

(continued)

Table 25.2 (continued)

Pulseless electrical activity	Patient is blue HR 50 over 2 min, PEA sinus; RR ventilator, BP 0/0, Sat 0%, $EtCO_2$ 10, CVP 0, T 35	Perform proper advanced cardiac life support (ACLS) protocol for PEA rhythm. Identify cause of PEA	End scenario
Debriefing: Immediate debriefing after a simulated educational experience is a critical part of the learning process. The debriefing session after this scenario should start with a general discussion of what went well and what aspects could use improvement. A brief lecture should ensue focusing on pathophysiology of VAE, intraoperative methods to monitor for VAE, and treatment steps for VAE. Constant reflection on the experience throughout the debriefing will help participants identify strengths and weaknesses of their clinical management. One may provide learners with a recent manuscript on VAE from the literature to reinforce the key concepts from the session and encourage more in-depth study of the topic [5]			

familiarize the participant with the signs and symptoms of acute air embolism in a high-fidelity simulated setting. The simulation will start with the induction, intubation, and positioning of the patient for resection of a posterior fossa tumor. The surgery will be performed at 180 degrees from the anesthesia machine ("head away") with the patient lateral and 30 degrees head up (patient sitting up and feet to anesthesia machine). The participant should determine a plan for monitoring (i.e., arterial line (a-line), precordial Doppler, central venous pressure (CVP), etc.), access, and maintenance of anesthesia (somatosensory-evoked potentials (SSEP) monitoring will be present). Upon incision of the dura by the surgeon, the patient will have a rapid decrease in end-tidal carbon dioxide ($EtCO_2$) and blood pressure (BP). A CVP (if placed) will increase. The participant will be forced to identify the cause for the symptoms and treat accordingly. The endpoints for this scenario include communication with the surgeon, maneuvers to stop entrainment of air, and initiation and escalation of supportive therapies. If these steps are taken, the patient will recover (facilitator-dependent); if not the symptoms will worsen, and pulseless electrical activity (PEA) will result. The scenario will be followed by a facilitator/peer-directed debriefing and didactic session. If time is limited, the facilitator may choose to have the learner assume control of the case following induction, intubation, and positioning with a-line and CVP already in place. After several minutes the patient will decompensate due to VAE. The endpoints for this version are the same. At the start of the simulation experience, the learner is brought into the simulation OR and briefly oriented to the patient and case. Patient history and hand-off documents are provided to the learner at the start of the simulation (Fig. 25.1).

Scenario 2: Intracranial Aneurysm

Similar to Case 1, the objectives of this simulation are for the participant to take a thoughtful, systematic approach to the patient presenting for surgical management of an intracranial aneurysm who develops intraoperative rupture of the aneurysm (Tables 25.3 and 25.4). This situation must be quickly recognized, and anesthesiologists should be prepared to work closely with the surgeon until the aneurysm is clipped. This simulation is designed to train the participant to quickly react in a high-fidelity simulated setting. The patient is a 32-year-old female who requires emergent clipping of an intracranial aneurysm. The patient will be full stomach (most recent meal 2 hours ago) due to the emergent nature of the procedure. The simulation will start with the induction of the patient. The participant will have the opportunity to obtain additional lines/monitors prior to the surgical procedure. The participant will need to take appropriate precautions during induction and intubation to maintain hemodynamic stability while minimizing risk for aspiration. Following intubation, the patient will become tachycardic and hypertensive. As the surgeon is dissecting the brain to get access to aneurysm, the patient will develop hemodynamic changes consistent with Cushing's triad. The surgeon will communicate that the brain is swelling and that the aneurysm has ruptured. The participant will then be tasked with optimizing hemodynamics for successful clipping of the aneurysm. The primary endpoints for completion of the simulation include successful clipping of aneurysm and (time permitting) emergence and extubation of the patient. Although the simulation is scripted, omissions of critical steps may be unpredictable but should result in appropriate response by patient. For example, failure to do a rapid sequence induction (RSI) will result in aspiration and hypoxia. At the start of the simulation experience, the learner in brought into the simulation OR and briefly oriented to the patient and case. Patient history and hand-off documents are provided to the learner at the start of the simulation (Fig. 25.2).

Scenario 3: Autonomic Hyperreflexia

The objective of this simulation is for the participant to take a thoughtful, systematic approach to the patient who experiences autonomic hyperreflexia (AH) while undergoing a cystoscopy (Tables 25.5 and 25.6). The scenario

Fig. 25.1 Document provided to participant at start of simulation for Scenario 1: venous air embolism

Your patient is a 60-year-old male presenting for resection of a posterior fossa brain tumor. He has experienced ataxia and vertigo for two weeks, and MRI yesterday showed aforementioned tumor. He has a past medical history significant only for mild hypertension and type II insulin-dependent diabetes. He has no history of anesthetic complications. He currently has an 18 g IV in the right hand. Your job is to come up with a plan for induction, intubation, and emergence for this patient. Patient has been NPO for 10 hours. You may ask additional questions.

General Information:
- **Name**: **TC**
- **Age**: 60
- **Weight:** 62 kg
- **Height**: 5'9"
- **Vital Signs**: HR 88, BP 122/80, RR 14, SpO2 98%

Patient History:
- **History of Present Illness**: symptomatic posterior fossa tumor
- **Allergies**: NKDA
- **Medications**: lisinopril, insulin
- **Past Medical / Surgical History**: inguinal hernia repair (uneventful general anesthesia)
- **Intake/outputs**: Foley will be placed

Symptoms:
- **Events leading up to Illness**: onset of ataxia and vertigo
- **Onset of symptoms**: 2 weeks
- **Provocation / provokes**: movement
- **Severity of pain**: N/A

Review of Systems
- **CNS**: alert but responds slowly, ataxia, vertigo
- **Cardiovascular**: normal, no chest pain
- **Pulmonary**: mild dyspnea with exertion, no wheezing, cough
- **Abdominal**: within normal limits

Physical Exam:
- **Airway**: Mallampati class 1, normal TM distance, oral opening and neck mobility
- **Chest**: regular rate and rhythm (RRR), no murmurs, mild diffuse rhonchi
- **Abdominal**: within normal limits
- **Neuro**: Ataxia but no focal weakness, numbness, no cranial nerve (CN) deficits, pupils equal, round, reactive to light (PERRL)

Laboratory, Radiology, and Other Relevant Studies: Labs:
- **Labs**: hematocrit 36, platelets 360 on admission
- **Chemistry**: within normal limits
- **Type and Cross**: negative antibody screen; 2 packed red blood cell units available
- **PT, PTT, INR**: within normal limits
- **CT scan**: large tumor at cerebellopontine angle
- **ECG**: normal sinus rhythm, no S-T changes

is designed to familiarize the participant with anesthetic options available for cystoscopy and to train the participant to respond appropriately to AH in a high-fidelity simulated setting. The patient is a 58-year-old male undergoing cystoscopy with laser lithotripsy and possible stent placement. He has a history of a spinal cord injury with T5 transection and quadriplegia. The scenario will start prior to arrival in the operating room where the participant can ask pertinent questions regarding the patient's medical history and discuss anesthetic options. The participant will decide between monitored anesthesia care (MAC), spinal, or general anesthesia. Ideally, they will choose either MAC or a general anesthetic (the patient will report he would prefer to avoid spinal as it would be difficult and uncomfortable to obtain optimum positioning). Following induction of the chosen anesthetic technique and upon initiation of the surgical stimulus, the patient's vital signs will fluctuate wildly, and the patient will become extremely hypertensive and bradycardic (which will resolve if participant asks surgeon to stop stimulus). Patient will also become erythematous and diaphoretic, which can be evidenced by the surgical team's commentary. The scenario will be followed by a facilitator/peer-directed debriefing and didactic session. At the start of the simulation experience, the learner is in brought into the simulation OR and briefly oriented to the patient and case. Patient history and handoff documents are provided to the learner at the start of the simulation (Fig. 25.3).

Table 25.3 Setup for Scenario 2: intracranial aneurysm

Monitors available to participant	Additional required equipment	Audiovisual equipment needed	Supporting files
Code cart with pacing/defibrillation pads	Anesthesia machine that has passed the checkout with circuit and $EtCO_2$ tubing extensions	Computer or smart board with images and sounds for debriefing lecture	Patient preoperative report
Five-lead electrocardiogram (ECG) monitoring	Airway equipment (laryngoscope and blades, endotracheal tubes, empty 10 mL syringe)		Debriefing lecture on intracranial aneurysm management and complications
Noninvasive blood pressure cuff, a-line (if requested)	Two prepared 1000 mL intravenous fluid bags on blood infusion lines		Recent manuscript about anesthesia for intracranial aneurysm to distribute to participants
Pulse oximetry, capnography	Pharmacologic agents available upon request: Propofol, etomidate, ketamine, succinylcholine, vecuronium, midazolam, fentanyl, atropine, ephedrine, phenylephrine, epinephrine, norepinephrine, vasopressin, neostigmine, glycopyrrolate, metoprolol, esmolol, dexmedetomidine, nitroprusside, mannitol, remifentanil		
Temperature probe	Yankauer suction		
CVP (if requested)	Record keeping material (computer or paper)		
Precordial Doppler (if requested, mocked-up device)	Pumps for continuous delivery of intravenous (IV) anesthetics		
	Central line (right internal jugular)		
	Surgical instrumentation and draping to mock up a neurosurgery case		

Table 25.4 Scenario 2: intracranial aneurysm

Title: Intracranial aneurysm			
Audience: Anesthesia resident, patient, surgeon, circulating nurse/scrub technician			
Objectives-medical knowledge: Demonstrate proper preoperative precautions for intracranial aneurysm clipping during induction to prevent rupture of aneurysm (appropriate IV access and hemodynamic monitoring, immediate access to vasopressors, and antihypertensives), recognize the signs of intraoperative rupture of aneurysm, rapidly manage hemodynamic instability, respond appropriately, and work with the surgical team to get control of bleeding			
Patient care: Management of intraoperative rupture of intracranial aneurysm until aneurysm is clipped. Manage induction, intubation, and emergence for this patient			
Communication: Utilize crew resource management skills to successfully manage an intraoperative emergency			
Case stem: KG is a 32-year-old female who presents for emergent clipping of an intracranial aneurysm. She presented to the emergency room with severe headache and stiff neck and was found on CT scan to have small intracranial hemorrhage. A subsequent angiography demonstrated an aneurysm of the middle cerebral artery. She had some solid food about 2 hours ago. She has no significant past medical history and takes no medications. She has never had surgery. Your job is to come up with a plan for induction, intubation, and emergence for this patient. You may ask additional questions			
Scenario setup: (see Table 25.3)			
Patient will have 18 g IV in her right hand. She will have ECG, BP cuff, pulse oximeter, and temperature probe			
An anesthesia machine will be 180 degrees from patient's head with induction drugs and airway equipment available. Learner may elect to turn head back towards the machine for induction			
State	**Patient status**	**Learner actions**	
Baseline	Awake, c/o headache, oriented appropriately HR 80, NSR; RR 14, BP 145/88, Sat 98% on 40%, $EtCO_2$ 35, CVP 5, T 37	Obtain additional access and monitors. CVP and invasive arterial monitoring will not be immediately available unless requested. Failure to do RSI will result in aspiration and hypoxia	If learner successfully intubates, go to hypertension

Table 25.4 (continued)

Hypertension	Anesthetized, paralyzed, mechanically ventilated Patient will have dramatic hypertensive response to intubation over about 30 seconds HR 120, Sinus tachycardia ST depression; RR 14 (ventilator), BP 175/100, Sat 98% on 40%, $EtCO_2$ 39, CVP 5, T 37	Quickly treat hypertension and tachycardia with short acting agents (i.e., esmolol, nicardipine).	If learner treats hypertension, go to maintenance If learner does not treat hypertension, go to rupture. If RSI not performed, go to RSI not performed
Maintenance (BP managed)	Anesthetized, paralyzed, mechanically ventilated HR 86, NSR, resolution of ECG changes; RR 14 (ventilator), BP 115/72, Sat 98% on 40%, $EtCO_2$ 30, CVP 5, T 37	The surgeon will continue. Surgeon will ask for mannitol and furosemide for brain relaxation. Communicate with surgeon regarding brain relaxation. Administration of mannitol, furosemide. Maintain normo- to hypocapnea and normotension. Check ABG after mannitol administration	When mannitol is administered, go to rupture
Rupture	Anesthetized, paralyzed, mechanically ventilated HR 40s, Sinus bradycardia; RR ventilator, BP 185/110, Sat 97% on 40%, $EtCO_2$ 35, CVP 5, T 37	As surgeon is dissecting, patient becomes hypertensive/bradycardic over 2 minutes. Surgeon states he sees brain swelling. Surgeon will ask for decreased BP. Learner should recognize possible aneurysm rupture. Communicate with surgeon. Call for help. Decrease the BP with mean around 50 mm hg to get control of bleeding. Administration of propofol for possible neurological protection (burst suppression). Hyperventilation to reduce ICP. Obtain blood products	After 3 minutes and additional BP medication is given, go to further deterioration
Further deterioration (bleeding)	Anesthetized, paralyzed, mechanically ventilated. Patient should now be hypotensive and tachycardic from intervention in "rupture" state HR 130, Sinus tachycardia; RR ventilator, BP 80/40, Sat 98%, $EtCO_2$ 28, CVP 0, T 37.6	Surgeon has not yet controlled the bleeding. Learner should communicate with surgeon to discuss other options (intravenous adenosine, bilateral carotid compression, temporary clip). After 1 minute the surgeon will get control of bleeding with resolution of vital signs	When aneurysm is clipped, go to maintenance
RSI not performed	Anesthetized, paralyzed, mechanically ventilated. Patient should now be hypertensive, hypoxic, and tachycardic due to RSI not being performed HR 110, Sinus tachycardia; RR ventilator, BP 170/100, Sat 85%, $EtCO_2$ 30, T 37.6	Recognize hypoxia and manage BP	If learner resolves hypoxia and BP is managed, go to stage maintenance
Recovery	Anesthetized, paralyzed, mechanically ventilated HR 100, NSR; RR ventilator, BP 100/55, Sat 98%, $EtCO_2$ 35, T 37.6	End scenario	End scenario

Debriefing: The debriefing session after this scenario should start with a guided reflection for participants, facilitating awareness of key clinical issues and turning points in the scenario and proficiencies and deficiencies in the participant's management. A didactic lecture on anesthetic concerns for intracranial aneurysm clipping, including timely recognition of intraoperative complications and review of crisis management for life-threatening hemorrhage, is an important component of the debriefing. This scenario can be especially useful for exploring effective communication with the surgical team during a chaotic intraoperative patient decompensation from aneurysm rupture. Advanced mastery of the information and skills targeted by this simulation can be encouraged by providing learners with a recent review article on anesthetic management of intracranial aneurysm [6]

Fig. 25.2 Document provided to participant at start of simulation for Scenario 2: intracranial aneurysm

Your patient is a 32-year-old female who presents for emergent clipping of an intracranial aneurysm. She presented to the emergency room with severe headache and stiff neck and was found on CT scan to have small intracranial hemorrhage. A subsequent angiography demonstrated an aneurysm of the middle cerebral artery. She had some solid food about 2 hours ago. She has no significant past medical history and takes no medications. She has never had surgery. She currently has an 18 g IV in the right hand. Your job is to come up with a plan for induction, intubation, and emergence for this patient. You may ask additional questions.

General Information:

Name: **KG**
Age: 32
Weight: 70 kg
Height: 5'4"
Vital Signs: HR 92, BP 140/85, RR 20, SpO2 98%

Patient History:

History of Present Illness: intracranial aneurysm with sentinel bleed
Allergies: NKDA
Medications: none
Past Medical / Surgical History: none, smokes 1PPD x 12 years
Intake/outputs: N/A

Symptoms:

Events leading up to Illness: severe headache and stiff neck
Onset of symptoms: several hours
Provocation / provokes: N/A
Severity of pain: N/A

Review of Systems

CNS: Awake, alert; in acute distress and severe pain
Cardiovascular: normal, no chest pain
Pulmonary: normal
Abdominal: within normal limits

Physical Exam:

Airway: Mallampadi class 1, good neck extension, normal thyromental distance, good oral opening
Chest: RRR, no murmurs, mild diffuse rhonchi
Abdominal: within normal limits
Neuro: Severe headache, but no focal deficits; PERRL, CNs normal

Laboratory, Radiology, and Other Relevant Studies: Labs:

Hematocrit: 33%
Chemistry: within normal limits
Type and Cross: negative antibody screen; 2 red blood cell units available
PT, PTT, INR: within normal limits.
ECG: 1mm ST depression in leads I, II, aVF.
CT scan: small intracranial hemorrhage in distribution of right middle cerebral artery. No mass effect.

Table 25.5 Setup for Scenario 3: autonomic hyperreflexia

Monitors available to participant	Additional required equipment	Audiovisual equipment needed	Supporting files
Five-lead electrocardiogram (ECG) monitoring	Anesthesia machine that has passed the check out	Computer or Smart Board with images and sounds for debriefing lecture	Patient preoperative report
Noninvasive blood pressure cuff	Airway equipment on the cart (Macintosh 3 and Miller 2, endotracheal tube 7.0 with stylet, and empty 10 mL syringe)		Debriefing lecture on autonomic hyperreflexia
Pulse oximetry	Two prepared 1000 mL intravenous fluid bags on blood infusion lines		Recent manuscript about AH to distribute to participants

Table 25.5 (continued)

Monitors available to participant	Additional required equipment	Audiovisual equipment needed	Supporting files
Temperature probe	Pharmacologic agents available upon request: propofol, etomidate, ketamine, succinylcholine, vecuronium, midazolam, fentanyl, atropine, ephedrine, phenylephrine, epinephrine (in syringe and prepared in 100 mL saline bag), norepinephrine (in syringe and prepared in 100 mL saline bag), vasopressin, nitroglycerin (in syringe and prepared 100 mL bag)		
Capnography	Yankauer suction		
Invasive arterial pressure monitoring	Record keeping material (computer or paper) (IHIS)		
Central venous pressure monitoring			
Pulmonary artery catheter			

Table 25.6 Scenario 3: autonomic hyperreflexia

Title: Autonomic hyperreflexia

Audience: Anesthesia resident, patient, surgeon

Objectives-medical knowledge: Demonstrate the ability to choose an appropriate anesthetic technique for cystoscopy, describe the pathophysiology of autonomic hyperreflexia (AH), demonstrate treatment steps for autonomic hyperreflexia

Patient care: Management of patient who experiences autonomic hyperreflexia while undergoing a cystoscopy manage induction, intubation, and emergence for this patient

Communication: Utilize crew resource management skills to successfully manage an intraoperative emergency

Case stem: JW is a 58-year-old male presenting for cystoscopy with lithotripsy and possible stent placement. His medical history is significant for a motor vehicle crash in 1993, which left him a T5 quadriplegic. He has a history of chronic sacral decubitus ulcer currently being followed and treated by a home health nurse. He also has a history of recurrent nephrolithiasis with several episodes resulting in pyelonephritis and urosepsis requiring prolonged hospitalization. Patient also has a history of asthma that is well controlled with infrequent use of albuterol and hypertension (HTN) that is well controlled with hydrochlorothiazide. He currently has an 18 g IV in his right arm. Your job is to come up with a plan for induction and emergence for this patient. You may ask additional questions

Scenario setup: (see Table 25.5)

Patient will have 18 g IV in his right arm. He will have ECG, BP cuff, pulse oximeter, and temperature probe

State	Patient status	Learner actions	
Baseline	Awake and alert, no apparent distress (NAD), answers questions appropriately Patient: "Hi Doc! What's the plan for the anesthesia? I'm really nervous about a spinal, they tried on me in the past and it was really difficult and uncomfortable for me to get in the right position, they struggled for a long time; couldn't you just sedate me a little? I won't feel the surgeons anyway because of my injury." Surgeon: "Ok, lets get going here, we need to get started. What's the plan?" HR 82, NSR; RR 16, BP 132/70, Sat 98% on RA	Acquire patient history, demonstrate an anesthetic plan, communicate effectively with patient, and surgical team regarding plan	Go to induction
Induction	Asleep or sedated depending on mode of anesthesia, supine position. Surgeon: "Ok, looks like we're set to start, anesthesia-are you ready for me to get going?" HR 90, NSR; RR 14, BP 110/68, Sat 96%	Proficient direct laryngoscopy with endotracheal tube placement or placement of laryngeal mask airway vs. initiation of MAC anesthesia, communication with surgeon when ready to get started with procedure. Goal is a normal "drift" of vital signs after induction of anesthesia. BP decreases to within 20% of baseline, HR increases slightly during laryngoscopy	At initiation of surgical stimulus, go to AH

(continued)

Table 25.6 (continued)

AH	Supine/lithotomy, if MAC anesthesia then patient would respond to verbal stimulus. Surgeon: "What's going on? We're just getting started and he's really hypertensive. Is everything ok up there?" HR 42, RR 14, BP 186/94, Sat 98%	Recognize labile cardiovascular status, communicate with surgeon re: patient clinical status, mitigate hemodynamic changes by deepening anesthetic, or using direct vasodilators If learner asks surgeon to stop or pause with the surgical stimulus, then vital signs can promptly to baseline. If learner fails to ask surgeon to stop, continue hypertension and bradycardia	If learner chose MAC anesthesia and repeatedly gives additional propofol, fentanyl, midazolam, etc., then go to respiratory failure
			If learner chose a general anesthetic, go to herniation after surgeon announces that patient is very erythematous and diaphoretic
			If scope is removed, go to induction
Respiratory failure	Supine/lithotomy, unresponsive Initially set mode into cannot ventilate (patient did not receive paralytic, likely making hand ventilation more difficult) HR 56, Sinus bradycardia; RR 0, BP 120/64, Sat 86%,	With repositioning and/or two-handed technique, learner should be able to hand ventilate the patient. Patient should be able to be intubated without difficulty. Consider calling for help from colleagues, communicate with the surgeon regarding deteriorating clinical picture, recognize need for and place controlled airway	At instructor's cue, go to herniation
Herniation	Unresponsive and posturing, unequal pupils, blown left pupil HR 72, BP 190/105, Sat 86%	End scenario	End scenario
Debriefing: This scenario should be followed by a debriefing session that includes participant's strengths and weaknesses of management. Constructive feedback is critical for participants to improve their clinical skills. An informative lecture about anesthetic techniques for cystoscopy, pathophysiology of AH, and treatment of AH should also be included. Reflecting on the clinical decisions made by the participants will allow them to recognize their strong points and where they have room for improvement. Furthermore, a recent review article on management of AH is provided to encourage additional proficiency [7]			

Fig. 25.3 Document provided to participant at start of simulation for Scenario 2: autonomic hyperreflexia

Your patient is a 58-year-old male presenting for cystoscopy with lithotripsy and possible stent placement. His medical history is significant for a motor vehicle crash in 1993, which left him a T5 quadriplegic. He has a history of chronic sacral decubitus ulcer currently being followed and treated by a home health nurse. He also has a history of recurrent nephrolithiasis with several episodes resulting in pyelonephritis and urosepsis requiring prolonged hospitalization. Patient also has a history of asthma that is well controlled with infrequent use of albuterol and hypertension (HTN) that is well controlled with hydrochlorothiazide. He currently has an 18 g IV in his right arm. Your job is to come up with a plan for induction and emergence for this patient. You may ask additional questions.

General Information:

Name: JW
Age: 58
Weight: 80 kg
Height: 5'8"
Vital Signs: HR 85, BP 138/74, RR 12, SpO2 99%

Patient History:

History of Present Illness: Recurrent nephrolithiasis
Allergies: NKDA
Medications: hydrochlorothiazide, Albuterol, baclofen
Past Medical / Surgical History: T5 quadriplegia, asthma, HTN, sacral decubitus ulcer, recurrent nephrolithiasis and pyelonephritis, Thoracic fusion (1993), laparoscopic cholecystectomy (1998), multiple cystoscopies with stent placement
Intake/outputs: N/A

Symptoms:

Events leading up to Illness: N/A
Onset of symptoms: N/A
Provocation / provokes: N/A
Severity of pain: N/A

Review of Systems

CNS: No HA, dizziness, or loss of consciousness, loss of sensation and motor function inferior to the xiphoid process.
Cardiovascular: Limited functional status due to quadriplegia, denies chest pains, palpitations, syncope, orthopnea, and LE swelling.
Pulmonary: No shortness of breath, dyspnea, or hemoptysis.
Abdominal: No heartburn, dysphagia, jaundice, easy bleeding, or bruising
Renal: Recurrent pyelonephritis and nephrolithiasis
Psychiatric: No symptoms of anxiety or depression

Physical Exam:

Head: Normal
Chest: Normal
Abdominal: Normal
Arms: Loss of sensation
Legs: Loss of sensation
Back: Normal

Laboratory, Radiology, and Other Relevant Studies: Labs:

CBC: WBC 12.1, Hgb 13.4 Plt 210
Chemistry: Na 134, K 3.7, Cl 106, C02 26, BUN 32, Cr 1.2
ECG: normal sinus rhythm

Conclusions

Neurosurgical and neurological emergencies require anesthesiologists to have functional knowledge of physiology and pharmacology that can be employed rapidly to respond to intraoperative complications. Fortunately, most life-threatening complications are rare, but this can limit exposure to these cases during training. Here we present two neurosurgical scenarios and one neurological scenario for use with a high-fidelity simulation mannequin to train anesthesia providers. In addition to the VAE, intracerebral aneurysm, and autonomic hyperreflexia cases presented, other topics appropriate for simulation-based education include dystonic reactions, delayed emergence, seizure in the post-operative anesthesia recovery unit, spinal cord injury, and traumatic brain injury. Simulation can be a high-yield educational experience, and use of this technology allows for cost-effective accruement of clinical expertise and confidence in a safe environment, with no risk of harm to patients.

References

1. Rajan S, Khanna A, Argalious M, Kimatian SJ, Mascha EJ, Makarova N, Nada EM, Elsharkawy H, Firoozbakhsh F, Avitsian R. Comparison of 2 resident learning tools—interactive screen-based simulated case scenarios versus problem-based learning discussions: a prospective quasi-crossover cohort study. J Clin Anesth. 2016;28:4–11.
2. One Brain Neuroanesthesia (2019) http://www.onebrain.org.uk/.
3. UCSD Department of Anesthesiology Neuroanesthesia Goals and Objectives [Internet]. UCSD Department of Anesthesiology. [cited 8 September 2016]. Available from: https://healthsciences.ucsd.edu/som/anesthesia/education/residency-program/curriculum/Documents/Neuro%20I%20GO%202.11.pdf.
4. The American Board of Anesthesiology – About MOCA 2.0 [Internet]. Theaba.org. 2016 [cited 8 September]. Available from: http://theaba.org/MOCA/About-MOCA-2-0.
5. Mirski MA, Lele AV, Fitzsimmons L, Toung TJ. Diagnosis and treatment of vascular air embolism. Anesthesiology. 2007;106(1):164–77.
6. Abd-Elsayed AA, Wehby AS, Farag E. Anesthetic management of patients with intracranial aneurysms. Ochsner J. 2014;14(3):418–25.
7. Krassioukov A, Warburton DE, Teasell R, Eng JJ, The SCIRE Research Team. A systematic review of the management of autonomic dysreflexia following spinal cord injury. Arch Phys Med Rehabil. 2009;90(4):682–95.

Simulation in Perioperative Medicine: From Preoperative Clinics to Postoperative Wards

26

Scott C. Watkins, Christopher Cropsey, and Matthew D. McEvoy

Introduction

Perioperative medicine (POM) is an emerging field of medicine that aims to reduce variability and improve coordination across the entire perioperative care continuum [1, 2]. POM has been proposed as a solution to solving some of the problems plaguing our current health system, namely, excessive cost associated with and fragmentation of perioperative care [3]. There are a number of synonymous care models that share aspects of perioperative medicine, including enhanced recovery after surgery, fast-track surgery, and the perioperative surgical home. These models share the same mission: improve clinical care and reduce cost through coordination and collaboration among care providers and across the entire perioperative care timeline [4]. The focus of POM is to reduce variability by treating the entire perioperative experience as one care episode, as opposed to the traditional model of multiple, discrete encounters that are sequential but not necessarily purposefully coordinated (i.e., preoperative, intraoperative, postoperative, and recovery) [3]. POM has an opportunity to substantially impact overall population health and healthcare costs as many patients have limited exposure to healthcare prior to presenting for surgery, i.e., deferred preventative health maintenance, and a disproportionate share of overall health expenditures are associated with elective surgery [1]. While the practice of POM is best adapted to local practice, resources, and patient populations, the evidence base for POM as a medical specialty has occurred globally [5]. The rapid endorsements by the Royal College of Anaesthetists (RCOA) in the United Kingdom and the American Society of Anesthesiologists (ASA) in North America are but two examples of the global commitment to POM as a medical specialty of the future [2, 4, 6]. In recent years, the RCOA and ASA have each launched a large multi-institutional collaborative to further explore and advance the specialty of POM [4, 6]. However, the best methods by which to train the next generation of anesthesiologists and other perioperative care providers in the skills needed to accomplish many of the aims of POM remain to be elucidated [7–9].

Chapter Objectives

The objective of this chapter is twofold: to highlight the competencies needed for anesthesiologists to evolve into perioperative physicians and to identify opportunities for SBET in the development of these specialists. SBET affords an opportunity to educate perioperative clinicians and assess competencies through the upper levels of Miller's pyramid, i.e., knows how, shows how, and demonstrates [10]. Many of the competencies required for the delivery of perioperative medicine are inherent in the practice of anesthesiology, such as multidisciplinary team training during resuscitations; use of advanced life support measures, e.g., extracorporeal membranous oxygenation; and the use of ultrasound for vascular access and performance of regional anesthetic blocks and are discussed in more detail in other chapters of this text.

S. C. Watkins
Department of Anesthesiology and Critical Care Medicine, Johns Hopkins University School of Medicine, Johns Hopkins All Children's Hospital, Saint Petersburg, FL, USA

C. Cropsey
Cardiovascular Anesthesiologists, P.C., Nashville, TN, USA

M. D. McEvoy (✉)
Division of Multispecialty Anesthesia, Department of Anesthesiology, CIPHER (Center for Innovation in Perioperative Health, Education, and Research), Vanderbilt University School of Medicine, Vanderbilt University Medical Center, Nashville, TN, USA
e-mail: matthew.d.mcevoy@vanderbilt.edu

B. Mahoney et al. (eds.), *Comprehensive Healthcare Simulation: Anesthesiology*, Comprehensive Healthcare Simulation,
https://doi.org/10.1007/978-3-030-26849-7_26

Training Physicians in Perioperative Medicine

The path to becoming a perioperative physician does not fit any one medical specialty or training curriculum. Physicians from many specialties including internal medicine, hospital medicine, intensive care medicine, primary care medicine, geriatric medicine, and cardiovascular medicine have all associated their specialties with POM [1]. However, the medical specialty with the most knowledge, skills, and training overlaps with those required for POM is anesthesiology [4, 6]. The existing structure of anesthesiology postgraduate training provides for a foundation on which to build that of POM [6]. Recently, the ASA commissioned a task force to identify core competencies needed for the practice of POM. The group identified more than 50 competencies spanning 7 domains that would be added to traditional anesthesiology training to meet the needs of POM (see Table 26.1) [4]. This is the most comprehensive attempt by any group to define the knowledge, skills, and core competencies necessary for perioperative physicians [3, 4]. At present, anesthesiologists are trained in many aspects required for the care of perioperative patients including unparalleled training in preoperative and intraoperative medicine and the management of pain and intensive care of perioperative patients [6]. In addition, as the largest hospital specialty, anesthesiologists possess a unique systems-level view of both perioperative care and clinical operations that are a natural segue for leading the development of POM [6]. For most residency programs, there remain several important gaps in the training of anesthesiologists that would need to be met before assuming the role of perioperative physicians, including full perioperative management of chronic disease states and common postoperative complications which tend to be medical in nature, training in the facilitation of collaborative or shared decision-making, advanced communication, team development and leadership skills, and training in quality improvement, value-based care, and implementation sciences. While many anesthesiology programs are beginning to incorporate POM rotations into their core residency training and while advanced fellowships in POM are emerging, these training opportunities are unlikely to be sufficient to meet the demands for perioperative physicians in the near term [7, 9, 11]. Until a critical mass of future anesthesiologists with POM training emerges, alternative forms of training in POM are needed to meet the growing educational demand.

SBET has an opportunity to fill training gaps in POM for physicians and to augment the education offered by existing training programs (see Table 26.2). Many healthcare institutions, including nonteaching facilities, have embraced the use of simulation for establishing and maintaining provider competencies in other areas of clinical medicine. Thus the incorporation of POM into course offerings would appear logical [12–14]. In recent years, the use of "boot camps," a form of intensive SBET training for onboarding and preparing new clinicians for practice, has increased in popularity and are being used in almost every specialty of medicine [15–18]. SBET lends itself well to the training of nontechnical skills, e.g., teamwork, communication, decision-making, leadership, etc., which are often the mainstay of team-based simulation exercises and a focus of many post-simulation debriefs [19–21]. These skills are consonant with those

Table 26.1 Proposed competencies for perioperative medicine

Domain	Competency
Patient care	EBM-based preoperative risk reduction and optimization strategies
	Practices EBM intraoperative management
	Primary consultant in general medical issues that commonly present in surgical patient population
Technical skills	Advanced interpretation skills – electrocardiogram, surface ultrasound, pulmonary function tests, coronary artery stents management, cardiac pacemakers and implantable cardioverter defibrillator
	management including bedside interrogation, thoracostomy tube placement
Medical knowledge	Expertise in evaluation, risk reduction, and postoperative management of the following medical conditions – congestive heart failure, diabetes, pneumonia, sepsis Chronic obstructive pulmonary disease, acute kidney injury, urinary tract infection, venous thrombus embolus, stroke, asthma, acute coronary syndrome, delirium, goal-directed therapy and blood management, deep vein thrombosis, acute renal failure, skin and wound breakdown, postoperative prevention/management falls, myocardial infarction
Practice-based learning and improvement	Ability to evaluate EBM and use of practice guidelines
	Use of continuous quality management tools and change management
	Understanding of practice models and current payment models
System-based practice	Systems approach to patient management and improvement
	Principles of operating rooms management
	Principles of process flow and perioperative care coordination
	Transition of care
	Principles of patient safety
Communication and interpersonal skills	Patient-centered communication skills
	Conflict resolution
	Task management, teamworking, and situational awareness
	Transitions of care
	Skills to supervise healthcare extenders
Professionalism	Patient-centered care
	Transparency of practice
	Focus on collaborative relationships with patients and other clinicians

Adapted from Kain et al. [4]
EBM evidenced-based medicine

Table 26.2 Simulation-based modalities for training and assessing perioperative medicine competencies

Domain	Competency	SBET example
Patient care	EBM-based preoperative risk reduction and optimization strategies Primary consultant in general medical issues that commonly present in surgical patient population	Standardized patient scenarios for preoperative evaluation, risk stratification, and counseling Screen-based exercises involving risk assessment and clinical decision-making, e.g., decision-making regarding preoperative cardiac testing and management of pain in chronic opioid users Mannequin-based simulations for managing critical events including acute complications and cardiopulmonary resuscitation
Technical skills	Advanced diagnostic, interpretive, and procedural skills	Partial task trainers – e.g., thoracostomy tube placement, ultrasound-guided regional blocks, and vascular access, bronchoscopy, etc. Screen-based simulations – Interpretation and management of mechanical ventilators, cardiac stress tests, ultrasound images, etc.
Medical knowledge	Expertise in evaluation, risk reduction, and postoperative management of chronic and systemic medical conditions	Standardized patient scenarios for preoperative risk stratification, optimization and counseling. Development of comprehensive perioperative care plans Screen based simulations – Knowledge assessment for managing specific disease states Mannequin based simulations – Measuring knowledge of chronic diseases at the upper levels of Miller's pyramid. Training in the management of acute physiological changes
Practice-based learning and improvement	Ability to evaluate EBM and use of practice guidelines Use of continuous quality management tools and change management Understanding of practice models and current payment models	Screen-based and tabletop exercises – e.g., *Night at the ER©* for teaching systems-based practice and red bead experiment for teaching continuous quality improvement Multidisciplinary team training for introducing new policies and practices (change management) and general leadership skills Standardized patients/actors for training in counseling and managing patient expectations using EBM and practice guidelines
System-based practice	Systems approach to patient management and improvement Principles of operating rooms management Principles of process flow and perioperative care coordination Transition of care Principles of patient safety	Screen based and tabletop exercises – *Night at the ER©* for teaching systems-based practice and red bead experiment for teaching continuous quality improvement Standardized patients/actors for training in error disclosure Mannequin-based simulations for detecting and managing medical errors, complications, and adverse events Training in debriefing skills for facilitating post-event debriefs and safety huddles
Communication and interpersonal skills	Patient-centered communication skills Conflict resolution Task management, team working, and situational awareness Transitions of care Skills to supervise healthcare extenders	Standardized patient/actor simulations to teach skills for conducting difficult conversations, conflict management, breaking bad news, and bedside teaching/counseling Multidisciplinary team training for training handovers and safe transitions of care Mannequin-based simulations and multidisciplinary team training for advanced crisis management and leadership skills
Professionalism	Patient-centered care Transparency of practice Focus on collaborative relationships with patients and other clinicians	Standardized patient/actor simulations to teach skills for advanced training in patient-centered communication including counseling and conducting difficult conversations Mannequin and multidisciplinary team training for managing conflict between providers, communicating during times of high workload, and role reversal exercises for better understanding of systems-based practice

Adapted from Kain et al. [4]
EBM evidenced-based medicine

required to be an effective perioperative physician and are not readily taught or assessed in clinical practice or didactic education [22, 23].

Knowledge and Competencies That Span the Continuum of Perioperative Medicine

POM may be thought of as *the practice of patient-centered, multidisciplinary, and integrated medical care of patients from the moment of contemplation of surgery until full recovery* [2]. Two aspects of POM that are integral to this definition are the continuous scope and patient-centered focus of practice, which encompass a patient's journey through the entire perioperative care process [2]. POM defines the future of perioperative care as physician-led, extends the role of anesthesiologists into the hospital and ambulatory care settings, and focuses care delivery on the patient and engages the patient as an active participant in his or her care (patient-centered care) [2]. The practice of POM is one of continuous care from the time the need for surgery is determined through hospital discharge and best recovery from surgery. Throughout this continuum of care, the role of the perioperative physician must change to meet the needs of the patient.

Patient-Centered Communication

It has been suggested that the nontechnical aspects of POM, i.e., communication, shared decision-making, interprofessional team leadership, etc., have a larger impact on improving patient outcomes than the technical interventions [24]. In other words, the real value in patient-centered *care* may be patient-centered *communication*. Patient-centered communication skills are difficult to teach and assess at the bedside but are routinely taught and assessed using SBET using standardized actors and mannequin-based simulation exercises [25]. During the early stages of preoperative care when the patient and caregivers are contemplating surgery (especially for high-risk complex cases and patients), the POM physician should engage the patient in shared decision-making processes to determine which strategies might improve the perioperative experience for the patient, mitigate risk of complications, and optimize outcomes [26–28]. The goal of shared decision-making is to ensure that patients have a comprehensive picture of the risks and benefits of surgical treatment so that they may make personalized decisions regarding their care [2]. Standardized patients may be used to teach clinicians how to facilitate shared decision-making. This might include training or assessment in how to carry out difficult conversations including frank discussions of risk or management of unreasonable expectations, demonstrate competency in performing comprehensive preoperative patient consultations, practice counseling patients on lifestyle modifications such as smoking cessation, and practice challenging conversations such as those about end-of-life care [29]. Standardized actors may be used to teach and assess inter-professional skills including conflict management, difficult conversations with colleagues, supervision of mid-level providers, and the demonstration of professionalism as a consultant physician [30, 31]. One can envision a scenario involving standardized patients with complex medical problems (e.g., a chronic opioid user with complex cardiac disease), in which the perioperative physician is tasked with creating an individualized preoperative risk assessment and risk reduction and optimization strategy, a comprehensive care plan that incorporates evidence-based medicine (EBM), and to demonstrate appropriate patient education and counseling (Table 26.3).

There is an extensive body of literature on simulation-based team training in healthcare which can be called upon to augment the training of perioperative physicians [32, 33]. SBET can be used to teach clinicians of all levels how to lead teams in crisis situations, maintain situational awareness and vigilance during times of high workload, avoid and overcome diagnostic errors, delegate and assign tasks to team members, triage clinical care during times of high patient census, and handle disagreements when co-managing patients with other providers [33]. SBET may incorporate individuals from different professions and disciplines allowing clinicians to practice communication skills in settings that reflect the interprofessional and multidisciplinary nature of perioperative care. POM is multidisciplinary in nature, so clinicians require advanced skills in interacting with and leading multidisciplinary teams including managing disagreements between teams, transitioning care between providers, and making collaborative team decisions. Many of these skills can be enhanced using SBET [34, 35].

Systems-Based Practice and Improvement

There is data to suggest that the variation in outcomes observed between patients is a function of the variability between providers and care delivery systems and not due to individual patient factors [2]. Recognizing this and reducing provider and system variability are a fundamental tenet of POM. Thus perioperative physicians require a strong foundation in systems-based practice, systems-level awareness, and application of the improvement sciences including quality improvement, value-based care, EBM, change management, and implementation science [4, 36]. The teaching and assessment of many of these skills can be augmented using SBET. A library of small group exercises is available for teaching clinicians quality improvement principles including developing change, testing and making change, and team cooperation [37]. Tabletop exercises such as *Friday Night at the ER*© [Breakthrough Learning, Inc., Portland, Oregon] can be used to teach systems-based healthcare delivery and the interplay between microsystems within an organization. Screen-based simulations (SBS) can be created to teach and evaluate the application of EBM, value-based care, and operating room management including value stream mapping and components of human resources such as simulations of patient schedules and staffing models [38].

Preoperative Patient Optimization

In addition to promoting shared decision-making, preoperative management involves ensuring fitness for the planned procedure, which may entail optimizing chronic disease processes, e.g., diabetes, and physiological functioning through lifestyle modification, including weight reduction, smoking cessation, and nutrition/exercise pre-habilitation [2]. SBS may be used to advance anesthesiologists' knowledge of chronic disease management and optimization, preoperative

Table 26.3 Sample perioperative anesthesia scenario

Title: PACU arrest

Audience: Anesthesia care provider

Objectives: Medical knowledge: Identify signs and symptoms of myocardial ischemia

Patient care: Diagnosis and management of myocardial ischemia

Communication: Utilize crew resource management skills to manage a clinical emergency

Case stem: Mr. Smith is a 56-year-old male with a history of morbid obesity, coronary artery disease, OSA, hyperlipidemia, and non-insulin-dependent diabetes status-post a partial colectomy for colon cancer.

Room setup: Post-anesthesia care unit (PACU) bay with patient lying in bed with no monitors attached, chart bundled, apparently prepared for transfer to the post-surgical inpatient unit. Preoperative and intraoperative record available to the learner

Pulse oximetry, noninvasive blood pressure, and five-lead electrocardiography available upon learner request. A PACU nurse will serve as the main confederate. The learner is called to the PACU to evaluate a patient complaining of severe pain just prior to transfer to the floor

State	**Patient status**	**Learner actions**	
Baseline	In acute distress (vital signs only available if the learner applies monitors or requests them reapplied) HR, 127; RR, 25; BP, 179/97; SpO_2, 94% (RA). ECG: ST depressions visible	The learner will introduce him/herself to the patient and PACU nurse Assess patient for pain or discomfort Apply monitors to the patient	The patient will indicate difficulty breathing due to severe surgical pain The nurse will claim that opioid analgesics were limited intraoperatively due to OSA
Anxiety and dyspnea	Increasingly uncomfortable and dyspneic *(over 2 minutes)* HR, 135; RR, 30; BP, 145/87; SpO_2, 92% (RA)	Recognize signs of acute coronary syndrome (ACS) Initiate management including beta-blockers, nitroglycerin, aspirin, oxygen, and opioid analgesics	If the learner does not recognize ACS, the patient will indicate increasing chest pressure and dyspnea misattributed to surgical pain
Unresponsive	Less responsive *(over 2 minutes)* HR, 130 with ectopy; RR, 30; BP, 98/78; SpO_2, 89% (RA). ECG reveals ST elevations	Request preparation for patient transport to the interventional cardiology unit Prepare for potential supportive care including airway support	If learner actions are performed, end the scenario. If the learner has not recognized ACS and initiated the appropriate care, continue to the next state (arrest)
Arrest	Unconscious/unresponsive *(over 2 minutes)* HR, PEA at 130 → ventricular tachycardia; RR, 0; BP, pulseless; SpO_2, pulseless	Initiate ACLS	Following a round of ACLS, end the scenario

Discussion points: Differential diagnosis severe chest pain and dyspnea in the immediate postoperative period. Management of ACS in the postoperative setting and pathophysiology. Postoperative pain management in the setting of CAD and OSA

risk assessment, and stratification. SBS may be used to teach and assess advanced clinical skills including electrocardiogram interpretation, cardiac risk stratification, management of antiplatelet therapy, management and interrogation of cardiac pacemakers and implantable cardioverter defibrillators, interpretation of advanced diagnostic tests including pulmonary function tests, sleep studies, and cardiac stress evaluations, and to assess knowledge of current evidence-based guidelines [39].

Additionally, the perioperative physician should be able to demonstrate technical proficiency in several diagnostic and therapeutic procedures. These skills include diagnostic ultrasound, transthoracic echocardiography, advanced cardiac physical examination skills, and management of implanted pumps, e.g., intrathecal and insulin pumps. Many of these procedural skills can be taught and assessed using partial task trainers and high-fidelity mannequins [40, 41].

Immediate Preoperative and Intraoperative Management

During the immediate preoperative phase (i.e., day of surgery) and during the intraoperative phase, the perioperative physician is focused on mitigating risk and optimizing the patient's physiological response to the stress of surgery in order to optimize the postoperative recovery. Management of pain is inherent in the practice of POM and is often focused on limiting the use of opioid-based analgesics through multimodal analgesia plans, which frequently include regional anesthesia blocks. These blocks require varying degrees of technical proficiency which may be taught and assessed using partial task trainers, live human models, and cadavers [42, 43]. POM physicians should be proficient in managing complications associated with performance of regional anesthetic techniques which can be demonstrated using partial task trainers and models, e.g., placement of chest tubes for pneumothorax, and through participation in mannequin-based simulations, such as management of high spinal blocks and local anesthetic toxicity [44, 45]. In addition to using ultrasound for regional anesthesia procedures, POM clinicians should be proficient in the use of ultrasound for vascular access for patients with difficult vascular access [46–49]. High-fidelity partial task trainers also exist for less common, but nonetheless useful, procedures such as bronchoscopy and transesophageal echocardiography.

Postoperative Management

The majority of postoperative complications are related to patients' coexisting or preexisting medical conditions and not to surgical or anesthetic insults [6]. Perioperative physicians should be able to identify and develop risk mitigation strategies for numerous chronic diseases and manage associated postoperative complications, which may affect every organ system and include both acute and chronic processes. SBET provides an avenue for teaching and assessing the perioperative clinician's ability to manage complex disease processes and complications. Simulation-based clinical scenarios may be developed for both commonly encountered and rare diseases to train and prepare POM physicians for clinical practice and to provide assessments for defining entrustable professional activities for purposes of credentialing perioperative physicians [50]. The list of competencies identified by the ASA taskforce includes a list of medical conditions, the management of which can be taught and assessed using SBET (see Table 26.1). SBET can be employed for teaching and assessing technical skills necessary for managing postoperative patients. Partial task trainers and SBS can be used to augment clinicians' skills in respiratory therapy (e.g., noninvasive and invasive ventilation methods) and critical care interventions (e.g., placement of invasive monitors, drains and bedside procedures) [38, 51]. SBET can be utilized to train and prepare POM physicians to recognize and manage decompensating patients early in order to prevent "failure to rescue" events [52, 53]. It is important to note that this training is likely to involve both the technical aspects as well as the nontechnical aspects of management.

Postoperative Care after Discharge and the Transition to Recovery

The role of the perioperative physician does not diminish as the patient nears discharge from the acute care setting, i.e., hospital, and should continue until the patent has obtained best possible recovery. This aspect of POM is likely to be the least familiar to anesthesiologists and more familiar to other specialties such as internal medicine. SBET has an opportunity to significantly improve the competencies of anesthesiologists in carrying out these less-familiar tasks. SBS and standardized actors may be used to train clinicians to manage patients following discharge including the remote management of chronic medical conditions and postoperative complications, maintaining open communication with patients and providers and providing ongoing patient and caregiver education and counseling [54–57].

Future Directions

As the value of perioperative services becomes more widely recognized by health systems, POM physicians will be called upon to play an increasing role in the management of surgical patients. The expansion of POM will require POM physicians to evolve as the demand for their services grow. This may entail leveraging the services of mid-level providers, expanding the role of information technology and exploring opportunities for telemedicine in managing patients post-discharge or remotely. These opportunities will place increasing demands on the skill set of POM physicians who will need to evolve as their specialty evolves. Training programs and clinicians will need to explore alternatives means of education, training, and competency assessment to keep pace with the demands of the evolving specialty. This presents a unique opportunity for SBET to play a critical role in the future of an emerging medical specialty.

Conclusion

The knowledge and training of anesthesiologists will need to expand as opportunities for anesthesiologists outside the operating room grow. SBET has an opportunity to play an increasing role in the training of anesthesiologists as perioperative physicians, especially since current postgraduate anesthesiology training, while actively evolving, is not yet keeping pace with the patient and clinical demands for POM. In addition, the existing anesthesiology workforce will look for opportunities to grow as perioperative physicians through continuing medical education, intensive hands-on courses, and workshops. Much of the knowledge and skills, both technical and nontechnical, required for the practice of perioperative medicine may be taught using experiential learning modalities.

References

1. Grocott MP, Pearse RM. Perioperative medicine: the future of anaesthesia? Br J Anaesth. 2012;108(5):723–6.
2. Grocott MP, Mythen MG. Perioperative medicine: the value proposition for anesthesia?: A UK Perspective on Delivering Value from Anesthesiology. Anesthesiol Clin. 2015;33(4):617–28.
3. Kain ZN, et al. The perioperative surgical home as a future perioperative practice model. Anesth Analg. 2014;118(5):1126–30.
4. Kain ZN, et al. Future of anesthesiology is perioperative medicine: a call for action. Anesthesiology. 2015;122(6):1192–5.
5. Cannesson M, et al. Anaesthesiology and perioperative medicine around the world: different names, same goals. Br J Anaesth. 2015;114(1):8–9.
6. Group, P.M.L.T.a.F. Perioperative medicine – the pathway to better surgical care. London: The Royal College of Anaesthetists; 2014.
7. McEvoy MD, Lien CA. Education in anesthesiology: is it time to expand the focus? A A Case Rep. 2016;6(12):380–2.
8. Alem N, et al. Transforming perioperative care: the case for a novel curriculum for anesthesiology resident training. A A Case Rep. 2016;6(12):373–9.
9. King AB, et al. Disruptive education: training the future generation of perioperative physicians. Anesthesiology. 2016;125(2):266–8.
10. Miller GE. The assessment of clinical skills/competence/performance. Acad Med. 1990;65(9 Suppl):S63–7.
11. Vanderbilt University Medical Center Perioperative Medicine Fellowship. Available from: https://ww2.mc.vanderbilt.edu/1anesthesiology/49807.
12. Rosen MA, et al. In situ simulation in continuing education for the health care professions: a systematic review. J Contin Educ Health Prof. 2012;32(4):243–54.
13. Zigmont JJ, et al. Utilization of experiential learning, and the learning outcomes model reduces RN orientation time by more than 35%. Clin Simul Nurs. 2015;11(2):79–94.
14. Will KK, et al. Interprofessional orientation for health professionals utilising simulated learning: findings from a pilot study. J Interprof Care. 2016;30(2):254–6.
15. Ceresnak SR, et al. Pediatric cardiology boot camp: description and evaluation of a novel intensive training program for pediatric cardiology trainees. Pediatr Cardiol. 2016;37(5):834–44.
16. Blackmore C, et al. Effects of postgraduate medical education "boot camps" on clinical skills, knowledge, and confidence: a meta-analysis. J Grad Med Educ. 2014;6(4):643–52.
17. Fernandez GL, et al. Boot cAMP: educational outcomes after 4 successive years of preparatory simulation-based training at onset of internship. J Surg Educ. 2012;69(2):242–8.
18. Smith ME, Trinidade A, Tysome JR. The ENT boot camp: an effective training method for ENT induction. Clin Otolaryngol. 2016;41:421.
19. Undre S, et al. Multidisciplinary crisis simulations: the way forward for training surgical teams. World J Surg. 2007;31(9):1843–53.
20. Nicksa GA, et al. Innovative approach using interprofessional simulation to educate surgical residents in technical and non-technical skills in high-risk clinical scenarios. JAMA Surg. 2015;150(3):201–7.
21. O'Dea A, O'Connor P, Keogh I. A meta-analysis of the effectiveness of crew resource management training in acute care domains. Postgrad Med J. 2014;90(1070):699–708.
22. Semler MW, et al. A randomized trial comparing didactics, demonstration, and simulation for teaching teamwork to medical residents. Ann Am Thorac Soc. 2015;12(4):512–9.
23. Lerner S, Magrane D, Friedman E. Teaching teamwork in medical education. Mt Sinai J Med. 2009;76(4):318–29.
24. Grocott MP, Martin DS, Mythen MG. Enhanced recovery pathways as a way to reduce surgical morbidity. Curr Opin Crit Care. 2012;18(4):385–92.
25. Epstein RM. Assessment in medical education. N Engl J Med. 2007;356(4):387–96.
26. Oresanya LB, Lyons WL, Finlayson E. Preoperative assessment of the older patient: a narrative review. JAMA. 2014;311(20):2110–20.
27. Moonesinghe SR, Walker EMK, Bell M. Design and methodology of SNAP-1: a Sprint National Anaesthesia Project to measure patient reported outcome after anaesthesia. Perioper Med. 2015;4(1):1.
28. Glance LG, Osler TM, Neuman MD. Redesigning surgical decision making for high-risk patients. N Engl J Med. 2014;370(15):1379.
29. Schmitz CC, et al. Learning by (video) example: a randomized study of communication skills training for end-of-life and error disclosure family care conferences. Am J Surg. 2016;212:996.
30. Marken PA, et al. Human simulators and standardized patients to teach difficult conversations to interprofessional health care teams. Am J Pharm Educ. 2010;74(7):120.
31. Chiarchiaro J, et al. Developing a simulation to study conflict in intensive care units. Ann Am Thorac Soc. 2015;12(4):526–32.
32. Boet S, et al. Transfer of learning and patient outcome in simulated crisis resource management: a systematic review. Can J Anesth. 2014;61(6):571–82.
33. Eppich W, et al. Simulation-based team training in healthcare. Simul Healthc. 2011;6 Suppl:S14–9.
34. Gaffney S, et al. The Modified, Multi-patient Observed Simulated Handoff Experience (M-OSHE): assessment and feedback for entering residents on handoff performance. J Gen Intern Med. 2016;31(4):438–41.
35. Starmer AJ, et al. Development, implementation, and dissemination of the I-PASS handoff curriculum: a multisite educational intervention to improve patient handoffs. Acad Med. 2014;89(6):876–84.
36. Vetter TR, et al. The perioperative surgical home: how anesthesiology can collaboratively achieve and leverage the triple aim in health care. Anesth Analg. 2014;118(5):1131–6.
37. Institute, N.Y.S.D.o.H.A. The game guide: interactive exercises for trainers to teach quality improvement in HIV care. New York: National Quality Center, New York State Department of Health AIDS Institute; 2006.
38. Nelson CK, Schwid HA. Screen-based simulation for anesthesiology. Int Anesthesiol Clin. 2015;53(4):81–97.
39. McEvoy MD, et al. A smartphone-based decision support tool improves test performance concerning application of the guidelines for managing regional anesthesia in the patient receiving antithrombotic or thrombolytic therapy. J Am Dent Soc Anesthesiol. 2016;124(1):186–98.
40. Bose RR, et al. Utility of a transesophageal echocardiographic simulator as a teaching tool. J Cardiothorac Vasc Anesth. 2011;25(2):212–5.
41. Ramsingh D, et al. Impact assessment of perioperative point-of-care ultrasound training on anesthesiology residents. J Am Dent Soc Anesthesiol. 2015;123(3):670–82.
42. Kessler J, et al. Teaching concepts in ultrasound-guided regional anesthesia. Curr Opin Anesthesiol. 2016;29(5):608–13.
43. Burckett-St Laurent D, et al. Teaching ultrasound-guided regional anesthesia remotely: a feasibility study. Acta Anaesthesiol Scand. 2016;60:995.
44. Cropsey CL, McEvoy MD. Local anesthetic systemic toxicity in a nonoperative location. Simul Healthc. 2015;10(5):326–8.
45. Vetrugno L, et al. Phantom model and scoring system to assess ability in ultrasound-guided chest drain positioning. Crit Ultrasound J. 2016;8(1):1.

46. Barsuk JH, et al. Simulation-based mastery learning reduces complications during central venous catheter insertion in a medical intensive care unit. Crit Care Med. 2009;37(10):2697–701.
47. Evans LV, et al. Simulation training in central venous catheter insertion: improved performance in clinical practice. Acad Med. 2010;85(9):1462–9.
48. Duran-Gehring P, et al. Ultrasound-guided peripheral intravenous catheter training results in physician-level success for emergency department technicians. J Ultrasound Med. 2016;35(11):2343–52.
49. Adhikari S, Schmier C, Marx J. Focused simulation training: emergency department nurses' confidence and comfort level in performing ultrasound-guided vascular access. J Vasc Access. 2015;16(6):515–20.
50. Wagner SJ, Reeves S. Milestones and entrustable professional activities: the key to practically translating competencies for interprofessional education? J Interprof Care. 2015;29(5):507–8.
51. Lino JA, et al. A critical review of mechanical ventilation virtual simulators: is it time to use them? JMIR Med Educ. 2016;2(1):e8.
52. Connell CJ, et al. The effectiveness of education in the recognition and management of deteriorating patients: a systematic review. Nurse Educ Today. 2016;44:133.
53. Liaw SY, et al. Effectiveness of a web-based simulation in improving nurses' workplace practice with deteriorating ward patients: a pre-and postintervention study. J Med Internet Res. 2016;18(2):e37.
54. Patel B, et al. Interprofessional communication of clinicians using a mobile phone app: a randomized crossover trial using simulated patients. J Med Internet Res. 2016;18(4):e79.
55. Cunningham NJ, et al. Telephone referrals by junior doctors: a randomised controlled trial assessing the impact of SBAR in a simulated setting. Postgrad Med J. 2012;88(1045):619–26.
56. Ajaz A, David R, Bhat M. The PsychSimCentre: teaching out-of-hours psychiatry to non-psychiatrists. Clin Teach. 2016;13(1):13–7.
57. Carter K, et al. Results from the first year of implementation of CONSULT: consultation with novel methods and simulation for UME longitudinal training. West J Emerg Med. 2015;16(6):845.

27 Simulation in Low-Resource Settings: A Review of the Current State and Practical Implementation Strategies

Mary DiMiceli, Arna Banerjee, Mark W. Newton, and Matthew D. McEvoy

Simulation Pearls

1. Challenges to development, implementation, and maintenance of a simulation program are similar to those in improving healthcare in low-resource settings.
2. Education of technical and non-technical skills received by simulation training may enhance quality of healthcare provided in LMICs.
3. Low to middle fidelity simulation programs may be more cost-effective than high fidelity simulation with little to no difference in outcomes, and they are easier to organize and implement in low-resource countries.
4. Development, implementation, and maintenance of a simulation program is best accomplished by following a structured approach similar to that offered by Kern's six-step approach to curriculum design.
5. Reflection of the simulation experience should take into consideration communication and cultural differences in order to enhance the learning solidifying during debriefing sessions.

M. DiMiceli (✉)
Anesthesia Medical Group, Inc., Nashville, TN, USA
e-mail: mary.dimiceli@vanderbilt.edu

A. Banerjee
Division of Critical Care, Medical Education and Administration, Simulation in Medical Education, Vanderbilt University Medical Center, Vanderbilt University School of Medicine, Nashville, TN, USA
e-mail: arna.banerjee@vanderbilt.edu

M. W. Newton
Department of Anesthesiology and Pediatrics, Vanderbilt University Medical Center, Nashville, TN, USA
e-mail: mark.w.newton@vanderbilt.edu

M. D. McEvoy
Division of Multispecialty Anesthesia, Department of Anesthesiology, CIPHER (Center for Innovation in Perioperative Health, Education, and Research), Vanderbilt University School of Medicine, Vanderbilt University Medical Center, Nashville, TN, USA
e-mail: matthew.d.mcevoy@vanderbilt.edu

Introduction

Simulation in medical education has its roots in the aviation industry but has grown substantially within healthcare, particularly anesthesia and other acute care fields, over the past three decades [1]. Although computer-based simulation has been in existence since the 1960s [2], high fidelity mannequin-based simulation did not emerge until the 1980s [3]. In their comprehensive review of medical simulation, Cooper and Taqueti suggested that it is important to realize that the term "simulator" is used to refer to all technologies that imitate task [4]. As noted by Gaba, "simulation is a technique—not a technology—to replace or amplify real experiences with guided experiences that evoke or replicate substantial aspects of the real world in a fully interactive manner" [5]. This understanding of simulation is especially important as we consider simulation in the setting of low- and middle-income countries (LMICs) or simulation for the austere environment.

Despite a greater than 50-year history of development and implementation in well-resourced areas, medical simulation is just breaking ground in low-resource settings. Although many perceived barriers exist, nongovernmental organizations (NGOs) and medical personnel funded by charitable organizations have been able to perform research studies or develop neonatal simulation programs in low-resource countries with some success [6–9]. However, there is a paucity of literature describing practical components of longitudinal program development, design, and implementation. Towards this end, we present this chapter divided into two main sections. First, a brief review of the use of medical simulation

B. Mahoney et al. (eds.), *Comprehensive Healthcare Simulation: Anesthesiology*, Comprehensive Healthcare Simulation,
https://doi.org/10.1007/978-3-030-26849-7_27

in low-resource settings including existing evidence on its utility in improving medical knowledge, clinical practice, self-efficacy and, ideally, clinical outcomes. The second section will describe best practices on the development, implementation, and maintenance of a successful simulation program in low-resource areas based on both current literature and the experience of the authors.

Chapter Objectives

This chapter focuses on the role of medical simulation in meeting educational and healthcare needs in low-resource settings, reviews current strides being made towards developing simulation programs, and discusses best practices in program development. There is a great deal of heterogeneity found between countries and regions in the clinical scenarios commonly encountered, availability of medical personnel and resources, health policies, and standards of medical knowledge and training. This chapter was developed to offer expert advice and evidence-based suggestions for those developing and implementing simulation in healthcare education in these low-resource settings.

History of Simulation in Low-Resource Settings

Medical simulation extends back to seventeenth–eighteenth-century France where M. Gregoire created the first obstetric simulator using a mannequin he created and a dead fetus in order to demonstrate techniques for assisted and complicated deliveries to midwives [10]. In 1748, the midwife for the Queen of France provided instruction on management principles of childbirth to other midwives using her own mannequin made from leather and bone [11]. While well-resourced countries have taken the lead in advancing technological development, knowledge, and experience in medical simulation since the 1960s, in low- to middle-income countries (LMICs) over the last decade, simulation training has increasingly been utilized as a means to provide medical education, improve knowledge gaps, and identify systems problems in order to enhance efficiency, efficacy, and outcomes of currently available medical care. In 2009, a systematic review of clinical interventions associated with reduced intrapartum deaths concluded that obstetric drills and safety checklists were among a limited number of strategies shown to improve provision of emergency obstetric care [12]. The authors suggest that simulation with "significantly lower cost, durable, easy to disassemble and sanitize, high-fidelity mannequins with culturally appropriate features" could reduce perinatal deaths in low-resource settings.

There are a variety of challenges to improving healthcare in low-resource settings: lack of financial support/funding, shortage of skilled healthcare workers, poor local and national infrastructure, availability and cost of transportation, and limited health supplies [13]. These features of some LMICs contribute to the "three-delay model," the components of which can be interdependent. These three delays are (1) a delay to first seeking medical care, (2) a delay in reaching medical care, and (3) a delay in receiving adequate healthcare (Fig. 27.1). This phenomenon was first described in explaining pregnancy-related mortality in the areas of Ghana, Sierra Leone, and Nigeria [14]. Barnes-Josiah et al., in examining the causes of maternal mortality in Haiti through the lens of the three-delay model, found, similar to Thaddeus and Maine, that the three delays contributed to maternal mortality in 12 cases and were intimately intertwined as opposed to being a sequence of discrete events [15]. They concluded that the first two delays were in large part due to an apparent lack of faith in the Haitian healthcare system and a perception that available obstetric care was inadequate or ineffective. Simulation training may be able to play a role in directly addressing the third delay by improving healthcare providers' knowledge, skills, and attitudes, identifying and addressing systems errors, and enhancing multidisciplinary teamwork and communication. Improved outcomes could, in turn, positively impact the first and second delay through a change in public perception of healthcare delivery with improved efficiency, efficacy, and safety of healthcare. In consideration of the healthcare disparities present in low-resource settings, the Lancet Commission in Global Surgery, the third Edition of the World Bank's Disease Control Priorities (DCP), and the World Health Assembly have identified "access to safe emergency and essential surgical care and anesthesia" as a primary goal as part of the initiative to achieve universal health coverage [16]. As part of this initiative, the World Health Organization (WHO) identified three "bellwether procedures" or essential surgeries that are most commonly performed and most likely to predict the ability of the healthcare delivery system to perform other WHO primary care package procedures: [17] cesarean delivery, laparotomy, and open fracture repair. According to the DCP, through improvements in the provision of healthcare for these essential surgeries in low- to middle-income countries (LMIC), 3.2% of annual deaths and 3.5% of disability-adjusted life years could be prevented [18]. Given this emphasis, it is appropriate that the majority of current simulation literature in LMICs reviews training of neonatal, maternal, and trauma resuscitation scenarios [6–8, 19, 20].

Simulation courses designed for training in obstetric and neonatal emergencies include the Pacific Emergency Obstetric Course, the WHO Essential Newborn Care Course [21], the Life Saving Skills Course, the Practical

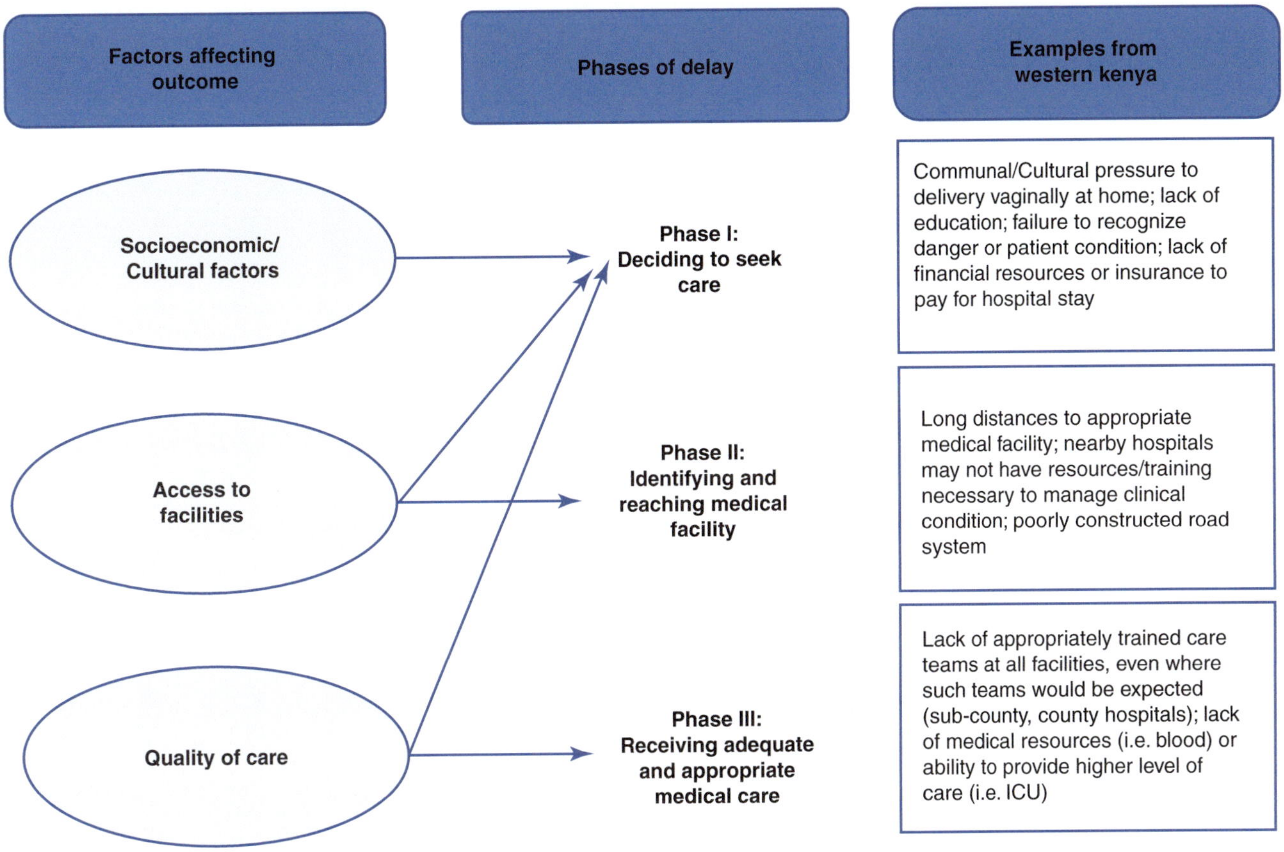

Fig. 27.1 The three delay model. First described in Ghana, Sierra Leone, and Nigeria, the three delay model offers an insight into the challenges that contribute to pregnancy mortality in low-resource countries. These factors are often interdependent, which makes seeking and obtaining medical care more of a challenge. (Based upon Barnes-Josiah et al. [15])

Obstetric Multi-Professional Training (PROMPT) Course, the PRONTO International Simulation Course [19, 20, 22–24], the IMPACT Africa Simulation Course (developed and directed by the authors of this chapter), and Helping Babies Breathe (Table 27.1). An evaluation following the implementation of the WHO Essential Newborn Care Course identified improvements in midwife skill and knowledge and demonstrated a reduction in perinatal deaths following its introduction in Zambia [21, 25]. While a randomized control trial assessing the impact of this course across multiple sites failed to demonstrate similar effects, it did reveal a significant decrease in the rate of stillbirths [26]. The simulation course led by PRONTO (Programa de Rescate Obstetrico y Neonatal: Tratamiento Optimo y Oportuno) International was reported to lead to improvements in inter-professional knowledge, self-efficacy [22–24], teamwork, and communication [19, 23] in two low-resource areas.

Helping Babies Breathe [HBB] is an American Academy of Pediatrics global neonatal resuscitation initiative that employs simulation training to improve neonatal resuscitation in low-resource countries and has been successfully implemented in more than 77 countries. In 2014, a report on perinatal mortality in Tanzania following implantation of HBB documented a decrease in early neonatal mortality (from 13.4 to 7.1 deaths per 1000 live births), stillbirths (from 19 to 14.5 per 1000 births), and early perinatal mortality (from 32.2 to 21.6 per 1000 births) [27]. Similar results have been reported from other countries following introduction of this training [28, 29]. A separate clinical trial evaluating the effectiveness of reducing perinatal mortality and resuscitation practices in three low-resources areas is currently underway [9].

PRONTO International conducted a randomized controlled trial with perinatal mortality at 12-month follow-up as the primary outcome in 12 government hospitals in Mexico [20]. Six hospitals were randomly selected to receive simulation training using a low-cost hybrid simulator (PartoPants™, or modified surgical scrubs on a simulated patient and Laerdal Neonatalie™). Simulation training consisted of scenarios focused on teamwork, communication, neonatal resuscitation, and obstetric emergencies (e.g., shoulder dystocia, hemorrhage, and preeclampsia/eclampsia). The authors reported a lower incidence of postpartum complications following cesarean delivery at 12-month follow-up but no other statistically significant results. Effecting improvements in maternal and neonatal outcomes through a

Table 27.1 Simulation courses

Program	Target population	Content focus	Training components	Course length	Scenarios	Type of simulator	Outcomes
Pacific Emergency Maternal & Neonatal Training	Nurses/midwives Selected clinical staff of those facilities delivering and providing postnatal care more than 200 women a year All staff of provincial labor and postnatal wards Reproductive health educators in the pre-service and post-basic training institutions	OB/ neonatal	Manual, lectures, in situ simulation	3 days for TOT	Preeclampsia/eclampsia; neonatal resuscitation; maternal collapse	Partial task trainer/actors; mannequin	NP
WHO Essential Newborn Care Course	Nurses/midwives	Neonatal	Manual, lectures, demonstrations, skills training, role play	5 days +6–7 days for TOT	Newborn resuscitation; breastfeeding	Mannequin; actors	Improved midwife skill and knowledge (McClure 2007 [21]); decreased perinatal deaths in Zambia (Carlo 2009 [25]); decreased stillbirth rate (Carlo 2010 [26])
Life Saving Skills Course	Nurses/midwives, obstetricians, anesthesiologists, medical assistants	OB/ neonatal	Lectures, scenario and skills teaching, demonstrations, workshops	3 days +1–2 days for TOT	Manual placental extraction; vacuum-assisted delivery; neonatal resuscitation	Partial task trainer/ mannequin	NP
Practical Obstetric Multi-Professional Training Course	Nurses/midwives, obstetricians, anesthesiologists/ anesthetists, medical assistants, pediatricians, nurse/midwife/ medical students	OB/ neonatal	Manual, lectures, in situ workshops	4×/year, 1 day for TOT course	PPH; cord prolapse; eclampsia; instrumental delivery	High-tech simulator (SimMom)	Reduction in neonatal hypoxic injuries, injuries from shoulder dystocia and improvements in emergency CDs and organizational culture [ref]
PRONTO International Simulation Course	Nurses/midwives, obstetricians, anesthesiologists/ anesthetists, medical assistants, pediatricians	OB/ neonatal	In situ simulation, team, and CRM training; debriefing; skills sessions; team building exercises; lectures	2 modules 2–3mo apart: Module I-2 days Module II-1 day	PPH; neonatal resuscitation; shoulder dystocia; preeclampsia/ eclampsia	Partial task trainer/actress NeoNatalie newborn simulator	Improved interdisciplinary knowledge, self-efficacy, communication, and teamwork [Cohen, Walker]; achieved more than 60% of the goals set during training; decreased number of cesarean deliveries performed in hospitals in Mexico that received PRONTO training
Helping Babies Breathe	Nurses, midwives, birth attendants	Neonatal	Simulation, visual guidebooks, flipcharts, and posters; skills training; OSCE	1–2 days; 3 days for TOT	Neonatal resuscitation	NeoNatalie newborn simulator	Decreased early neonatal mortality, stillbirths, and early perinatal mortality (Msemo 2013 [27], Goudar 2013 [28], Hoban 2013 [29])
IMPACT Africa Simulation Course	Nurses/midwives, obstetricians, anesthesiologists/ anesthetists, pediatricians, pediatric nurses, medical assistants/hospital staff	OB/ neonatal	Simulation, team, and CRM training; debriefing; manual, lectures	2 days +1–2 days for TOT	PPH, preeclampsia/ eclampsia; high spinal; difficult airway; obstructed labor/fetal distress; neonatal resuscitation	High-tech simulator (SimMom and NeoNatalie)	Adherence to best practices in safe CD Checklist[a]

Pacific Emergency Obstetric Course: https://www.psrh.org.nz; accessed Dec 8, 2016
Life Saving Skills Course: https://www.rcog.org.uk/en/global-network/global-health.../life-saving-skills-course; accessed Dec 8, 2016
Practical Obstetric Multi-Professional Training (PROMPT) Course: http://www.promptmaternity.org/au/training; accessed Dec 8, 2016
OSCE Observed Structured Clinical Evaluation, *TOT* train the trainer, *NP* not published
[a]Study Ongoing. Study design: pre- and post- training clinical observations. This best practice checklist was developed

simulation-based training program without a means to financially maintain a simulation center or the associated training program may prove pointless. At the Society in Europe for Simulation Applied to Medicine Conference in 2011, Msemo stated, "You need commitment to be there from the government side, because training without support for the trainee to have equipment [in order] to do resuscitation is useless." Professor Vanessa Burch of the University of Cape Town also warns against the impetus to pursue simulation in healthcare without considering the "hidden costs" of maintaining a center, equipment, and skills [30]. Given that simulation centers with advanced simulation technology, high fidelity mannequins, and software requiring trained personnel are the most financially intensive to maintain [31], some programs have used lower fidelity models with success to decrease cost [7, 20, 32]. A low-cost simulation course for trauma using only medical equipment and resources locally available demonstrated not only improvement in knowledge acquisition but also increase in number of tasks completed and a decrease in time in which critical actions were completed. The authors were able to develop their course for 33 participants for $2844.00 with a total maintenance cost for all participants of $8.82 as compared to using a single high fidelity chest tube simulator which may cost as much as $3000 [7]. Multiple studies have failed to demonstrate superior improvement in performance of trainees after high fidelity simulation training versus low fidelity [33–37], supporting the claim that low to moderate fidelity simulation programs are more cost-effective and can yield comparable outcomes in a low-resource country.

Development and Implementation of a Simulation Program

The currently existing models reviewed here provide examples of successfully implemented and sustained healthcare simulation programs. The following discussion will focus on development and implementation of an LMIC healthcare simulation program based on existing models including the ImPACT Africa project (ImProving Perioperative Anesthesia Care & Training in Africa) simulation program in East Africa which was created and implemented by the authors of this chapter. This capacity-building program involved the creation of two self-sustaining simulation centers of excellence in Kenya which function as components in a wider nurse anesthesia training program in Kenya.

Livingston et al. outlined key steps undertaken to develop and implement a sustainable simulation center-based training program in Rwanda. These include engaging multidisciplinary partners with a shared vision, identifying feasible short- and long-term goals, obtaining a viable funding source, recruiting local staff, developing site-appropriate curricula, training of local leaders, constructing a physical space, cultivating sustainable partnerships while engaging the wider community, and finally monitoring and evaluating use following program implementation [38]. Kern's Six-Step Approach to Curriculum Development offers a broader outline for application to the design and implementation of a simulation program [39]. Adaptation of the above two approaches alongside methods undertaken by these authors are represented in Fig. 27.2.

Prior to incorporating simulation training into medical education in an LMIC, an understanding of the healthcare environment is critical to the development of common clinical scenarios appropriate for achieving practical learning objectives. For example, there are 5.1 million trauma-related deaths worldwide each year, 90% of which occur in LMICs, with a majority resulting from road traffic collisions [7]. Against this backdrop, identification of the need to improve response time and trauma skill competency in Managua, Nicaragua, led to the development of a low-cost simulation program using Advanced Trauma Life Support (ATLS) principles and procedure stations made from local material. In another example, given that laparoscopic surgery is becoming more widely accessible to LMICs while laparoscopic simulation technology remains cost prohibitive, a teaching hospital in Northern Haiti provided simulation training for surgical residents using a box trainer (made from cardboard, plastic, a small webcam, and laparoscopic handles) alongside a structured modular curriculum [40]. Both of these courses addressed the needs of their medical community and targeted learners through the creation of programs that were reproducible and sustainable in a low-resource setting.

Assessment of local resources is a critical component of any needs assessment in the creation of a simulation training program. Croft and colleagues warn that we should heed the recommendations published by the WHO to avoid development of training models based on those created in high-income countries. They suggest that the success of any training model depends primarily on "appropriately skilled instructors in sufficient numbers and suitable, locally adapted training materials." They go on to state that "Care must be taken to ensure that areas with the highest maternal and neonatal mortality, and perhaps, with the most need for training are given appropriate support to develop and evaluate sustainable, clinically effective training programmes" [11]. A successful training program must be customized to fit the clinical ecosystem, resources, culture, language, and local leadership of the target environment.

During the initiation of a LMIC simulation training program, infrastructure, expertise, and funding from high-resourced educational institutions may be necessary. However, the relationship between the medical leaders in the LMIC and the high-resourced institution must be one

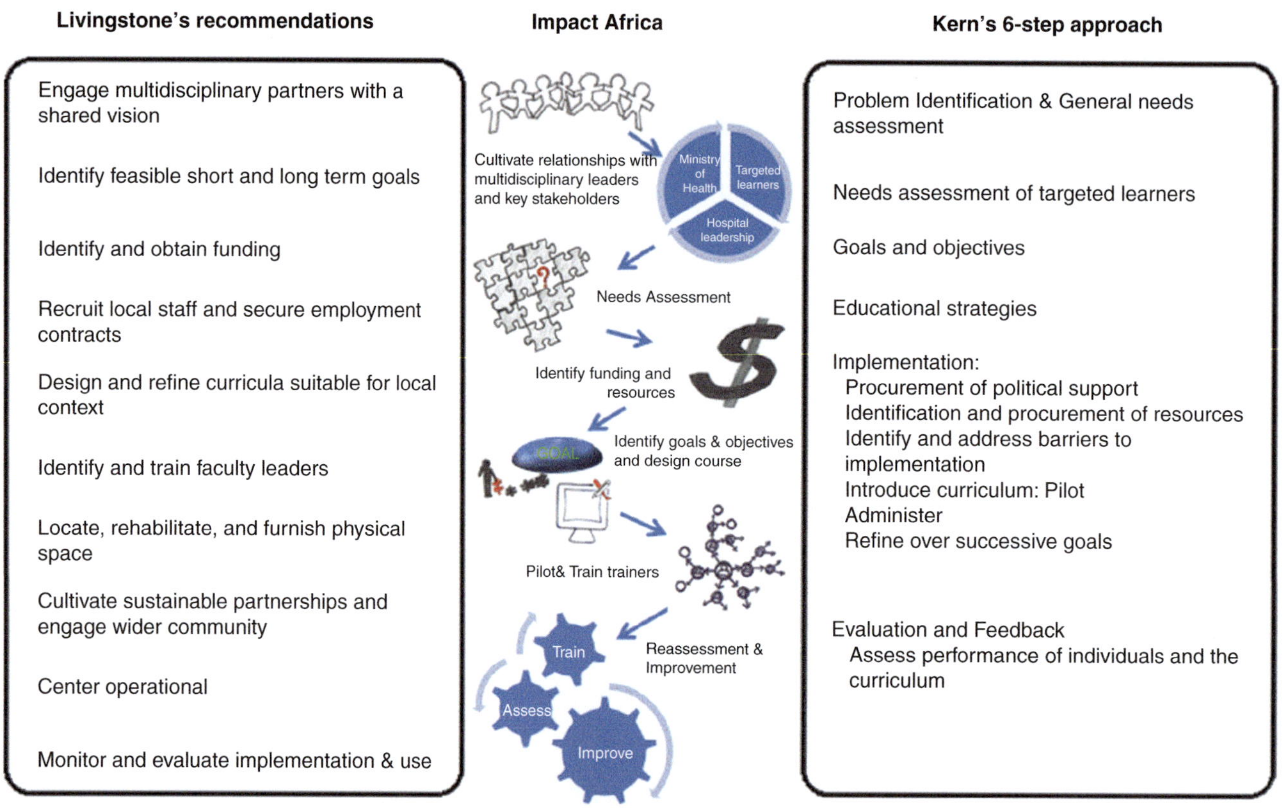

Fig. 27.2 Stepwise and dynamic approach to developing and implementing a simulation course in low-resource settings. This image illustrates a practical implementation of recommendations from two well-known curriculum development guidelines [38, 39] in an ongoing simulation training program in East Africa

of mutual respect and partnership. In the experience of the authors and of Livingston et al., this is more easily facilitated when there is a preexisting *relationship that has been cultivated with the principles of trust and support. Identification of both key stakeholders* (i.e., government officials from Ministry of Health, hospital leadership, targeted learners, and patients) *and potential barriers* is vital to ensure operability and sustainability.

Dependent upon both the resources and goals for a simulation program, one must address specific questions to identify the appropriate setting for instruction: "Are there sufficient resources available to construct a simulation center?" "Is in situ simulation a suitable model for meeting program goals?" "Can the objectives be accomplished utilizing a low technology center while still providing a high level of fidelity?"

A simulation center should be located at a site accessible to participants and in close proximity to a health facility to ensure consistent and ongoing participation, reduced travel costs, and improved security. Depending on the degree of technology employed, it may be necessary to train local staff as simulation technologists. An ideal simulation center would include both a simulation theater designed to maximize scenario fidelity and a separate space for safe and effective debriefing.

In situ simulation occurs in the clinical environment (e.g., hospital) with participants composed of on-duty personnel. Performing simulation in the actual clinical environment provides a realism that cannot be replicated in a simulation center, while also allowing the simulation program to meet goals less realizable through use of a de novo center. Center-based simulation, often associated with a prescribed set of learning objectives, is more often focused on the practice of technical and non-technical skills, whereas in situ simulation is more likely to identify system deficiencies and preexisting team dynamics. While it is difficult to compare outcomes between programs utilizing in situ or center-based simulation, one randomized controlled trial comparing NRP programs demonstrated improved technical scores (based on number of correct interventions performed), team performance scores, and greater efficiency of neonatal resuscitation based on mannequin heart rate at 3 and 5 minutes in an in situ simulation intervention group [42].

In Kern's Six-Step Approach, a learner's needs assessment must be performed in order that the *goals and objectives* of the course addresses the group targeted [39]. However, given the variable knowledge base within groups and over time, Kern emphasizes the dynamic nature of the Six-Step Approach. The learning objectives and goals, while initially developed to address the general needs of the group as a whole, adapt and evolve to meet the growing and changing needs of the targeted learners as discovered through repeated evaluative processes. Therefore, goals and objectives for a simulation program should result from a review of basic knowledge on a specific clinical topic (i.e., epidemiology, clinical presentation, management), reasons the topic is clinically relevant for targeted learners, and the relevant technical and non-technical skills. Furthermore, the information presented and the clinical scenarios practiced as part of a simulation course must be culturally and contextually relevant. This requires an understanding of current local practices, available resources (medical equipment and medications), and local health policy. For example, our Kenyan learners stated that they may respond better if the simulation mannequin had a greater resemblance to their patient population. Also, it is inappropriate to expect learners from low-resource settings to respond to certain emergencies with interventions available to those in a high-resource area, such as the initiation of a massive transfusion for an obstetric hemorrhage. Treatment protocols presented through simulation curricula must integrate context-appropriate interventions or the functional utility of the program would be compromised.

Results obtained from a needs assessment of the local environment and learners will guide simulation course design and decisions on logistics such as choosing among a de novo simulation center, in situ simulation, or a lower-cost hybrid to achieve the predetermined goals and objectives. The IMPACT Africa (Improving Perioperative Anesthesia Care and Training in Africa) Simulation Course for Obstetric Emergencies was developed with input from over 70 anesthesia and obstetric care providers practicing in East Africa (see curriculum description in Table 27.2). The IMPACT Africa simulation course provided didactic training on those obstetric emergencies determined to be the most common and critical based on learner input (obstetric hemorrhage, preeclampsia/eclampsia, obstructed labor/fetal distress, and high spinal) followed by an introduction to team training and crisis resource management principles. The knowledge and skills were incorporated into a series of simulation scenarios with structured debriefing. Soon after implementation, the importance of sharing common language to facilitate effective team dynamics and crisis management was discovered. This issue was compounded by the diversity of clinical backgrounds found among our learners (midwives, nurses, obstetricians, and anesthetists/anesthesiologists), and it became clear that an introductory didactic session was needed to build a common language which could be reinforced through simulation. This cycle of feedback and redesign through both and initial and repeated needs assessment is crucial to program success.

The goals of any simulation-based training program include improvements in individual and team knowledge, team performance, the culture of safety, and patient outcomes. Key characteristics that have been identified among obstetric simulation programs associated with improvement in clinical outcomes [41] include institution-level incentives,

Table 27.2 This describes the initial preparation and organization of the IMPACT Africa OB emergency simulation training course

Course preparation: An initial assessment was made by the course directors of each of eight government hospitals in Western Kenya to assess the need for the course and the type and frequency of obstetric emergencies encountered, in addition to the direct needs of the participants.	
Course registration: Agreement to participation was provided after supplementing a description of the course, its goals, and expected outcomes. Registration was opened to multidisciplinary members (including nurses/midwives, obstetricians, anesthesiologists, registered nurse anesthetists (KRNAs), student nurse anesthetists, security personnel, and administrators) that would be involved in delivering care to the pregnant patient.	
Course structure: An average of 20 participants were enrolled at each facility. The duration of the course spanned 2 days, for a total of 4 days. Each cohort was divided into two groups of ten, and during the course each group was further divided into two groups of five to facilitate efficient simulation sessions and in order to ensure each member was able to actively participate in each scenario.	
Participant preparation: At this time, preparation of the participants was not performed, but the ultimate goal is to provide each course member with a soft cover book reviewing all essential information regarding the most frequent obstetric emergencies encountered in Western Kenya, team training, and an introduction into simulation techniques and debriefing.	
Course curriculum	
Day 1	**Day 2**
Introductions	Overview of the day
Review basic obstetric and anesthetic principles	Review management of high spinal
Review of high-risk obstetrics	High spinal scenario
Break	Group debrief
Review neonatal resuscitation	Break
Review team training and simulation/simulator	Preeclampsia/eclampsia scenario
Introduction to mannequin	Group debrief
Lunch	Obstetric hemorrhage scenario
"Ice breaker" faculty simulation scenario and debrief	Group debrief
Peripartum hemorrhage scenario	Lunch
Group debrief	Review management of obstructed
Preeclampsia/eclampsia scenario	Labor/fetal distress
Group debrief	Obstructed labor/fetal distress scenario Group debrief

The course curriculum is outlined below

multidisciplinary training of all hospital staff within the unit in which they work, integration of teamwork principles into clinical teaching, and the use of a high-fidelity (though not high-tech) simulation model. In the authors' experience, offering institution level *and* individual incentives can aid in garnering initial interest and while also sustaining high rates of participation. Multidisciplinary training of all relevant hospital staff can also enhance participants' shared commitment to providing exemplary patient care.

In addition to incorporating a feedback mechanism to allow for simulation program revisions based on interval needs and program assessments, sustainability and contextual relevance is maximized through efforts at "training the trainers." As participants are trained as instructors, the needs of the health workers, facility, and community targeted by the program are likely to evolve. Finally, an assessment of needs and curriculum effectiveness based on outcome measures and participant feedback will allow for program improvements and potential expansion, at the regional or national level.

Debriefing and Cultural Influence

Debriefing is an exercise in facilitated reflection which helps to solidify the technical and non-technical skills gained during a simulation experience and ideally result in the restructuring of one's approach to real-life clinical scenarios [43]. When led by a trained facilitator, post-simulation debriefing plays a critical role in experiential learning. As Chung et al. have acknowledged, while simulation in healthcare has spread worldwide, the practice of debriefing and all related literature originate from Western culture with little consideration of cultural differences in learning and pedagogy. A deep understanding of the local culture and its bearing on learning and communication can play a decisive factor in ensuring a safe and effective learning environment in which learners feel capable of sharing their thoughts and gain from the simulation experience. The non-judgmental, objective nature of effective feedback provided as a component of facilitated debriefing [44] delivered with knowledge of the local culture will be more readily accepted by cultures prone to shame brought on by criticism or negative attention. More research is needed to understand efficacious and culturally appropriate debriefing methods and can be highly specific to cultural context.

Conclusion

Local and effective partnership with stakeholders, creation of simulation facility infrastructure appropriate for program goals and objectives, and curriculum development based on initial and repeated needs assessments performed in parallel with the training of local simulation faculty represent the critical initial steps in the implementation of a sustainable simulation program in an LMIC. While evidence demonstrating improvement in patient outcomes is largely lacking, guided debriefing of common and critical emergency scenarios can help identify individual and system deficiencies. In the experience of these authors, an effective simulation program can motivate local leaders to advocate for improvements to local infrastructure. Identification of each culture's unique modes of learning and communication and integrating these features into the simulation program can enhance the educational experience during the simulation experience and post-simulation debriefing.

References

1. Rosen K. The history of medical simulation. J Crit Care. 2008;23:157–66.
2. Denson JS, Abrahamson S. A computer-controlled patient simulator. JAMA. 1969;208(3):504–8. https://doi.org/10.1001/jama.1969.03160030078009.
3. Gaba DM, DeAnda A. A comprehensive anesthesia simulation environment: rec-creating the operating room for research and training. Anesthesiology. 1988;69(3):387–94.
4. Cooper J, Taqueti V. A brief history of the development of mannequin simulators for clinical education and training. Qual Saf Health Care. 2004;13(Suppl 1):i11–8.
5. Gaba DM. The future vision of simulation in healthcare. Simul Healthc. 2007;2(2):126–35. https://doi.org/10.1097/01.SIH.0000258411.38212.32.
6. Tansley G, Bailey JG, Gu Y, Murray M, Livingston P, Georges N, Hoogerboord M. Efficacy of surgical simulation training in a low-income country. World J Surg. 2016;40(11):2643–9.
7. Pringle K, Mackey JM, Modi P, Janeway H, Romero T, Meynard F, Perez H, Herrera R, Bendana M, Labora A, Ruskis J, Foggle J, Partridge R, Levine AC. A short trauma course for physicians in a resource limited setting: is low-cost simulation effective? Injury. 2015;46:1796–800.
8. Pammi M, Dempsey EM, Ryan CA, Barrington KJ. Newborn resuscitation training programmes reduce early neonatal mortality. Neonatology. 2016;110(3):210–24. https://doi.org/10.1159/000443875.
9. Bang A, Bellad R, Gisore P, Hibberd P, Patel A, Goudar S, Esamai F, Goco N, Meleth S, Derman RJ, Liechty EA, McClure E. Implementation and evaluation of the Helping Babies Breathe curriculum in three resource limited settings: does Helping Babies Breathe save lives? A study protocol. BMC Pregnancy Childbirth. 2014;14:116–21.
10. Buck GH. Development of simulators in medical education. Gesnerus. 1991;48:7.
11. Crofts JF, Winter C, Sowter MC. Practical simulation training for maternity care-where we are and where next. BJOG. 2011;118:11–6.
12. Hofmeyr GJ, Haws RA, Bergstrom S, Lee AC, Okong P, Darmstadt GL, Mullany LC, Shwe Oo EK, Lawn JE. Obstetric care in low-resource settings: what, who and how to overcome challenges to scale up? Int J Gynaecol Obstet. 2009;107(Suppl 1):S21–44.
13. Abass OA, Samuel BO, Odufeko GT. Medical simulation a tool yet untapped in most developing nations in Africa. Int J Comput Appl. 2014;97(5):1–4.

14. Thaddeus S, Maine D. Too far to walk: maternal mortality in context. Soc Sci Med. 1994;38(8):1091–110.
15. Barnes-Josiah D, Myntti C, Augustin A. The “three delays” as a framework for examining maternal mortality in Haiti. Soc Sci Med. 1998;46(8):981–93.
16. O’Neill KM, Greenberg SL, Cherian M, Gillies RD, Daniels KM, Roy N, Raykar NP, Riesel JN, Spiegel D, Watters DA, Gruen RL. Bellwether procedures for monitoring and planning essential surgical care in low and middle income countries: caesarean delivery, laparotomy, and treatment of open fractures. World J Surg. 2016;40(11):2611–9.
17. Meara JG, Leather AJ, Hagander L, et al. Global surgery 2030: evidence and solutions for achieving health, welfare, and economic development. Lancet. 2015;386:569–624.
18. Mock CN, Donkor P, Gawande A, et al. Essential surgery: key messages from disease control priorities, 3rd edition. Lancet. 2015;385:2209–19.
19. Walker DM, Cohen SR, Estrada F, Monterroso ME, Jenny A, Fritz J, Fahey JO. PRONTO training for obstetric and neonatal emergencies in Mexico. Int J Gynaecol Obstet. 2012;116:128–33.
20. Walker DM, Cohen SR, Fritz J, Olvera-Garcia M, Zelek ST, Fahey JO, Romero-Martinez M, Montoya-Rodriguez A, Lamadrid-Figueroa H. Impact evaluation of PRONTO Mexico: a simulation based program in obstetric and neonatal emergencies and team training. Simul Healthc. 2016;11:1–9.
21. Mcclure EM, Carlo WA, Wright LL, Chomba E, Uxa F, Lincetto O, Bann C. Evaluation of the educational impact of the WHO Essential Newborn Care course in Zambia. Acta Paediatr. 2007;96(8):1135–8.
22. Cohen SR, Cragin L, Wong B, Walker DM. Self-efficacy change with low-tech, high fidelity obstetric simulation training for midwives and nurses in Mexico. Clin Simul Nurs. 2012;8(1):e15–24. https://doi.org/10.1016/j.ecns.2010.05.004.
23. Walker D, Cohen S, Fritz J, Olvera M, Lamadrid-Figueroa H, Greenberg Cowan J, Gonzalez Hernandez D, Dettinger JC, Fahey JO. Team training in obstetric and neonatal emergencies using highly realistic simulation in Mexico: impact on process indicators. BMC Pregnancy Childbirth. 2014;14:367–76.
24. Walker D, Holme F, Zelek ST, Olvera-Garcia M, Montoya-Rodriguez A, Fritz J, Fahey J, Lamadrid-Figueroa H, Cohen S, Kestler E. A process evaluation of PRONTO simulation training for obstetric and neonatal emergency response teams in Guatemala. BMC Med Educ. 2015;15:117–24.
25. Carlo WA, Wright LL, Chomba E, Mcclure EM, Carlo ME, Bann CM, Collins M, Harris H. Educational impact of the neonatal resuscitation program in low-risk delivery centers in a developing country. J Pediatr. 2009;154(4):504–508.e5. https://doi.org/10.1016/j.jpeds.2008.10.005.
26. Carlo WA, Goudar SS, Jehan I Chomba E, Tshefu A, Garces A, Sailajanandan P, Althabe F, McClure EM, Derman RJ, Goldenberg RL, Bose C, Krebs NF, Panigrahi P, Buekens P, Chakraborty H, Hartwell TD, Wright LL, First Breath Study Group. Newborn care training and perinatal mortality in developing countries. N Engl J Med. 2010;362:614–23. https://doi.org/10.1056/NEJMsa0806033.
27. Msemo G, Massawe A, Mmbando D, Rusibamayila N, Maji K, Kidanto HL, Mwizamuholya D, Ringia P, Ersdal HL, Perlman J. Newborn mortality and fresh stillbirth rates in Tanzania after Helping Babies Breath training. Pediatrics. 2013;131:e353–60. https://doi.org/10.1542/peds.2012-1795.
28. Goudar SS, Somannavar MS, Clark R, Lockyer JM, Revankar AP, Fidler HM, Sloan NL, Niermeyer S, Keenan WJ, Singhal N. Stillbirth and newborn mortality in India after helping babies breathe training. Pediatrics. 2013;131(2):e344–52.
29. Hoban R, Bucher S, Neuman I, Chen M, Tesfaye N, Spector JM. ‘Helping babies breathe’ training in sub-Saharan Africa: educational impact and learner impressions. J Trop Pediatr. 2013;59:180. https://doi.org/10.1093/tropej/fms077.
30. Burch V. Does simulation based training have a future in Africa? Afr J Health Prof. 2014;6(2):117–8. https://doi.org/10.7196/AJHPE.534.
31. McIntosh C, Macario A, Flanagan B, Gaba DM. Simulation: what does it really cost? Simul Healthc. 2006;1(2):109.
32. Skelton T, Nshimyumuremyi I, Mukwesi C, Whynot S, Zolpys L, Livingston P. Low-cost simulation to teach anesthetists' non-technical skills in Rwanda. Anesth Analg. 2016;123:474–80.
33. Campbell DM, Barozzino T, Farrugia M, Sgro M. High-fidelity simulation in neonatal resuscitation. Pediatr Child Health. 2009;14(1):19–23.
34. King JM, Reising DL. Teaching advanced cardiac life support protocols: the effectiveness of static versus high-fidelity simulation. Nurse Educ. 2011;36(2):62–5.
35. Hoadley TA. Learning advanced cardiac life support: a comparison study of effects of low- and high-fidelity simulation. Nurs Educ Perspect. 2009;30(2):91–5.
36. Donoghue AJ, Durbin DR, Nadel FM, Stryjewski GR, Kost SI, Nadkarni VM. Effect of high-fidelity simulation on pediatric advanced life support training in pediatric house staff: a randomized trial. Pediatr Emerg Care. 2009;25(3):139–44.
37. Nimbalkar A, Patel D, Kungwarni A, Phatak A, Vasa R, Nimbalkar S. Randomized control trial of high fidelity versus low fidelity simulation for training undergraduate students in neonatal resuscitation. BMC Res Notes. 2015;8:636. https://doi.org/10.1186/s13104-015-1623-9.
38. Livingston P, Bailey J, Ntakiyiruta G, Mukwesi C, Whynot S, Brindley P. Development of a simulation and skills centre in East Africa: a Rwandan-Canadian partnership. Pan Afr Med J. 2014;17:315. https://doi.org/10.11604/pamj.2014.17.315.4211.
39. Kern DE, Thomas PA, Howard DM, Bass EB. Curriculum development for medical education: a six step approach. Baltimore: The John Hopkins University Press; 1998. Print
40. Damas E, Norceide C, Zephyr Y, William KL, Renouf T, Dubrowski A. Development of a sustainable simulator and simulation program for laparoscopic skills training in Haiti. Cureus. 2016;8(6):e632. https://doi.org/10.7759/cureus.632.
41. Siassakos D, Crofts JF, Winter C, Weiner CP, Draycott TJ. The active components of effective training in obstetric emergencies. BJOG. 2009;116:1028–32.
42. Rubio-Gurung S, Putet G, Touzet S, Gauthier-Mouliniere S, Jordan I, Beissel A, Labaune JM, Blanc S, Amamra N, Balandras C, Rudigoz RC, Colin C, Picaud JC. In-situ simulation training for neonatal resuscitation: a RCT. Pediatrics. 2014;134:e790–7.
43. Chung HS, Dieckmann P, issenberg SB. It is time to consider cultural differences in debriefing. Simul Healthc. 2013;8:166–70.
44. Rudolph JW, Simon R, Rivard P, Dufresne RL, Raemer DB. Debriefing with good judgment: combining rigorous feedback with genuine inquiry. Anesthesiol Clin. 2007;25:361–76.
45. Draycott TJ, Sibanda T, Owen L, Akande V, Winter C, Reading S, Whitelaw A. Does training in obstetric emergencies improve neonatal outcome? BJOG. 2006;113(2):177–82.
46. Draycott TJ, Crofts JF, Ash JP, Wilson LV, Yard E, Sibanda T, Whitelaw A. Improving neonatal outcome through practical shoulder dystocia training. Obstet Gynecol. 2008;112(1):14–20. https://doi.org/10.1097/AOG.0b013e31817bbc61.
47. Siassakos D, Hasafa Z, Sibanda T, Fox R, Donald F, Winter C, Draycott TJ. Retrospective cohort study of diagnosis-delivery interval with umbilical cord prolapse: the effect of team training. BJOG. 2009;116(8):1089–96. https://doi.org/10.1111/j.1471-0528.2009.02179.
48. Shoushtarian M, Barnett M, McMahon F, Ferris J. Impact of introducing practical obstetric multi-professional training (PROMPT) into maternity units in Victoria, Australia. BJOG. 2014;121(13):1710–8. https://doi.org/10.1111/1471-0528.12767.

Part V

Conclusion

A Translational Roadmap to Create the Future of Simulation in Healthcare

28

Samsun Lampotang

Introduction

This chapter started out as a request by the editors to predict the future of simulation as the closing bookend to the opening chapter about the history and past of simulation. One is reminded about the risks of forecasting in general from our shared experience that weather forecasting is sometimes about predicting what the weather *should* have been. With that cautionary experience in mind, rather than predict the future paths of simulation of healthcare which Gaba [1] has already envisioned along 11 dimensions and others have also addressed [2], a novel contribution is a proposed roadmap that may of assistance in navigating and creating the future of simulation of healthcare. The roadmap also identifies bottlenecks that may affect the paths that simulation will take in the future. Abraham Lincoln is credited with the saying "The best way to predict the future is to create it." Taking this advice, the chapter concludes with some concrete steps toward creating the future of simulation in healthcare.

The proposed roadmap is based on the author's privilege and honor to have been on the ground floor of the rebirth of simulation in healthcare in the late 1980s as a co-inventor of the Human Patient Simulator licensed technology [3, 4, 5, 6] developed at the University of Florida. The roadmap is a synthesis of the author's experience over three decades of designing, developing, evaluating, and teaching clinicians with simulators for acquiring affective [7], cognitive [8, 9], and psychomotor [10, 11] skills across the physicality-virtuality continuum [12]. The roadmap is also based on an updated literature search on translational science, the author's publications, and lectures and also as a formally trained simulation instructor during simulation-based training sessions, demonstrations, hands-on workshops, and Maintenance of Certification in Anesthesiology (MOCA) simulation sessions.

This exercise of creating a roadmap for the future of simulation in healthcare is based on some general principles:

Learn from the mistakes of the past; try not to repeat them.
An inefficient model is less likely to survive than a sustainable one.
Start with the desired end in mind.

We will not predict the times when identified bottlenecks will be cleared or new processes and metrics broadly adopted because timelines are harder to predict.

A sustainable model can be attained by simulation-based training that has been validated to yield at least a positive, and ideally a high, return on investment (ROI). Cost-effective, high-ROI models can convince influencers and decision- and policy-makers to promote and invest in simulation in healthcare.

The desired end is pervasive, lifelong, evidence-based, cost-effective simulation training that improves patient outcomes in terms of safety (reduced complications, morbidity, and mortality), quality, and cost of care. How do we get there? How do we create the future of simulation in healthcare?

Translational Simulation in Healthcare

In the future, to become even more clinically relevant by directly improving patient outcomes, simulation in healthcare must be aimed squarely at translational science. What is translational science?

S. Lampotang (✉)
Center for Safety, Simulation & Advanced Learning Technologies, Simulation Innovation, Office of Educational Affairs/Office of Medical Education, Simulation Core, Clinical & Translational Science Insitute, University of Florida, Gainesville, FL, USA
e-mail: slampotang@anest.ufl.edu

B. Mahoney et al. (eds.), *Comprehensive Healthcare Simulation: Anesthesiology*, Comprehensive Healthcare Simulation,
https://doi.org/10.1007/978-3-030-26849-7_28

The National Institutes of Health National Center for Advancing Translational Sciences (NIH NCATS) [13] defines "translation" as:

> The process of turning observations in the laboratory, clinic and community into interventions that improve the health of individuals and the public — from diagnostics and therapeutics to medical procedures and behavioral changes.

The previous definition is broad and encompasses simulation in healthcare as an "intervention" that produces "behavioral changes" to "improve the health of individuals and the public."

NIH NCATS [13] further describes "translational science" as:

> The field of investigation focused on understanding the scientific and operational principles underlying each step of the translational process.

The Kirkpatrick model [14, 15] for evaluating training programs is suited for defining each step of the translational process for simulation in healthcare that is proposed in this chapter. The original Kirkpatrick model consists of 4 levels that each builds upon the previous level in a crawl, walk, run manner. The 4 levels are (1) reaction, (2) learning, (3) behavior, and (4) results, depicted in Fig. 28.1 which has been customized to simulation in healthcare. Figure 28.1 includes an additional fifth level (return on investment, ROI) which has been attributed to Phillips [16] and is sometimes called Kirkpatrick-Phillips Level 5.

Simulation in healthcare is not an end in itself, but a means to the ultimate end: improving patient outcomes such as quality of care, safety, cost-efficiency, and reducing morbidity and mortality. Most of the research in simulation in healthcare, a still nascent field, has graduated at the time of writing to Kirkpatrick Level 2 (learning outcomes). While not yet at Kirkpatrick Level 3 or higher, this maturation step is a welcome and overdue transition from earlier simulation research that mainly concentrated on Level 1 evaluations (reaction) with studies where the reported metrics were subjective, evaluating reactions such as what participants thought of the simulator/simulation session and whether they *felt* that they had learned something from the simulation experience. The few exceptions are the inspirational work of pioneers like Draycott [17] and Barsuk [18] who performed Kirkpatrick Level 4 (patient outcomes) evaluations and Cohen [19] who performed a Kirkpatrick Level 5 (return on investment) study. It bears mentioning and seems revealing that the Cohen study demonstrating a 7:1 rate of return (also called return on investment) for every dollar spent on simulation-based training was reported to be the most often cited of all peer-reviewed papers published by the journal *Simulation in Healthcare*.

From the perspective of simulation as a means to improved patient outcomes, simulation in healthcare is evidently in alignment with translational science. To indicate that simulation in healthcare is being considered within the framework of translational science, the term *translational simulation in healthcare* is suggested.

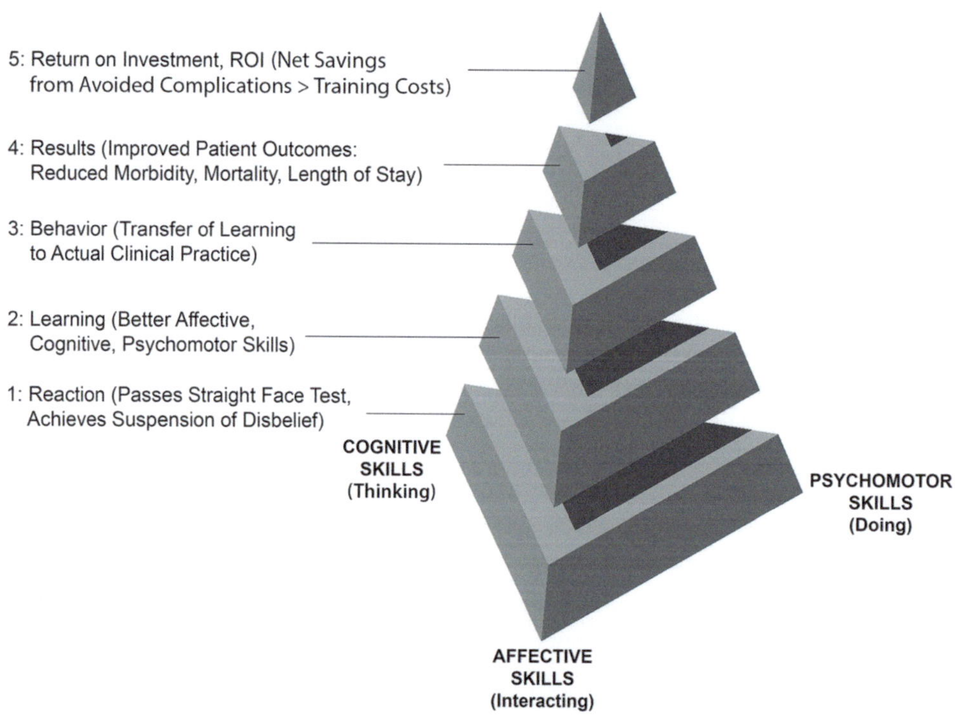

Fig. 28.1 The Kirkpatrick-Phillips model customized to simulation-based training for the acquisition and maintenance of affective, cognitive, and psychomotor skills in healthcare

In translational simulation in healthcare, the concepts of translational science are applied to simulation in healthcare. As an example, simulation-based training is considered and evaluated like other interventions such as a new drug [20, 21], process, or equipment.

Translational Science

Translational science was initially described by a roadmap that included three main translations T1, T2, and T3 between 4 stages [22] where T indicates translation from one phase to the next.

- T1 is translation from "basic biomedical science" to "clinical efficacy knowledge."
- T2 from "clinical *efficacy* knowledge" to "clinical *effectiveness* knowledge."
- T3 from "clinical effectiveness knowledge" to "improved healthcare quality and value and population health."

The T2 translation step clearly illustrates the important and sometimes unappreciated difference between "efficacy" and "effectiveness" because these two words are the only differences between the two stages bridged by T2. While in plain English and in lay dictionaries such as Oxford [23], the definitions of the two terms are very similar, it is not so in clinical English dictionaries such as Stedman's [24] where "efficacious" means that something works as intended in *ideal* conditions whereas "effective" delivers the desired results under *average and routine* conditions, a much tougher proposition. A concrete example is a new drug. A new drug that has received regulatory approval, e.g., by the FDA, is generally efficacious because it has been shown to work in controlled conditions; the newly approved drug's effectiveness is still to be determined. The post-market surveillance period, after the drug is approved for sale, is when its performance under routine conditions (the effectiveness) can be evaluated. This important distinction between, and the proper usage of, the two terms have also been recommended for simulation in healthcare [12]. In the future, we should evaluate simulation-based training first for efficacy and later effectiveness, with the latter being a desirable higher bar because facilities, logistics, and instructors do not have to be ideal to obtain the benefits of *effective* simulation-based training. As with drugs and evidence-based medicine, early adoption of simulation-based training should be predicated on demonstrated efficacy with post-market surveillance providing continued assessment of the adopted simulation-based training. If the assessment is positive, then the simulation-based training is considered effective and ready for widespread adoption.

The 3 T roadmap (circa 2008) formed the basis for subsequent mapping of medical education (including simulation) research as translational science by McGaghie [25] whereby the contributions of medical education interventions to outcomes are:

- T1: Improved knowledge, skills, attitudes, and professionalism
- T2: Patient care practices
- T3: Patient outcomes

The operational phases of the translational research spectrum have since been expanded from 3 to 5 translational steps between 6 stages: T0 to T4 [26, 27] where:

- T0: Basic biomedical research; identification of opportunities and approaches to health problems
- T1: Translation to humans; movement of fundamental discovery into health application, to provide clinical insights
- T2: Translation to patients; health application to implications for evidence-based practice guidelines
- T3: Translation to practice; transfer of practice guidelines to health practices
- T4: Translation to communities; impact of health practice on population health, to provide communities with the optimal intervention

An updated mapping for translational simulation in healthcare within the 5-step translational science framework is therefore proposed as in Fig. 28.2. The translational simulation in healthcare roadmap consists of 6 steps because T2

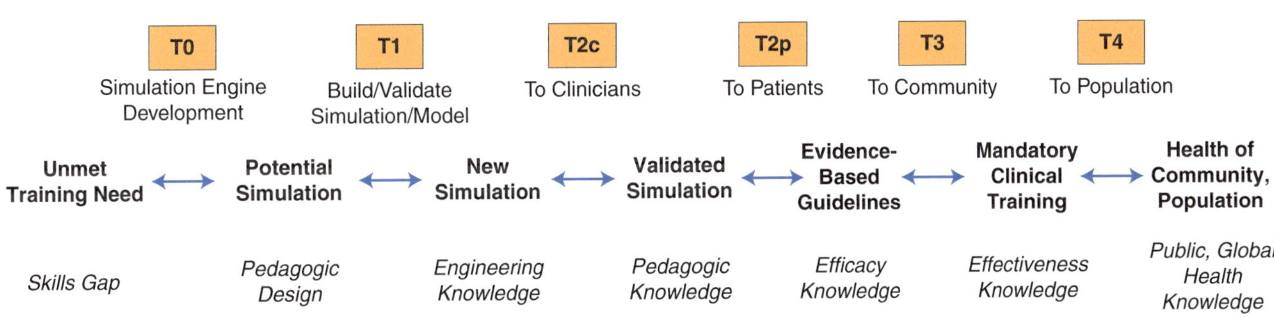

Fig. 28.2 A translational simulation in healthcare roadmap

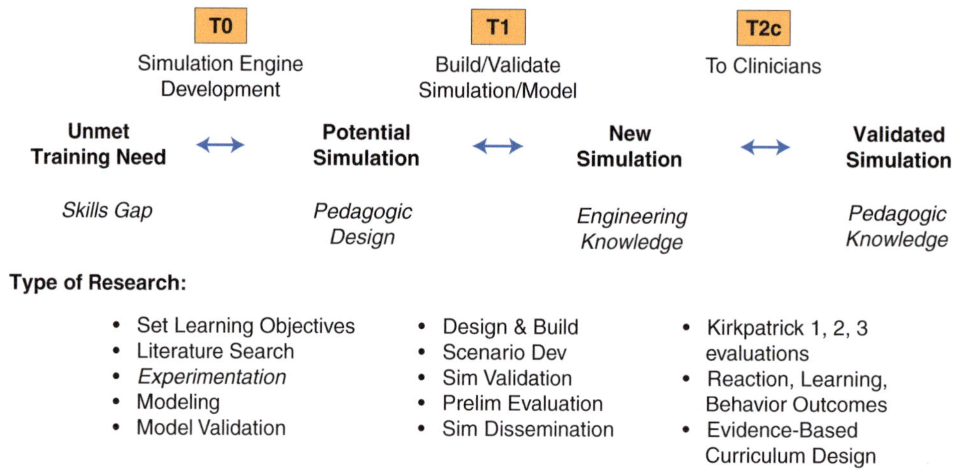

Fig. 28.3 Detailed T0–T2c steps of the translational simulation in healthcare roadmap

is split into 2 steps (T2c for clinicians and T2p for patients). Unlike a drug where the intervention is directly to the patient in terms of a straightforward administration according to prescribed dosing guidelines, in the usual case of simulation-based training of clinicians (simulation can also be used to train patients), the training intervention is mediated via clinicians; the T2c step must be accomplished before the intervention can be translated to patients.

The proposed translational simulation in healthcare roadmap is comprehensive encompassing the entire process from identifying an unmet training need to improving global health by addressing the training gap. Figure 28.3 is explored in detail as the entire roadmap is traversed; for brevity, the term "simulator" in that context going forward should be understood to also encompass scenarios, simulation-based training sessions, simulation-based curricula, and simulators across the physicality-virtuality continuum (including standardized patients).

Translation T0

The roadmap starts when an unmet training need is identified. During T0 translation, to avoid duplication of efforts, it is first determined via literature searches if a simulator that addresses the training need is already available. If the training need is truly unmet, the learning objectives that will be addressed by a new simulator are specified by a team consisting of clinicians, educators, and engineers. The resulting learning objectives then drive the design specifications of the simulator, including whether the simulation engine that drives the simulator should be a mathematical model, a script, instructor-driven, etc. A simulation engine and a simulator are not the same. One can think of a simulator as the externalization of an internal simulation engine to make the engine's output understandable and familiar to the intended trainees [28].

If a model, such as a pharmacokinetic and pharmacodynamic (PK/PD) model for a drug, is deemed necessary, a literature search may determine whether such models already exist. If models are already available, then they are used instead of developing new ones. If the model does not exist or does not match clinical experience, then the model will need to be developed or modified and may require experimentation to obtain data to build or modify the model. Irrespective of whether the model is preexisting or newly developed, once built, it will require validation, for example, by having a panel of clinicians and subject matter experts (SMEs) review the output of the model in steady and transient states as well as during normal and abnormal conditions.

At the conclusion of the T0 translation, we have a pedagogic design and a simulation engine (which could be a model among other options) that address an unmet training need, but we do not yet have a simulator; that is, we have not yet externalized the output of the simulation engine to make it familiar, readily understandable, and usable by the intended trainees. For example, the blood pressure numerical output of a mathematical model would be a list of numbers representing blood pressure in mmHg over time that is not intuitive and readily interpreted by clinicians. On the other hand, externalizing the blood pressure output of the model via a dynamic (scrolling) blood pressure waveform displayed in the same way as it usually appears on physiological monitors is more user-friendly and may facilitate interpretation and suspension of disbelief by the intended trainees.

Translation T1

In translation T1, we design and build the simulator that will wrap around the simulation engine, thereby externalizing the latter's output via a familiar and user-friendly user interface for both output (vital signs and waveforms from physiological monitors) and input (trainee interventions such as administering drugs, venous access, ultrasound-guided regional anesthesia blocks, and prostate biopsy). At the successful conclusion of translation T1, a new simulator has been developed and we have the engineering knowledge to build that simulator but not always; for example, commercial off the shelf (COTS) technology may not be available to create an affordable or practical simulator that meets the learning objectives.

Reality gets in the way of learning. This is true from considerations that are, among others, statistical (e.g., rare dangerous events like MH occur rarely giving few opportunities to learn in reality), ethical (e.g., novices should not learn on patients or supervisors should intervene and not wait to see if a trainee picks up on early symptoms of a dangerous, labile complication), and physical (both the body and medical equipment, like anesthesia machines are essentially "black boxes" that we struggle to peek into). That is why we created simulators. Thus, simulation is not about mimicking reality: novices and those unfamiliar with simulation (including this author when he started in simulation in the late 1980s) initially believe and sometimes reflexively demand high fidelity, even though the effort and expense of added realism may not be justified.

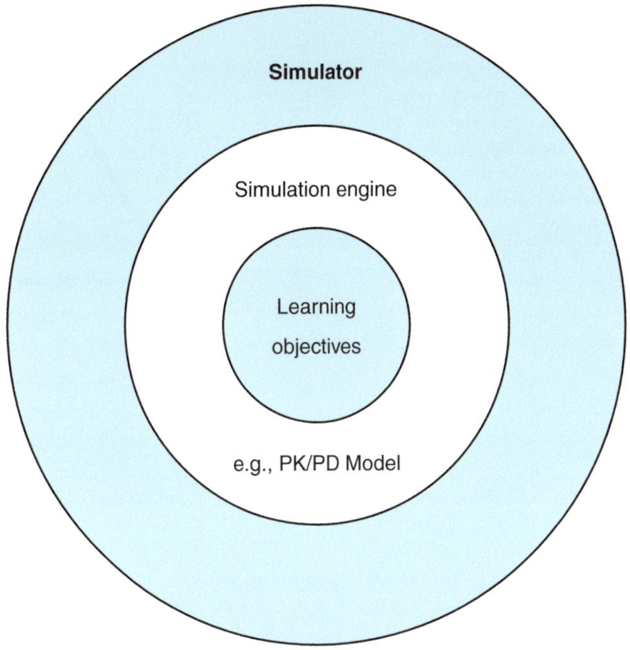

Fig. 28.4 A conceptual representation of the difference between a simulation engine and a simulator and the primacy of learning objectives as the core of the simulator design

The skills triangle From a different perspective such as that of a simulation designer or educator, simulation is a means to acquire and maintain skills. Therefore, one approach to designing a simulator is skills-driven selection of the technology to be used for the simulator. Skills can be classified into three main classes: affective (interacting), cognitive (thinking), and psychomotor (doing) that form the skills triangle [29]. The skills triangle also represents the three domains of educational activities or learning in Bloom's [30] taxonomy: "knowledge," "skills," and "attitudes" (KSA). In Fig. 28.4, terms related to Bloom's taxonomy are in italic font and in quotes in the skills triangle. "Knowledge," "skills," and "attitudes" correspond to "cognitive," "psychomotor," and "affective" skills, respectively. The term "skills" is used in its plain English meaning throughout this chapter and not as in Bloom's taxonomy where it is synonymous to psychomotor. The skills triangle is why the pyramid in Fig. 28.1 representing the Kirkpatrick-Phillips levels is three-sided.

Teamwork, leadership, delegation, bedside manners, professionalism, breaking bad news, apology, and speaking up are examples of affective skills pertinent to healthcare. Affective skills consist of receiving, responding, valuing, organization, and characterization. Cognitive skills encompass knowledge, analysis, synthesis, diagnosis, situation awareness, risk assessment, risk mitigation, application of knowledge, and spatial ability. The components of cognitive skills include remembering, understanding, applying, analyzing, evaluating, and creating. Examples of psychomotor skills include dexterity, hand-eye coordination, fine motor control, and depth perception. Components of psychomotor or kinesthetic skills are reflex movements, fundamental movements, perceptual abilities, physical abilities, and skilled movements.

While a simulator may address more than one class of skills since medical procedures do not generally fall neatly into only one single skill class, there should generally be a dominant class of skills that is prominent (such as psychomotor skills in an endotracheal intubation mannequin head or affective skills in a simulator for speaking up or teamwork) that can be used for initial selection of a corresponding simulator technology (Fig. 28.5).

The simulation triangle Simulator technology can similarly be classified into three main groupings: biologic, virtual, and physical forming the simulation triangle [29].

Biologic simulation includes humans as embedded simulated persons (ESPs, formerly known as confederates [2]) and standardized patients, cadavers, animal organs and tissues and any other biologic material. Because biologic simulation includes humans, it is indicated for affective skills training (trainees interacting with other humans such as patients and members of a clinical team) including teamwork skills such as closed-loop communication, leadership, and delegation.

Virtual simulation encompasses screen-based simulations including web-enabled simulations [8] that run on desktop computers, mobile devices such as smartphones and tablet

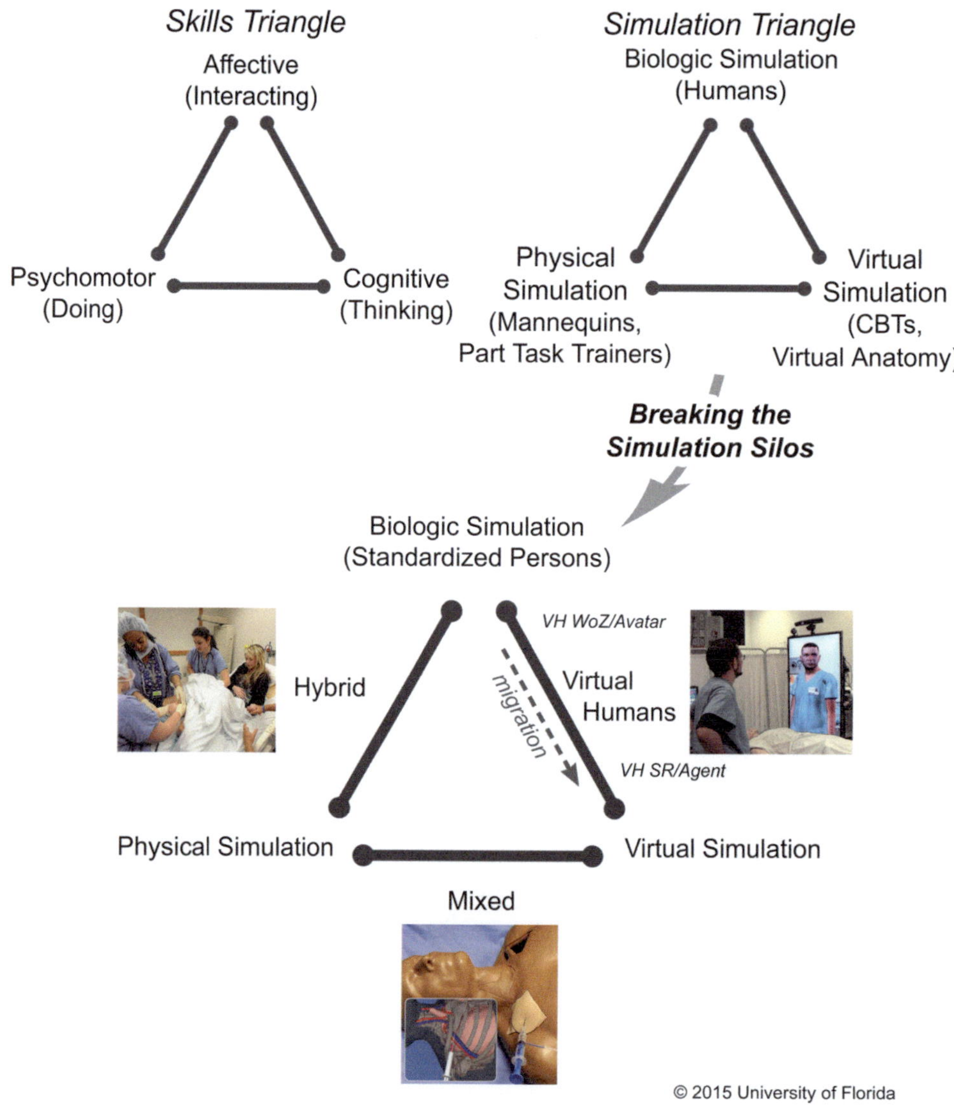

Fig. 28.5 Graphically depicts the concept of skills-driven selection of simulator technology. The skills and simulation triangles are arranged such that overlaying the triangles provides a guideline for the technology to consider based on the main set of skills that a new simulator will address

computers [31], and other forms of virtual displays like the HoloLens. Computer-based trainers (CBT) are examples of virtual simulation [32, 33, 34, 35].

Visualization, especially 3D visualization of complex anatomy, is a potent tool in the armamentarium of virtual simulation. There are two medical definitions of visualization: (a) formation of mental visual images and (b) making an internal organ visible during medical imaging by swallowing radiopaque substances. In the context of visualization in simulation in healthcare, we use both definitions. However, we are not using definition (b) in the strict sense of medical imaging but in the sense of illuminating "black box" objects, processes, and procedures by making internal, invisible, and/or hidden entities visible. Kosara [36] has proposed a criteria list in determining what is (and, conversely, what is not) a visualization: (a) Is it based on non-visual data? (b) Does it produce an image? (c) Is the result readable and recognizable? Two-dimensional visualization of invisible anesthetic gases and internal plumbing of an anesthesia machine is efficacious for learning about anesthesia machine function [8, 9]. Three-dimensional visualization of procedures (e.g., supraclavicular access to the subclavian vein) by creating 3D virtual representations of the relevant internal anatomy and tools (handheld needle and ultrasound probe) is efficacious as an aid to enhancing simulation-based training, whether the visualization is in real time (visualization provided while performing venous access) or delayed (after completing venous access, during debriefing) [11]. Real-time, 3D visualization is a form of augmentation, in this case visual augmentation, of a simulation experience.

Knowing what trainees know and don't know can be extremely helpful to instructors. If instructors are aware that the trainee's mental model of the subject matter is flawed, then a learning intervention can be designed. However, it can take time and effort to pry a mental model from a trainee and even then there is no guarantee that the instructor's understanding of the trainee's mental model is accurate. Visualization has the pedagogic advantage of providing an explicit, shared, visual mental model between instructors and trainees, which removes the guess work.

Virtual simulation is suited for imparting cognitive skills such as knowledge and the application of knowledge, especially if the subject matter is abstract (e.g., the body "compartments" in PK/PD compartmental models [37] that do not have an explicit physical or concrete existence compared to, e.g., the liver, a distinct, localized organ), invisible (e.g., the flow of anesthetic gases [8]), or internal organs, tissues, vessels, or parts generally hidden from sight (e.g., the anatomy below the skin of the patient [10] or the plumbing of an anesthesia machine [8]).

Examples of virtual simulation are screen-based or display-based, augmented reality (AR), mixed reality (MR), and VR simulations. Computer-based trainers such as GasMan, AneSoft, and the Virtual Anesthesia Machine are examples of screen-based simulators, the latter being also web-enabled. AR simulators overlay virtual graphics or information over the real world or a depiction of the real world. There is no interaction between the physical world and the virtual overlay in AR.

An example of an AR simulator is the Augmented Anesthesia Machine that was validated as an efficacious tool for undergraduate psychology students to learn about the anesthesia machine and detect machine faults [9]. A hand-held tracked tablet working in "magic lens" mode displayed an abstract, 2D conceptual representation of the internal plumbing, gas flows, and function of the specific part of the anesthesia machine being viewed through the magic lens. There was no interaction between real-world elements and the virtual overlay. For example, if the trainee manually turned the oxygen flowmeter knob, a hand would not appear in the virtual overlay. As a lay example, in pure AR, the yellow first-down line when viewing American football on TV would be incorrectly overlaid over football players because there is no interaction between the physical and virtual worlds.

In mixed reality, users can interact and manipulate both physical and virtual items with the virtual items behaving appropriately in real time in response to what is happening in the real or physical world. Using the lay example of the yellow first-down line again, in mixed reality, the yellow line disappears when a football player steps over it, as it should. So, although the yellow first-down line or the black line sweeping an Olympic swimming pool that visually indicates an Olympic record pace may be thought of as AR applications, technically they are MR.

An example of an MR simulator is the central venous access simulator described in this chapter [10, 11].

Virtual reality (VR) is not synonymous with virtual simulation. In the broadest common language definition, a virtual simulation is any non-physical simulation when we consider virtual as the opposite of physical. Thus, VR-based simulations belong to a subset of virtual simulation. Increasingly, digital or computer simulations or graphics are used in virtual simulations. VR-based simulators are totally immersive; there is no physical component to the simulated environment compared to AR and MR.

Physical simulation runs the range from high-integration life-size mannequins to part task trainers, intubation heads, and even bananas and eggs.

A subset of physical simulation is stimulation (with two "t"s) [28] where real equipment such as physiological monitors are used in the simulated environment and stimulated by appropriate signals (CO_2, O_2, volatile anesthetic concentration time profiles, gas pressure, voltage, current, etc.) and waveforms generated by a simulator such as the CAE/METI HPS (disclosure: the author is an inventor of the HPS). The physiological monitor or other stimulated equipment is unmodified. While this approach can be costly if the stimulated equipment is expensive, an advantage is that a simulator such as the HPS can be used to conduct simulator-based usability studies with the actual intended users of new equipment prior to finalizing the design and seeking regulatory (such as FDA) approval. The author has conducted multiple usability studies using the HPS for numerous multinational companies. From his experience, simulator-based usability studies generate timely, valuable clinical feedback without putting patients at risk, importantly while the design team is still intact. Given that up to 80% of the major flaws in equipment design can be identified with a well-designed simulator-based usability study, this under-used application and contribution of simulation to patient safety is expected to increase in the future. We hope that simulation-based usability studies will become standard operating procedure when designing new medical equipment.

The term silos has been used to indicate the separation and lack of communications between different stakeholders in patient care. Simulation technology was not only in silos initially (think early mannequins, screen-based simulators, standardized patients), but there was even competition between the silos such as papers comparing mannequin simulators to screen-based simulators. Comparing simulation technologies is a technology-centric exercise like comparing a saw to a hammer while in a learning/skills-centered perspective, we consider simulators as merely tools to an end. Thanks to the work of pioneers like Kneebone (hybrid simulation), Lok (virtual humans), and our DoD-funded work in MR simulators for "blind" and guided procedures, simulation technology silos are being broken and merged and this trend should continue in the future.

Translation T2c

At the beginning of translation T2c, we have a simulator and the engineering knowledge to build it but we do not yet know whether the simulator is efficacious in conveying to trainees (usually clinicians) the learning objectives it was designed to address. In a traditional translational medicine roadmap, the evaluation of efficacy is performed on patients, not clinicians, such as evaluating a new drug by administering it to patients with the disease or condition that the drug treats or cures. However, in simulation in healthcare, the effect of the intervention on patients is mediated through clinicians such as simulation-based training of clinicians in managing shoulder dystocia directly resulting in reduced brachial plexus injury in newborn patients [17]. The efficacy of a new simulator can be evaluated during step T2c by using Levels 1–3 of the Kirkpatrick model. At Level 1, the reaction of trainees to the simulator is evaluated. Are users generally able to suspend disbelief when training on the simulator? At Level 2, a simulator is evaluated in terms of learning outcomes. Do trainees acquire better skills (affective, cognitive, psychomotor) after training with the simulator? Transfer to actual patient care of the new skills and techniques acquired during simulation-based training is evaluated at Level 3. This can be a challenging translation because it may require unlearning decades of ingrained practice. As an example, will a clinician who has used an outward spiral scrubbing technique for skin prepping for decades readily adopt the now recommended to and fro scrubbing technique on patients after training with a skin prep simulator or will ingrained practice prevail? During step T2c, if the simulator produces the intended outcomes under ideal conditions, a simulator is validated for training of clinicians. Patient privacy rights such as HIPAA are needed and justified. They are also a constraint in monitoring and evaluating the adoption and application of skills learned on the simulator to actual patients. Reconciling HIPAA and the need to monitor Kirkpatrick 3 outcomes (transfer of simulation-based learning to clinical practice) is a bottleneck that we need to address and find creative ways to solve.

The translational simulation in healthcare roadmap may be of assistance to authors and reviewers of manuscripts in quickly defining the scope of work addressed by studies described in peer-reviewed papers. Reviewers are beginning to ask why manuscripts do not include the effect of simulation-based training on patients. It is a pertinent question that can be pre-empted by authors of simulation-related manuscripts if they frame their study as a learning outcome study that is a self-contained step in a methodical crawl, walk, run manner to eventually conducting patient or even ROI outcome studies.

Translation T2p

Translation T2p evaluates if simulation-based training of clinicians affects the outcomes of the patients of the trained clinicians (Kirkpatrick 4) (Fig. 28.6). The work of Draycott [17] and Barsuk [18] are prime examples of T2p research.

Electronic Heath Record (EHR) systems like Epic hold the potential of facilitating T2p research by providing ready access to patient outcomes and complications both pre- and post-intervention where the intervention is simulation-based training. However, EHRs are not living up to the slogan and promise that "every patient encounter will be a research encounter." The data is hard to mine and the quality and grouping of the data often does not meet the needs of T2p

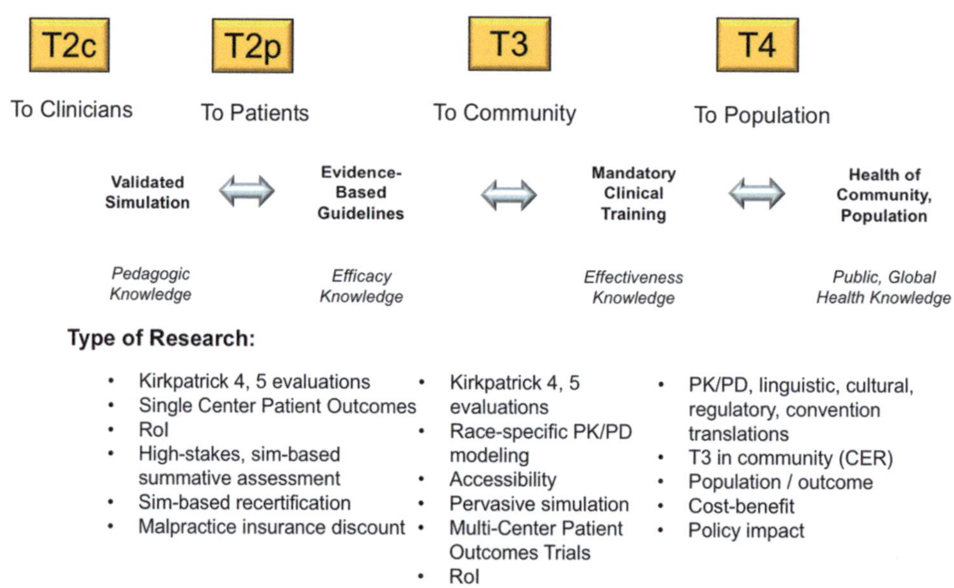

Fig. 28.6 Detailed T2c–T4 steps of the translational simulation in healthcare roadmap

research, including in some cases temporal resolution. If we are to conduct more T2p patient outcome studies with high-quality patient data that we can mine from EHRs, much work still needs to be done in this author's experience with a well-known EHR system. This is another fundamental roadblock that we may solve if the simulation and patient safety communities can obtain a seat at the table to work with EHR companies to upgrade their capabilities.

Translation T3

During translation step T3, we have determined that the simulator-based training is efficacious in the group in which it was evaluated but we do not know if the simulator will work in average conditions for clinicians with different training, skill sets, and backgrounds and patients of different genders, health status, and race. During translation, we may need to, for example, develop a race-specific model of drug PK/PD such as a race-specific PD model of propofol-induced LOC [38]. At the end of T3, effectiveness or lack thereof has been established and program directors and professional society boards now have the necessary evidence to determine whether the simulation-based training should be made mandatory.

Translation T4

During the final translation step T4, the simulator has been proved to be effective, and it is ready to be disseminated widely with the potential to positively affect global health. During step T4, we address diversity in practices (societal and clinical), culture, and climate and any other differences such as race-specific PK/PD as already mentioned. A concrete example of the need to localize or customize a simulation is a recent experience of the author when he was part of a US delegation of simulationists helping to inaugurate a new obstetric simulation center in China. One of the findings during simulation-based training was that due to elder respect that is prevalent in Asian countries such as Japan, Korea, and China, the leader in managing a crisis is the senior clinician, irrespective of the skill or updated knowledge base or how recently the senior person had a refresher course in crisis management. Portability of validated scenarios [39] means that we can share these scenarios rather than having to reinvent them. The caveat is that we need to adapt or customize the scenario or even the learning objectives to the local context. Generally, the best persons to localize a scenario validated elsewhere are the local simulationists as they would know their societal and clinical culture best as well as the prevailing climate at their clinical facility.

Kirkpatrick/Phillips Level 5

The formula for evaluating Kirkpatrick/Phillips Level 5, i.e., calculating the return on investment (ROI; also called the rate of return, ROR) on simulation-based training is mathematically simple.

$$ROI = \frac{\textbf{Net}\text{ savings from complications avoided via simulation training}}{\text{Cost of simulation training}}$$

$$ROI = \frac{\text{Savings from avoided complications} - \text{Cost of simulation training}}{\text{Cost of simulation training}}$$

As a concrete example, Cohen et al. [19] estimated the cost savings from avoiding, as a result of simulation training, 9.95 catheter-related bloodstream infections (CRBSI) at \$823,164 and the cost of simulation training at \$111,916. Thus:

$$\mathrm{ROI} = \frac{823{,}164 - 111{,}916}{111{,}916} = \frac{711{,}248}{111{,}916} = 6.4$$

An ROI greater than 0 (positive ROI) is desirable because it indicates that the simulation-based training is cost-effective for the bottom line of the healthcare institution; the more the ROI is larger than 0, the better the return on the investment in simulation-based training. The pioneering work of Cohen et al. in simulation-based prevention of central line-associated bloodstream infection (CLABSI) has established that ROI levels greater than 6 are attainable.

Benefit cost ratio (BCR) can also be used [40] to determine the effectiveness of a simulation investment. The benefit is simply divided by the cost. In the case of the Cohen study used above, BCR = 823,164/111,916 = 7.4. Summarizing, an ROI > 0 or a BCR > 1 is desirable as both indicate that the simulation-based training being evaluated is effective in improving patient outcomes.

ROI and BCR could become established metrics in the future for determining which simulator model and make to acquire, all else being equal, for a given learning objective or skill, especially for expensive simulators, just like miles per gallon can be a metric (possibly obsolete in the future with electric cars) when currently selecting a car model.

Creating the Future of Simulation in Healthcare

We can use ROI as a design input when developing a simulator.

The mathematical simplicity of the ROI equation facilitates two simple strategies for developing high-ROI simulators: (a) increase the numerator (net savings from avoided complications) and (b) decrease the denominator (reduce training costs). To increase the numerator, select processes, drugs, and equipment where errors are likely and/or expensive or outcomes are suboptimal such as a false-negative rate reportedly as high as 47% during prostate biopsy. This low hanging fruit approach will ensure that frequent and/or severe (expensive) errors are addressed first with simulation instead of lower severity (expense) or lower-frequency incidents.

To decrease the denominator, reduce the cost of training which consists of two main components: a one-time (or acquisition) cost and an operating cost (cost of instructor time, maintenance contracts, depreciation (replacement cost usually spread over 5 years), disposables, etc.).

Instructor time can be both expensive and rare if the instructor is a clinician who has competing time demands from patient care. The unavailability of instructors can be exacerbated if compensation incentivizes patient care over simulation-based teaching. Often, simulators are idle more than half of the time, i.e., more often than not. Part of the reason may be the lack of instructors. Many simulators are implicitly designed to have an instructor present just like cars were traditionally designed to have a driver at the steering wheel. The expense and unavailability of clinical instructors provide compelling arguments to minimize or eliminate the need for instructors, where appropriate, when designing new simulators. Similar to driverless cars, a simulator designed for self-study and self-debriefing in central venous access has been validated to be non-inferior to an average human instructor for specific CVA techniques [41]. Instructor-less simulators facilitate competency-based training and on-demand-training. Trainees can take as long as needed to reach competency. Trainees can cancel a scheduled session if not ready, rested, or receptive for training such as being inadvertently scheduled for a training session in the morning after a call night. No instructor is inconvenienced if the trainee cancels an early morning self-study, self-debriefing simulator-based training session. Systems that teach without a human instructor have been called virtual coaches or integrated tutors. The term "intelligent tutor" is often misused and should be avoided if the tutor does not have artificial intelligence but simply regurgitates "intelligence" that has been codified and integrated into a simulator by humans. The key term in intelligent tutor is *intelligent*. An example of an intelligent tutor would be one that can analyze the data from trainees independently without help from humans and, for example, develop a better way to teach that is, for example, faster.

One can reduce acquisition costs by scrutinizing the cost of goods (Is there a less expensive alternative? Is that expensive sensor accuracy overkill or justified?) and focusing on specific learning objectives, avoiding mission creep and the temptation to design a simulator that does everything but possibly not so well. Acquisition cost can also be reduced by reducing development time and effort. A way to reduce development cost is to design modular sets of simulators, for example, a set of simulators for simulating different medical procedures that all use ultrasonography-guided or ultrasonography-assisted needling such as ultrasound-guided regional anesthesia (USGRA), central venous access (CVA) and prostate biopsy (PBx). Common mechanical elements in this modular design are then a tracked needle and a tracked ultrasound probe. A modular design concept can also be extended to software for running a simulator in the form of a software development kit (SDK) and in the process facilitate development of simulators for new applications or procedures by third parties [42]. BioGears and Kitware are other examples of SDKs that third parties can use to develop new simulators.

Reducing or eliminating the cost of disposables is good not only for reducing cost of ownership but also the environment. We need a better model than the tired "razor/razor blade" model, from an environmental as well as an economic perspective.

Simulator idleness is the elephant in the room. This author has visited multiple simulation centers worldwide and has always been struck that more often than not, training was not occurring during the visits. Considering idle simulators as wasteful simulators, we can work to increase ROI by decreasing the idle time of simulators. A simulator as a tangible asset depreciates over time whether it is used or not. As an example, using the "straight line" method, a $300,000 simulator that will have a residual value of $0 after 5 years is depreciated by a constant amount, $60,000, each year whether it is used or not. An accelerated depreciation scheme can also be used whereby depreciation is higher during the earlier years, as with a car, in the planned lifetime of a tangible asset. The term amortization is similar to depreciation but used for intangible assets such as a patent for a simulator and is therefore not indicated for a physical, tangible simulator. Also, amortization is almost always performed using the "straight line" method, whereas depreciation can be accelerated.

Assuming that a simulator is effective with a positive ROI and there are clinicians requiring training, an idle simulator then decreases ROI. The numerator (net savings from avoided complications) is decreased due to idleness on the expectation that idleness implies less clinicians are trained and therefore less complications are avoided; the net savings from avoided complications are not as high as they could be if the simulator was less idle, an opportunity cost.

However high the ROI of a given simulator-based training, its effective ROI is negative if the simulator is totally idle (not used at all for training) after purchase, a not uncommon situation in the early days of simulation in healthcare, e.g., if allowance was not made in the budget for a simulation engineer or technician to run the simulator. Factoring simulator idleness into the simple ROI equation modifies the ROI equation to:

$$\textit{Modified ROI} = \left(\frac{\textbf{Net}\text{ savings from complications avoided via simulation training}}{\text{Cost of simulation training}}\right) * \left(1 + \text{idleness allowance} - \text{idleness proportion}\right)$$

$$\text{Modified ROI} = \text{ROI} * \text{idleness factor}$$

where

$$\text{Idleness factor} = \left(1 + \text{idleness allowance} - \text{idleness proportion}\right)$$

The idleness allowance accounts for the fact that most simulators are not used 100% of the time, maybe not even 50% of the time. The idleness allowance can be adjusted by end users (individual researchers, simulation center directors, professional societies if adopted, others). An idleness allowance of 0 is aspirational currently because it means that a simulator is never idle and is in use during all times at which the simulator is available. A default value of the idleness allowance of 0.5 is more realistic and means mathematically that if a simulator is idle more often than not, i.e., > 50% of the time, then the idleness factor is below 1.0. Multiplying the ROI by an idleness factor less than 1.0 reduces the modified ROI. As a concrete example, if a simulator is idle 60% of the time, then the idleness proportion is 0.6 and the idleness factor (using an idleness allowance of 0.5) becomes 1 + 0.5–0.6 = 0.9. As a result, assuming an ROI of 7, the modified ROI becomes 6.3, less than 7.

$$\text{Modified ROI} = \text{ROI} * \text{idleness factor} = 7 * 0.9 = 6.3$$

Conversely, an idleness proportion greater than 0.5 (simulator is used more often than it is idle) is rewarded by making the modified ROI larger than the simplified ROI.

The idleness proportion is the time the simulator is actually used for training divided by the time the simulator is available for training. If a simulator is used for 16 hours out of 40 available hours, then it is idle for 24 hours and the idleness proportion is 24/40 = 0.6.

Idleness proportion can be calculated on different usage models for estimating simulator availability. A simple availability model is based on a 40-hour workweek. Other models may choose to calculate availability by including weekends or on a 24/7 model especially for expensive simulators and facilities. Where the simulator availability is dependent on support personnel such as instructors and simulation technicians, the available work days in a year can be reduced to take into account scheduled downtime such as for maintenance, public holidays, vacation days, and sick days.

If the idleness allowance is set to 0, then the idleness factor of a 100% idle simulator will be (1 + 0 – 1) = 0 such that the ROI becomes 0 for a 100% idle simulator, however high the ROI may be when it is actually used.

While the modified ROI equation is presented here for a simulator or simulator-based training, the scope of the modified ROI equation can be readily enlarged when applied to larger entities like a modular simulator, a simulation lab, or a simulation center.

Conclusion

We conclude by reiterating the desired future we might want to create: pervasive, lifelong, evidence-based, cost-effective simulation training that improves patient outcomes in terms of safety (reduced complications, morbidity, and mortality), quality, and cost of care. We described some general approaches that might help us create a more ideal future of simulation in healthcare and ways to get there more quickly.

References

1. Gaba DM. The future vision of simulation in health care. Qual Saf Health Care. 2004;13:i2–i10. https://doi.org/10.1136/qshc.2004.009878.
2. Palaganas JC, Maxworthy JC, Epps CA, Mancini ME, editors. Defining excellence in simulation programs (DESP). 1st ed: Lippincott, Williams & Wilkins, Wolters Kluwer; 2015.
3. Lampotang S, Gravenstein N, Banner MJ, Jaeger MJ, Schultetus RR. A lung model of carbon dioxide concentrations with mechanical or spontaneous ventilation. Crit Care Med. 1986;14:1055 1057.

4. Lampotang S, Good ML, Gravenstein JS, Carovano RG: Method and apparatus for simulating neuromuscular stimulation during medical surgery. US Patent 5,391,081 issued February 21, 1995.
5. van Meurs WL, Good ML, Lampotang S. Functional anatomy of full-scale patient simulators. J Clin Monit. 1997;13:317–24.
6. Palaganas JC, Maxworthy JC, Epps CA, Mancini ME, editors. Lampotang DESP memoirs. In: Defining excellence in simulation programs (DESP). 1st ed: Lippincott, Williams & Wilkins, Wolters Kluwer; 2015.
7. Robb A, Kleinsmith A, Cordar A, White C, Wendling A, Lampotang S, Lok B. Training together: how another human trainee affects behavior during virtual human-based team training. Front Inform Commun Technol. 2016;3 https://doi.org/10.3389/fict.2016.00017.
8. Fischler I, Kaschub CE, Lizdas DE, Lampotang S. Understanding of anesthesia machine function is enhanced with a transparent reality simulation. Simul Healthcare. 2008;3:26–32.
9. Quarles J, Lampotang S, Fischler I, Fishwick P, Lok B. Tangible user interfaces compensate for low spatial cognition. In: Proceedings of the IEEE symposium on 3D user interfaces 2008, 978-1-4244-1972-2/08; 2008. p. 11–8.
10. Robinson AR, Gravenstein N, Cooper LA, Lizdas D, Luria I, Lampotang S. A mixed reality part-task trainer for subclavian venous access. Simul Healthc. 2014;9:56–64.
11. Sappenfield JW, Smith WB, Copper LA, Lizdas D, Gonsalves DB, Gravenstein N, Lampotang S, Robinson AR. Visualization improves supraclavicular access to the subclavian vein in a mixed reality simulator. Anesth Analg. 2018;127(1):83–9. https://doi.org/10.1213/ANE0000000000002572. PMID: 29200069.
12. Lampotang S, Nelson DR, Hamstra SJ, Naik V. Efficacious vs effective: what's in an adjective? Simul Healthc. 2013;8(3):191–2.
13. Visited 12/29/2016. https://ncats.nih.gov/translation/spectrum.
14. Kirkpatrick DL. Evaluation of training. In: Craig RL, editor. Training and development handbook. New York: McGraw-Hill; 1976.
15. Kirkpatrick DL. Evaluating training programs: the four levels. San Francisco: Berrett-Koehler; 1994.
16. Phillips JJ. Measuring return on investment (Vol 2). American Society for Training and Development; 1997. ISBN 1-56286-065-8.
17. Draycott TJ, Crofts JF, Ash JP, Wilson LV, Yard E, Sibanda T, Whitelaw A. Improving neonatal outcome through practical shoulder dystocia training. Obstet Gynecol. 2008;112:14–20.
18. Barsuk JH, Cohen ER, Feinglass J, McGaghie WC, Wayne DB. Use of simulation-based education to reduce catheter-related bloodstream infections. Arch Intern Med. 2009;169:1420–3.
19. Cohen ER, Feinglass J, Barsuk JH, Barnard C, O'Donnell A, McGaghie WC, Wayne DB. Cost savings from reduced catheter-related bloodstream infection after simulation-based education for residents in a medical intensive care unit. Simul Healthc. 2010;5(2):98–102. https://doi.org/10.1097/SIH.0b013e3181bc8304.
20. Weinger MB. The pharmacology of simulation: a conceptual framework to inform progress in simulation research. Simul Healthc. 2010;5(1):8–15. https://doi.org/10.1097/SIH.0b013e3181c91d4a.
21. Gaba DM. The pharmaceutical analogy for simulation: a policy perspective. Simul Healthc. 2010;5(1):5–7. https://doi.org/10.1097/SIH.0b013e3181c75ddb.
22. Dougherty D, Conway PH. The "3T's" road map to transform US health care: the "how" of high-quality care. JAMA. 2008;299(19):2319–21. https://doi.org/10.1001/jama.299.19.2319.
23. Pearsall J, Trumble B. The Oxford encyclopedic English dictionary. 3rd ed. New York: Oxford University Press; 1996.
24. Spraycar M, Randolph E. Stedman's medical dictionary. 26th ed. Baltimore: Williams & Wilkins; 1995.
25. McGaghie WC. Medical education research as translational science. Sci Transl Med. 2010;2(19):19cm8. https://doi.org/10.1126/scitranslmed.3000679.
26. Committee to Review the Clinical and Translational Science Awards Program at the National Center for Advancing Translational Sciences; Board on Health Sciences Policy; Institute of Medicine; Leshner AI, Terry SF, Schultz AM, Liverman CT, editors: The CTSA program at NIH: opportunities for advancing clinical and translational research. Washington (DC): National Academies Press (US); 2013.
27. Surkis A, Hogle JA, DiazGranados D, Hunt JD, Mazmanian PE, Connors E, Westaby K, Whipple EC, Adamus T, Mueller M, Aphinyanaphongs Y. Classifying publications from the clinical and translational science award program along the translational research spectrum: a machine learning approach. J Transl Med. 2016;14(1):235. https://doi.org/10.1186/s12967-016-0992-8.
28. Lampotang S. Unlike history, should a simulator not repeat itself? Simul Healthc. 2015;10(6):331–5.
29. Lampotang S, Lizdas D, Rajon D, Luria I, Gravenstein N, Bisht Y, Schwab W, Friedman W, Bova F, Robinson A. Mixed simulators: augmented physical simulators with virtual underlays. Proceedings of the IEEE Virtual Reality 2013 meeting. 2013;978-1-4673-4796-9/13:7–10.
30. Bloom BS, Engelhart MD, Furst EJ, Hill WH, Krathwohl DR. Taxonomy of educational objectives, handbook I: the cognitive domain. New York: David McKay Co Inc.; 1956.
31. Lizdas DE, Gravenstein N, Luria I, Lampotang S. An iPad simulation of skin prepping. Simul Healthc. 2012;7(6):564–5.
32. Smith NT, Starko KR. The physiology and pharmacology of growing old, as shown in body simulation. Stud Health Techno Inform. 2005;111:488–91.
33. Philip JH. Gas Man—an example of goal oriented computer-assisted teaching which results in learning. Int J Clin Monit Comput. 1986;3(3):165–73.
34. Schwid HA, O'Donnell D. The anesthesia simulator consultant: simulation plus expert system. Anesthesiol Rev. 1993;20(5):185–9.
35. Lampotang S. Computer and web-enabled simulations for anesthesiology training and credentialing. J Crit Care. 2008;23:173–8.
36. Kosara R. Visualization criticism – the missing link between information visualization and art. Proceedings of the 11th International Conference on Information Visualisation (IV). 2007:631–6. http://kosara.net/papers/2007/Kosara_IV_2007.pdf.
37. Yavas S, Lizdas D, Gravenstein N, Lampotang S. Interactive web simulation for propofol and fospropofol, a new propofol pro-drug. Anesth Analg. 2008;106:880–3.
38. Lampotang S, Lizdas DE, Derendorf H, Gravenstein N, Lok B, Quarles JP. Race-specific pharmacodynamic model of propofol-induced loss of consciousness. J Clin Pharmacol. 2016;56(9):1141–50. https://doi.org/10.1002/jcph.716.
39. Sidi A, Gravenstein N, Lampotang S. Construct validity and generalizability of simulation-based objective structured clinical examination scenarios. J Graduate Medical Education. 2014;6(3):489–94.
40. Asche CV, Kim M, Brown A, Golden A, Laack TA, Rosario J, Strother C, Totten VY, Okuda Y. Communicating value in simulation: cost-benefit analysis and return on investment. Acad Emerg Med. 2018;25(2):230–7. https://doi.org/10.1111/acem.13327; PMID: 28965366.
41. McGough E, Sappenfield J, Gravenstein N, Cooper LA, Lizdas DE, DeStephens A, Gifford A, Zeng D, Lampotang S. Non-inferiority assessment of a self-study, self-debriefing mixed reality simulator for central venous access. San Antonio: IMSH, 01/27/19 Poster presentation.
42. Johnson WT, Andre B, Lizdas DE, Lampotang S. Using modular principles to efficiently design and build new simulators for different healthcare procedures. San Antonio: IMSH. 01/27/2019 Poster, invited and oral presentation.

Index

B. Mahoney et al. (eds.), *Comprehensive Healthcare Simulation: Anesthesiology*, Comprehensive Healthcare Simulation,
https://doi.org/10.1007/978-3-030-26849-7

N

O

P

Q

R

S

MIX
Papier aus verantwortungsvollen Quellen
Paper from responsible sources
FSC® C105338

If you have any concerns about our products,
you can contact us on
ProductSafety@springernature.com

In case Publisher is established outside the EU,
the EU authorized representative is:
Springer Nature Customer Service Center GmbH
Europaplatz 3, 69115 Heidelberg, Germany

Printed by Libri Plureos GmbH
in Hamburg, Germany